MRI of the Pituitary Gland

Jean-François Bonneville
Fabrice Bonneville
Françoise Cattin
Sonia Nagi

MRI of the Pituitary Gland

With a Foreword by A. Beckers

Springer

Jean-François Bonneville, MD
Department of Endocrinology
CHU Sart-Tilman
Liège
Belgium

Fabrice Bonneville, MD, PhD
Department of Neuroradiology
University Hospital Paul Sabatier
Toulouse
France

Françoise Cattin, MD
Department of Neuroradiology
and Endovascular Therapy
University Hospital of Besançon
Besançon
France

Sonia Nagi, MD
Faculty of Medicine
National Institute of Neurology
University of Tunis El Manar
Tunis
Tunisia

ISBN 978-3-319-29041-6 ISBN 978-3-319-29043-0 (eBook)
DOI 10.1007/978-3-319-29043-0

Library of Congress Control Number: 2016935498

Printed on acid-free paper

This Springer imprint is published by Springer Nature
The registered company is Springer International Publishing AG Switzerland

Foreword

The pituitary is a tiny and fascinating gland of extreme importance biologically, surrounded by an array of vital structures. Correct decision-making about the pituitary is of the utmost clinical importance. While we can infer pathology from hormonal profiles and clinical symptoms, neuroradiological images often provide us with the key information in planning correct treatment. Thankfully, this potentially confusing experience for the uninitiated is made far easier with the publication of *MRI of the Pituitary Gland* by Prof. Jean-Francois Bonneville and his co-authors. This new book is aimed at an audience far wider than just neuroradiologists, although they too will find much of interest therein. It is for all of us, particularly endocrinologists, who find ourselves faced regularly with clinical problems that may be related to pituitary pathology. The book covers all of the major topics of importance, building from the foundations of normal appearance and characteristics of the pituitary and surrounding structures to cover tumors and related disorders. It is remarkable how many differential diagnoses must be entertained when assessing disorders of pituitary appearance on MRI. The pituitary gland is not only the site of primary pathologies but also can act as an important site of secondary systemic pathology of immune, inflammatory, or infectious diseases. Prof. Bonneville guides us through these various possibilities and carefully shows us how they may be distinguished from one another. Furthermore, he integrates his long experience as a diagnostician and researcher by adding information on how the appearance of pituitary tumors can determine aspects of their clinical behavior (e.g., acromegaly). Prof. Bonneville is an acknowledged world-leading authority in neuroradiology of the pituitary and surrounding structures who gained this experience through a lifetime of clinical and teaching work in France. Since he retired from his hospital position in France, happily he has agreed to continue sharing his experience with us having swapped the Jura for the Ardennes of Belgium. So I have now had the personal pleasure of benefiting from his input on clinical neuroradiology on my own patients and undertaking new research working together as colleagues in Liège. I was delighted on many occasions to attend lectures and courses given by Prof. Bonneville on the topic of pituitary neuroradiology. These events never fail to be informative and interesting, given his wide breadth of knowledge and experience. However, these are not entirely relaxed encounters, as Prof. Bonneville always ends with a quiz on what he has just been teaching and illustrating. I have often seen quite experienced senior endocrinologists squirming under questioning when interpreting pituitary imaging! This is, for me, one of the important reasons why this book is so welcome. Pituitary neuroradiology is complex and there are many pitfalls of which we can become victims. With this book we can learn to identify those elements that can confound correct interpretations, and with the copious illustrations and images we can visualize the pathology clearly and memorably.

Albert Beckers MD, PhD
Chief, Department of Endocrinology
Centre Hospitalier Universitaire de Liège
University of Liège, Liège, Belgium

Preface

Magnetic resonance imaging (MRI) is currently considered as a major keystone of the diagnosis of diseases of the hypothalamic-hypophyseal region. However, the relatively small size of the pituitary gland, its deep location at the skull base, and the numerous physiological variants present in this area impede the precise assessment of the anatomical structures and, particularly, of the pituitary gland itself.

The diagnosis of the often tiny lesions of this region, such as pituitary microadenomas, is thus difficult if the MRI technology is not optimized and if potential artifacts and traps are not recognized. Advanced MRI technology is able not only to depict small lesions with greater reliability, but also helps in the differential diagnosis of large tumors, particularly for which defining the presence or absence of invasion of the cavernous sinus is an important task.

This book describes and illustrates the role of MRI in the diagnosis of the different lesions of the sellar region, from the common prolactinoma, to the nonfunctioning adenoma and the Rathke cleft cyst, to the less frequent lymphocytic hypophysitis or pituitary corticotroph adenoma in Cushing disease, and other neoplastic and non-neoplastic entities.

Finally, the book emphasizes the necessity of adapting the MRI sequences to the symptoms of each particular patient and of working in close collaboration with all specialists involved in the pathology of the sellar area.

Jean-François Bonneville
Fabrice Bonneville
Françoise Cattin
Sonia Nagi

Contents

Abbreviations

3D TOF	3-dimensional time-of-flight
AC	arachnoid cyst
ACTH	adrenocorticotropic hormone
ADC	apparent diffusion coefficient
ADH	antidiuretic hormone
AIP	aryl hydrocarbon receptor interacting protein
CE T1WI	contrast-enhanced T1-weighted image
CISS	constructive interference in steady state
CNS	central nervous system
CPC	craniopharyngeal canal
CSF	cerebrospinal fluid
CT	computed tomography
DWI	diffusion-weighted image
FLAIR	fluid-attenuated inversion recovery
FSH	follicle-stimulating hormone
GCT	granular cell tumor
GE	gradient echo
GH	growth hormone
LH	luteinizing hormone
MEN 1	multiple endocrine neoplasia type 1
MRA	magnetic resonance angiography
MRI	magnetic resonance imaging
PCNSL	primary central nervous system lymphoma
rCBV	relative cerebral blood volume
RCC	Rathke cleft cyst
ROI	region of interest
T1WI	T1-weighted image
T2WI	T2-weighted image
TSH	thyroid-stimulating hormone
WHO	World Health Organization

Collaborators

Michael Buchfelder, MD, PhD Professor of Neurosurgery, University of Erlangen-Nürnberg, Erlangen, Germany

Cyrine Drissi Faculty of Medicine, University of Tunis El Manar, Department of Neuroradiology, Institut National de Neurologie, Tunis, Tunisia

Julie Kreutz Department of Radiology, Centre Hospitalier Universitaire de Liège, Liège, Belgique

Maha Mahmoud Faculty of Medicine, University of Tunis El Manar, Department of Neuroradiology, Institut National de Neurologie, Tunis, Tunisia

Iulia Potorac Department of Endocrinology, Centre Hospitalier Universitaire de Liège, Liège, Belgique

Sven-Martin Schlaffer, MD Neurosurgeon, Department of Neurosurgery, University of Erlangen-Nürnberg, Erlangen, Germany

MRI Technique and Radiological Anatomy of the Pituitary Gland

1

Françoise Cattin

1.1 Basic MRI Sequences

Three basic sequences are indicated in all clinical situations. These sequences are often adequate for the diagnosis, particularly in the search for microprolactinomas. Additional sequences may be obtained according to the clinical and biological status and after reading the basic sequences.

Sagittal T1W sequence focused on the pituitary region constitutes the first step of the MR examination: this sequence is rarely informative in the diagnosis of intrasellar lesions, but allows one to draw an anatomical plane, for example the sub-callosal plane, which will allow perfect reproducibility of the coronal cuts for serial MRI (Fig. 1.1). This sagittal T1W sequence is essential in the evaluation of lesions with suprasellar extension to analyze the anatomical surroundings. At 3.0 T, sagittal spin echo T1WI are obtained with the following parameters: TR/TE: 425/14, BW: 31,25 kHz, FOV/matrix: 23 cm/416 × 256, 3.0 mm thk/0.3sp, 3NEX, AT: 5:29. Standard protocol includes a coronal fast spin-echo T2W sequence (TR/TE: 3500/140, BW: 25 kHz, FOV/matrix: 20 cm/384 × 384, 2 mm thk/0.2sp, 4 NEX, AT: 5:15 and a coronal spin-echo T1W sequence (TR/TE: 700/14, BW: 31,25, FOV/matrix: 23 cm/416 × 256, 3 mm thk/0.2sp, 3 NEX, AT: 6:53) (Fig. 1.2).

When an intrasellar lesion is suspected on the sequences without contrast, the diagnosis can be confirmed by the realization of coronal T1WI after gadolinium injection (CE T1WI). A low dose of contrast medium (0.05 mmol/k) is recommended to avoid a too intense enhancement, which may hide a small intraglandular lesion. Nevertheless, it is our own policy to spare gadolinium administration when the clinical situation is clear and confirmed by the noncontrast T1 and T2WI, for instance when searching for microprolactinomas. Delayed imaging 45 min after gadolinium injection can have some interest, mainly in Cushing disease, in revealing a very small microadenoma ("picoadenoma") when T1, T2, and CE T1WI are not informative.

In the case of a lesion with suprasellar extension, coronal and sagittal T1W sequence after gadolinium injection and, if necessary, a 3D gradient echo T1W acquisition with gadolinium for neurosurgical planning are performed.

1.2 Additional Sequences

Axial TWI, preferentially with fat saturation is the best sequence to evaluate the storage of vasopressin and is thus highly recommended for the exploration of diabetes insipidus. This sequence will also be extremely useful to consolidate the diagnosis of intrasellar Rathke cleft cyst even when associated with pituitary microadenoma.

In the exploration of Cushing disease, if the standard sequences including the sequences after gadolinium injection are negative, a dynamic imaging is obtained (Fig. 1.3). A 3D T1W gradient-echo sequence with inframillimetric section

J.-F. Bonneville et al., *MRI of the Pituitary Gland*, DOI 10.1007/978-3-319-29043-0_1

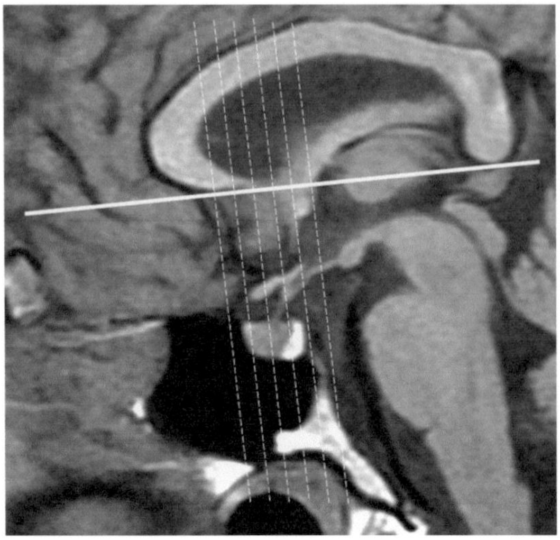

Fig. 1.1 Sagittal T1WI. The coronal cuts are obtained perpendicularly to the sub-callosal plane

thickness may demonstrate a tiny ACTH-secreting pituitary microadenoma.

3D TOF MRA is useful in the lesions affecting the cavernous sinus, particularly in the diagnosis of aneurysm of the intracavernous internal carotid artery, ectasic carotid siphons, and dural fistula, or to confirm anatomical variations such as persistent trigeminal artery.

1.3 Advanced MRI Techniques

Diffusion imaging, perfusion imaging, and proton MR spectroscopy (MRs) can be helpful in differentiating various types of lesions involving pituitary gland and hypothalamus. These techniques require the positioning of a region of interest (ROI) with a sufficient size, and thus may have a role only in the evaluation of large lesions.

Diffusion imaging can have an interest in early detection of pituitary infarction or pituitary apoplexy and in differentiation of abscess from hemorrhage, the ADC value being considerably decreased in pituitary ischemia and abscess. The relationship between diffusion imaging and apparent diffusion coefficient on one hand, and consistency of the pituitary adenoma on the other, is controversial. For some authors, macroadenomas with hypersignal on diffusion imaging and a low ADC value present a soft consistency, while those with hyposignal and a high ADC value are firmer: these data may have been useful for the neurosurgeon but are not confirmed in recent studies. It is generally admitted today that there is no correlation between the ADC and both the consistency and secretory type of the pituitary adenoma.

MRs has a limited interest in the diagnosis of pituitary lesions. However, some MRs patterns can help to confirm a diagnosis evoked on standard sequences. Hypothalamic gliomas demonstrate increased choline peak and decreased N-acetylaspartate (NAA) peak. In craniopharyngiomas and germinomas, a high level of lipids is usually observed with only some traces of other metabolites. Hypothalamic hamartomas are characterized by decreased NAA and increased myo-inositol. Pituitary adenomas can show only a choline peak; in the case of hemorrhagic complications, no metabolites are found.

1.4 Radiological Anatomy

1.4.1 The Anterior Lobe of the Pituitary Gland

In adults, the upper pole of the anterior lobe can be plane, concave, or convex. The signal of the normal anterior lobe is homogeneous, similar to that of the white matter of the temporal lobe on T1WI. A possible discrepancy between the size of the sella turcica and that of the pituitary gland can lead to mistakes. When the sella turcica is unusually small, the pituitary gland may appear bulky, overflowing frankly the theoretical plan of the sellar diaphragm in the manner of a brioche leaving its mold.

The size and morphology of the anterior lobe of the pituitary gland are variable according to age and sex (Fig. 1.4).

In the newborn and up to the end of the second month of life, the pituitary gland is rounder and larger than in the older child : 63 % of infants aged less than 1 month present a convex pituitary gland against only 4 % of the children older than 2 months.

Before 2 months, the anterior lobe of the pituitary gland appears hyperintense on T1WI in 75 % of the cases if compared with the brainstem. This hypersignal is never observed beyond the second month. This hypersignal is related to an increase of endoplasmic reticulum and intense activity of protein synthesis. The relatively large size of the pituitary gland at birth is correlated with hyperplasia of prolactin cells, an intense endocrinal activity and an important protein synthesis. Lack of high signal or discovery of a small pituitary gland in a

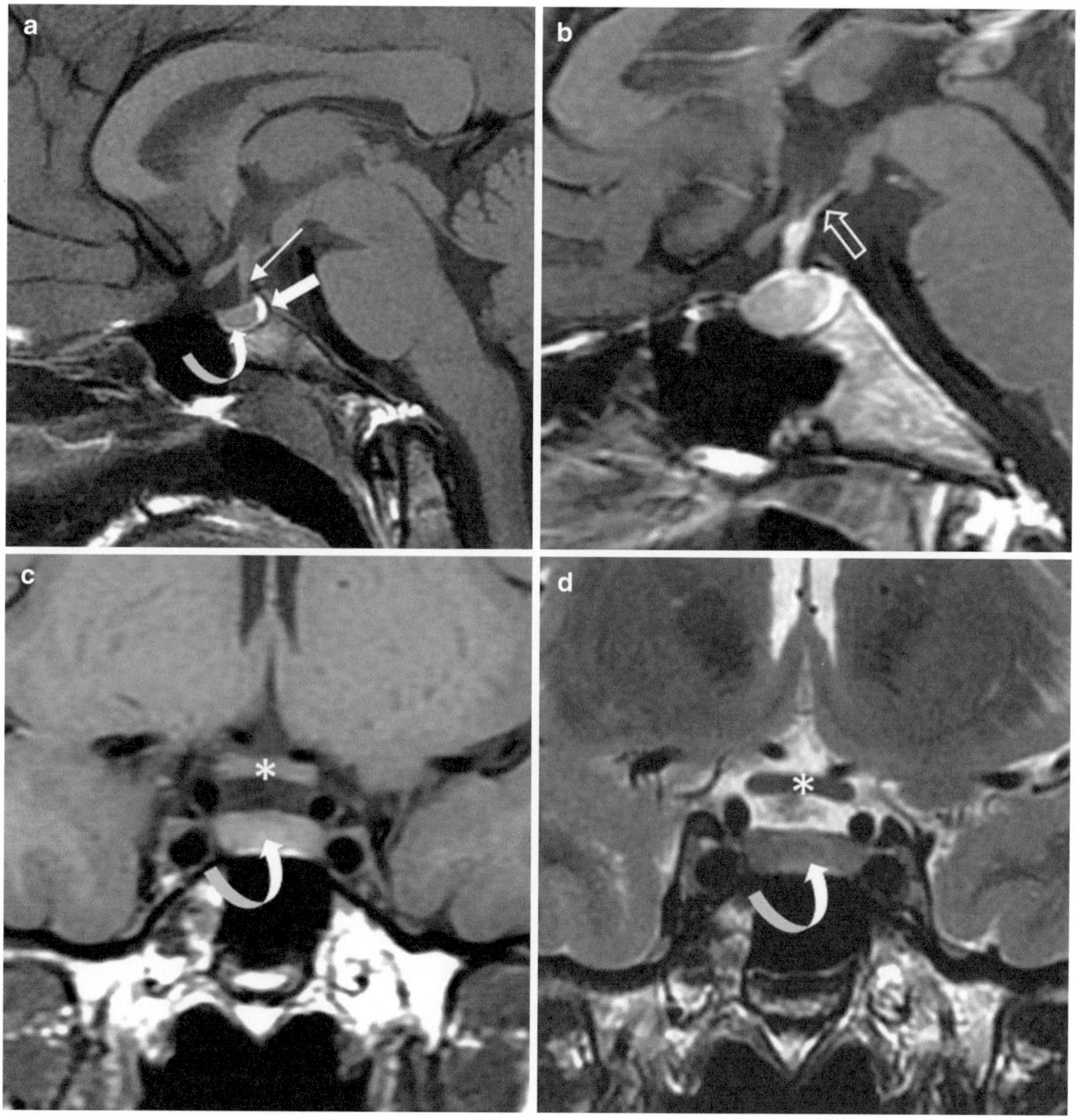

Fig. 1.2 Normal pituitary gland. (**a**, **b**) Sagittal T1 and CE T1WIs. (**c**, **d**) Coronal T1 and T2 WIs at the anterior part of the pituitary gland. (**e**, **f**) Coronal T1 and T2 WIs, 2 mm posterior to (**c**) and (**d**). Anterior lobe (*curved arrow*). Posterior lobe (*thick arrow*). Pituitary stalk (*thin arrow*). On T2WI, a flow artifact in the suprasellar cistern blurs the pituitary stalk. Optic chiasm (*asterisk*). After gadolinium injection (**b**), enhancement of anterior lobe, pituitary stalk, and tuber cinereum (*open arrow*)

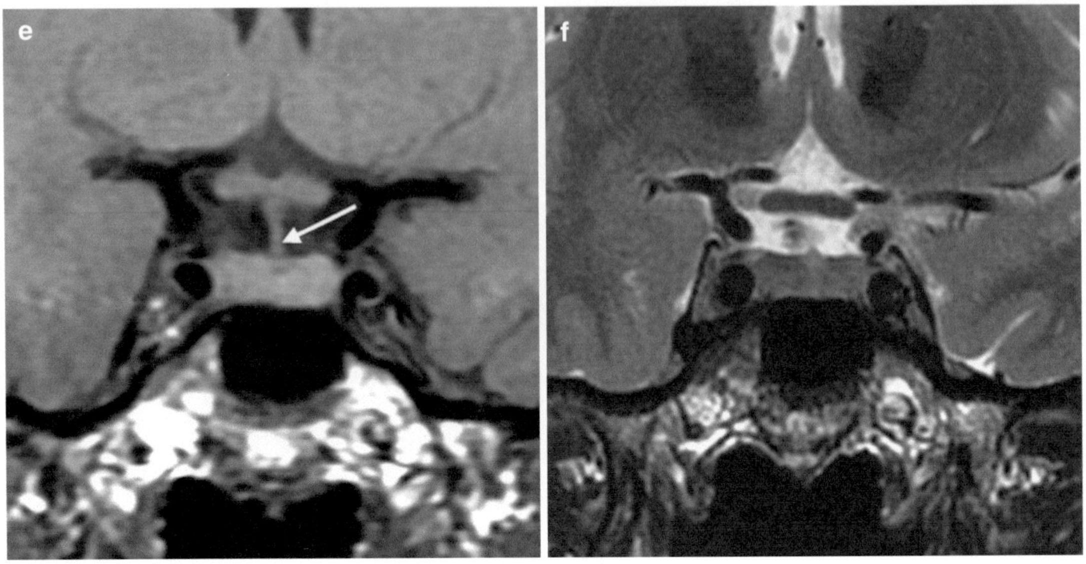

Fig. 1.2 (continued)

neonate should alert one to the possibility of pituitary malformation or dysfunction such as hypoglycemia. The usual hypersignal of the posterior lobe on T1WI is detectable from birth, so that the pituitary gland of the newborn appears entirely hyperintense.

Beyond 2 months of age, the pituitary gland tends to flatten and the signal of the anterior lobe becomes similar to that seen in the adult; the posterior lobe only remains hyperintense on T1WI. The height of the pituitary gland measured on the midsagittal plane is usually between 2 and 6 mm, and there is no difference between males and females.

At puberty, a physiological hypertrophy of the gland is visible in females and males, but is definitively more marked in females. Before 12 years, the pituitary gland does not measure more than 6 mm in height. At puberty, a pituitary gland height from 8 to 10 mm is not rare in females. In males, a height higher than 7 mm must be regarded as suspect. The upper pole of the pituitary gland is upwardly convex in 56 % of females at puberty versus 18 % in the other age groups. Thus, the increase in volume and T1 hypersignal of the pituitary gland occurs during the maximal hormonal secretion period.

In women less than 50 years old, the pituitary gland is larger than in men and is more often upwardly convex. The height of the pituitary gland is more than 7 mm in 1 out of 4 women; between 20 and 40 years, 58 % of women have a pituitary gland more than 7 mm in height. In men, the height of the pituitary gland decreases regularly between 20 and 65 years; only 10 % of men have a pituitary gland more than 6 mm in height, and only 3 % a pituitary height greater than 7 mm. In the elderly population, interstitial and perivascular fibrosis can lead to an empty sella, most of the time without major influence on pituitary function. Small deposits of amyloid and iron may be observed.

After gadolinium injection, the enhancement of the anterior lobe of the pituitary gland is usually intense and homogeneous. On dynamic imaging, the anterior lobe is opacified later than in the posterior lobe because of its predominantly portal blood supply. Temporal resolution of dynamic imaging of the pituitary gland is longer than that of a dynamic CT scan. The first image is obtained 20–30 s after the beginning of gadolinium injection, and shows opacification of the pituitary stalk and upper

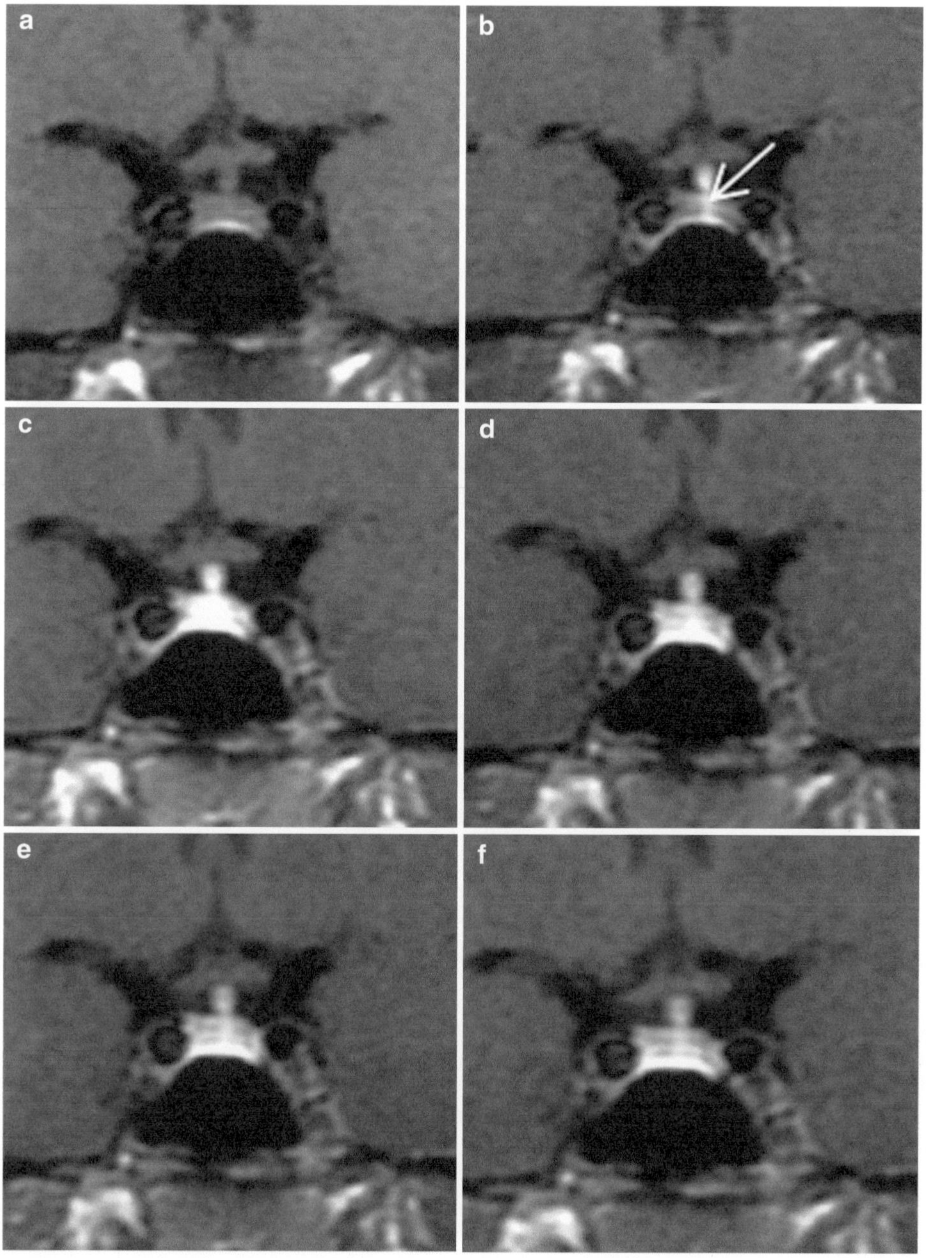

Fig. 1.3 Dynamic MRI of the normal pituitary gland. (**a**) Before contrast injection. (**b**) About 30 s later, opacification of the pituitary stalk and the secondary capillary bed (*arrow*). (**c**) At 60 s, the enhancement of the pituitary gland is intense and homogeneous. (**d–f**) Slow decrease of enhancement intensity

part of the pituitary gland corresponding to the secondary pituitary capillary bed ("tuft") and the adjacent glandular parenchyma already contaminated by gadolinium. On the second image at 40–60 s after gadolinium, the pituitary gland is intensely and homogeneously opacified, after which a slow decrease of intensity is observed.

1.4.2 The Pituitary Stalk

Under normal conditions, the diameter of the upper part of the pituitary stalk is thicker than the lower part. Thus, a tube-like pituitary stalk may be an indicator of an abnormal pituitary stalk. A physiological elongation of the infundibular recess of the third ventricle can simulate an enlarged stalk. The maximal diameter of the pituitary stalk measured on the axial plane is about 3 mm. The pituitary stalk is not always vertical: a more or less marked tilting is not infrequent. This anatomical variation confirms that the displacement of the pituitary stalk is not a highly reliable sign for the diagnosis of pituitary microadenoma.

1.4.3 The Posterior Lobe of the Pituitary Gland

It is currently well established that the hypersignal visible on T1WI and located at the poste-

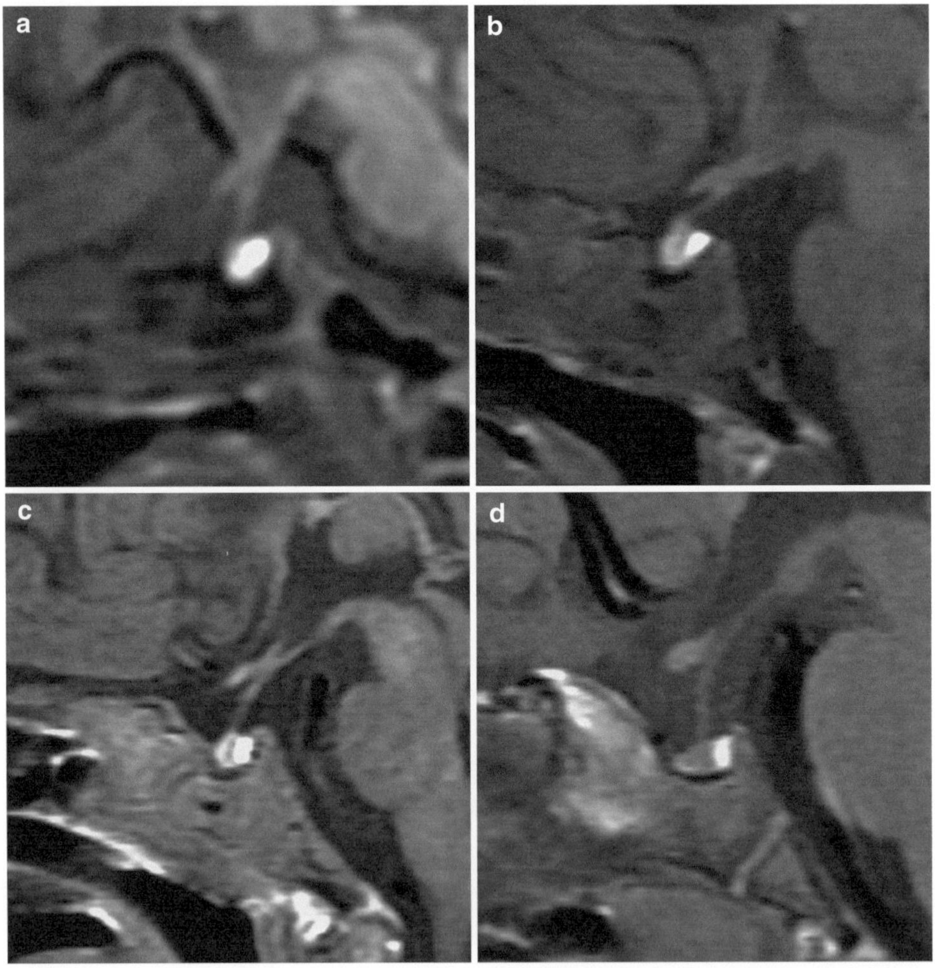

Fig. 1.4 Pituitary gland in children, sagittal T1WIs. (**a**) 5-day-old newborn. Round and globulous pituitary gland. Anterior pituitary is markedly hyperintense and indistinguishable from the posterior lobe. (**b**) 12-day-old newborn. The convex anterior pituitary is hyperintense but slightly less so than the posterior pituitary. (**c**) 7-week-old infant. Convex upper pole of the pituitary gland. Hyperintensity of the anterior pituitary is less marked than that of the posterior pituitary. (**d**) 21-month-old child. The anterior pituitary gland is no more hyperintense. The posterior lobe is proportionally larger than in adult. (**e**) 7-year-old boy. No change when compared with (**d**). (**f**) 15-year-old girl. Normal convex pituitary gland of the adolescent

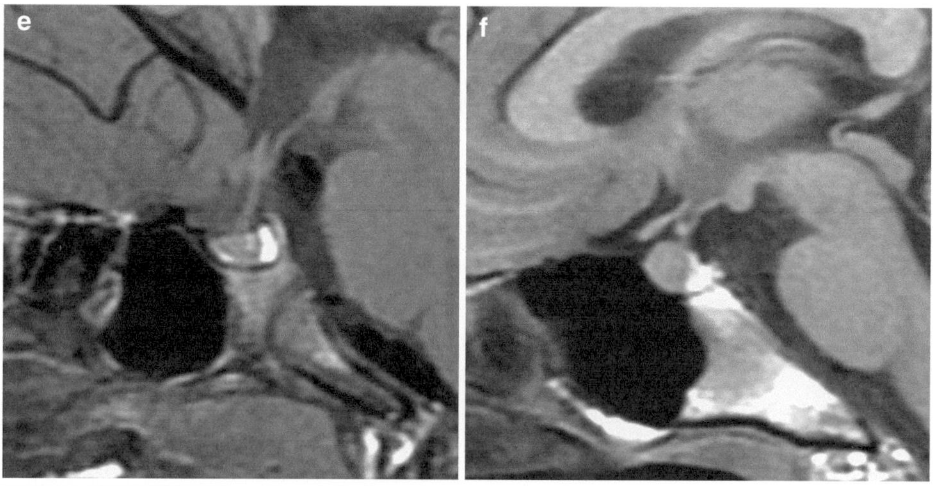

Fig. 1.4 (continued)

rior part of the sella turcica corresponds to the storage of vasopressin in the posterior lobe. This T1 hypersignal indicates a normal functional state of the posterior lobe. The T1 hypersignal disappears in patients with central diabetes insipidus. An exact explanation of this T1 hypersignal is as yet not available. For some authors, the hypersignal is in relation with lipidic droplets present in the pituicytes. For others, the hypersignal corresponds to the antidiuretic hormone (ADH) granules or to a complex of ADH and neurophysin. A third theory states that the hypersignal is related to the presence of phospholipids in the posterior lobe of the pituitary gland.

Lack of visualization of the posterior lobe on the sagittal plane in normal subjects is generally due to an inappropriate technique, or to anatomical reasons such as a fatty or thick dorsum sellae. Realization of axial cuts allows one to reach a rate of detection of the posterior lobe close to 100 %. Classically, the posterior lobe is described on sagittal images as a hyperintense and homogeneous structure with regular anterior convexity, in contact with the dorsum sellae (Fig. 1.5). In fact, this pattern is not always seen: heterogeneous signal and irregularities of the anterior aspect of the posterior lobe, which could suggest an irregular distribution of the neurosecretory granules, are frequently observed. In the elderly, the signal of the posterior lobe is less intense and often heterogeneous, as a result of the persistently raised plasmatic osmolality (Fig. 1.6). For the same reason, lesser T1 hyperintensity can be observed during pregnancy, in patients undergoing hemodialysis or with uncontrolled diabetes mellitus, severe anorexia nervosa, and in a stressed condition.

Cysts are rarely encountered in the posterior lobe. They appear on axial T1WI without contrast as T1-hypointense clefts surrounded by a T1-hyperintense rim corresponding to normal vasopressin storage (Fig. 52.4).

1.4.4 The Cavernous Sinus

Before gadolinium injection, the internal carotid arteries present a hyposignal in T1 and T2 related to fast flow; this lack of signal is known as "flow void."

Most venous elements of the cavernous sinus are located below and laterally to the internal carotid artery. When the internal carotid artery is remote to the wall of the sphenoid sinus, the vacant space is always filled by a vein, the vein of the carotid sulcus, or by several small veins.

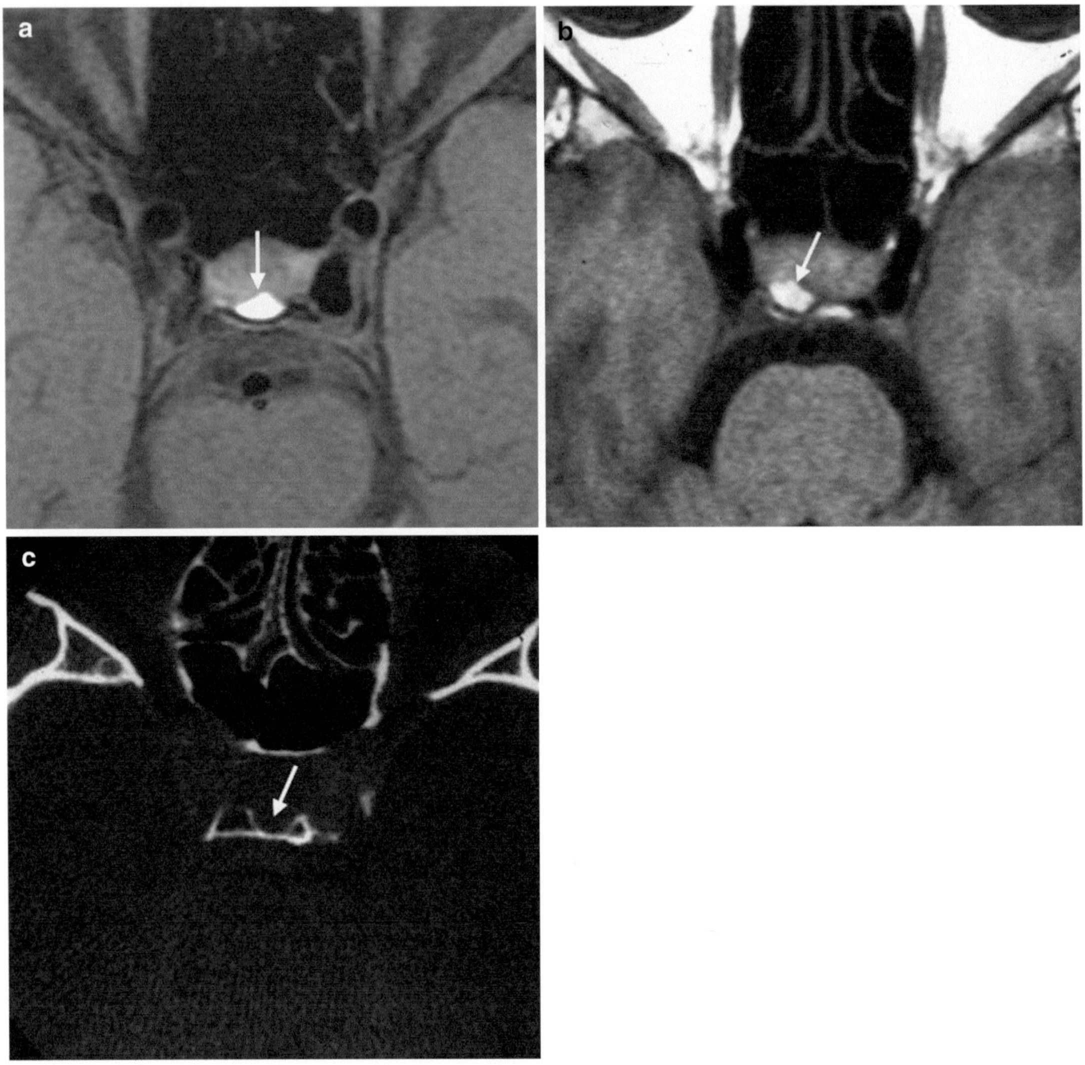

Fig. 1.5 Normal posterior lobe of the pituitary gland. (**a**) Axial Fat-Sat T1WI at 3.0 T. Suppression of the fat signal of the dorsum sellae allows good delineation of the hyperintense posterior lobe (*arrow*). (**b**) Axial T1WI at 1.5 T. Lateralized posterior lobe. (**c**) Axial CT scan, bone window demonstrating the imprint of the posterior lobe in the dorsum sellae (fossula hypophyseos) (*arrow*)

Lack of visualization of the vein of the carotid sulcus can be considered a reliable sign of invasion of the cavernous sinus by a pituitary adenoma.

The large veins with fast flow are hypointense on T1WI while the smaller veins with slow flow are hyperintense. Often one or more venous structures are visualized between the intracavernous internal carotid artery and the pituitary gland, indicating the medial limit of the cavernous sinus. The inferior intercavernous sinus is frequently demonstrated in normal children. In adults, a prominent inferior intercavernous sinus leads to a search for an intracranial hypotension syndrome or a vascular malformation of the sellar region.

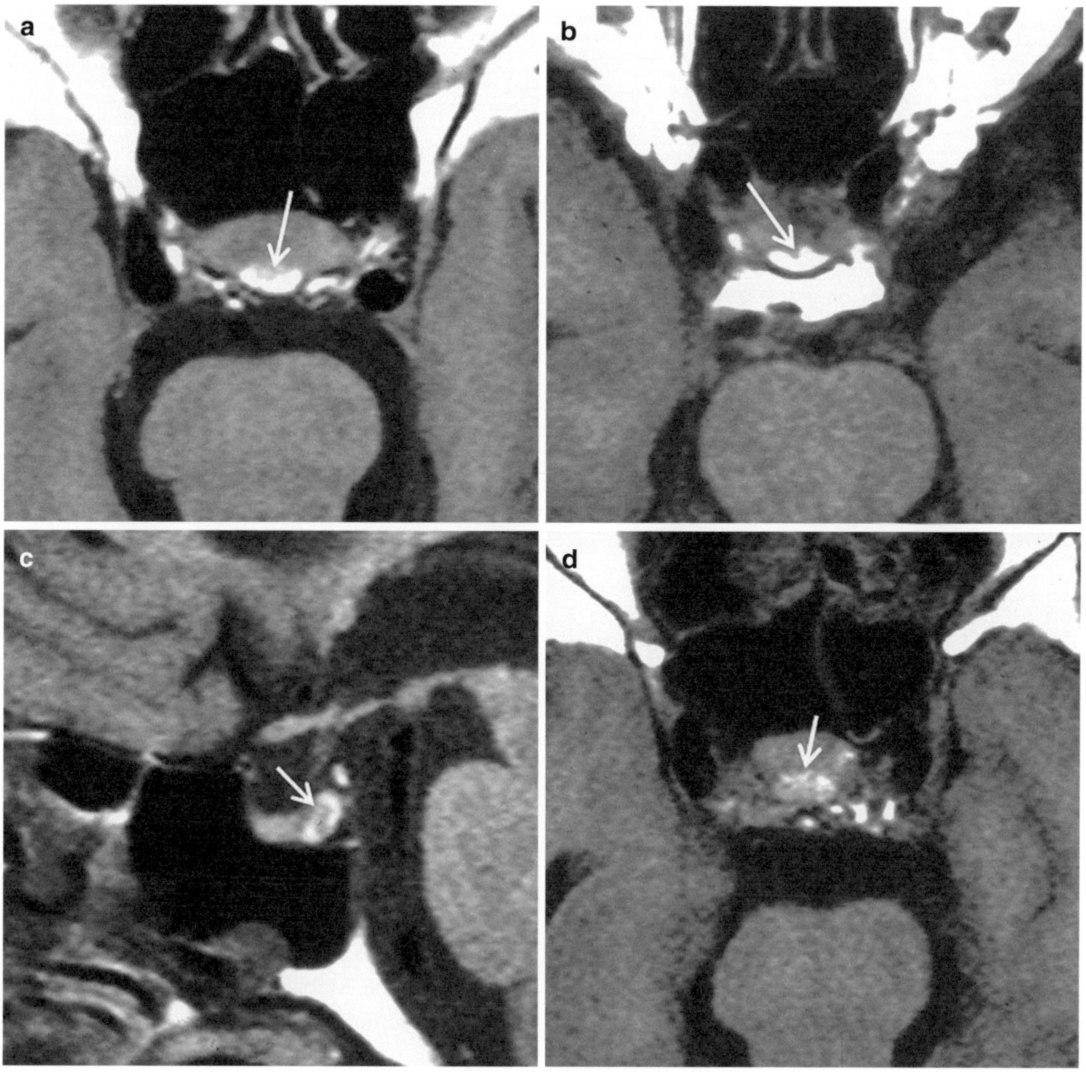

Fig. 1.6 Variants of posterior lobe. (**a**, **b**) Axial T1WIs in two elderly subjects. Heterogeneous appearance and irregularities of the anterior aspect of the posterior lobe (*arrow*). (**c**, **d**) Axial T1WIs in a 78-year-old woman. The posterior lobe is faintly hyperintense (*short arrow*)

The intracavernous cranial nerves appear hypointense on T1WI relative to the other elements of the cavernous sinus, and are thus better visible when underlined by hyperintense veins. The oculomotor nerve is always identified in the upper compartment of the cavernous sinus. On T2WI, a hyperintense thin layer of CSF is often observed around the cranial nerves, in particular the oculomotor nerve. The dural layer separating the pituitary gland from the cavernous sinus is extremely thin, particularly in the posterior part of the sella turcica. This layer is frequently visible on the coronal and, sometimes, axial T2WI at 3.0 T. The rupture of this membrane constitutes a direct sign of invasion of the cavernous sinus by a pituitary adenoma. The thicker lateral dural wall of the cavernous sinus is always identified, and markedly hypointense on T1WI and T2WI.

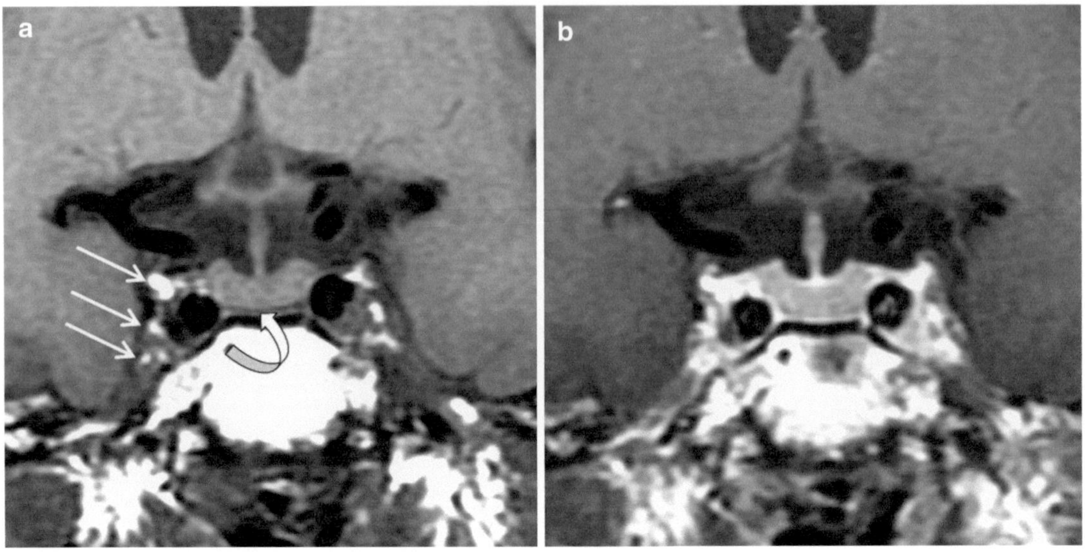

Fig. 1.7 Normal cavernous sinus. (**a**) Coronal T1WI and (**b**) CE T1WI. The low-flow veins appear hyperintense on T1WI and CE T1WI (*arrows*). A thin inferior intercavernous sinus is demonstrated in contact with the sellar floor (*curved arrow*)

After gadolinium injection, the lumen of the intracavernous internal carotid arteries does not enhance on spin-echo T1WI. The T1-hypointense large veins usually enhance while there is no change of the spontaneously T1-hyperintense veins (Fig. 1.7). The dural lateral wall of the cavernous sinus intensely enhances. Later after gadolinium injection, the intracavernous internal carotid artery and the cranial nerves appear as hypointense structures within the quite homogeneous hyperintense cavernous sinus.

High-resolution spin-echo T1WI and fast spin-echo T2WI allow the visualization of the internal architecture of the Meckel cave. The tracts of nervous fibers that constitute the trigeminal nerve in the Meckel cave can be identified within the CSF, especially on T2WI (Fig. 1.8). In general, the trigeminal ganglion is visible laterally in the anterior part of the Meckel cave, as a semilunar or nodular structure taking up contrast. In the other cases, the trigeminal ganglion is incorporated with the lateral dural wall of the Meckel cave.

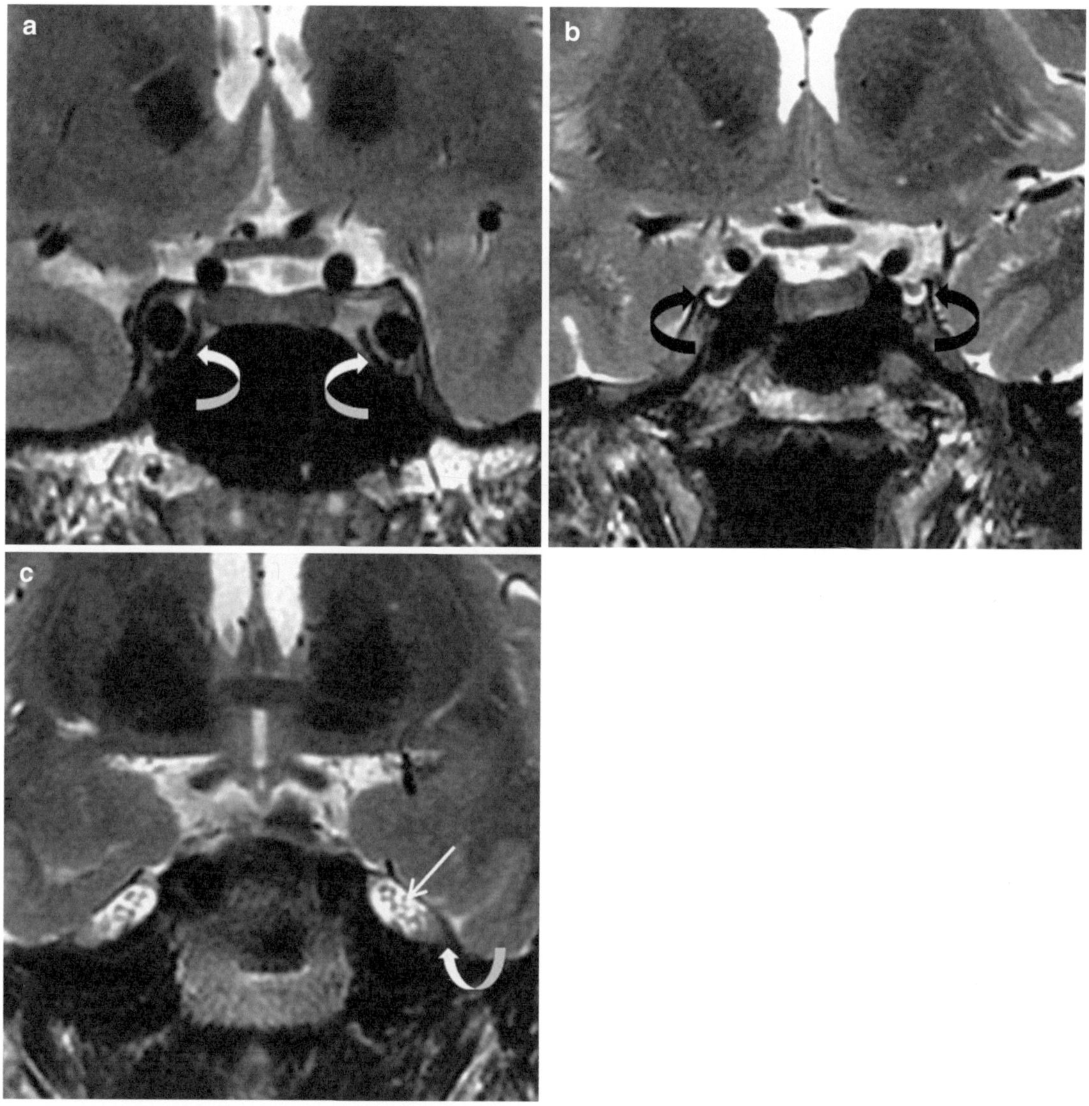

Fig. 1.8 Normal cavernous sinus. Coronal T2WIs. (**a**) Bilateral veins of the carotid sulcus located between the sphenoid sinus lateral wall and the intracavernous internal carotid artery (*curved arrows*). (**b**) The oculomotor nerves, well delineated by their CSF-filled sheaths, are identified at the upper compartment of the cavernous sinus (*black curved arrows*). (**c**) Posterior cut through the Meckel cave. The tracts of nervous fibers constituting the trigeminal nerve (*arrow*) are seen in the CSF of both the Meckel cave and the trigeminal ganglia (*curved arrow*)

Further Reading

Doraiswamy PM, Potts JM, Axelson DA et al (1992) MR assessment of pituitary gland morphology in healthy volunteers: age- and gender-related differences. AJNR Am J Neuroradiol 13:1295–1299

Kucharczyk W, Lenkinski RE, Kucharczyk J, Henkelman RM (1990) The effect of phospholipid vesicles on the NMR relaxation of water: an explanation for the MR appearance of the neurohypophysis? AJNR Am J Neuroradiol 11:693–700

Tien RD, Kucharczyk J, Bessette J, Middleton M (1992) MR imaging of the pituitary gland in infants and children: changes in size, shape and MR signal with growth and development. AJR Am J Roentgenol 158:1151–1154

2 Traps and Artifacts

Jean-François Bonneville

Artifacts and traps constitute a daily source of difficulties and mistakes when reading MR images of the sellar region. If not recognized they can mimic intrasellar lesions, in particular pituitary microadenomas.

Partial volume artifacts occur when a 3-mm-thick section, for instance, includes different anatomical structures such as the anterior pituitary gland and the sphenoid sinus anteriorly, the dorsum sellae posteriorly, or the intracavernous internal carotid arteries laterally. The computer calculates the intensity average of the different components of the section and makes an image that can simulate an intrasellar tumor (Fig. 2.1). Partial volume effects can be eliminated by coupling orthogonal projections or by using 1 mm-thick cuts, for instance with a gradient-echo 3D technique. *Magnetic susceptibility artifacts* are responsible for geometrical distortion and localized signal intensity changes at the interface of anatomical structures of different signal intensities, mainly in the case of a curved interface. Magnetic susceptibility artifacts are often present at the planum sphenoidale or at the sellar floor level; they are more pronounced at 3.0 T (Fig. 2.2) but can be cleared up with technical ploys. *Chemical shift artifacts* and ghosting are related to the high signal of fat; they can compromise the visualization of vasopressin storage in the posterior lobe on axial T1W sections when the dorsum sellae is fatty, particularly at 3.0 T. In this case fat saturation is very useful (Fig. 2.3).

Flow artifacts arise mainly out of pulsating internal carotid arteries and CSF. They are more marked at 3.0 T and can blur or pollute images of the pituitary fossa or subarachnoid space (Fig. 2.4). *The posterior lobe and a deep fossula hypophyseos* are frequently mistaken for a posteriorly located pituitary adenoma on coronal T2WIs (Fig. 2.5); topography of the posterior lobe, which is half of the time off-midline, is ideally demonstrated on axial T1W fat-saturated imaging. *Dynamic imaging* should not be performed routinely but only in specific cases. Its interpretation must be rigorous or it can lead to false-positive diagnoses (Fig. 15.5).

J.-F. Bonneville et al., *MRI of the Pituitary Gland*, DOI 10.1007/978-3-319-29043-0_2

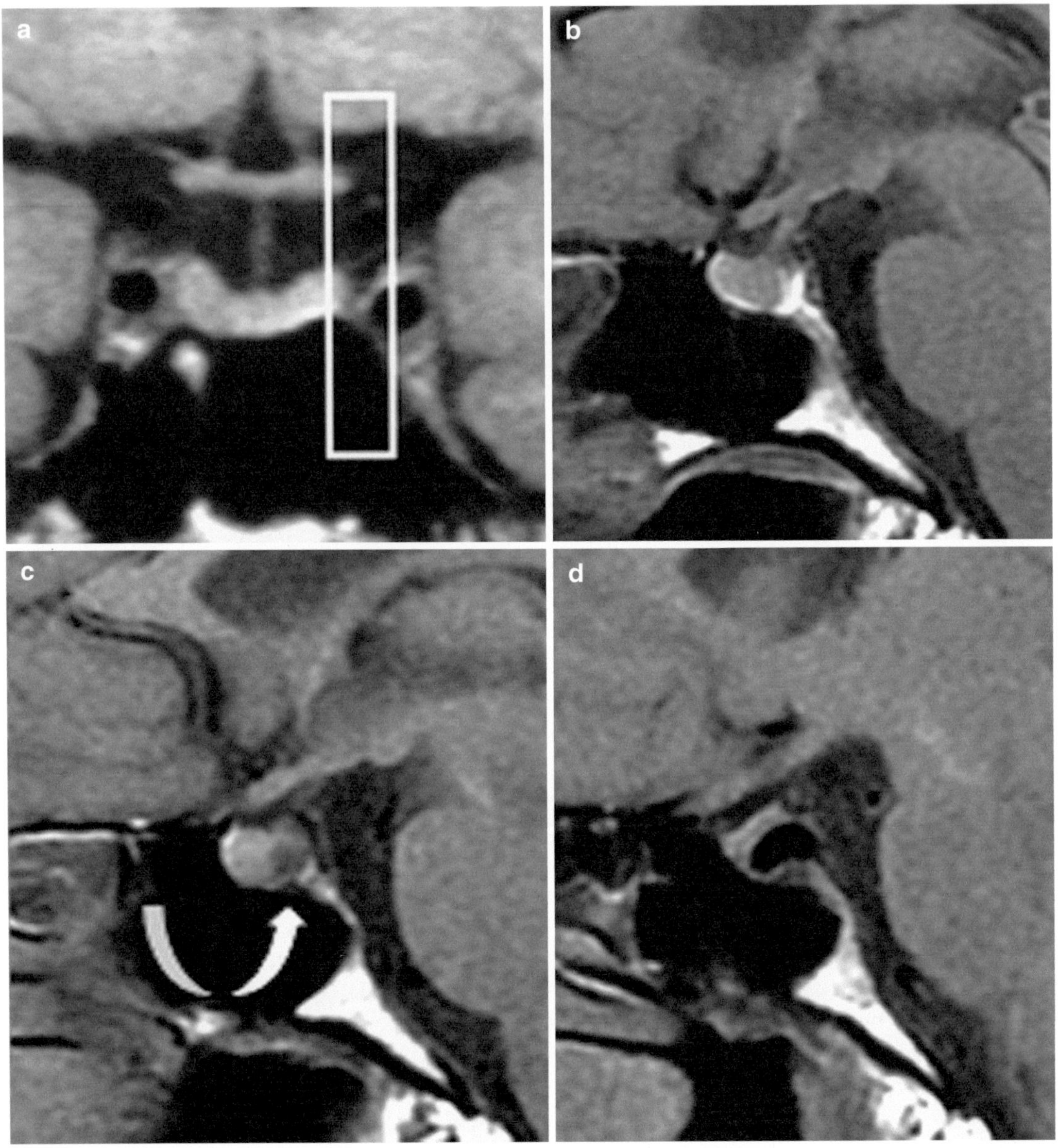

Fig. 2.1 Partial volume effect artifact. (**a**) Coronal T1WI. (**b–d**) Sagittal T1WIs. A thick section includes pituitary tissue and part of the intracavernous internal carotid artery, with a resulting image simulating a pituitary adenoma (*arrow*)

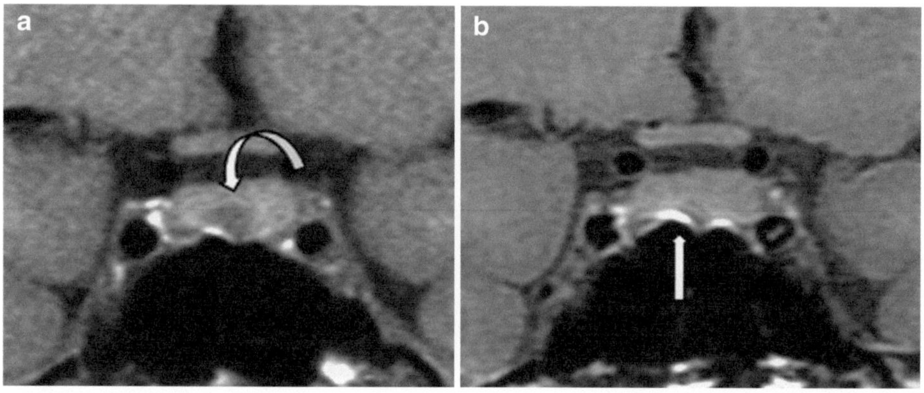

Fig. 2.2 Magnetic susceptibility artifact. (**a**) Coronal T1WI at 1.5 T demonstrates a 5-mm hypointense microadenoma (*curved arrow*). (**b**) T1WI at 3.0 T: the distortion of the sellar floor (*straight arrow*) masks the pituitary adenoma

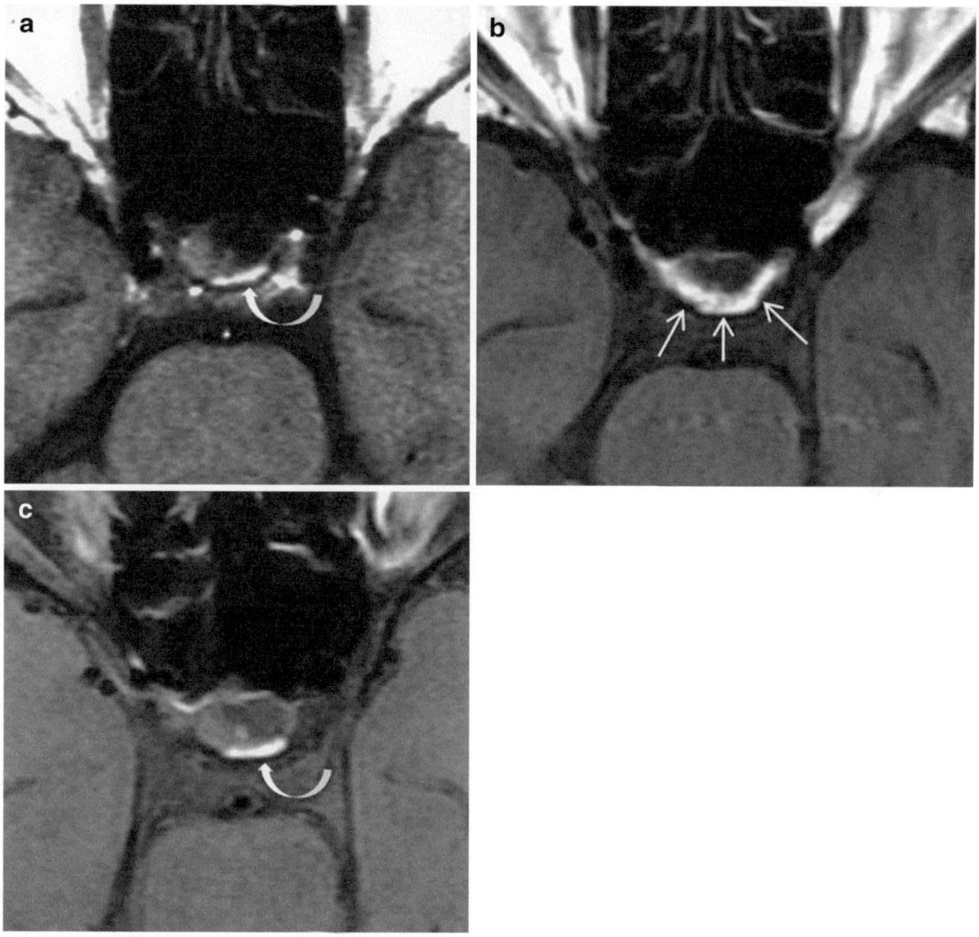

Fig. 2.3 Chemical shift artifact. (**a**) Axial T1WI at 1.5 T shows a normal T1-hyperintense posterior lobe (*curved arrow*). (**b**) Axial T1WI at 3.0 T fails to demonstrate the posterior lobe: the image of the fatty dorsum sellae is displaced forward and is superimposed on the posterior lobe: chemical shift artifact (*straight arrows*). (**c**) Axial T1W fat-saturated image at 3.0 T: this sequence eliminates fat and permits localization of the antidiuretic hormone storage in the posterior lobe

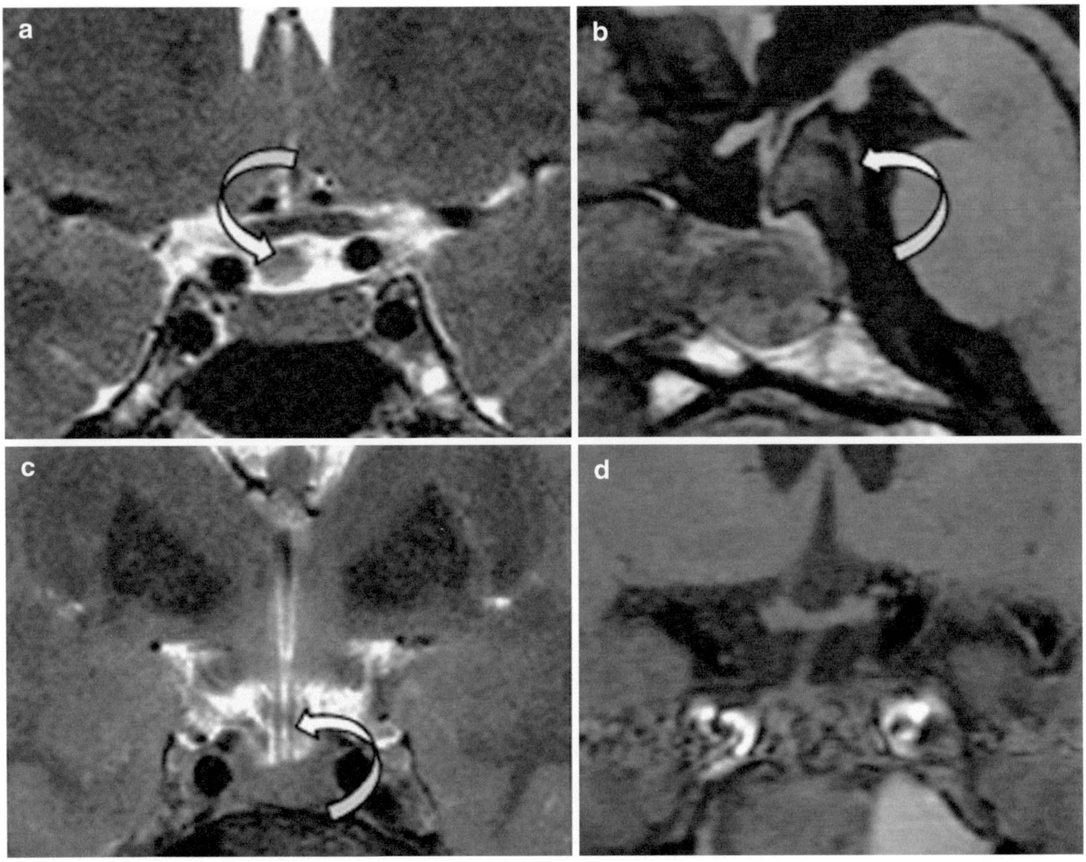

Fig. 2.4 Flow artifacts. (**a**) Coronal T2WI. (**b**) Sagittal TIWI. (**c**) Coronal T2WI. (**d**) Coronal T1WI. Flow artifacts from CSF (**a–c**) can be misleading, particularly in the optochiasmatic cistern (*arrows*). Flow artifacts from the internal carotid arteries (**d**) can hinder visualization of the pituitary gland

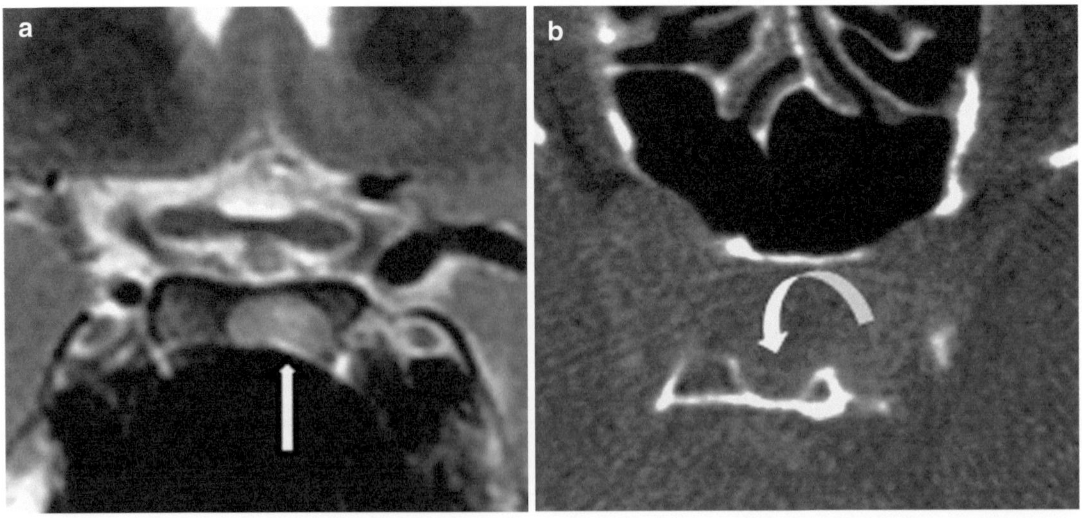

Fig. 2.5 Fossula hypophyseos and posterior lobe. (**a**) Coronal T2WI through the dorsum sellae. A rounded T2-hyperintense image (*arrow*) could mimic a pituitary adenoma. (**b**) axial CT, bone window. This image is the result of a deep imprint of the dorsum sellae serving as a bed for the posterior pituitary (*curved arrow*)

Further Reading

Bonneville JF, Bonneville F, Cattin F (2005) Magnetic resonance imaging of pituitary adenomas. Eur Radiol 15(3):543–548

Elster AD (1993) Sellar susceptibility artifacts: theory and implications. AJNR Am J Neuroradiol 14(1):129–136

Sakurai K, Fujita N, Harada K et al (1992) Magnetic susceptibility artifact in spin-echo MR imaging of the pituitary gland. AJNR Am J Neuroradiol 13(5):1301–1308

3 Small Sella and Convex Pituitary Gland

Jean-François Bonneville and Françoise Cattin

A small sella turcica is a normal anatomical variant responsible for an inadequacy between the sellar volume and its content, with a resultant bulging of the pituitary gland. It can mimic a pathological enlargement of the pituitary gland and, if not recognized, can lead to a false diagnosis of "pituitary hyperplasia" or even pituitary tumor. This is particularly true in teenage females with physiological enlargement of the pituitary gland.

In adults, a small sella turcica is frequently related to a hyperpneumatization of the sphenoid sinus. It feels like excessive pneumatization of the sphenoid sinus inhibits the complete development of the pituitary fossa. Hyperpneumatization of the sphenoid sinus may be associated with a flat or narrow sella and a resultant bulging of the pituitary gland.

A thick dorsum sellae, either pneumatized or fatty, can restrict the anteroposterior diameter of the pituitary fossa. The sella turcica can also be short transversally. This condition is difficult to apprehend: we must bear in mind that only 2 out of 100 adults have a sellar floor width of less than 10 mm. Therefore, an upward convex pituitary gland above a sella floor less than 10 mm wide is very likely to be an anatomical variant (Fig. 3.1).

In summary, in front of what looks like an enlarged pituitary gland with normal T1 and T2 signals and normal enhancement after gadolinium injection, a small sella has to be evoked: for instance, in the case of unusual hyperpneumatization of the sphenoid sinus, such as pneumatization extending beyond the spheno-occipital synchondrosis or deep in the pterygoid processes. Asymmetrical hyperpneumatization may be particularly misleading (Fig. 3.2). Blistering of the planum sphenoidale also accompanies sphenoid sinus hyperpneumatization (Fig. 3.3). The shape of the dorsum sellae and the sellar width must also be carefully scrutinized.

Differential diagnosis of an upward bulging of the pituitary gland includes mainly the holosellar pituitary adenoma. In the latter, the posterior lobe appears compressed on axial T1WI, but not in the case of a bulging normal pituitary gland above a small sella turcica. An ignored or masked pregnancy in women of child-bearing age must also be kept in mind: T1 hyperintensity of the pituitary gland, if compared with the pons on sagittal T1WI, will make the diagnosis beyond the second trimester of the pregnancy. The useful volume of a normal-sized sella can also rarely be reduced by an unusually large inferior coronary sinus, for instance, "kissing" internal carotid arteries (Fig. 56.5) or a sellar spine (Fig. 3.4). Finally, several factors can be associated with reduction in sellar volume (Fig. 3.5) Conversely, a small sella or a narrowed sellar volume are not necessarily associated with an upward bulging of the pituitary gland.

J.-F. Bonneville et al., *MRI of the Pituitary Gland*, DOI 10.1007/978-3-319-29043-0_3

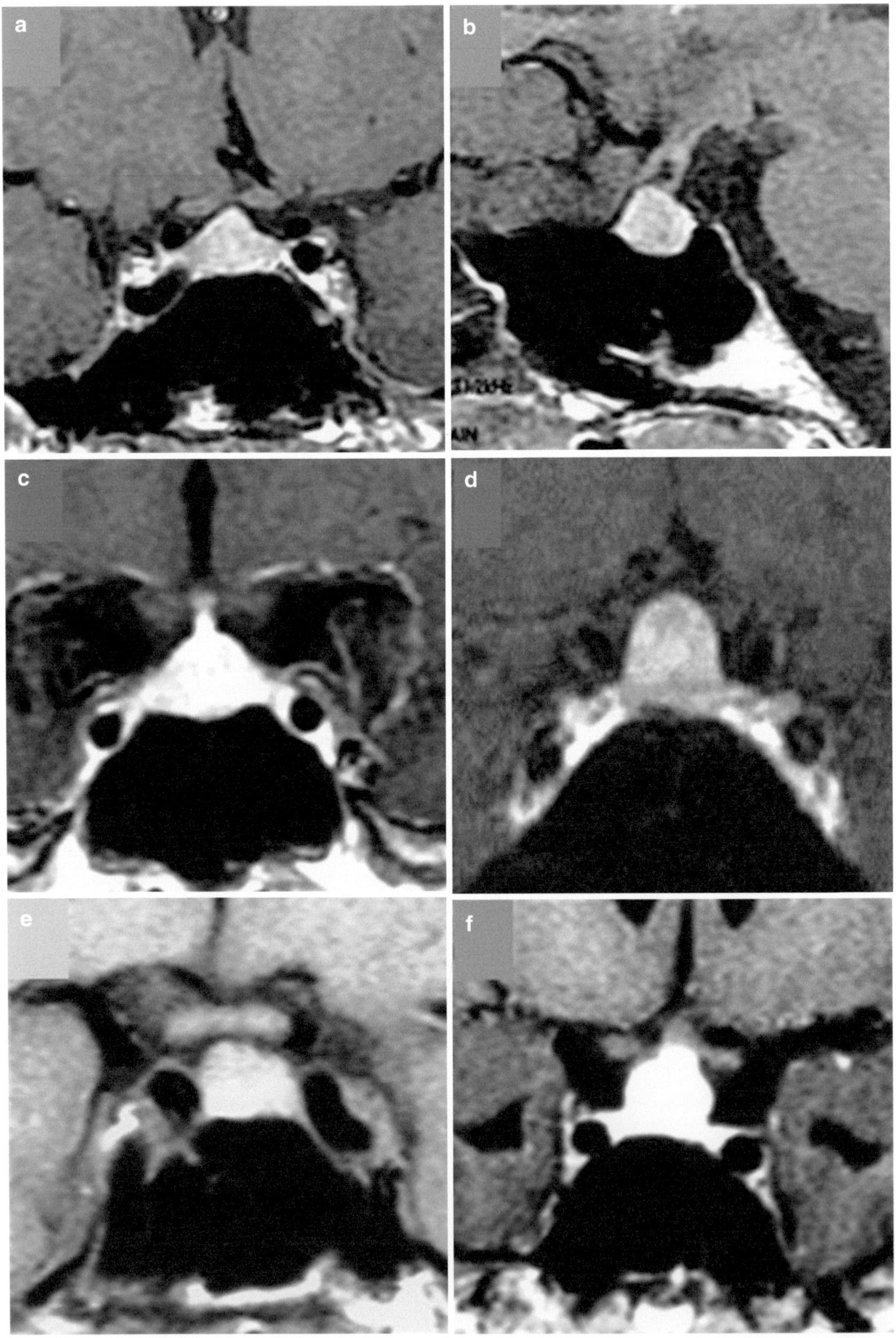

Fig. 3.1 (**a**, **b**) Physiological bulging of the pituitary gland on coronal and sagittal CE T1WI. (**c**–**f**) Coronal CE T1WI. Small sella, hyperpneumatization of the sphenoid sinus, and/or narrow sellar floor

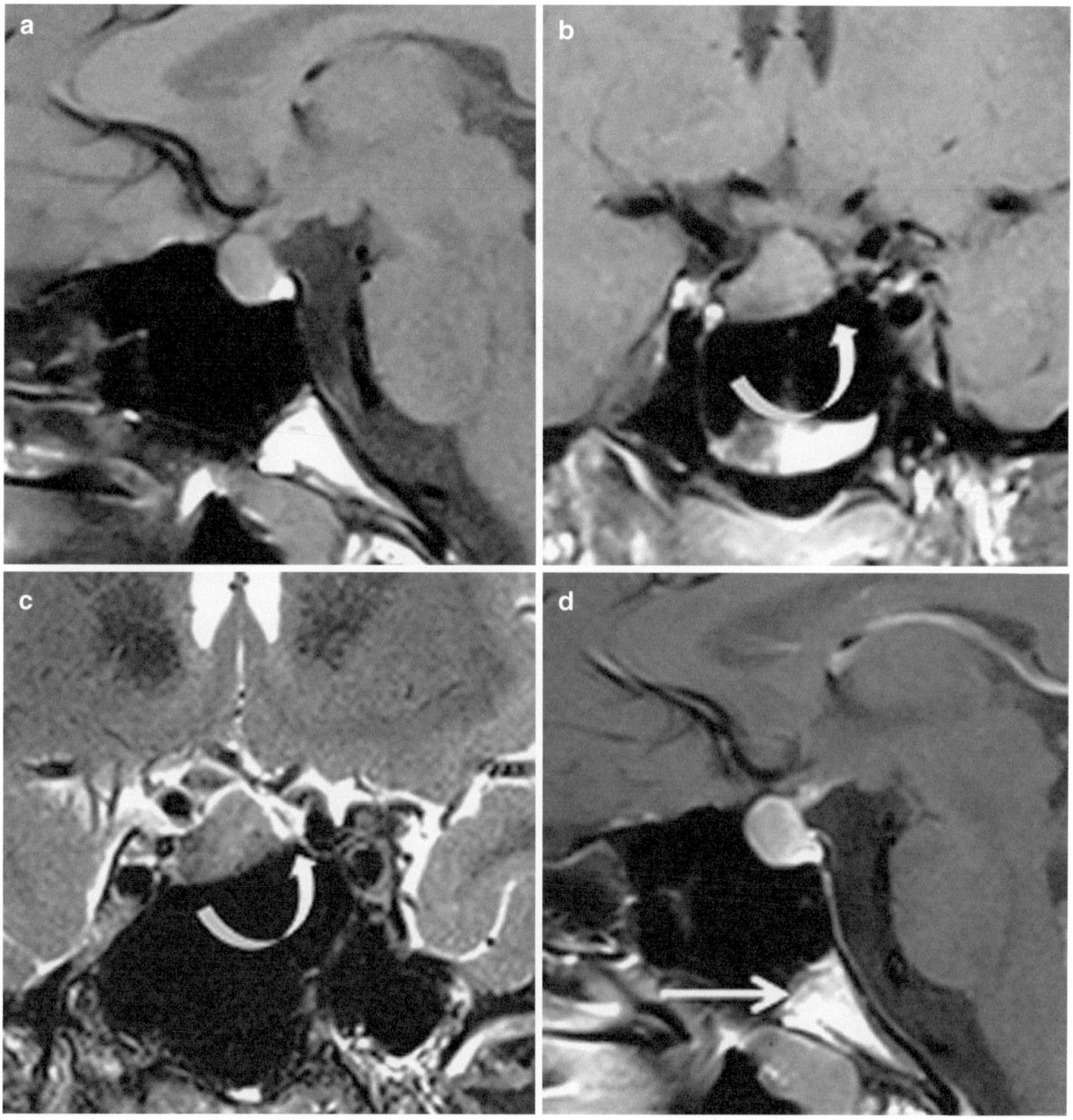

Fig. 3.2 Physiological bulging of the pituitary gland in a 16-year-old girl. Asymmetrical hyperpneumatization. (**a**, **d**) Sagittal T1 and CE T1WIs. (**b**, **e**) Coronal T1 and CET1WIs. (**c**) coronal T2WI. (**f**) Axial CE TIWI. Sphenoid sinus pneumatization reaches the spheno-occipital synchondrosis (*arrow*). Excessive pneumatization on the left side (*curved arrows*) pushes the pituitary gland upward and to the right

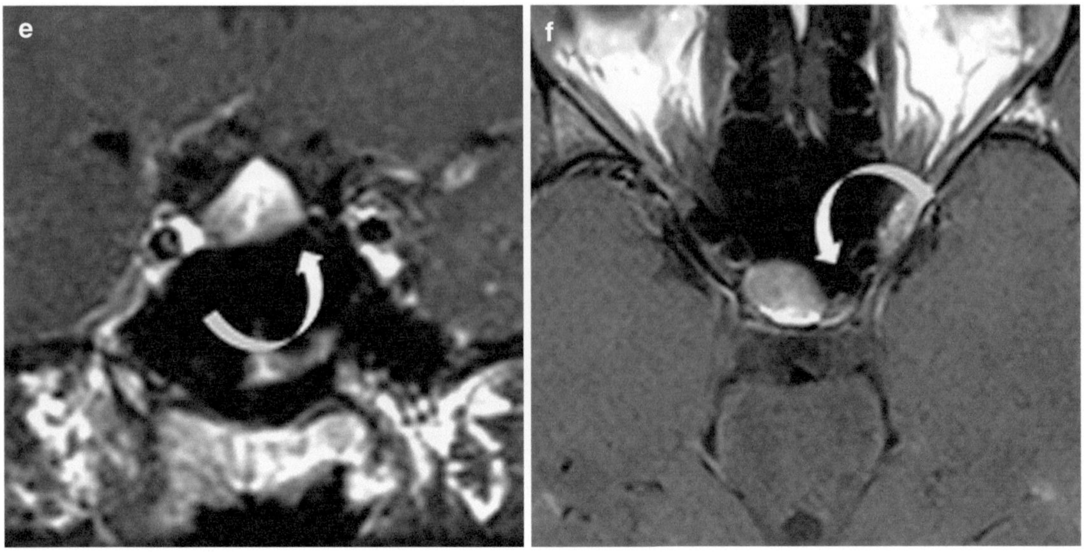

Fig. 3.2 (continued)

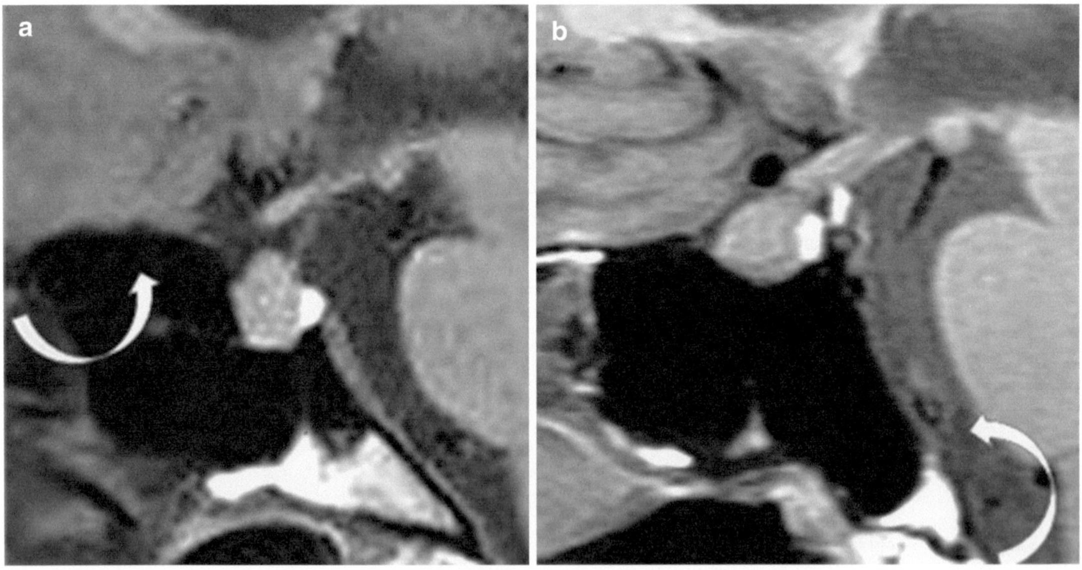

Fig. 3.3 Physiological bulging of the pituitary gland; small sella and hyperpneumatization of the sphenoid sinus. (**a**, **b**) Sagittal T1WI. (**a**) Blistering of the planum sphenoidale (*arrow*). (**b**) extension of the pneumatization beyond the spheno-occipital synchondrosis (*arrow*)

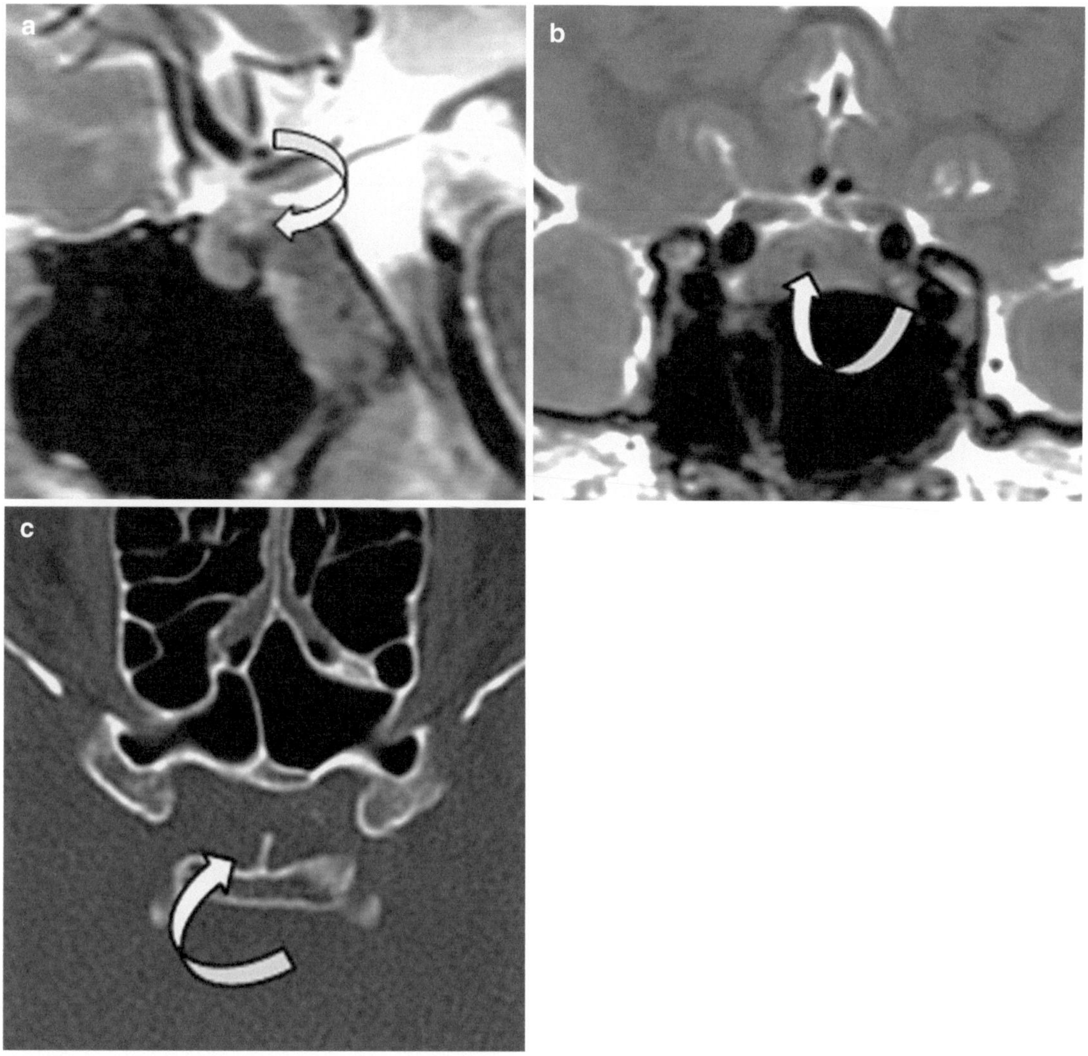

Fig. 3.4 Sellar spine (*arrow*) arising from the dorsum sellae and pushing the pituitary gland upward. (**a**, **b**) Sagittal and coronal T2WIs. (**c**) Axial CT

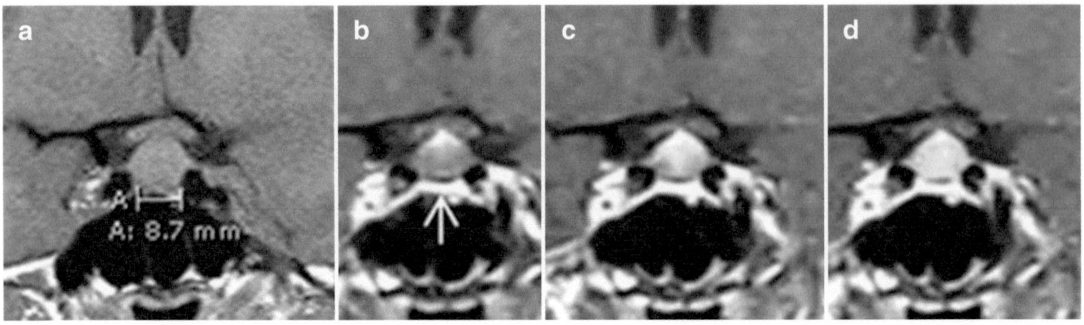

Fig. 3.5 Upward bulging of the upper surface of a normal pituitary gland resulting together from a narrow sellar width (**a**) coronal T1WI and from an unusual thick inferior coronary sinus, demonstrated with dynamic MRI (**b–d**) (*arrow*). Normal enhancement of the pituitary gland

Further Reading

Bonneville JF (2002) When the pituitary swells up a little. J Radiol 83(3):319–320

Cattin F, Bonneville JF, Tang YS (1990) Diagnostic d'une hypophyse convexe. Rev Inst Med 2:221–228

Nonfunctioning Pituitary Macroadenoma: General Points

4

Jean-François Bonneville

Nonfunctioning pituitary macroadenomas, also named nonsecreting adenomas, are frequently in fact gonadotropic adenomas, more rarely null-cell adenomas. They are responsible for neurologic symptoms (mainly visual field defect, headache) or endocrinologic symptoms (mainly anterior pituitary insufficiency). They are also very frequently discovered by chance and can be totally asymptomatic. In the latter case, a conservative approach can be proposed, particularly in the elderly, with a long-term MRI follow up. In young patients, finding a large, invasive pituitary adenoma—secreting or not—should prompt research of AIP and MEN1 gene mutations. Family history of pituitary adenomas or other features of the MEN1 syndrome in the patient and family should also be used to orient genetic research. In every case, a strict imaging protocol must be applied after surgery, the risk of recurrence being around 30 %. Pituitary nonfunctioning macroadenomas are usually centered by an enlarged sella turcica. Signal intensity is usually inhomogeneous, particularly on T2W images with disseminated areas of hyperintensities reflecting cystic or necrotic components. T1 hyperintensity indicates the presence of blood, as does fluid-fluid level (Figs. 4.1 and 4.2). Old hemorrhage may be detected on T2*WI only (Fig. 4.3). Gadolinium injection offers a more clear-cut demonstration of tumoral contours; it enhances the normal pituitary tissue, which is distorted and displaced laterally on one side, and superiorly, but quite never inferiorly (Fig. 4.4). Demonstration of the normal residual pituitary gland is of crucial importance for the neurosurgeon. Enhancement of the dura, the so-called dural tail (Figs. 4.4 and 4.5), previously described as specific of meningiomas, has been described with large pituitary adenomas, especially if hemorrhagic or soon after surgery, and with perisellar aneurysms and other sellar tumors. The degree of enhancement of the solid part of the pituitary adenoma does not reflect the vascular density of the tumor and is thus not predictable of a potential perioperative hemorrhage. Conversely, flow-void linear images on T1WI or T2WI indicate the presence of intratumoral arteries (Fig. 4.6). Nonfunctioning macroadenomas present usually with an extrasellar extension, upward into the suprasellar cistern, downward into the sphenoid sinus, or laterally into the cavernous sinus. Upward extension is present in more than 70 % of cases. The suprasellar component of the largest macroadenomas is often multilobular (Fig. 4.7). The sellar diaphragm can operate as a belt, giving the adenoma an hourglass shape. If the suprasellar extension is moderate, the T1-hyperintense posterior lobe is compressed and flattened, and best identified in axial T1 fat-saturated noncontrast WI. Aberrant storage of antidiuretic hormone, the so-called ectopic posterior lobe, occurs when the pituitary stalk is severely compressed, i.e., in practice with macroadenomas more than 20 mm in height (see Chap. 53). Various degrees of distortion or thinning of the optic chiasm can be observed. Its hyperintensity on T2WIs could indicate a poor visual prognosis, but the lesion can be

J.-F. Bonneville et al., *MRI of the Pituitary Gland*, DOI 10.1007/978-3-319-29043-0_4

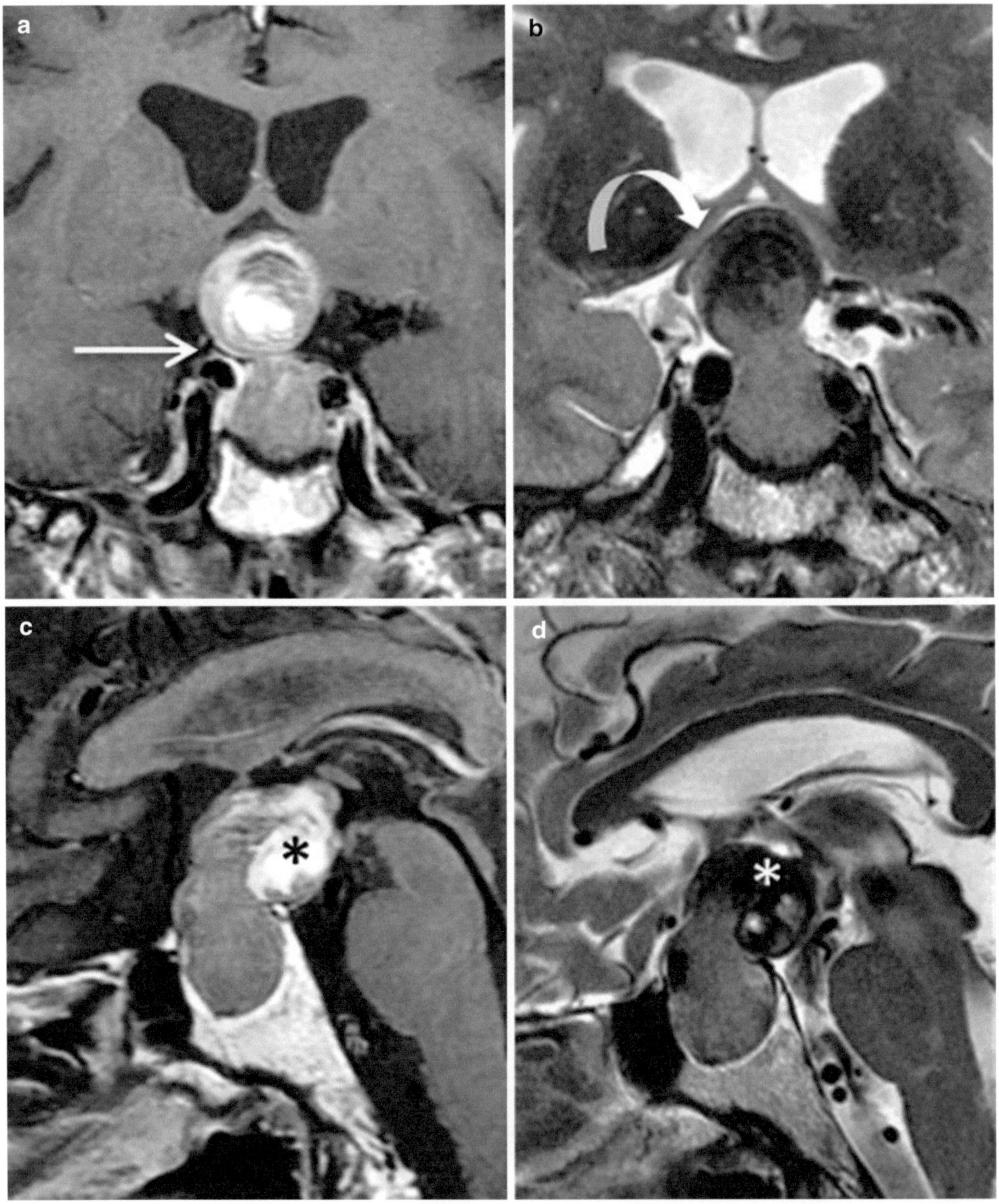

Fig. 4.1 Nonfunctioning pituitary adenoma with suprasellar extension and hemorrhagic component. (**a**, **b**) Coronal CE TI and T2 WIs. (**c**, **d**) Sagittal T1 and T2 WIs. The sellar diaphragm (*straight arrow*) separates as a waist the intra- and suprasellar tumoral compartments. The most superior and posterior part of the adenoma is hyperintense on T1WI and hypointense on T2WI, thus signaling a hemorrhagic event (*asterisk*). Note the extreme thinness of the displaced optic chiasm (*curved arrow*)

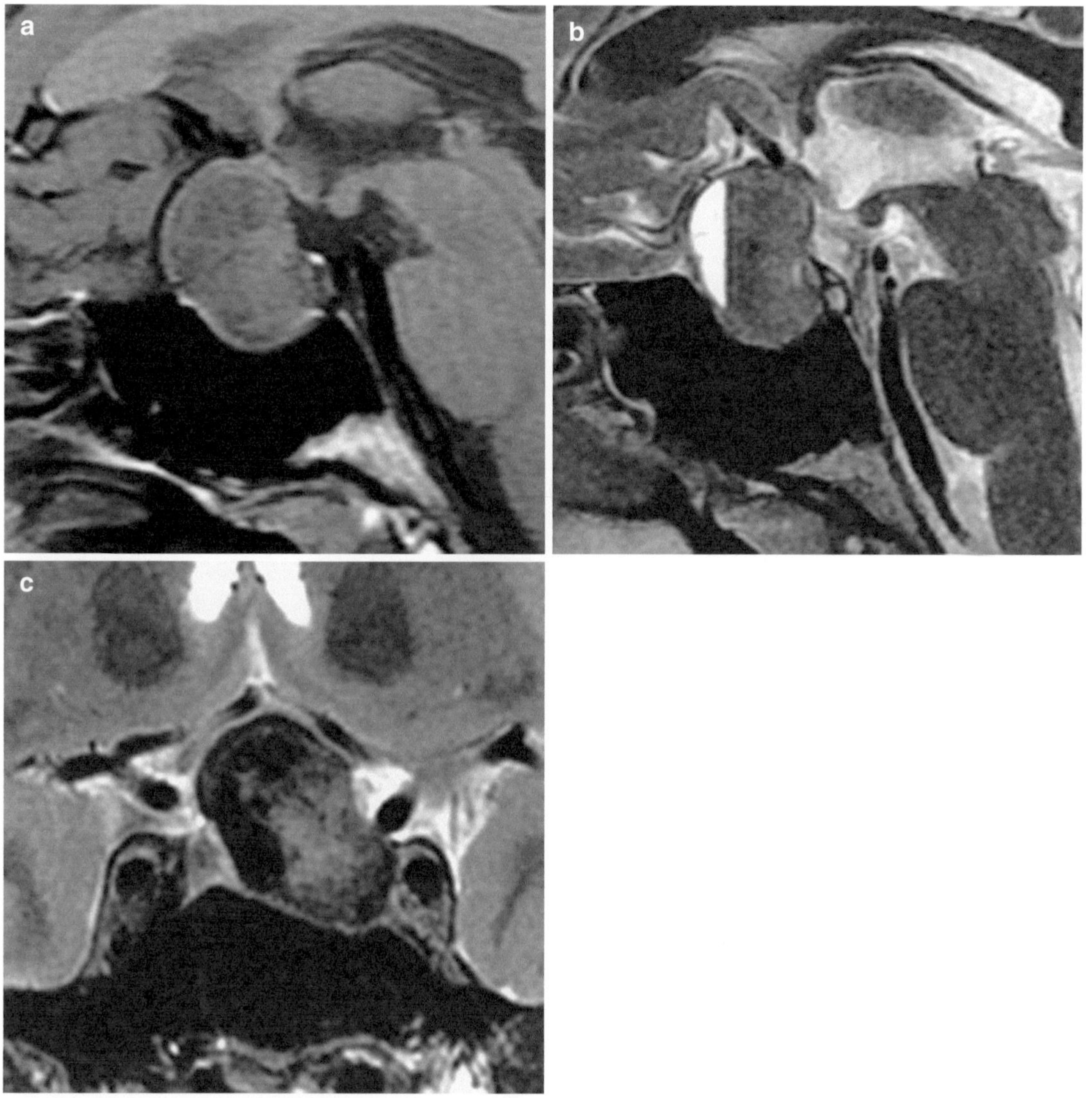

Fig. 4.2 Hemorrhagic macroadenoma with fluid-fluid level. (**a**) Sagittal T1WI. (**b**, **c**) Sagittal and coronal T2WIs. Heterogeneous signal in (**a**). In (**b**), fluid-fluid level shows old hemorrhage. (**c**) Coronal T2WI: predominant T2-hypointense signal

reversible if the responsible pituitary adenoma is quickly removed (Fig. 4.8). Ptosis of a V-shaped appearing optic chiasm within a secondary empty sella frequently occurs after surgery.

Downward extension of nonfunctioning pituitary adenomas is less frequent than in GH-secreting adenomas or prolactinomas. Special attention has to be paid to clival invasion, present in 8 % of macroadenomas, preferentially in females and with large-volume null-cell adenomas (Fig. 10.4). MRI or, better, CT demonstrate a focal or widespread defect of the more anterior cephalad portion of the clivus and decreased attenuation in underlying trabecular bone. Severe surgical complications can occur, especially if clival invasion is not recognized preoperatively .

Lateral extension in the cavernous sinus, usually unilateral, is present in about 30 % of cases. This is extensively described in Chap. 11.

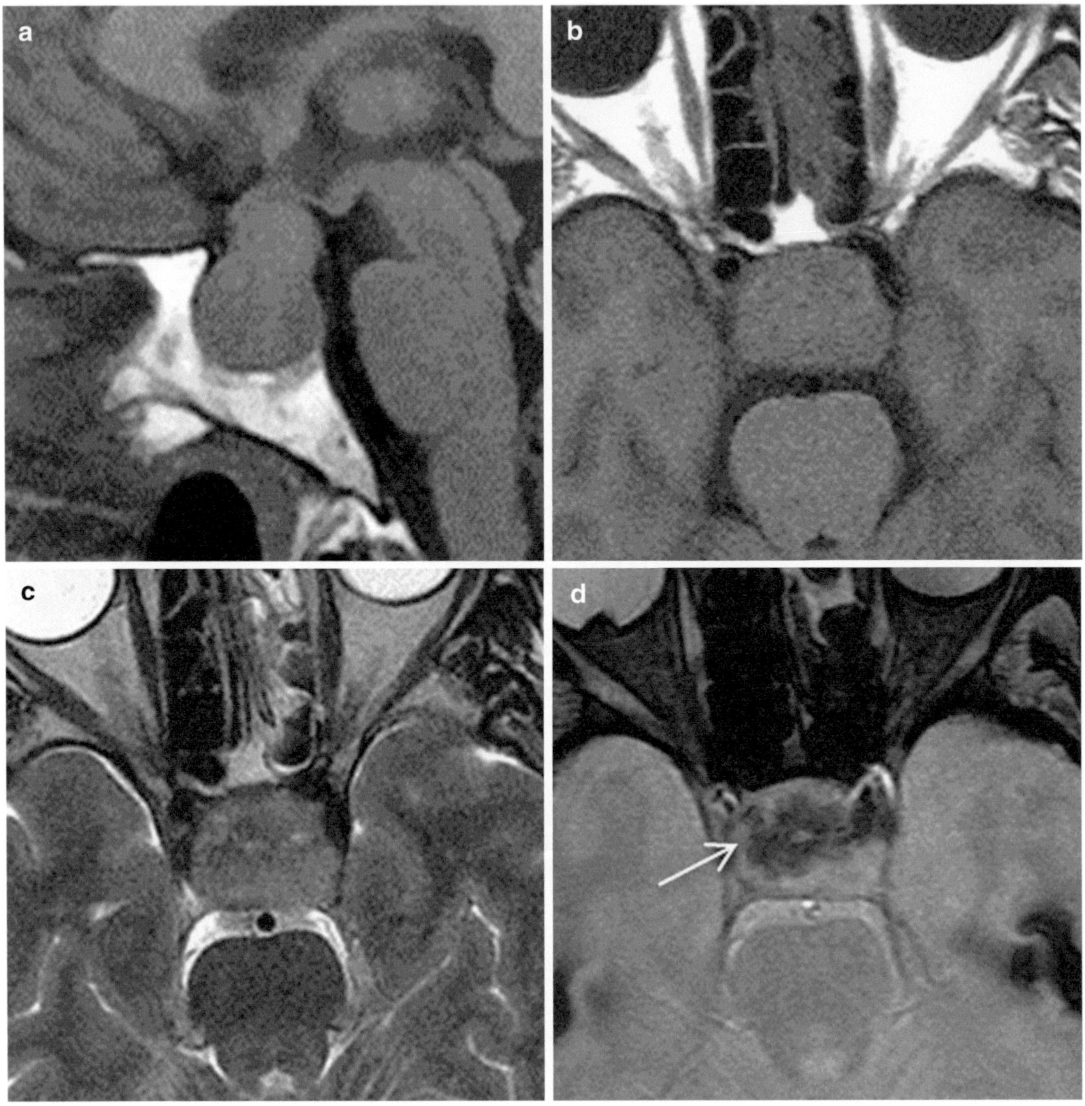

Fig. 4.3 Pituitary macroadenoma with suprasellar extension discovered fortuitously. (**a**) Sagittal T1WI. (**b–d**) Axial T1, T2 and T2* WIs. Intratumoral hypointensities reflecting old hemorrhage are demonstrated on T2*WI only (*arrow*)

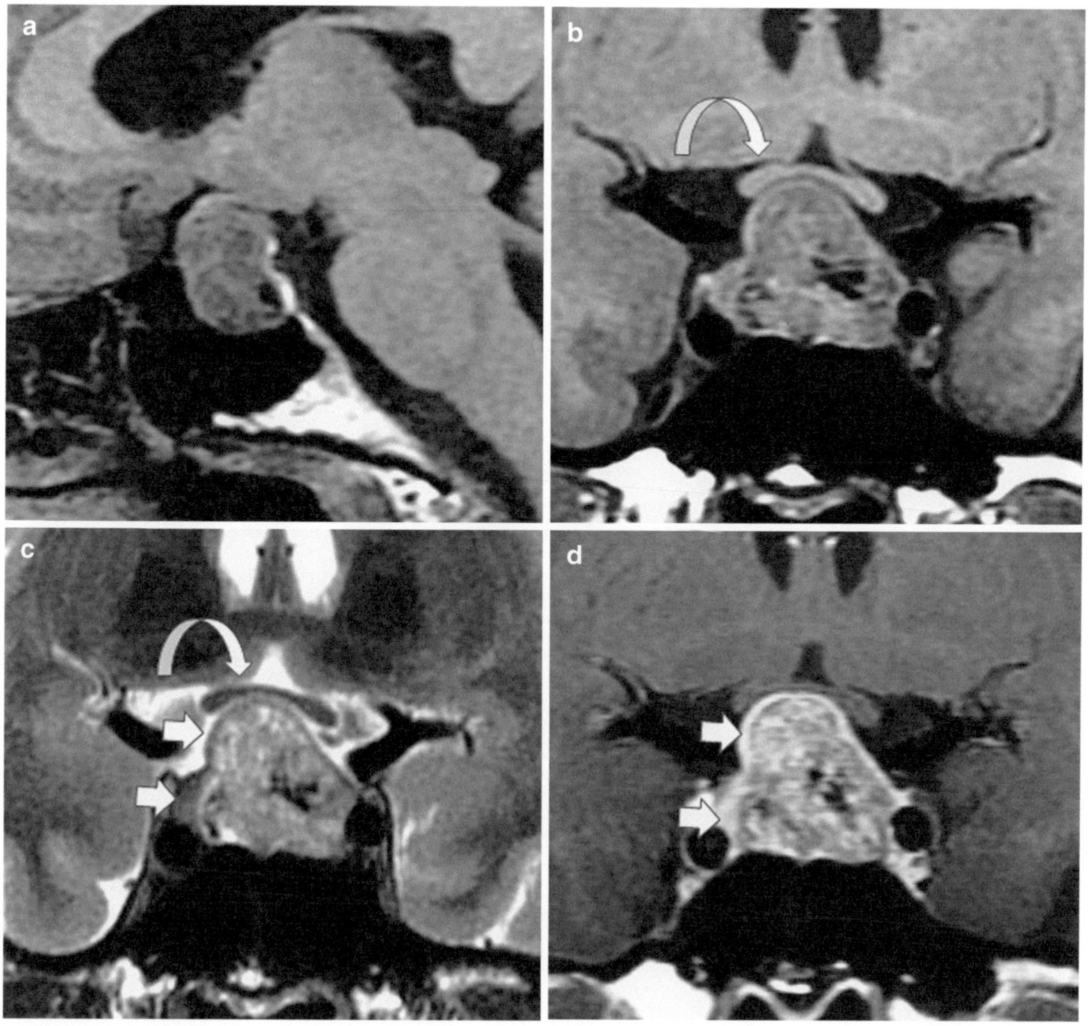

Fig. 4.4 Macroadenoma abutting the optic chiasm (*curved arrow*) (**a**, **b**) Sagittal and coronal T1WIs. (**c**, **d**) Coronal T2 and CE T1 WIs. The normal pituitary tissue is demonstrated on the right side (*thick arrows*)

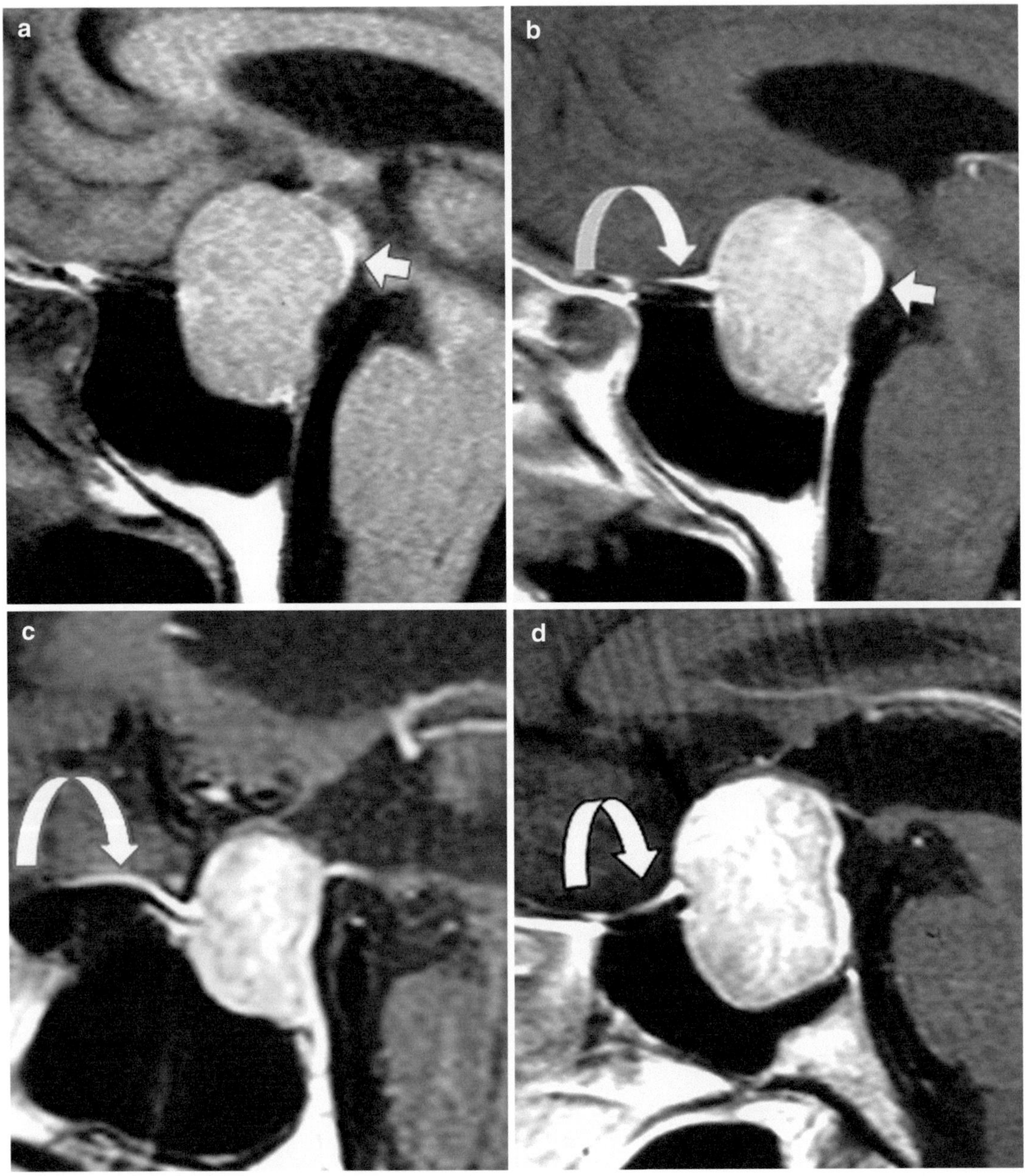

Fig. 4.5 Macroadenoma with ectopic posterior lobe (*short arrow*) and dural tail (*curved arrow*). (**a**, **b**) Sagittal TI and CE T1 WIs. (**c**, **d**) Sagittal CE T1WI: dural tail (*curved arrows*) in two cases of nonfunctioning macroadenomas

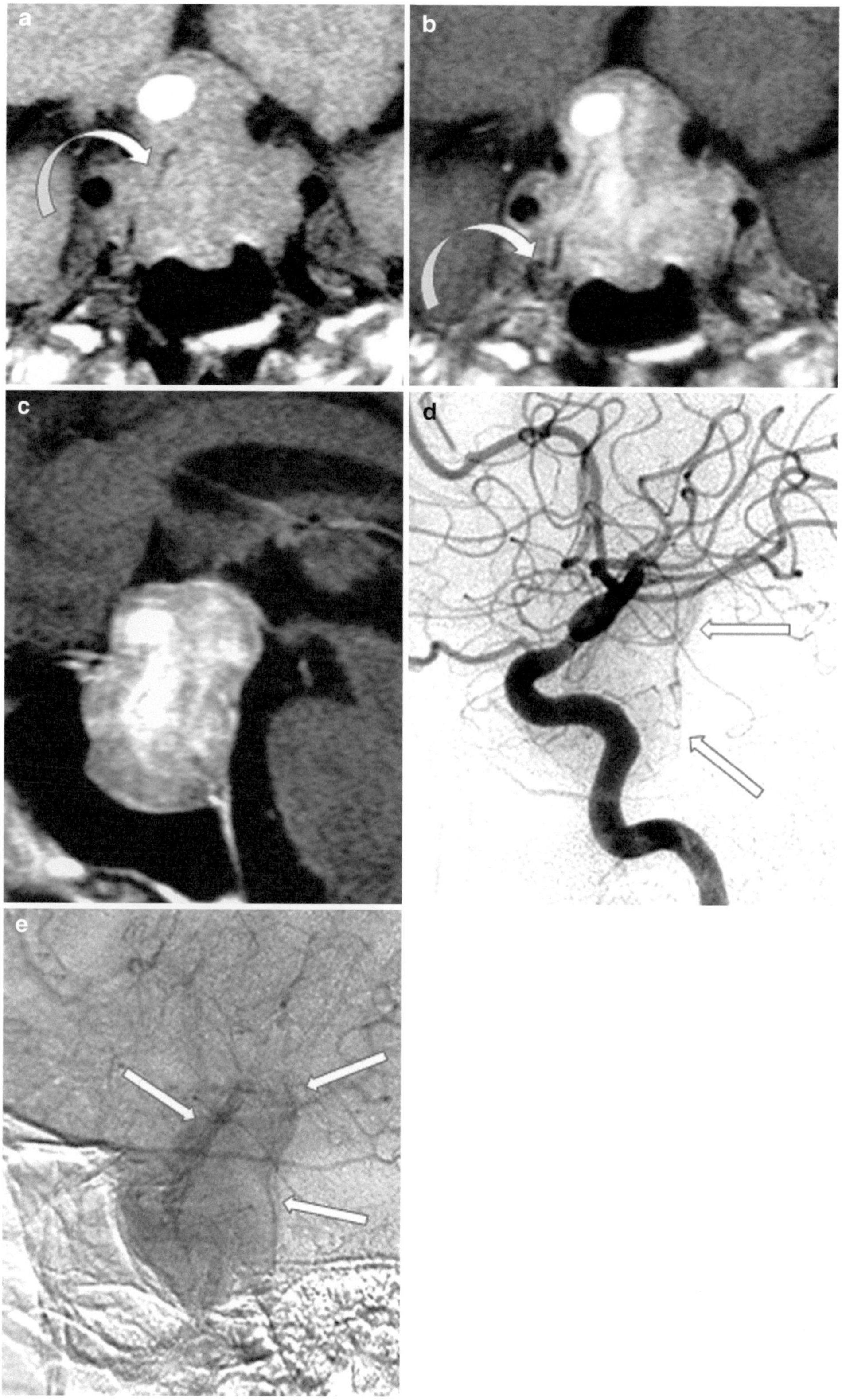

Fig. 4.6 Macroadenoma: unusual blood supply. (**a–c**) Coronal T1, CE T1, and sagittal CE T1 WIs. Hemorrhagic area at the top of the lesion; running artery (*curved arrow*) through the pituitary mass. (**d, e**) Carotid angiography, arterial and parenchymatous phases: arterial blush modeling the contours of the pituitary adenoma (*straight arrows*)

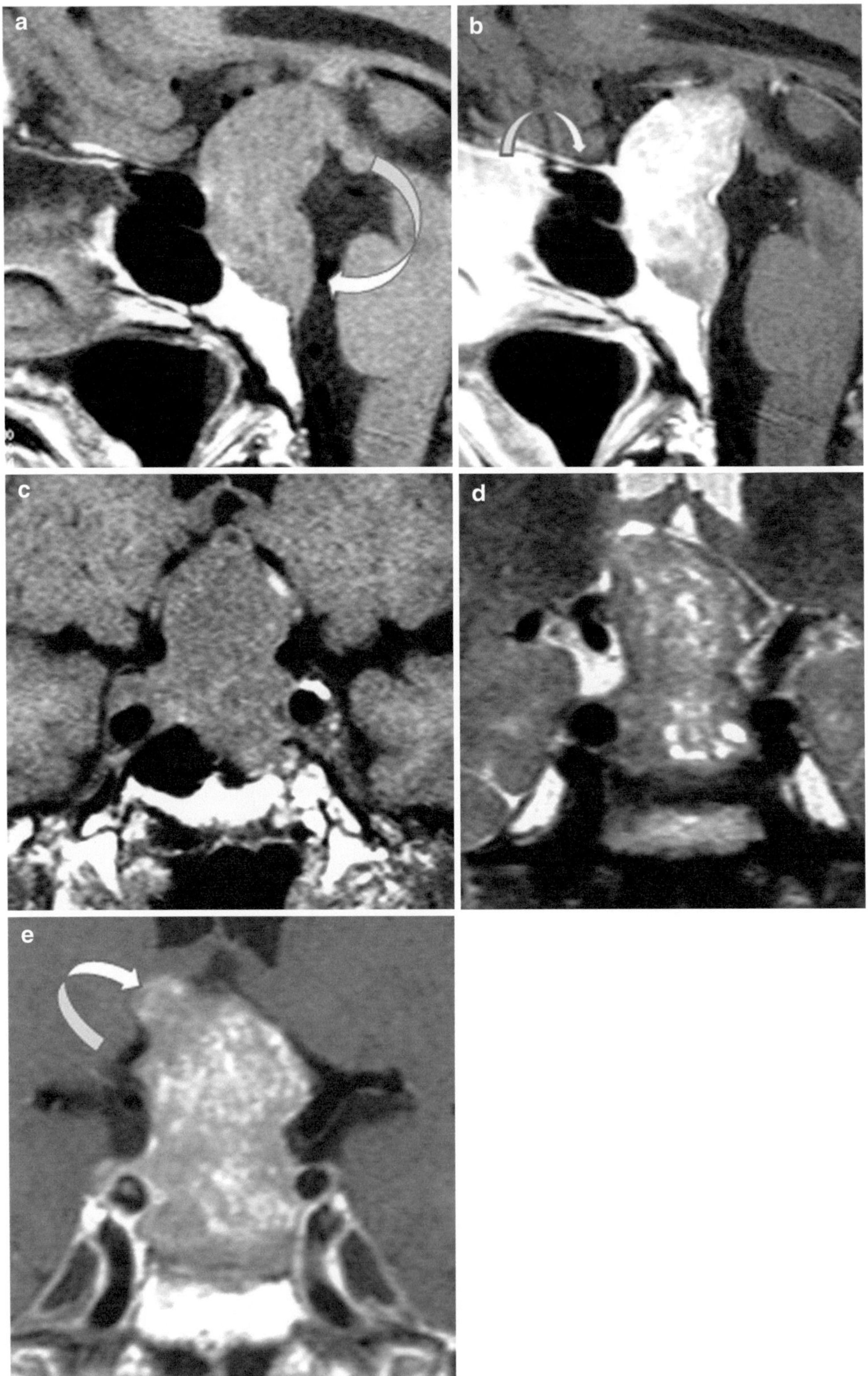

Fig. 4.7 Macroadenoma and clival invasion. (**a**, **b**) Sagittal T1 and CE T1 WIs. (**c**–**e**) Coronal T1, T2, and CE T1WIs. Erosion of the dorsum sellae and clivus (*large curved arrow*), dural tail (*small curved arrow*); lobulated contour (*curved arrow* in **e**)

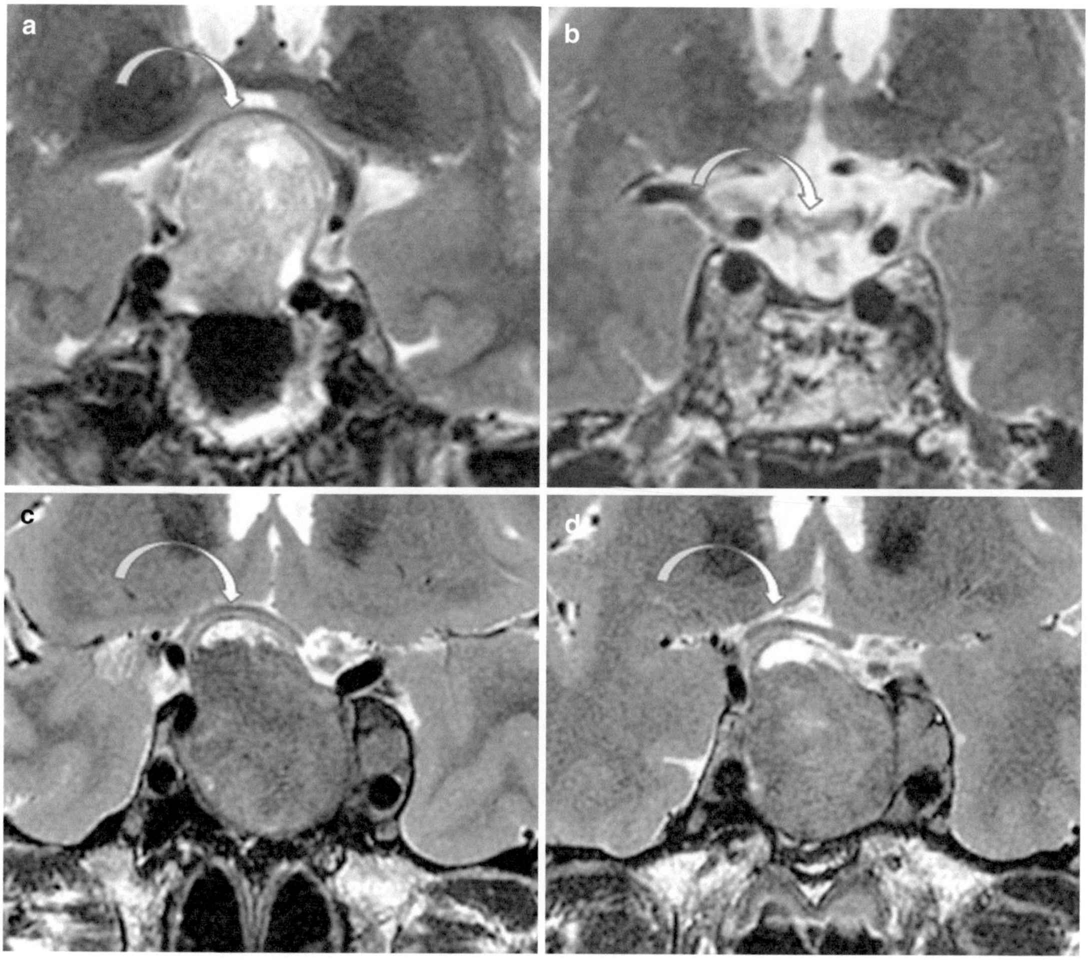

Fig. 4.8 Nonfunctioning pituitary adenomas with huge suprasellar extension and optic chiasm compression. (**a**) T2WI. The optic chiasm is compressed and thinned (*arrow*). Three months after surgery (**b**), the optic chiasm is now repositioned, but its T2 signal is heterogeneous and T2 hyperintense, indicating a chronic lesion of the optic nerve fibers and a poor long-term visual prognosis. (**c**, **d**) Pituitary macroadenoma with cavernous sinus and suprasellar extension on T2WI in a different patient. The optic chiasm is raised (*curved arrow*) with a rail-like pattern probably related to edema. Three weeks after partial debulking (**d**), the optic chiasm is less compressed and the rail-like pattern has vanished

Further Reading

Chen X, Dai J, Ai L et al (2011) Clival invasion in pituitary macroadenomas. Am J Neuroradiol 32: 785–789

Chen Y, Wang CD, Su ZP et al (2012) Natural history of postoperative nonfunctioning pituitary adenomas: a systematic review and meta-analysis. Neuroendocrinology 96(4):333–342

Molitch ME (2014) Nonfunctioning pituitary tumors. Handb Clin Neurol 124:167–184

5 Prolactinoma in Women

Jean-François Bonneville

Hyperprolactinemia is by far the most frequent indication of an MRI of the pituitary region. The typical situation is that of a young woman with infertility and hyperprolactinemia. Irregular or absent menses can be masked by a contraceptive pill. Galactorrhea is inconstant and not specific. Nonadenomatous hyperprolactinemias have to be ruled out, such as those related to some drugs or secondary to hypothyroidism. In our experience, a prolactinoma has very little chance of being demonstrated on MRI if the prolactin level is below 35 ng/ml. Most prolactinomas in women are microadenomas (less than 10 mm in diameter), and many are less than 5–6 mm or even less than 3 mm. We call these "picoadenomas" (Fig. 5.1). There is usually a good correlation between the adenoma size and the prolactin level: microprolactinomas are found when the prolactin level is roughly between 35 and 80 ng/ml; macroprolactinomas correspond to higher prolactin levels. A very high prolactin level, such as more than 200 ng/ml, is not consistent with a microprolactinoma and must raise the question of a macroprolactinemia, particularly if the clinical situation is unclear. Conversely, a mild elevation of the prolactin level is not consistent with a macroprolactinoma: in this case, a nonfunctioning pituitary adenoma has to be suspected. Nevertheless, the rule of a good correlation between prolactin level and adenoma size has exceptions : hemorrhagic adenomas (Fig. 5.2) proportionally display lower prolactin levels, as well as cystic or necrotic adenomas presenting areas of marked T2 hyperintensity (Fig. 5.3); just as the extremely rare calcified macroprolactinomas, at least in young women, which (may shrink) moderately after dopamine agonist treatment (Fig. 6.6). Unusual T2-hypointense noncalcified microprolactinomas proportionally display higher prolactin levels than the common T2-hyperintense ones (Fig. 5.4).

Microprolactinomas are round or oval, sometimes triangular in shape, or can present with irregular contours (Fig. 5.5) and are usually located off-midline. Mostly they are hypointense on T1 if compared with the normal anterior pituitary gland, and more or less hyperintense on T2WI. In other terms, most microprolactinomas present with a T1 signal very similar to that of the cerebral gray matter, while the normal anterior pituitary gland has the same T1 signal as the cerebral white matter. Microprolactinoma T1 hyperintensity resulting from subclinical hemorrhage is not uncommon and nearly always totally asymptomatic. Ancillary signs such as localized bulging of the upper surface of the pituitary gland or mild depression of the sellar floor are rarely absent if the microadenoma is more than 3 or 4 mm in diameter. Displacement and distortion of the posterior lobe are well appreciated on axial T1 sequence (Fig. 5.6) and can constitute a useful additional feature, for instance in cases of rare isointense microadenoma. Conversely, tilting of the pituitary stalk is not always a faithful sign. Gadolinium injection shows a lesser degree of

J.-F. Bonneville et al., *MRI of the Pituitary Gland*, DOI 10.1007/978-3-319-29043-0_5

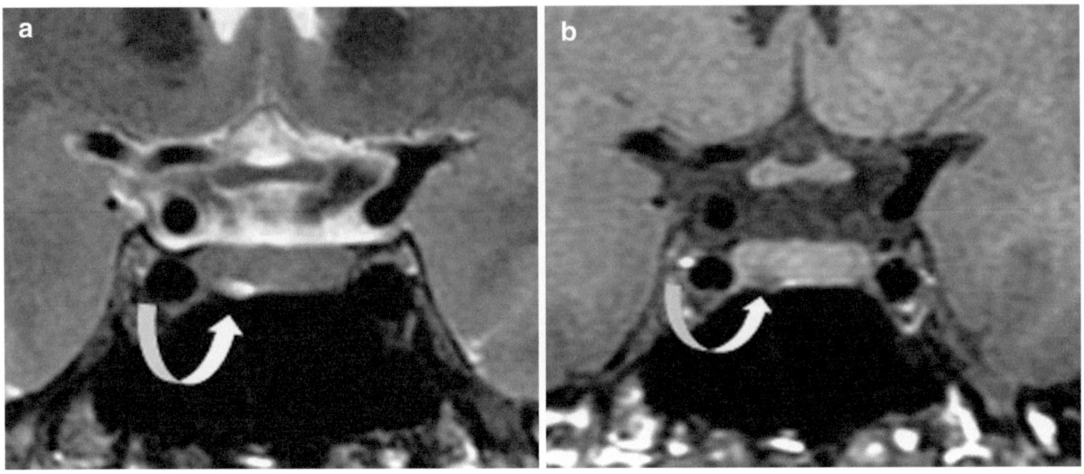

Fig. 5.1 Picoprolactinoma. Galactorrhea. PRL is 38 ng/ml. (**a**, **b**) Coronal T2 and T1 WIs. T2-hyperintense, T1-hypointense right-sided lesion. Note a subtle depression of the sellar floor below the adenoma (*arrow*)

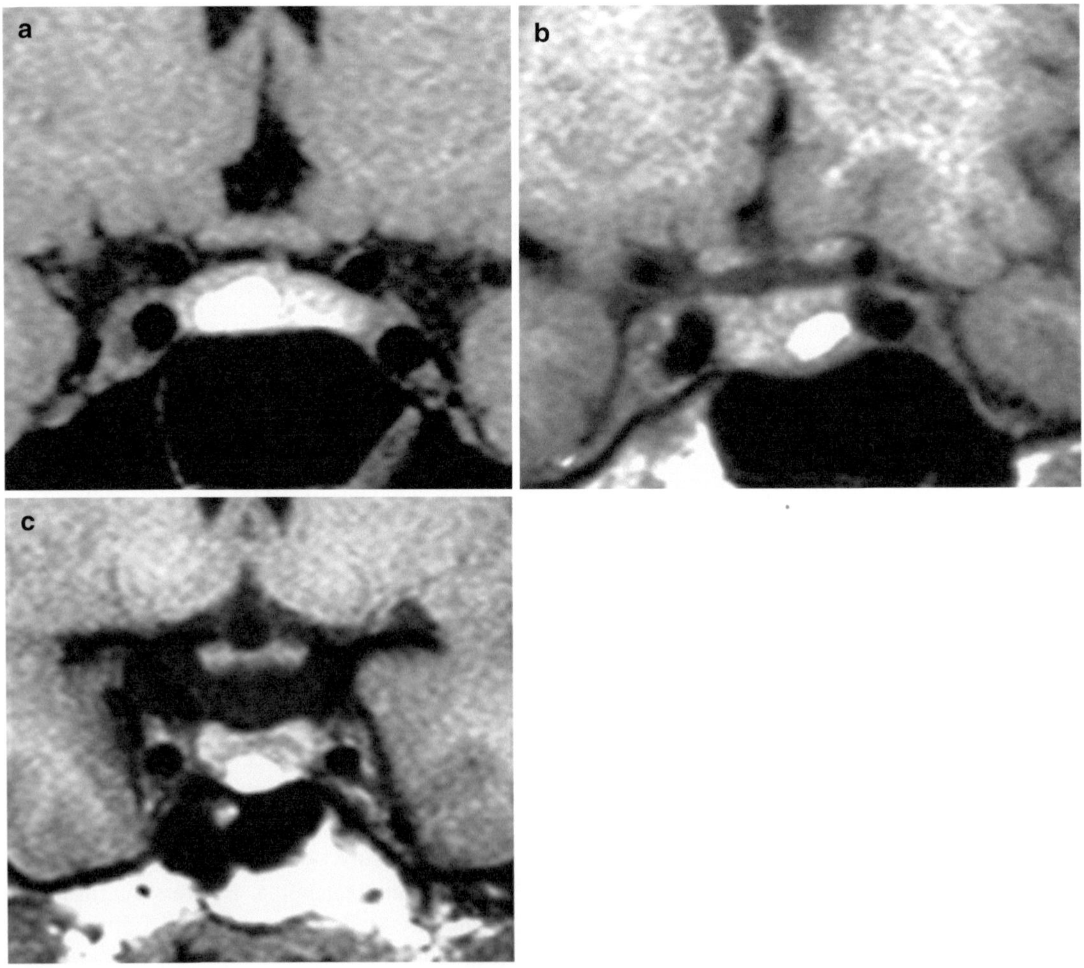

Fig. 5.2 Microprolactinomas with hemorrhagic component on coronal T1WIs (**a**–**c**). Prolactin levels are 42, 44, and 57 ng/ml, respectively

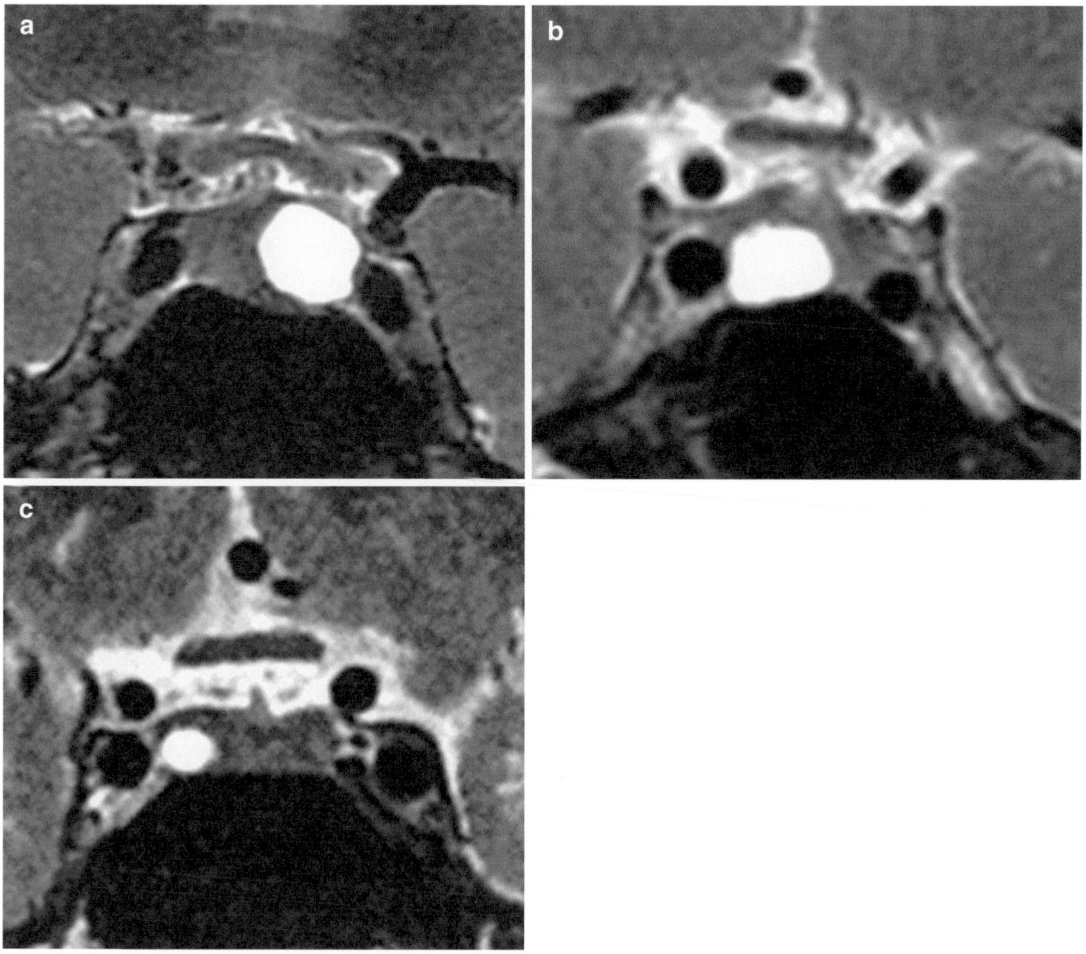

Fig. 5.3 T2-hyperintense prolactinomas on coronal T2WIs (**a**–**c**). Prolactin levels are 50, 47, and 39 ng/ml, respectively

enhancement of the adenoma compared with the normal pituitary gland (Fig. 5.7). Contrast injection is not mandatory if the diagnosis is, as is usual, obvious on high-quality T2WI (Fig. 5.8). Late enhancement of the prolactinoma itself can be observed if an additional T1W sequence is obtained 30 or 40 min after contrast injection (Fig. 5.9), especially with prolactinomas displaying a marked T2 hyperintensity. Dynamic MRI (Fig. 5.10) is usually unnecessary and can lead to false-positive diagnoses (Fig. 15.6). Differential diagnosis includes unrecognized artifacts, mainly partial volume effect artifacts, intrasellar cysts, and particularly Rathke cleft cysts, as well as the normal posterior lobe or a deep fossula hypophyseos thinning the dorsum sellae.

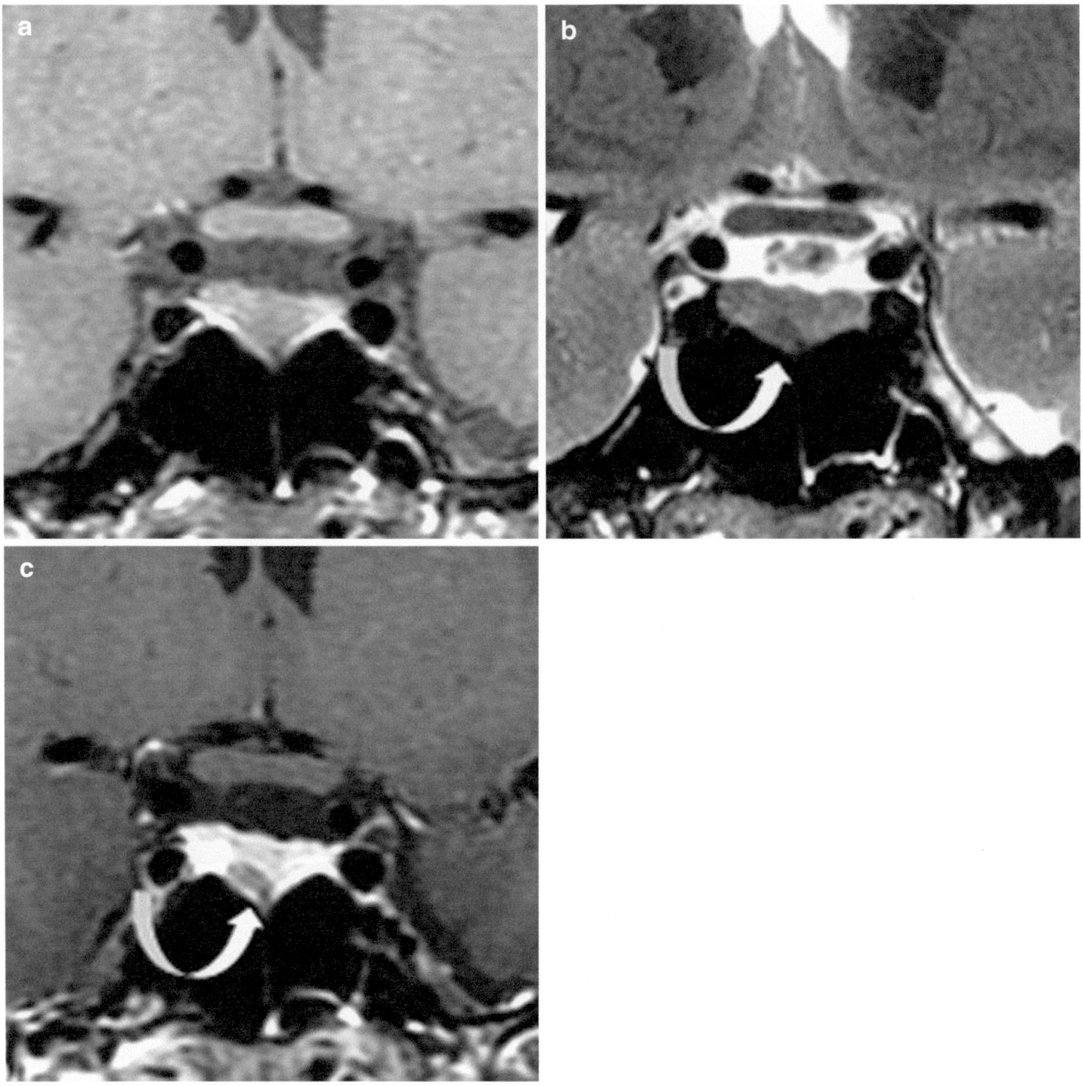

Fig. 5.4 T2-hypointense prolactinoma (*arrows*). (**a**–**c**) Coronal T1, T2 and CE T1WIs. Prolactin is 96 ng/ml. The microadenoma is faintly visible in (**b**) and well shown in (**c**)

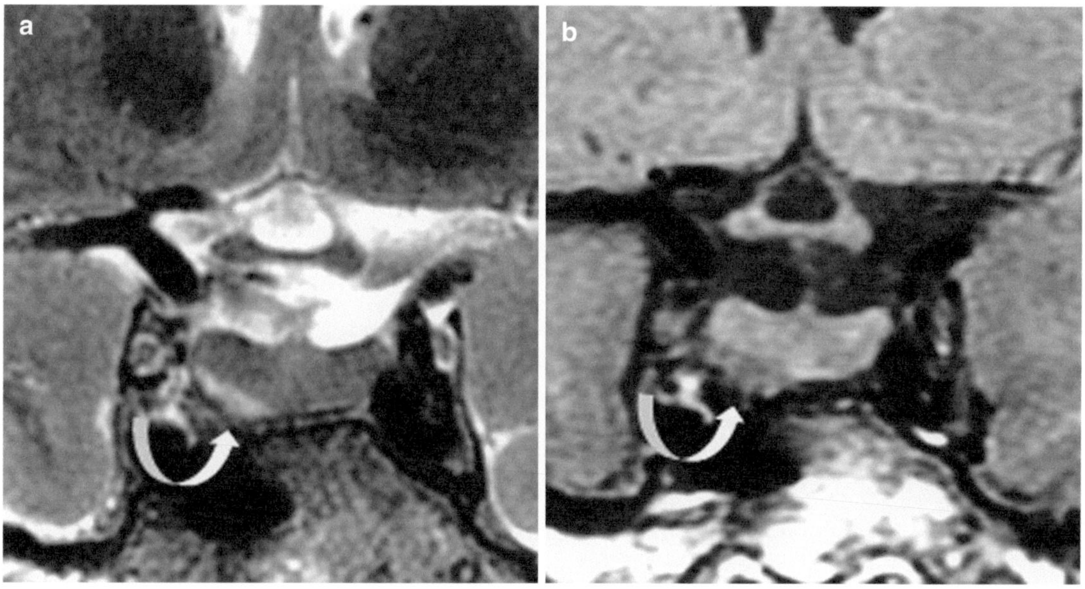

Fig. 5.5 T2 and T1 WIs (**a**, **b**) of a right-sided microprolactinoma irregular in shape (*arrow*)

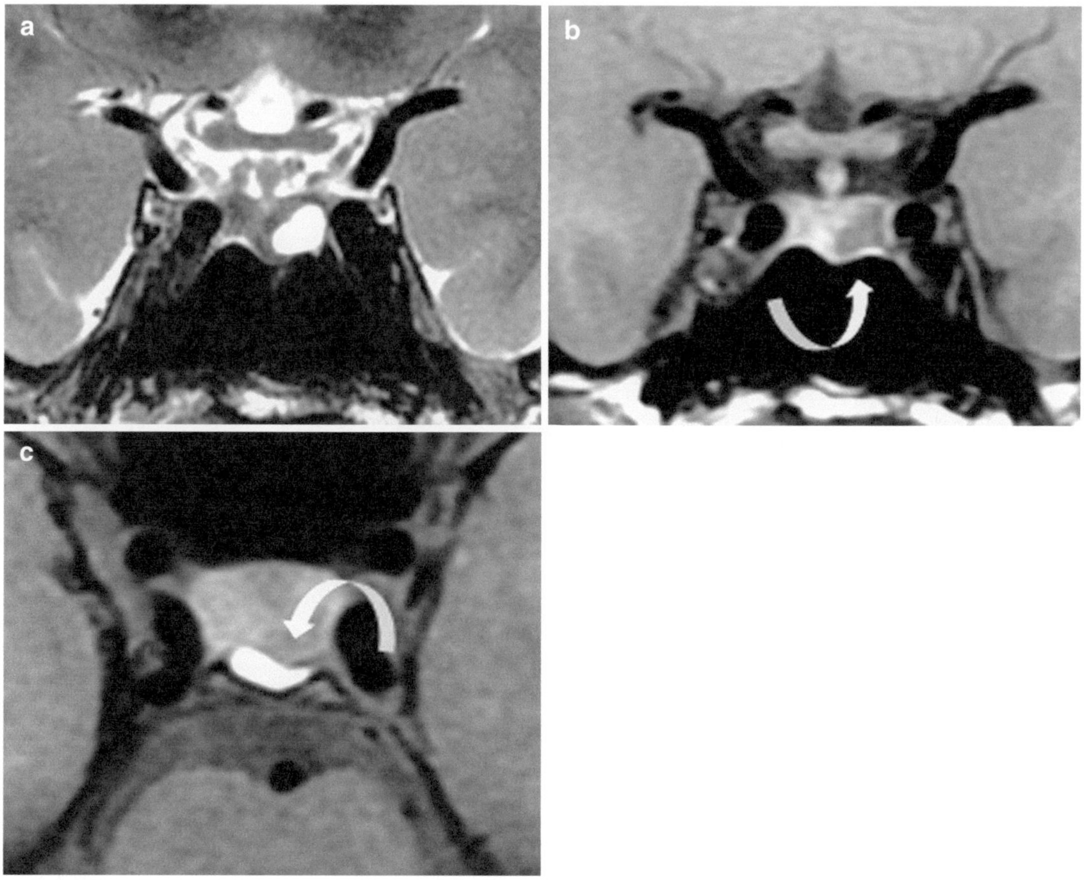

Fig. 5.6 Microprolactinoma on (**a**, **b**) coronal T2 and T1WIs, (**c**) axial T1 fat-saturated WI. The posterior lobe is compressed laterally (*arrow* in **c**)

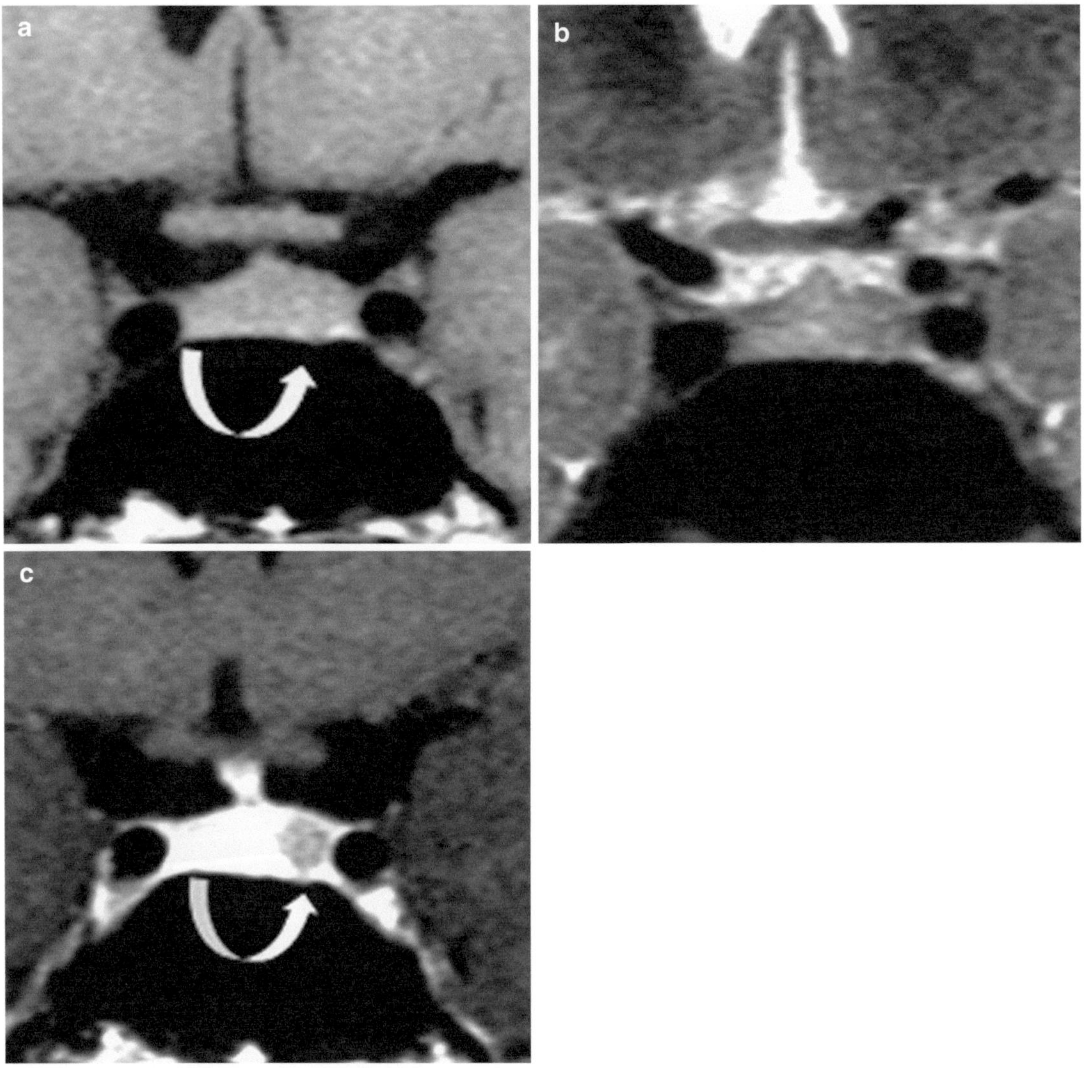

Fig. 5.7 Rare isointense prolactinoma demonstrated after gadolinium injection. (**a**–**c**) Coronal T1, T2, and CE T1 WIs. The pituitary stalk is paradoxically tilted toward the pituitary adenoma

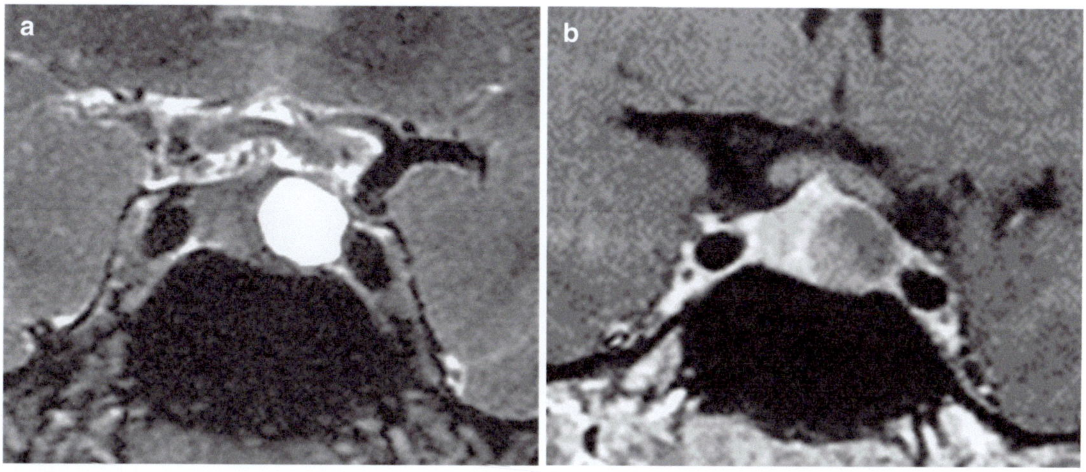

Fig. 5.8 Intrasellar prolactinoma. (**a**, **b**) T2 and CE T1 WIs: gadolinium injection is frequently unnecessary for the diagnosis of prolactinoma

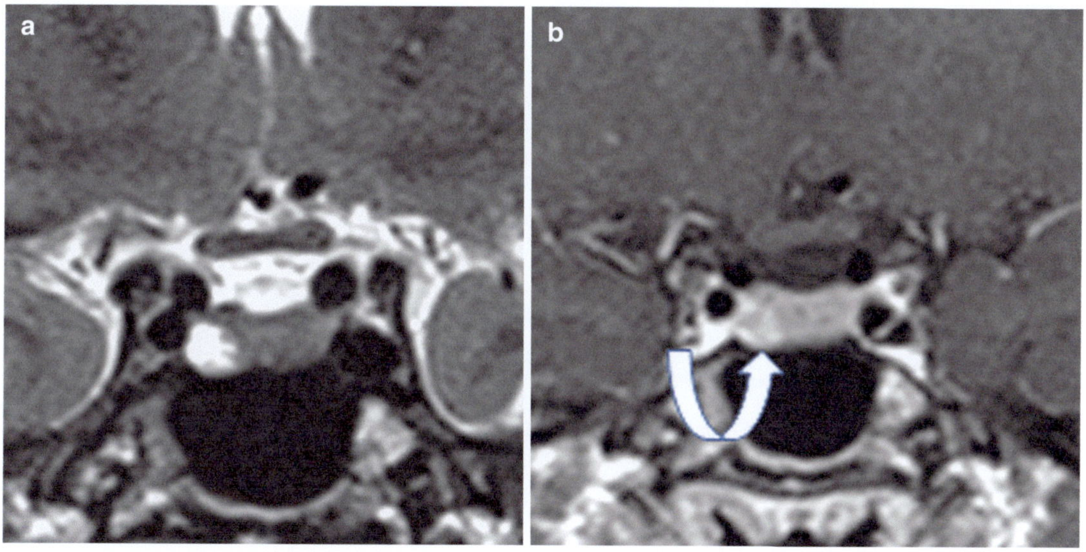

Fig. 5.9 Microprolactinoma. (**a**, **b**) T2 and CE T1 WIs 30 min after gadolinium injection. Delayed enhancement of the adenoma (*arrow*)

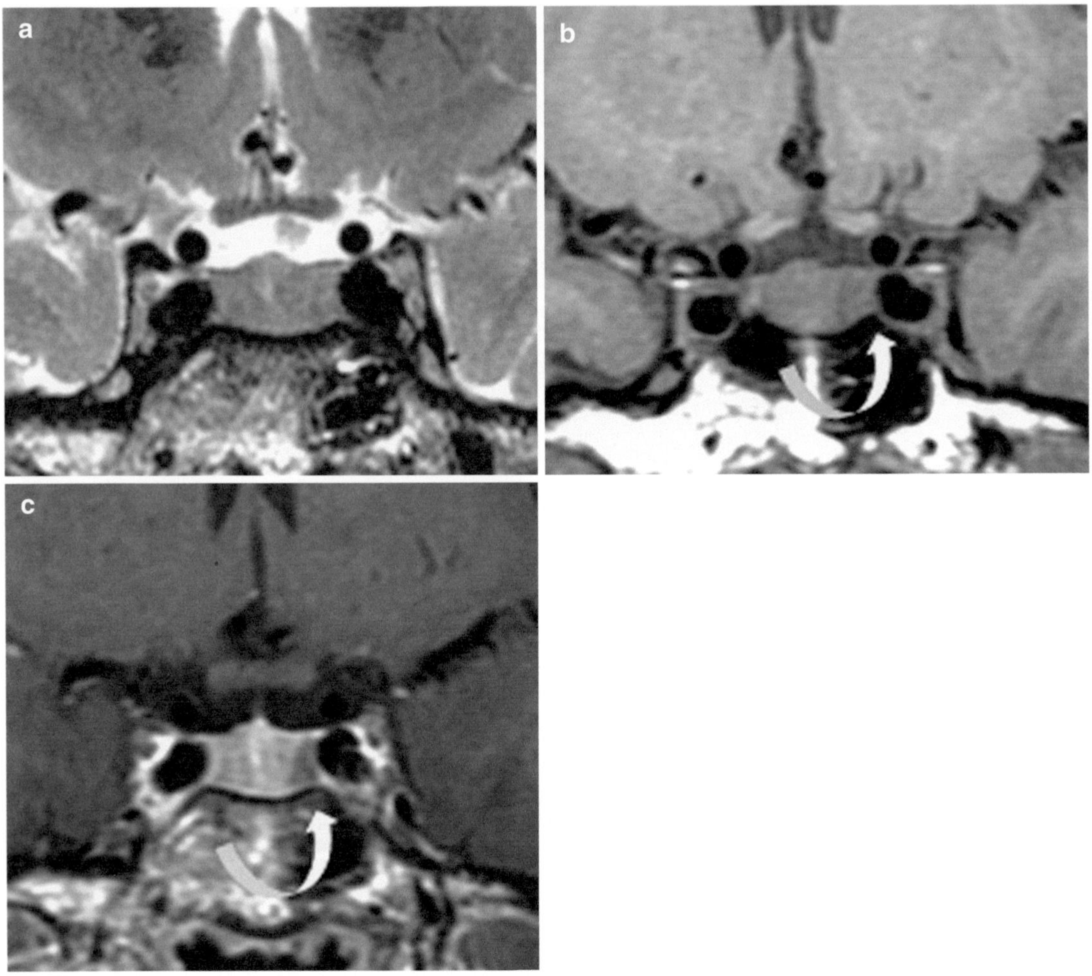

Fig. 5.10 Dynamic imaging. (**a–c**) Coronal T2, T1, and CE T1 WIs. (**d**) Dynamic imaging. The microprolactinoma (*arrow*) is well demonstrated in (**c**) (*arrow*). Dynamic imaging (**d**) does not bring more information

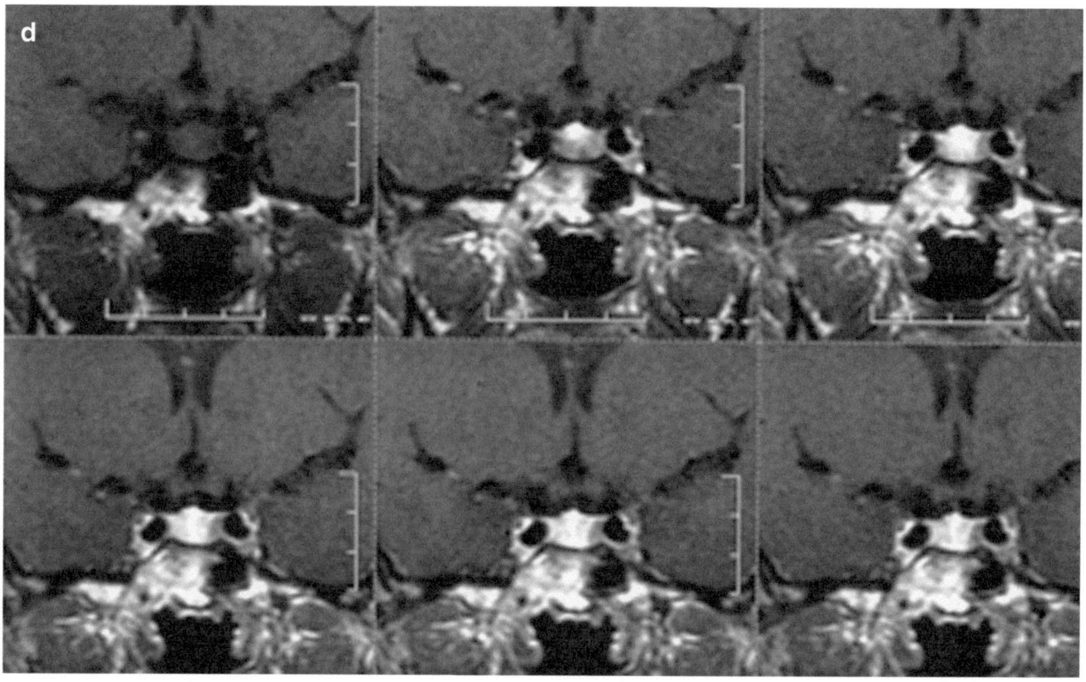

Fig. 5.10 (continued)

Further Reading

Bonneville JF, Bonneville F, Cattin F (2005) Magnetic resonance imaging of pituitary adenomas. Eur Radiol 15(3):543–548

Casanueva FF, Molitch ME, Schlechte JA et al (2006) Guidelines of the pituitary society for the diagnosis and management of prolactinomas. Clin Endocrinol (Oxf) 65(2):265–273

Kucharczyk W, Bishop JE, Plewes DB et al (1994) Detection of pituitary microadenomas: comparison of dynamic keyhole fast spin-echo, unenhanced, and conventional contrast-enhanced MR imaging. AJR Am J Roentgenol 163(3):671–679

6 Prolactinoma and Dopamine Agonists

Jean-François Bonneville

The long-acting dopamine agonist cabergoline is considered the first line therapy for both microprolactinomas and for macroprolactinomas. Tumor shrinkage starts very early (days or weeks) after initiation of medical treatment (Fig. 6.1). Therefore, cabergoline can be prescribed even for macroprolactinomas abutting the optic chiasm, but in such cases an early MR follow-up, for instance after 2 weeks, is strongly recommended to check that the optic chiasm is not further compromised. Importance of tumor shrinkage is variable and cannot be predicted in individual cases. Usually if a significant shrinkage of about 50 % is demonstrated in the first weeks after initiation of medical treatment, the maximum shrinkage of macroprolactinomas can be observed after 6 months or 1 year (Fig. 6.2). Conversely, observations of quick and complete tumoral shrinkage have been described, with a risk of rhinorrhea, meningitis, or abscess after opening a meningeal breach in macroprolactinomas invading the sphenoid sinus (Fig. 42.1). It is thus recommended to start cabergoline treatment at low dosage, and strictly assess tumoral shrinkage with MRI in those cases of macroprolactinomas invading the sphenoid sinus with skull base erosion. More frequently, shrinkage of macroprolactinoma leads to a partial or, more rarely, complete secondary empty sella with ptosis of the optic chiasm (Fig. 6.3). Tumoral shrinkage is mostly accompanied by MRI signal changes: accentuation of T2 hyperintensity of the adenoma is commonly observed (Fig. 6.4). Nevertheless, no T1 signal change is noted with hemorrhagic adenomas (Fig. 6.5) or T2 markedly hyperintense adenomas (Fig. 6.6). In these situations, tumoral shrinkage is less important than is generally seen in the more common T1 hypointense/T2 slightly hyperintense microprolactinomas.

Late changes of microprolactinomas with prolonged dopamine agonist treatment are variable (Fig. 6.7). Complete disappearance of the prolactinoma image is rare: when stabilization is obtained, it generally remains a T2-hyperintense, laterally located image, with no correlation with the prolactin level. A pathognomonic V-shaped appearance of the upper surface of the pituitary gland sometimes represents the late memory of the treated microprolactinoma (Fig. 6.8). Remodeling of the bony contours is often remarkable. Silent pituitary hemorrhage is frequently observed with medical treatment, but dopamine agonists do not seem to be a risk factor for true pituitary apoplexy. An increased T1 hyperintensity of the normal residual anterior pituitary has been noted in rare cases (Fig. 6.9); we have advanced the hypothesis of a compensatory mechanism of a localized increased hormonal synthesis of the residual anterior pituitary gland. Decision making of a therapeutic window may be proposed after 2 years of dopamine

J.-F. Bonneville et al., *MRI of the Pituitary Gland*, DOI 10.1007/978-3-319-29043-0_6

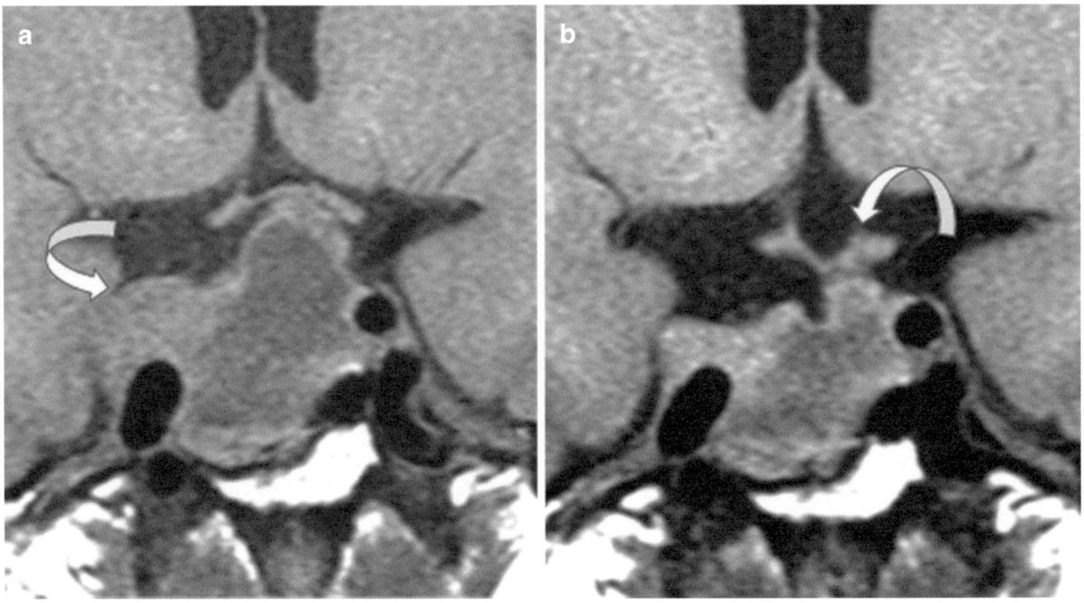

Fig. 6.1 Macroprolactinoma abutting the optic chiasm and invading right cavernous sinus (*arrow*). (**a**, **b**) Coronal T1WIs. Rapid shrinkage is visualized 10 days after cabergoline treatment initiation (**b**). Note that the shape of the optic chiasm is reversed (*arrow*)

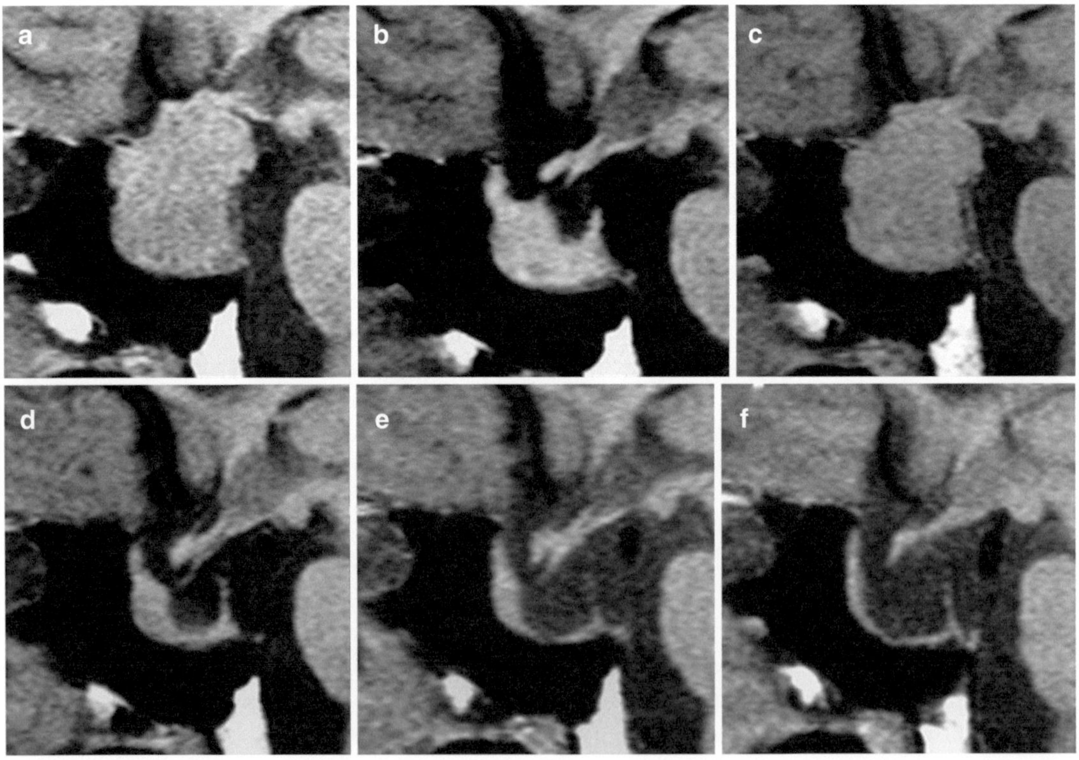

Fig. 6.2 Macroprolactinoma with suprasellar extension. (**a–f**) Sagittal T1WIs. (**a**) Before treatment. (**b**) Six weeks after dopamine agonist treatment. (**c**) The patient has stopped treatment: re-expansion of the tumor. (**d–f**) Shrinkage of the adenoma after reinstitution of medical treatment on sequential MRIs at 2 months, 1 year, and 2 years, respectively. Secondary empty sella

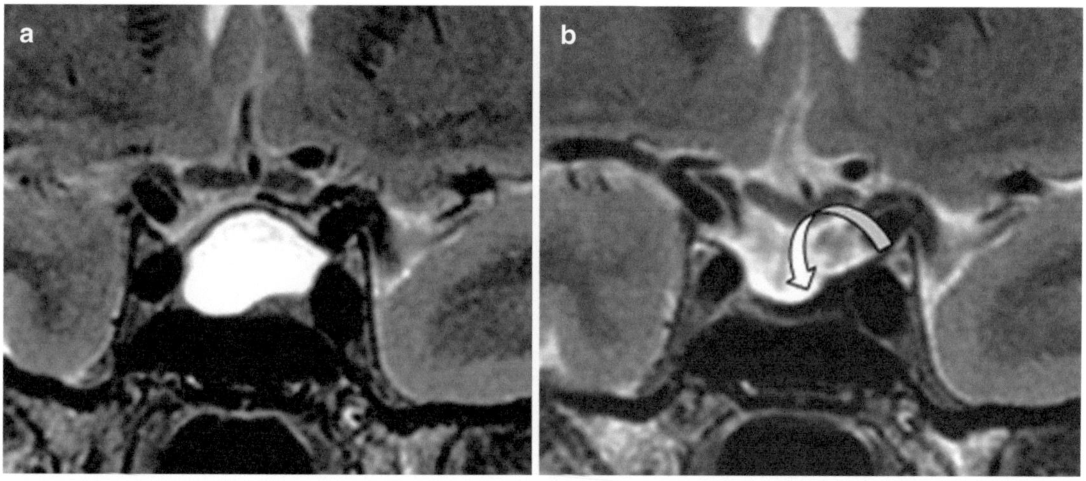

Fig. 6.3 Macroprolactinoma with old hemorrhage. (**a**, **b**) Coronal T2WIs. T2 tumoral hyperintensity. Six months after dopamine agonist treatment (**b**), complete shrinkage of the tumor is seen. A thin dark band doubling the sellar diaphragm is related to hemosiderin deposit (*arrow*)

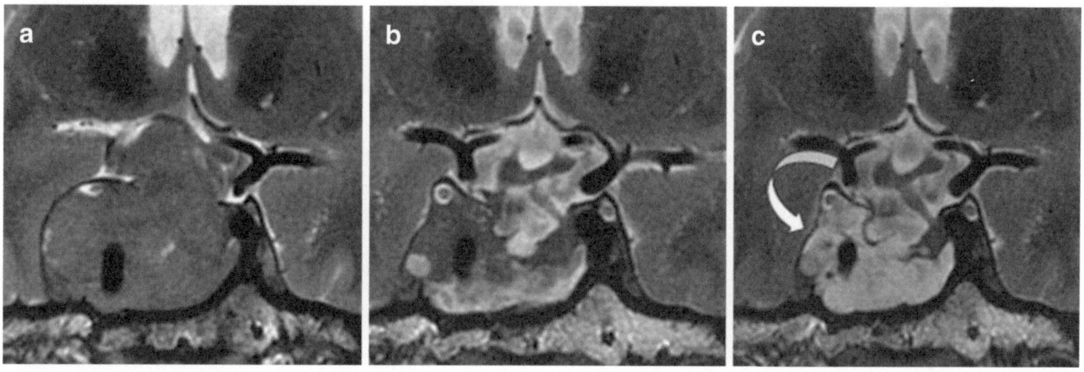

Fig. 6.4 Macroprolactinoma invading right cavernous sinus. (**a**–**c**) Coronal T2WIs. (**a**) Before treatment. Shrinkage and progressive T2 hyperintensity at 3 months (**b**) and 1 year (**c**) of dopamine agonist treatment. Shrinkage and signal changes affect cavernous sinus tumoral compartment (*arrow*) and intrasellar compartment

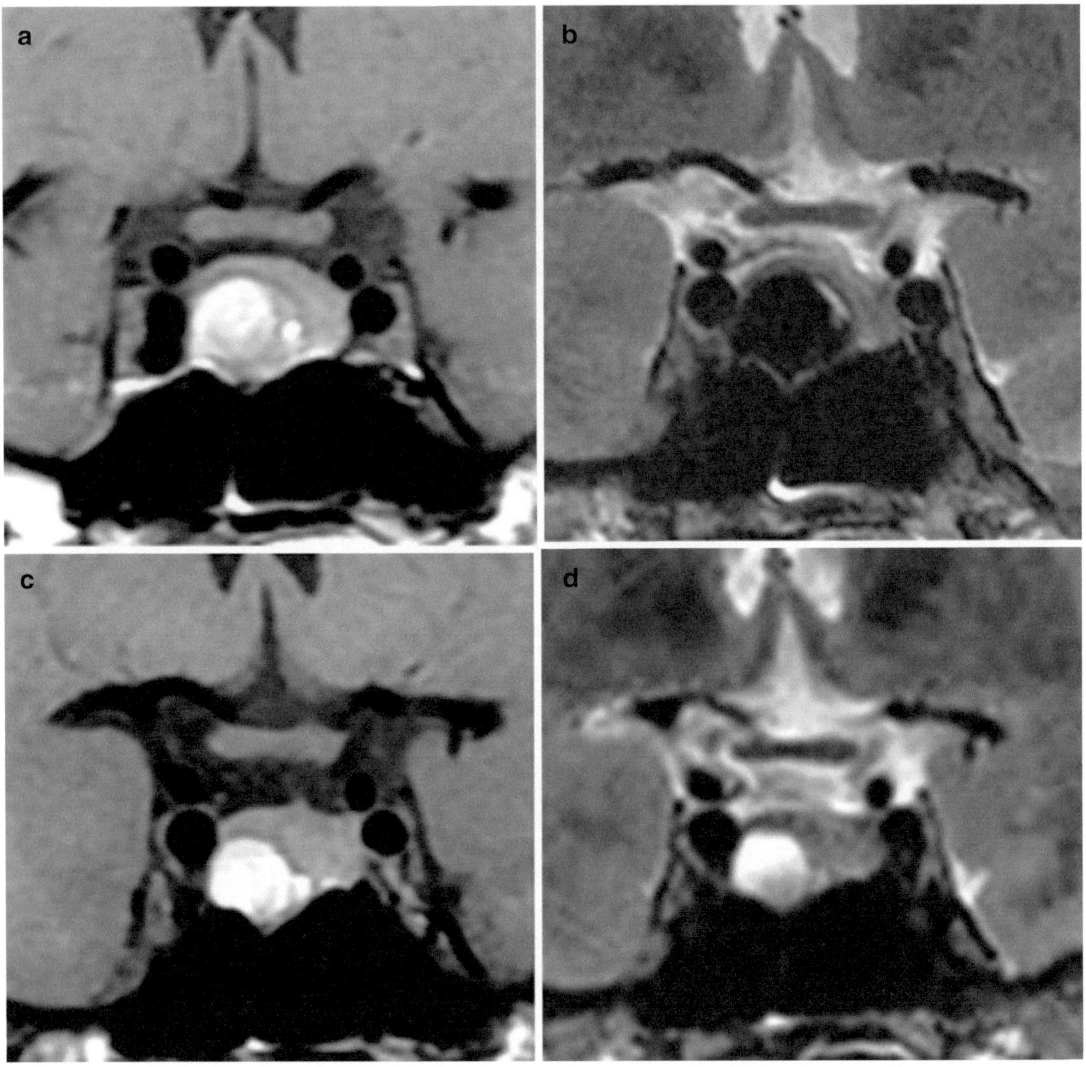

Fig. 6.5 Macroprolactinoma with fresh hemorrhage. (**a**, **c**) Coronal T1WIs. (**b**, **d**) Coronal T2WIs. Four months after treatment with dopamine agonists (**c**, **d**), T1 and T2 hyperintensity of the mass is observed. Mild tumoral shrinkage

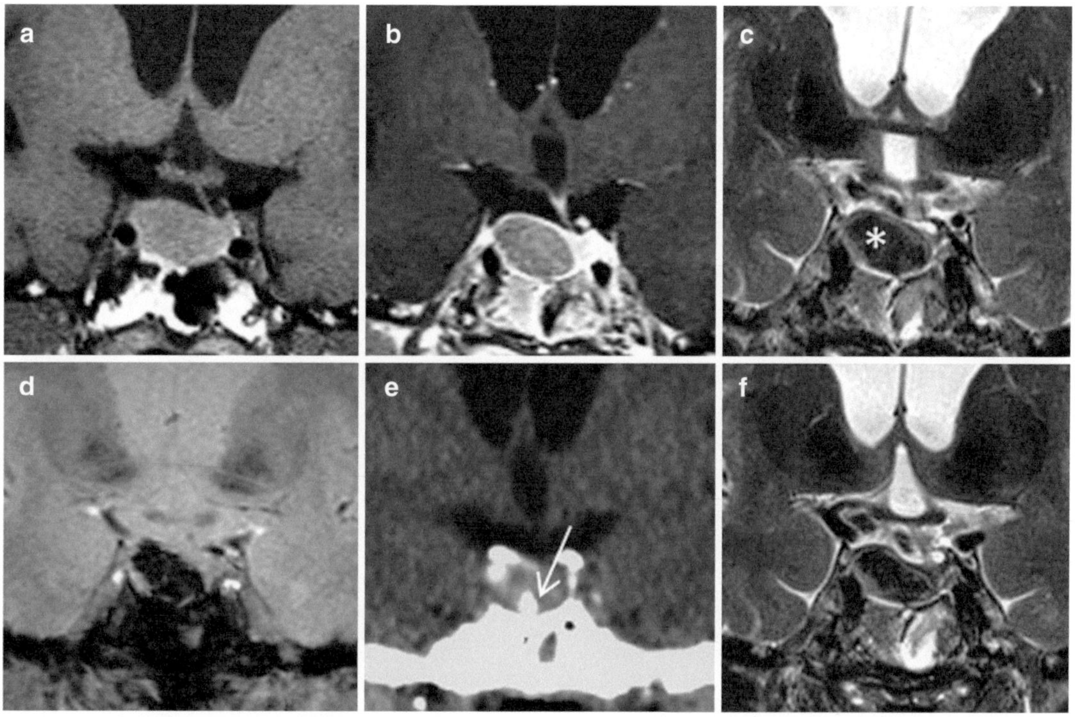

Fig. 6.6 Rare calcified prolactinoma in a 66-year-old woman before and after 6 months of cabergoline treatment. Prolactin level is 60 and 7 ng/ml, respectively. (**a–d**) Coronal T1, CE T1, T2, and T2* WIs. Marked T2 hypointensity of the intrasellar adenoma (*asterisk*). (**e**) Coronal CT. Confirmation of intrasellar calcifications (*arrow*). (**f**) Coronal T2WI. Moderate shrinkage after treatment

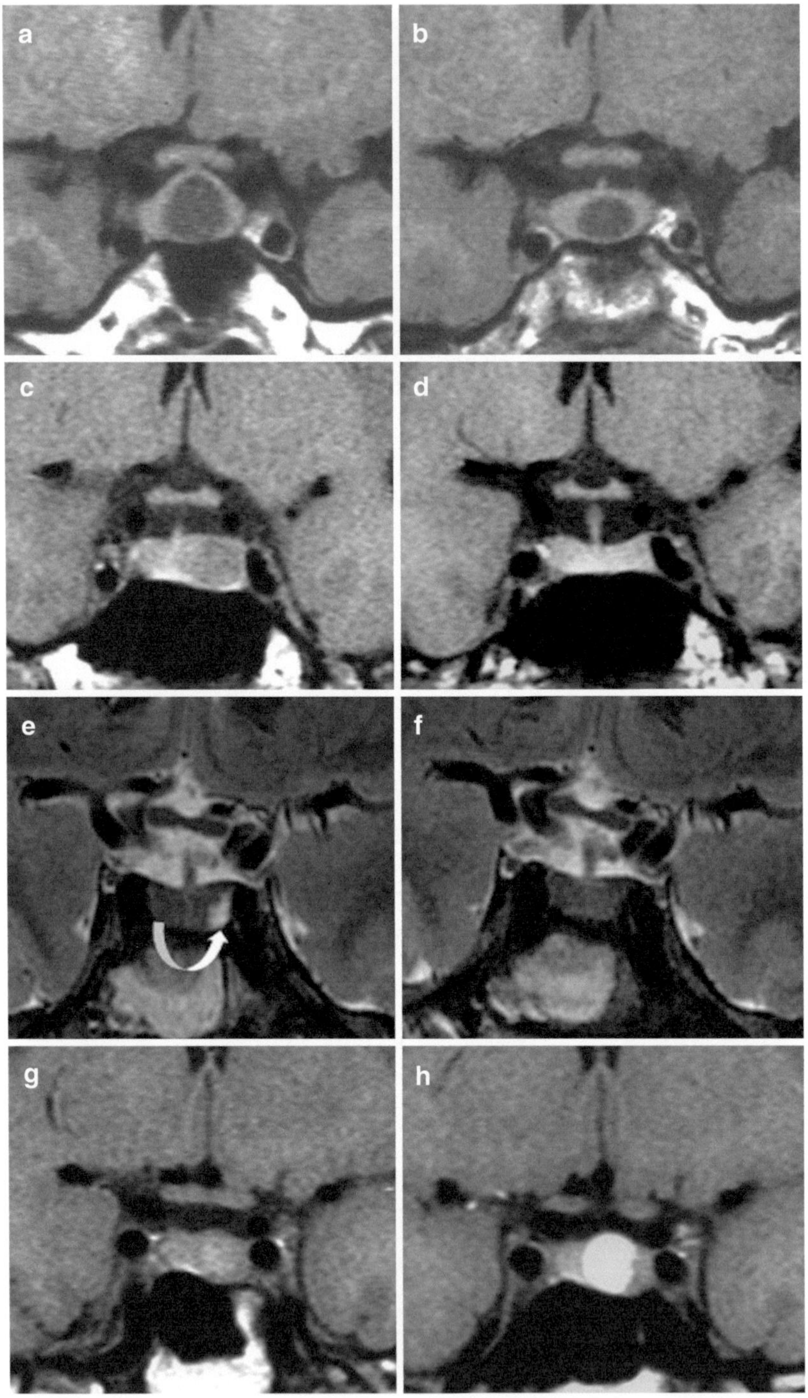

Fig. 6.7 Usual patterns of microprolactinomas before (*left column*) and a few months after dopamine agonist treatment (*right column*). (**a–d**) Coronal T1WIs. (**e**, **f**) Coronal T2WIs. (**g**, **h**) Coronal T1WIs. 50 % shrinkage in (**b**). Complete disappearance of the adenoma image and normalization of the sellar floor (rare) in (**d**). Disappearance of the prolactinoma on T2WI in (**f**): this evolution does not preclude the cure of the prolactinoma if cabergoline treatment is suspended. Hemorrhagic transformation (asymptomatic) in (**h**)

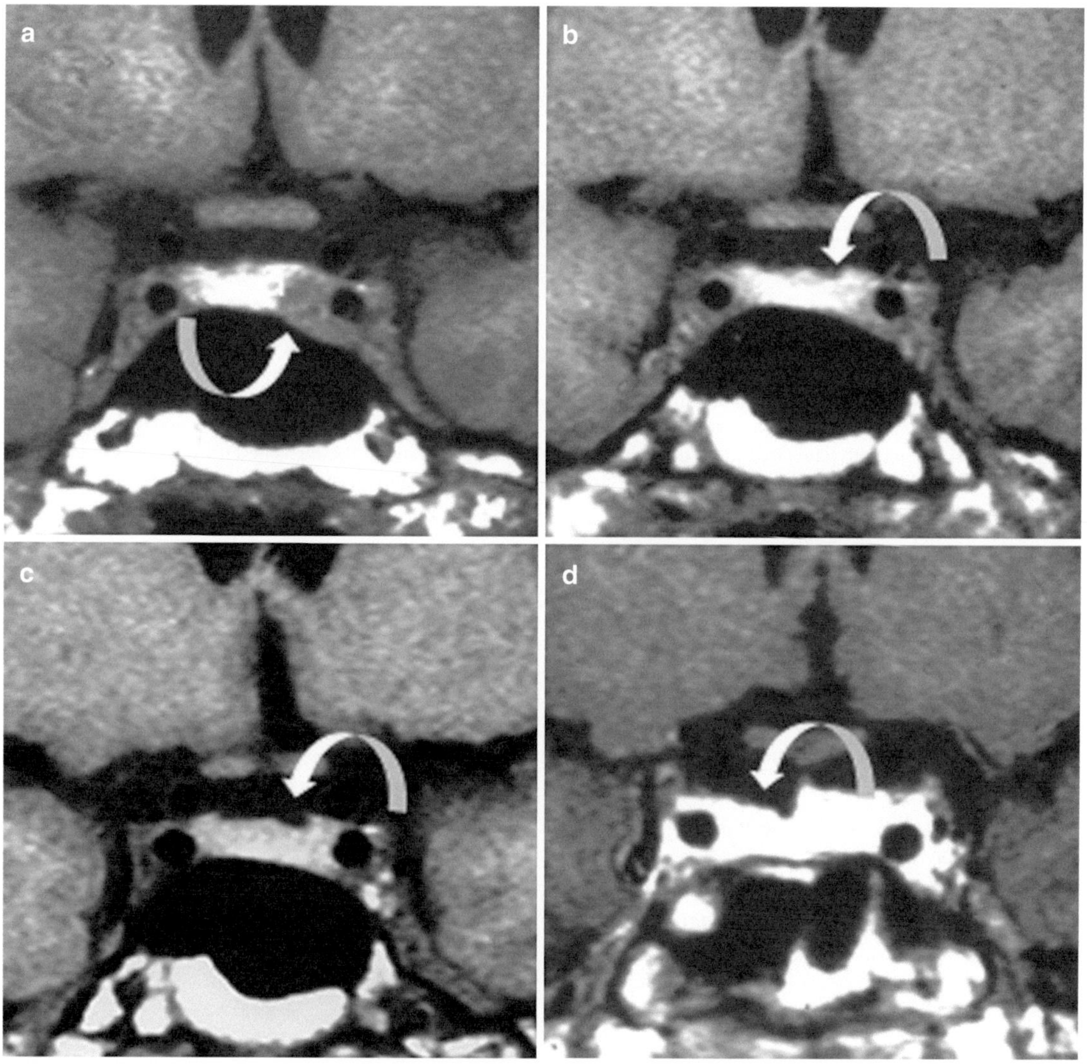

Fig. 6.8 V-shaped appearance of the upper surface of the pituitary gland in treated microprolactinomas. (**a–c**) Coronal T1WIs and (**d**) CE T1WI. (**a**) Left-sided prolactinoma invading left cavernous sinus (*arrow*). (**b**) Prolactinoma shrinkage and small indentation of the upper surface of the gland after cabergoline treatment (*arrow*). (**c, d**) V-shaped indentation of the upper surface of the pituitary gland in two patients with treated prolactinomas (*arrows*)

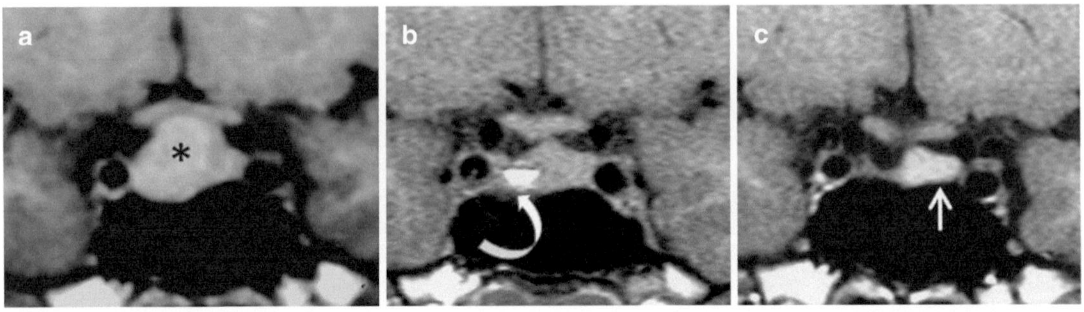

Fig. 6.9 T1W hyperintensity of normal residual anterior pituitary. (**a–c**) Coronal T1WIs. (**a**) Right-sided hemorrhagic macroprolactinoma (*asterisk*) deforming the sellar floor and abutting the optic chiasm; prolactin level is 520 ng/ml. (**b**) Six months after treatment there is tumor shrinkage, remodeling of the sellar floor, and small residual hemorrhagic component (*curved arrow*). Prolactin level is now 6 ng/ml. (**c**) One year later, there is marked atrophy of the sellar content on the right side with upward bulging of the sellar floor; T1 hyperintensity of the normal pituitary tissue on the left side (*straight arrow*) indicates possibly of compensatory increased hormonal activity

agonist treatment, especially if a pregnancy has been obtained or is not desired. Recurrence of hyperprolactinemia and tumor regrowth following discontinuation of dopamine agonist therapy in patients with prolactinoma occur on average at 6 months, and more commonly in macroprolactinoma (93 %) than in microprolactinoma (64 %). True resistance to dopamine agonist therapy is rare. It has been said that cavernous sinus invasion is a predictable factor of such resistance, but we do not share this assertion.

Further Reading

Barber TM, Kenkre J, Garnett C et al (2011) Recurrence of hyperprolactinaemia following discontinuation of dopamine agonist therapy in patients with prolactinoma occurs commonly especially in macroprolactinoma. Clin Endocrinol (Oxf) 75(6):819–824

Bonneville F, Cattin F, Barrali E et al (2001) Increased T1 signal of the residual normal anterior pituitary gland following medical treatment of pituitary prolactinoma. J Radiol 82(4):501–505

Cuny T, Chanson P (2013) Aggressive and resistant-to-treatment pituitary tumors. Ann Endocrinol (Paris) 74:S3–S12

7 Normal Pituitary Gland and Pregnancy

Jean-François Bonneville

The normal pituitary gland enlarges gradually during pregnancy because of estrogen-stimulated hyperplasia and hypertrophy of prolactin cells. In parallel, serum prolactin levels rise and can reach 40 ng/ml at the end of the first trimester, 150 ng/ml by the end of the second trimester, and 200 or even 400 ng/ml at term. MRI is considered safe to follow, if necessary, the changes of the pituitary gland during pregnancy. The precautionary principle dictates to avoid MRI in the first trimester. For the same reason, gadolinium injection is prohibited. The normal pituitary gland height increases linearly by 0.08–0.1 mm/week, i.e., by 3–4 mm at term. The upper surface of the gland becomes more convex superiorly (Fig. 7.1). The pituitary gland height can reach 10 mm during the last trimester and 12 mm in the immediate postpartum period, and approach the optic chiasm. This situation can be more sharply defined in the cases of small sella (Fig. 7.2). It has been said that the pituitary stalk width presents its highest value within the 3 days postpartum; if this is true, it could be related to some enlargement of the pars tuberalis of the anterior pituitary; more likely, this change of the infundibulum corresponds to a shortening of the pituitary stalk in relation to the upward bulging of the pituitary content—the reverse of what is observed in empty sella where the pituitary stalk attached to the hypoplastic pituitary gland is stretched. At the same time, T1 signal intensity of the pituitary gland increases, particularly during the last trimester; this is clear when comparing the T1 signal of the anterior pituitary with that of the temporal white matter on coronal views or with that of the pons on sagittal views. The mechanism of T1 shortening of the anterior pituitary gland during pregnancy has not been fully elucidated. It has been suggested that the mechanism may be related to high protein-synthesis activity, an increase in the bound fraction of water molecules, and/or an increase in the number of secretory granules. Visualization of the normally hyperintense posterior lobe on sagittal T1 view has previously been reported as much less frequent during pregnancy. In fact, by using axial T1 fat-saturation sequences, the posterior lobe is constantly demonstrated just as it is in young nonpregnant women. The reason explaining the poor rate of its visualization on sagittal T1WI during pregnancy in the literature is that the posterior lobe may be slightly compressed and thinned by the enlarged anterior pituitary and pressed against the dorsum sellae (Fig. 7.3). In this situation, the posterior lobe can be masked by the dorsum, especially if the dorsum is not aerated and contains fatty bone marrow; however, the compressed posterior lobe is routinely clearly defined on axial T1WI, preferentially with fat saturation. Another reason is that changes of serum osmolarity in pregnant women lead to an increase of vasopressin release and, consequently, to a decrease of the posterior lobe hyperintensity if compared with that of nonpregnant women of the same age group. In the postpartum period, shrinkage of the pituitary gland is initiated about 2 weeks after delivery (Fig. 7.4). The return of T1 signal of the anterior pituitary to that observed in the nonpregnant state is delayed if the mother is breast-feeding.

J.-F. Bonneville et al., *MRI of the Pituitary Gland*, DOI 10.1007/978-3-319-29043-0_7

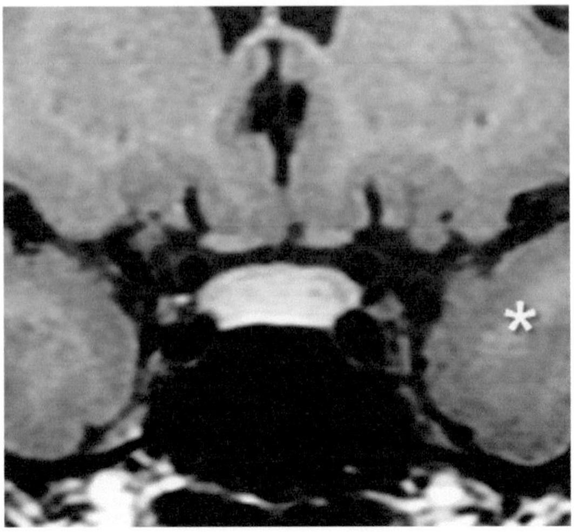

Fig. 7.1 Normal pregnancy, last trimester. Coronal T1W I. Upward bulging of the pituitary gland and increased T1 signal if compared with that of the cerebral white matter (*asterisk*)

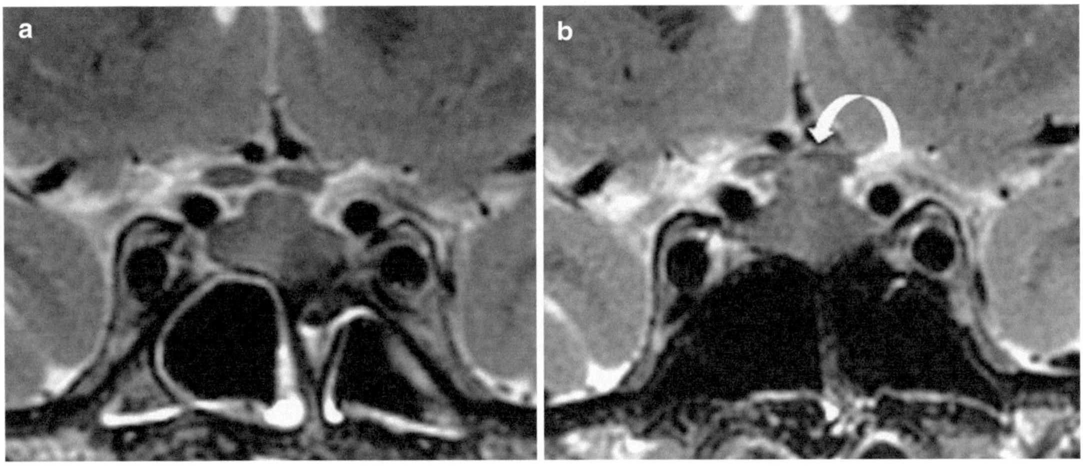

Fig. 7.2 Pregnancy and small sella in a normoprolactinemic 31-year-old woman. (**a**, **b**) Coronal T2WIs. (**a**) Before pregnancy; upward physiological bulging of the pituitary gland above a narrow sella. (**b**) Spontaneous pregnancy, 8 months. The enlarged pituitary gland abuts the optic chiasm without visual field impairment

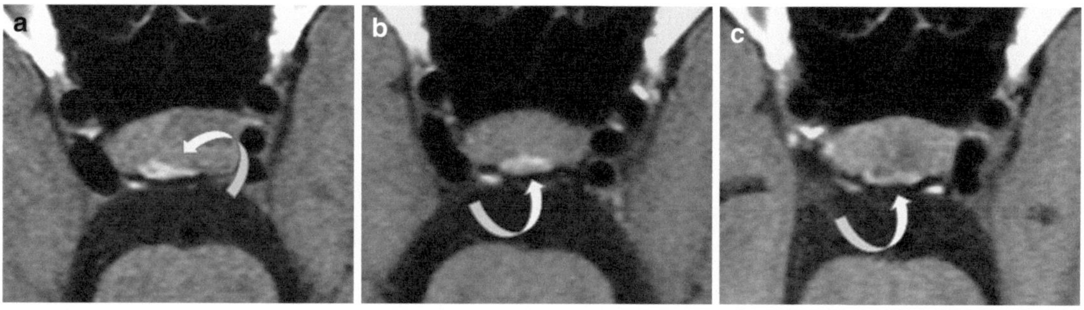

Fig. 7.3 Left-sided prolactinoma. (**a–c**) Axial T1WIs. (**a**) Before treatment: the posterior lobe is compressed laterally (*arrow*). (**b**) After 1 year with cabergoline treatment, the pituitary adenoma has shrunk; the posterior lobe is no longer compressed. (**c**) Pregnancy, last trimester: the posterior lobe is flattened again and its T1 signal is less intense than previously

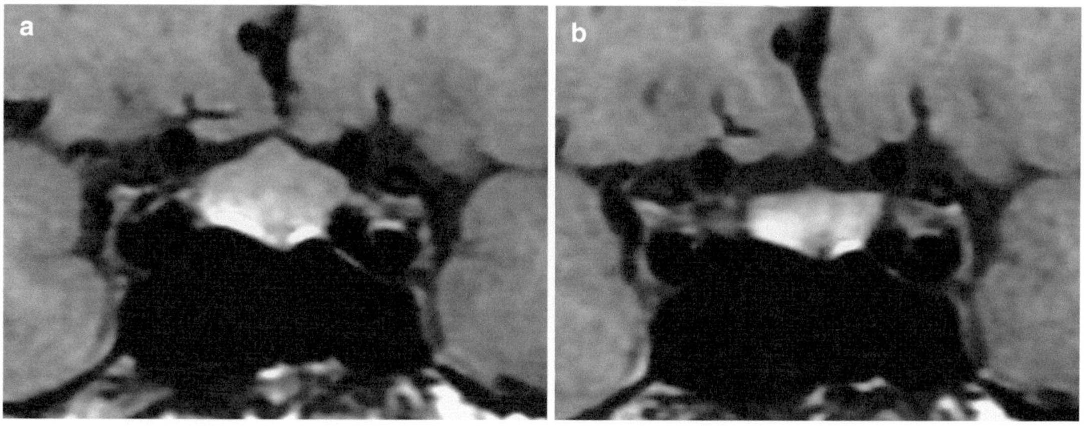

Fig. 7.4 Normal pregnancy and postpartum. (**a**, **b**) Coronal T1WIs. (**a**) Last trimester and (**b**) 10 days after delivery. Rapid pituitary gland shrinkage with persistent T1 hyperintensity

Further Reading

Bonneville JF, Bonneville F, Cattin F (2005) MRI of the pituitary gland: indications and results in gynaecology and in obstetrics. Gynecol Obstet Fertil 33(3):147–153

Elster AD, Sanders TG, Vines FS et al (1991) Radiology 181(2):531–535

Miki Y, Asato R, Okumura R et al (1993) Anterior pituitary gland in pregnancy: hyperintensity at MR. Radiology 187(1):229–231

8 Pituitary Tumors and Pregnancy

Jean-François Bonneville

As dopamine agonists are usually stopped as soon as a pregnancy is confirmed, prolactinomas increase in size during pregnancy (Fig. 8.1). The prolactinoma volume roughly doubles when measured during the last trimester of pregnancy, and the volume of normal pituitary tissue also increases (Fig. 8.2). Increase in volume involves the intrasellar tumoral component as well as the intracavernous one, if any (Fig. 8.3). According to the size of the tumor, the risk of complications is well defined: very rare with microprolactinomas, and rare and depending on the original size with macroprolactinomas. This means that the size of a prolactinoma has to be precisely known before any dopamine agonist treatment is instituted: dopamine agonists given blind, even for a few weeks, can change a macroprolactinoma into a microadenoma. The rule "MRI first" must never be broken. Moreover, apart from the size, the T2 signal of the prolactinoma can also have some interest: it seems that the unusual T2-hypointense prolactinomas have the propensity to increase their size in larger proportion than the hyperintense ones during pregnancy (Fig. 8.4). Practically, if MRI follow-up has no place during pregnancy for the usual T2 hyperintense microadenomas, such a place may be discussed at the onset of the third trimester for the rare T2-hypointense prolactinomas, mainly if their maximal diameter is at the upper limit of microadenomas (i.e., 10 mm). If necessary, MRI—without gadolinium injection—can be obtained. In the rare cases where medical treatment appears mandatory to avoid further enlargement of the adenoma during pregnancy, the oldest molecule, bromocriptine, is still preferred to cabergoline by some clinicians.

Prolactinomas with hemorrhagic component, demonstrating a T1-hyperintense signal, are frequently encountered without or with dopamine agonist treatment; the hemorrhagic prolactinoma increases during pregnancy but usually remains asymptomatic (Fig. 8.5). In a few cases, bleeding of a pituitary adenoma can be responsible for headache (Fig. 8.6). Coagulopathies and anticoagulation therapy have been stated as contributing factors (Fig. 8.7). It does not seem that intra-adenomatous hemorrhage predisposes to the occurrence of true pituitary apoplexia.

After delivery, the maximal height of the sellar content is reached 2 or 3 days postpartum, then decreases quickly, but with some delay in cases of breast-feeding. In about 20 % of patients harboring microprolactinoma, the prolactin level may remain normal without treatment after delivery. This situation could be favored by an intratumoral hemorrhagic event and seems to be observed more frequently after a second pregnancy.

Pregnancy can occur in acromegalic patients, most of the time with an uneventful outcome (Fig. 8.8). Safety of somatostatin analog treatment during pregnancy is not completely established. Pregnancy with Cushing disease is rare and risky for both the mother and the child. The issue here is not the risk induced by the adenoma size increase, the initial size of the tumor

J.-F. Bonneville et al., *MRI of the Pituitary Gland*, DOI 10.1007/978-3-319-29043-0_8

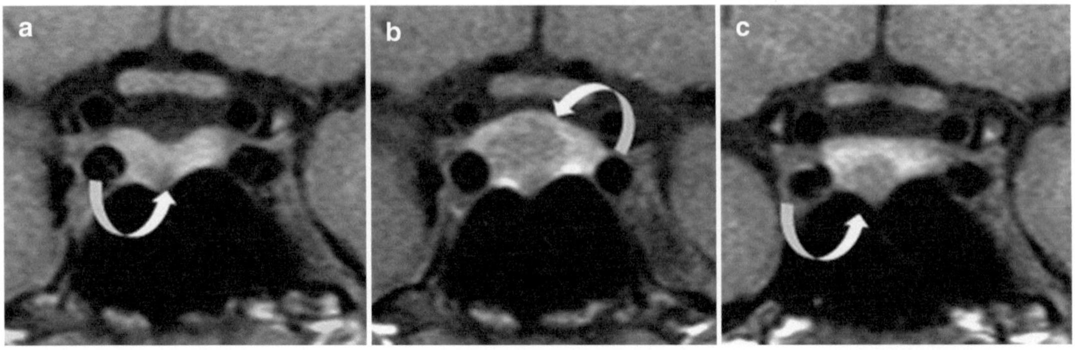

Fig. 8.1 Intrasellar prolactinoma seen first after dopamine agonist treatment given blindly. (**a–c**) Nonenhanced coronal T1WIs. (**a**) After dopamine agonist treatment (*arrow*). (**b**) At seventh month of first pregnancy. Cabergoline was withdrawn as soon as pregnancy was confirmed. Marked increase of adenoma size; slight T1 hyperintensity of the normal anterior pituitary. (**c**) At seventh month of a second pregnancy while dopamine agonist treatment was maintained during pregnancy. Similar increased T1 signal of the pituitary, but very slight increase in adenoma size

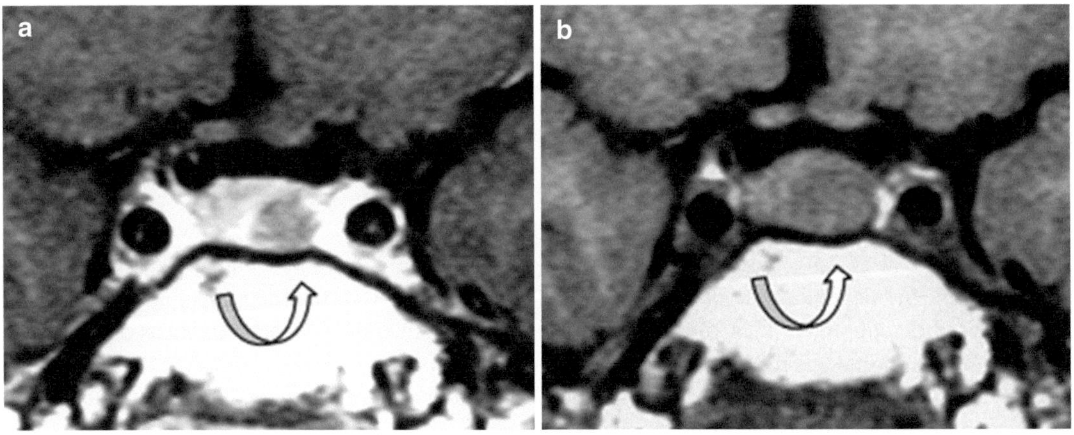

Fig. 8.2 Prolactinoma and pregnancy. (**a**) Coronal CE T1WI. Left-sided microadenoma (*arrow*). A pregnancy is obtained after cabergoline treatment. (**b**) Noncontrast coronal T1WI at the onset of the last trimester of pregnancy. Bulging of the upper surface of the pituitary gland and increased volume of the T1 hypointense pituitary adenoma

being usually moderate or small, but aggravation of hypercorticism. Nonfunctioning pituitary tumors occur infrequently in women of child-bearing age. In the cases where a pregnancy has been obtained through ovulation induction or in vitro fertilization, MRI follow-up to check on the tumoral volume increase is advisable.

Rathke cleft cysts are stable or can slightly increase their volume during pregnancy. In a few cases, pregnancy can reveal a Rathke cleft cyst previously nonsymptomatic (Fig. 8.9). Changes of T1 signal of the cyst during pregnancy, without fluid level, have been observed, and indicate more frequently a change in protein content than hemorrhage (Fig. 8.10).

Occurrence of an oculomotor nerve palsy during pregnancy may reveal a cavernous sinus meningioma.

Cases of Rathke cyst rupture have been described during pregnancy (Fig. 8.9).

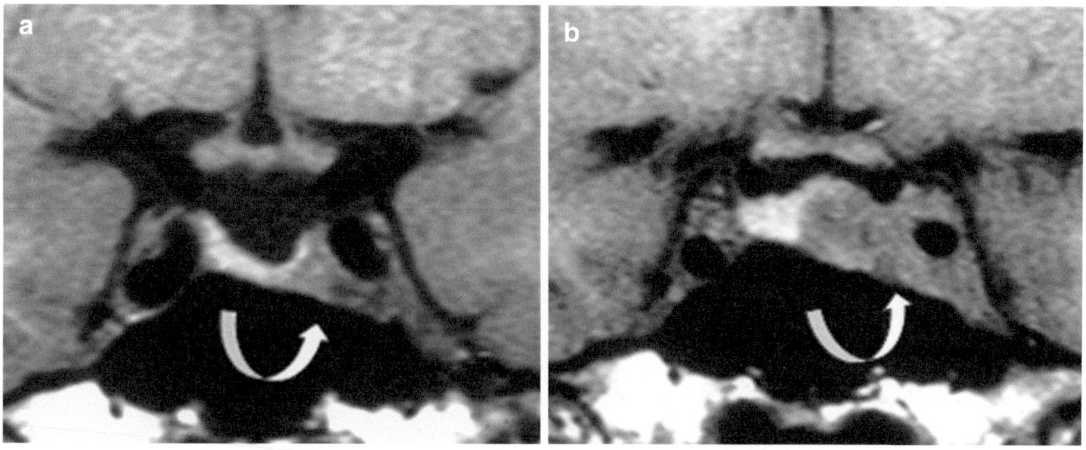

Fig. 8.3 Prolactinoma seen after cabergoline treatment. (**a**, **b**) Coronal T1WIs. (**a**) Residual T1 hypointense tumor occupying the left side of the sella and invading left cavernous sinus (*arrow*). (**b**) MRI follow-up at seventh month of pregnancy. Cabergoline was withdrawn as soon as the pregnancy was confirmed. Increased volume of the intrasellar and intracavernous compartments of the pituitary adenoma

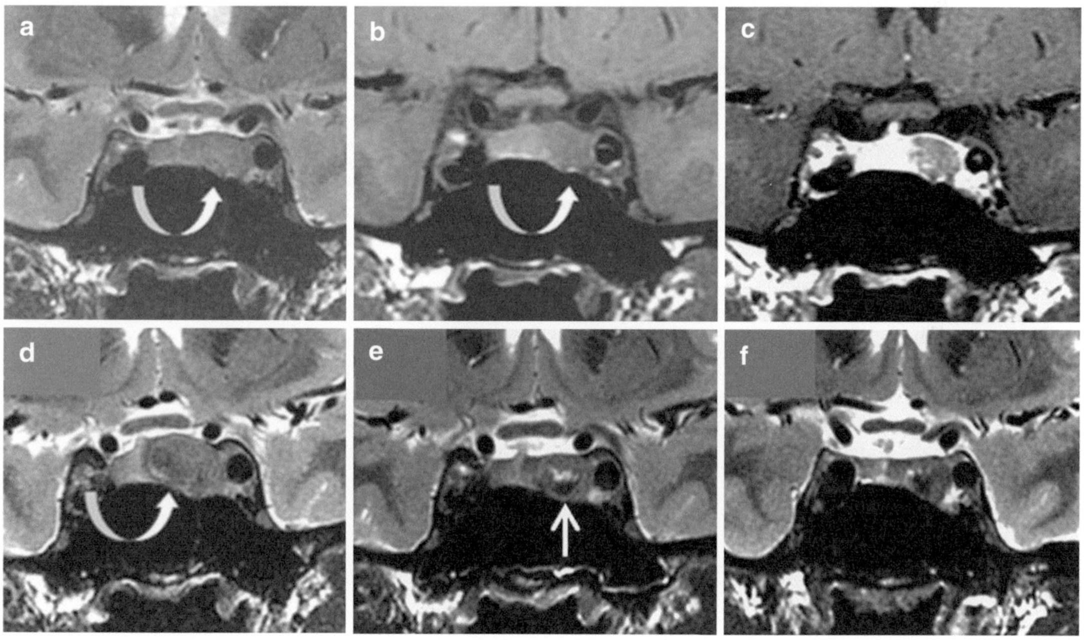

Fig. 8.4 27-year-old woman. Post pill amenorrhea. Prolactin is 4,000 mIU/l. (**a**–**c**) T1, T2, and CE T1 WIs. Left-sided prolactinoma with unusual T2-hypointense signal (*arrow*). A pregnancy occurred after dopamine agonist treatment, which was stopped as soon as the pregnancy was known. (**d**) Coronal T2WI at the eighth month of pregnancy. Clear enlargement of the adenoma (*arrow*) and tilting of the optic chiasm. Cabergoline was reintroduced and delivery occurred normally. (**e**) Coronal T2WI 4 months after delivery. Shrinkage and slight hemorrhagic transformation of the adenoma (*straight arrow*). (**f**) T2WI 1 year later: further tumoral shrinkage

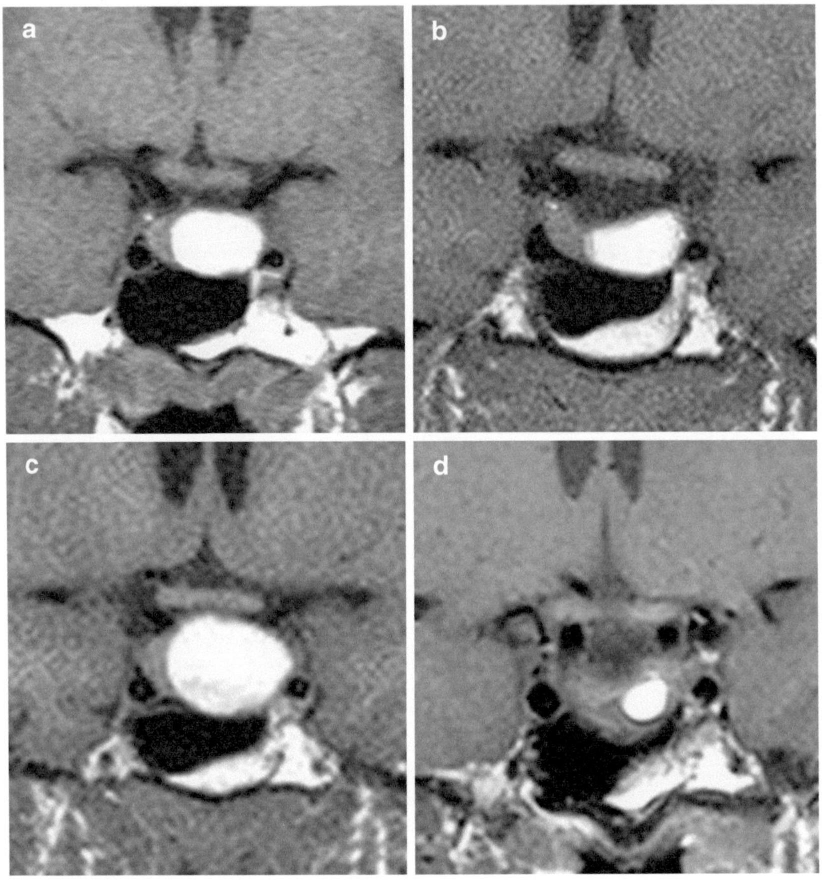

Fig. 8.5 22-year-old woman. Amenorrhea and galactorrhea. Prolactin is 1,400 mIU/l. (**a–d**) Coronal T1WIs. (**a**) At diagnosis. Intrasellar T1 hyperintense mass displacing the sellar floor and the pituitary stalk corresponding to a prolactinoma with spontaneous hemorrhagic transformation. (**b**) One year after cabergoline treatment. Prolactin level is normal. Partial shrinkage of the adenoma. (**c**) At third month of pregnancy (MRI made by mistake at this time). Marked increased size of the hemorrhagic prolactinoma. Cabergoline is reintroduced. (**d**) MRI follow-up 3 months after normal delivery. Massive shrinkage of the sellar content

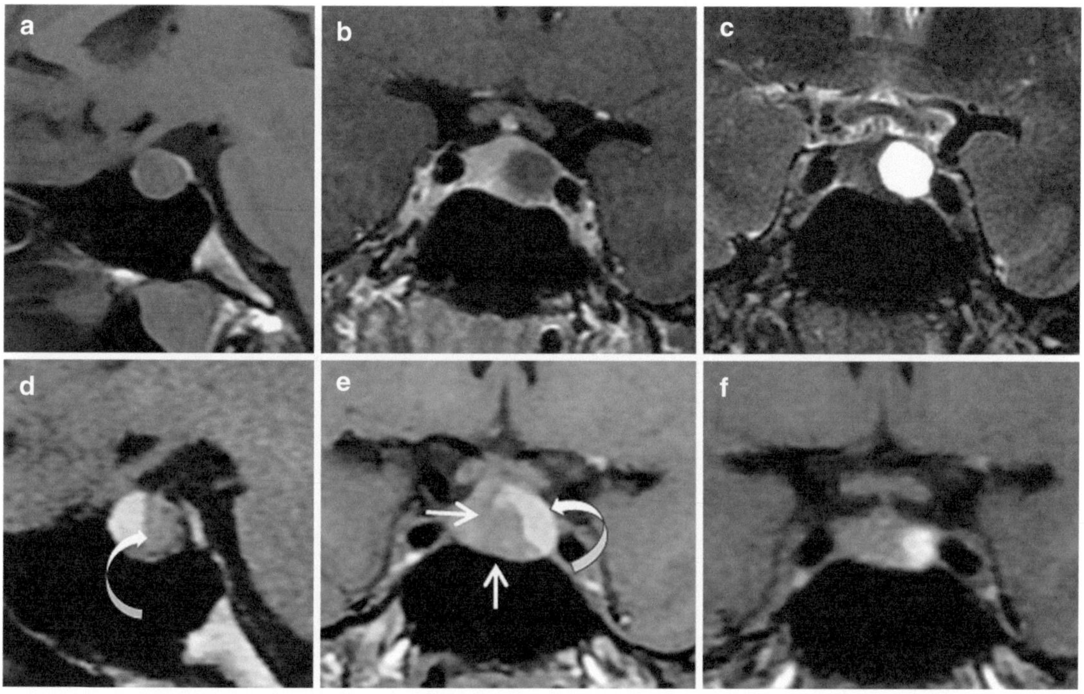

Fig. 8.6 25-year-old woman. Post pill amenorrhea and galactorrhea. Prolactin is 50 ng/ml. (**a–c**) Sagittal T1, coronal CE T1, and coronal T2 WIs at diagnosis. Left-sided 9 mm prolactinoma; the T2 signal is markedly hyperintense. A pregnancy was obtained as soon as 1 month after institution of cabergoline treatment. Cabergoline was immediately withdrawn. At 32 weeks of pregnancy, dizziness and altered vision. (**d**, **e**) Sagittal and coronal T1WIs. Increased volume of the adenoma (*arrows*) and partial hemorrhagic transformation with fluid-fluid level (*curved arrow*). Medical treatment was restored. (**f**) Coronal T1WI at 2 months postpartum. Shrinkage of the prolactinoma

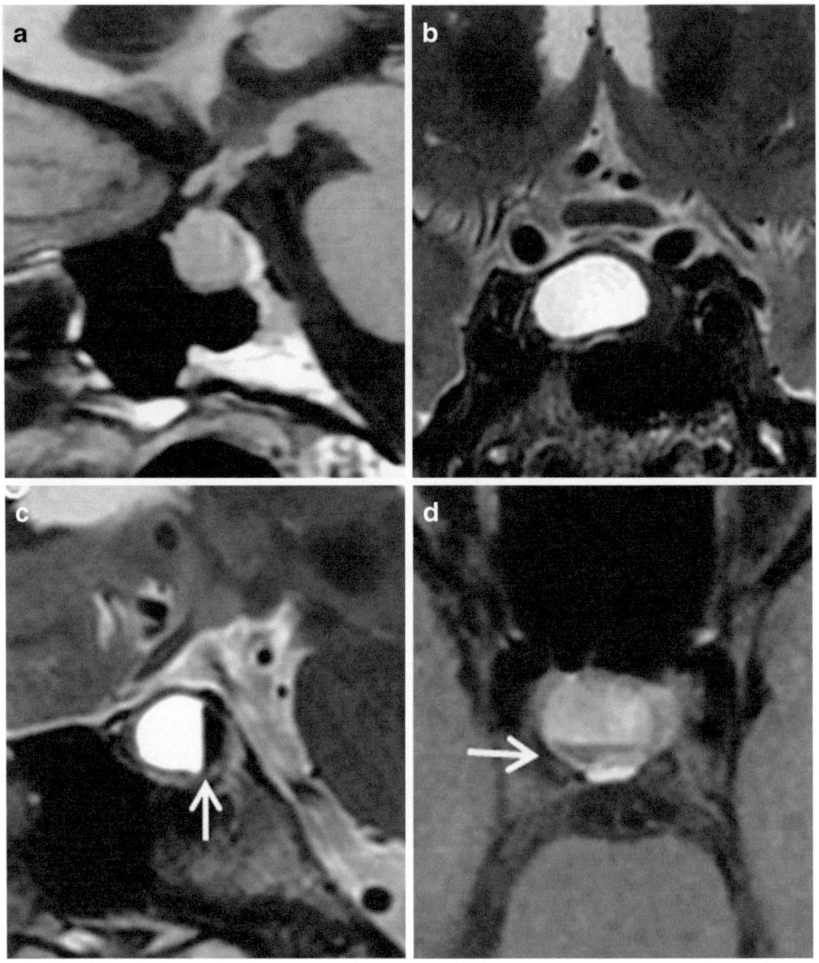

Fig. 8.7 33-year-old woman with factor V Leiden mutation. Treatment with aspirin. First pregnancy. Headache at fifth month. (**a**, **b**) Sagittal T1 and coronal T2 WIs. T1-isointense, T2-hyperintense lesion. (**c**, **d**) Sagittal T2 and axial T1 fat-saturated WIs at sixth month of pregnancy. The patient was now asymptomatic. Demonstration of a fluid-fluid level confirming hemorrhage within a nonfunctioning pituitary adenoma

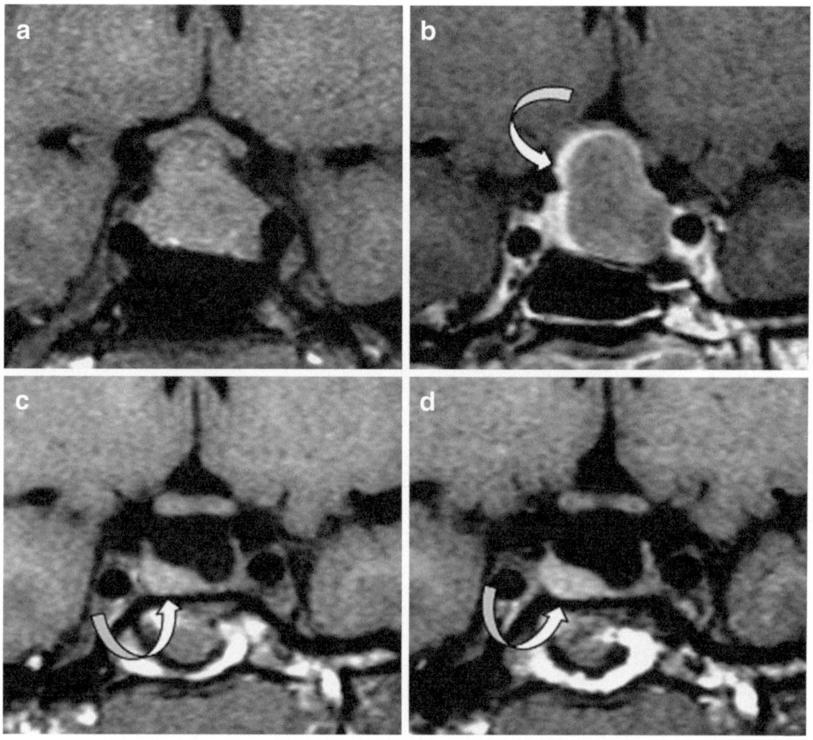

Fig. 8.8 24-year-old woman. Acromegaly. IGF-1 is 1,036 ng/ml. Pituitary adenoma with suprasellar extension. (**a**, **b**) Coronal T1 and CE T1 WIs. The normal pituitary tissue (*arrow*) is located on the right side and at the dome of the adenoma. (**c**) Coronal T1WI 18 months after surgery. Remodeling of the normal pituitary tissue (*arrow*). No tumoral remnant. (**d**) Coronal TIWI at sixth month of a spontaneous pregnancy 2 years later. TI hyperintensity of the normal pituitary tissue (*arrow*). No tumoral recurrence

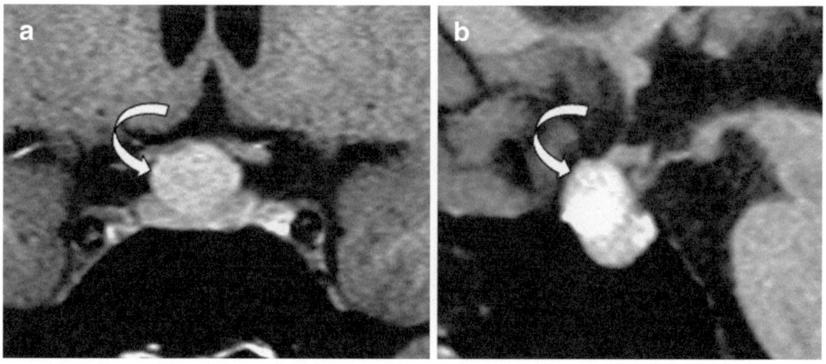

Fig. 8.9 Suprasellar Rathke cleft cyst. (**a**, **b**) Coronal and sagittal T1WIs. Visual field defect at the second month of an unknown pregnancy. Slightly T1 hyperintense cyst abutting the optic chiasm (*arrow*)

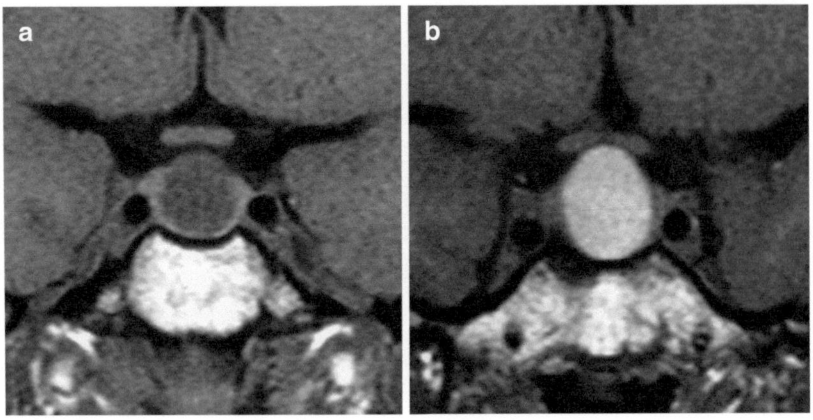

Fig. 8.10 25-year-old woman with Rathke cleft cyst. Galactorrhea. Prolactin is 43 ng/ml. Unknown 2 months pregnancy. (**a**, **b**) Coronal T1WIs. (**a**) At diagnosis, T1-hypointense Rathke cleft cyst. (**b**) MRI follow-up at 6 months of pregnancy. Increased cyst volume and T1 hyperintense signal without fluid-fluid level on sagittal T1 and T2 WIs (not shown). The patient is asymptomatic

Further Reading

Araujo PB, Vieira Neto L, Gadelha MR (2015) Pituitary tumor management in pregnancy. Endocrinol Metab Clin N Am 44(1):181–197

Domingue ME, Devuyst F, Alexopoulou O et al (2014) Outcome of prolactinoma after pregnancy and lactation: a study on 73 patients. Clin Endocrinol (Oxf) 80(5):642–648

Molitch ME (2010) Prolactinomas and pregnancy. Clin Endocrinol (Oxf) 73(2):147–148

9 Prolactinoma in Men

Jean-François Bonneville and Julie Kreutz

Macroprolactinomas predominate in males in comparison with microprolactinomas, with a greater tendency to invasiveness than in females. The clinical symptoms of decrease in libido and sexual potency are frequently misunderstood in men, with a consequent delay in diagnosis, but this cannot totally explain this gender difference. The responsibility of increased markers of cellular proliferation which have been reported to occur more often in men have confirmed that prolactinomas are more aggressive (Fig. 9.1). From a clinical point of view, the frequency of incidental diagnosis and the rarity of headache in men in comparison with women are noteworthy. It is suspected that many of these prolactinomas present a rapid growth in a relatively short period of time. Microprolactinomas represent 25 % of all prolactinomas in men and do not present different characteristics if compared with those found in women. Many macroprolactinomas are very large in size, which correlates with a very high serum prolactin level (up to thousands of nanograms per ml) almost never observed in women. The parallelism between serum prolactin level and maximal tumor diameter is present only if the volume of the cystic and/or hemorrhagic components are subtracted from the total volume of the tumor. Another point concerns the relative frequency of giant tumors preferentially invading the sphenoid sinus and sometimes referred for assessment of a "sphenoid tumor" (Fig. 9.2). A wise rule could be to systematically obtain the prolactin plasma level in every "sphenoid sinus tumor" (Fig. 9.3). The extracranial inferior extension could perhaps explain the usual absence of headache even in very large tumors in men. Similarly, optic chiasm compromise is observed in only 25 % of the cases. Cavernous sinus invasion is recognized in roughly one-third of cases. Macroprolactinomas in men are usually hypointense on T1WI and hyperintense on T2WI and, in at least half of the cases, heterogeneous, with large areas of T1 hyperintensity giving evidence of hemorrhage and T2 hyperintensity representing local necrosis or old hemorrhage. Calcifications or amyloid deposits are represented by T2-hypointense intratumoral nodules; they seem less rare than in other types of pituitary adenomas (Fig. 9.4). Cabergoline is, as a rule, rapidly efficient in normalizing the prolactin level; an increased T2 hyperintensity is noted on MRI, while the tumor shrinkage can be modest or delayed (Fig. 9.5). Intratumoral hemorrhage, possibly symptomatic, can occur in large prolactinomas under treatment (Fig. 9.6). A CSF fistula can exceptionally occur with high dosages of dopamine agonists.

Exceptionally, air from the sphenoid sinus can subsequently accumulate within the capsule of the necrosed macroadenoma through a one-way valve mechanism. If under pressure, this trapped air is called a "pneumatocyst," and exerts a significant mass effect on the adjacent cerebral structures (Fig. 9.7).

J.-F. Bonneville et al., *MRI of the Pituitary Gland*, DOI 10.1007/978-3-319-29043-0_9

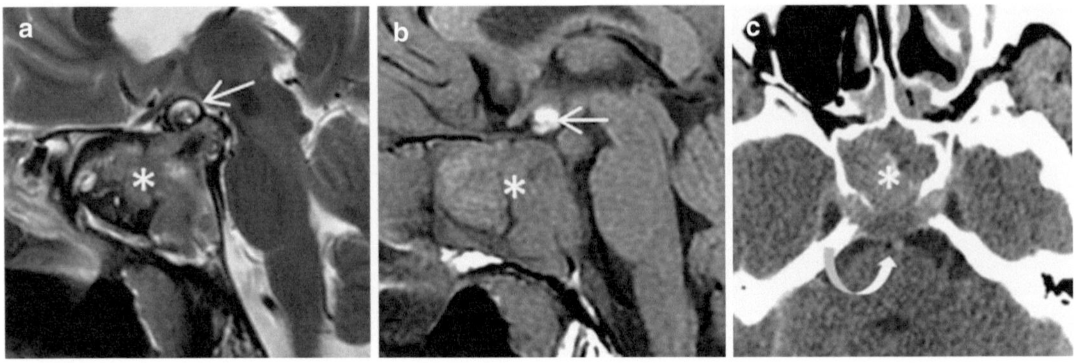

Fig. 9.1 57-year-old man. Impotence. Prolactin is 1590 ng/ml. (**a**, **b**) Sagittal T2 and T1 WIs. (**c**) Axial CT. Macroprolactinoma invading the sphenoid sinus (*asterisk*) and eroding the clivus (*curved arrow*). Small round hemorrhagic component in the upper part of the tumor (*straight arrow*)

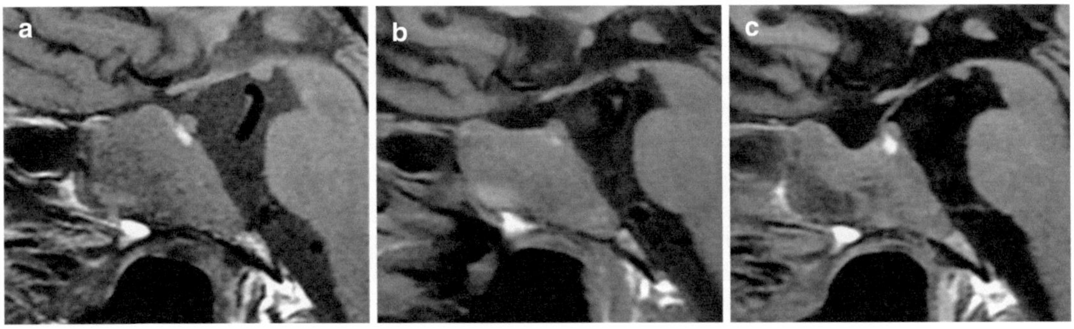

Fig. 9.2 52-year-old man. Prolactin is >100,000 mIU/l. Macroprolactinoma invading the sphenoid sinus. Follow-up with cabergoline treatment. Sagittal T1WIs at diagnosis (**a**), 3 months (**b**), and 1 year after treatment (**c**). Progressive tumoral shrinkage

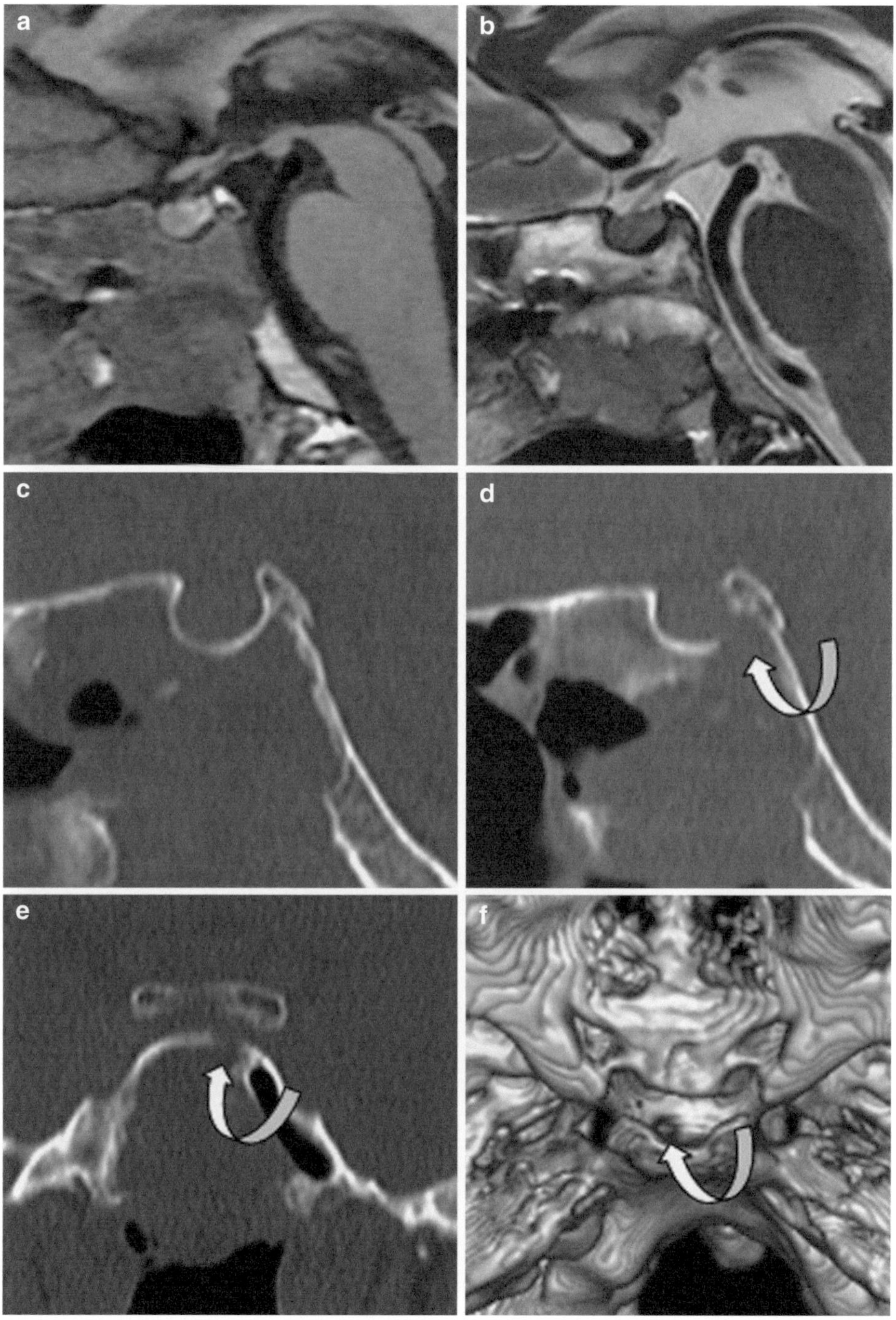

Fig. 9.3 53-year-old man. Intrasphenoidal macroprolactinoma diagnosed during surgery for "sphenoidal sinus tumor." Prolactin is 1820 ng/ml. (**a**, **b**) Sagittal T1 and T2 WIs. Sphenoidal sinus tumor. The sella turcica seems intact. (**c**) Midsagittal section, CT. Normal sella. (**d**–**f**) Parasagittal and coronal sections and 3D reformatted image reveal a tiny defect at the most posterior part of the sellar floor (*arrows*)

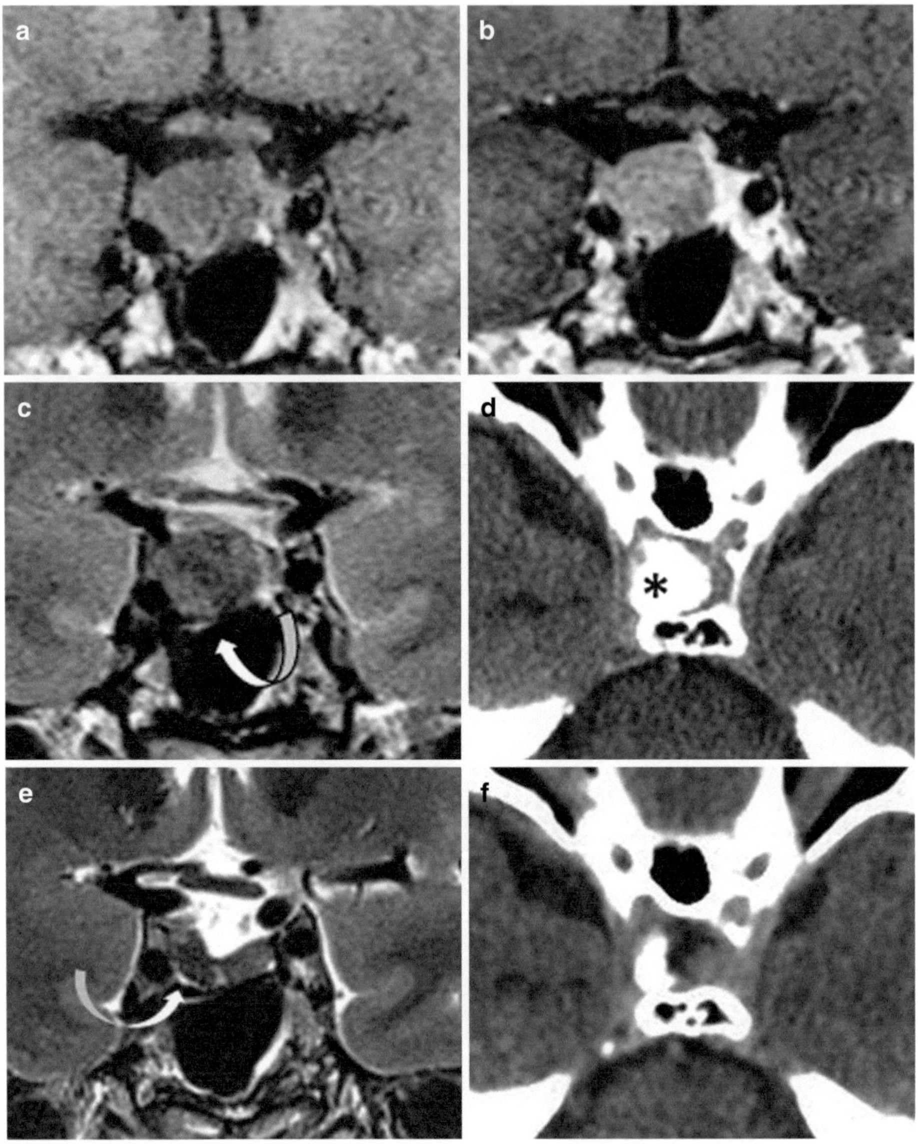

Fig. 9.4 43-year-old man. T1- and T2-hypointense prolactinoma. Prolactin is 5949 mIU/l. (**a–c**) Coronal T1, CE T1, and T2 WIs. (**d**) Axial CT. Tumoral T2 hypointensity (*arrow*) corresponding to calcifications or amyloid deposits on CT (*asterisk*). (**e**) Coronal T2WI after 2 years of cabergoline treatment (*arrow*). Adenoma shrinkage and, in parallel, decreased size of the calcification or amyloid deposit on CT (**f**)

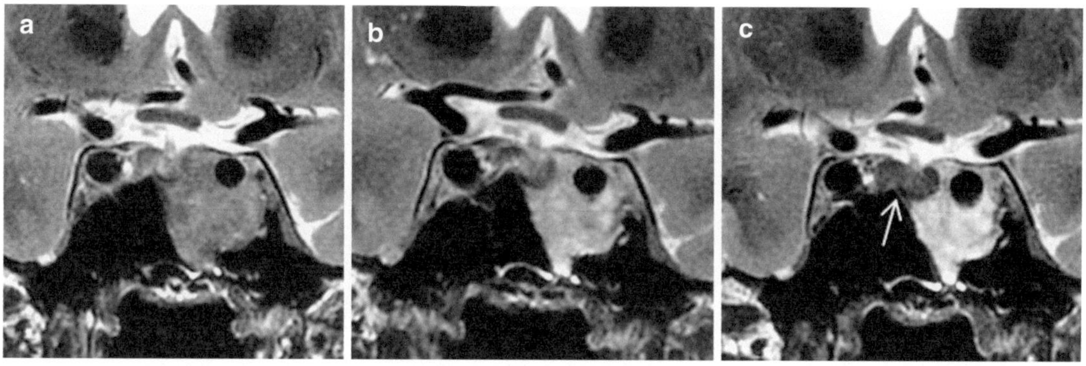

Fig. 9.5 55-year-old man. Hyperprolactinemia (1100 ng/ml) discovered on the occasion of a wrist fracture with osteoporosis. (**a–c**) Coronal T2WIs. Prolactinoma invading the sphenoid sinus and the cavernous sinus. (**a**) At diagnosis. (**b**, **c**) One and 2 years after cabergoline treatment. Slight shrinkage and T2 tumoral hyperintensity. The prolactin level is normalized. The anterior pituitary gland appears normal (*arrow*)

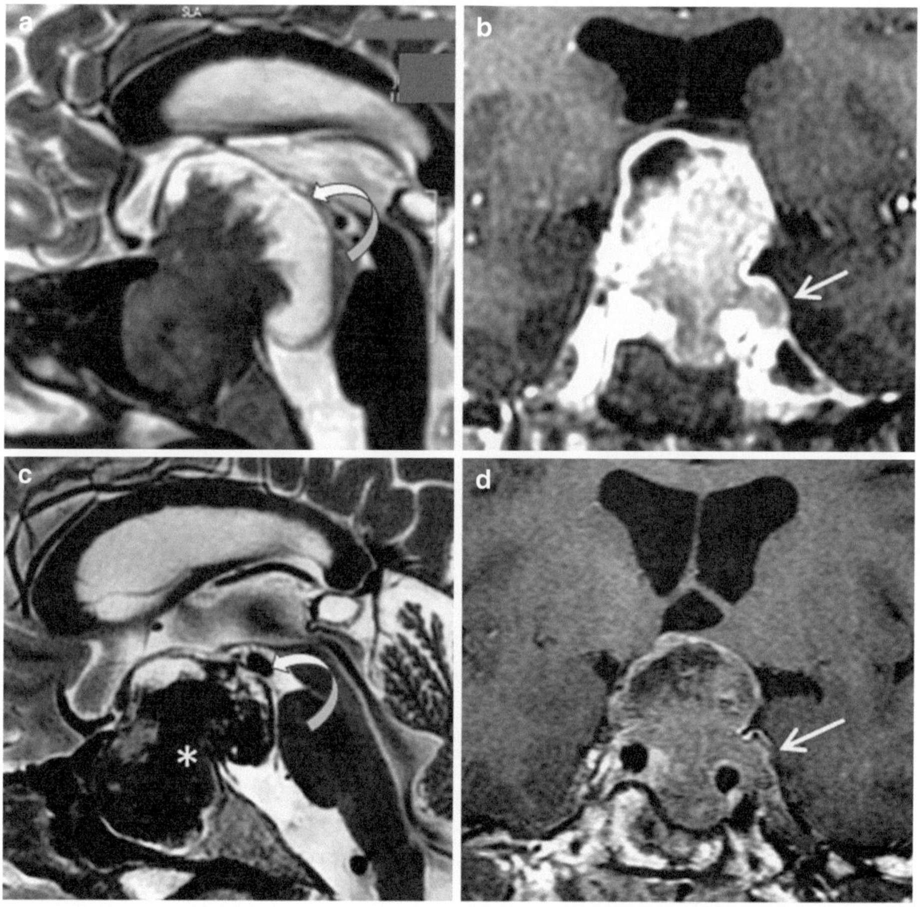

Fig. 9.6 38-year-old man. Headache and bitemporal hemianopia. Prolactin is 6000 ng/ml. Normal sexual activity. Sagittal T2 and coronal CE T1WIs at diagnosis (**a**, **b**) and 6 weeks after cabergoline (**c**, **d**). Huge necrotic pituitary macroadenoma with suprasellar extension (*curved arrow*) and invasion of left cavernous sinus (*straight arrow*). Six weeks after treatment, hemorrhagic transformation of the tumor recognized by the hypointense T2 signal (*asterisk*). Prolactin is now 18 ng/ml. Vision was improved as soon as 1 day after institution of cabergoline treatment

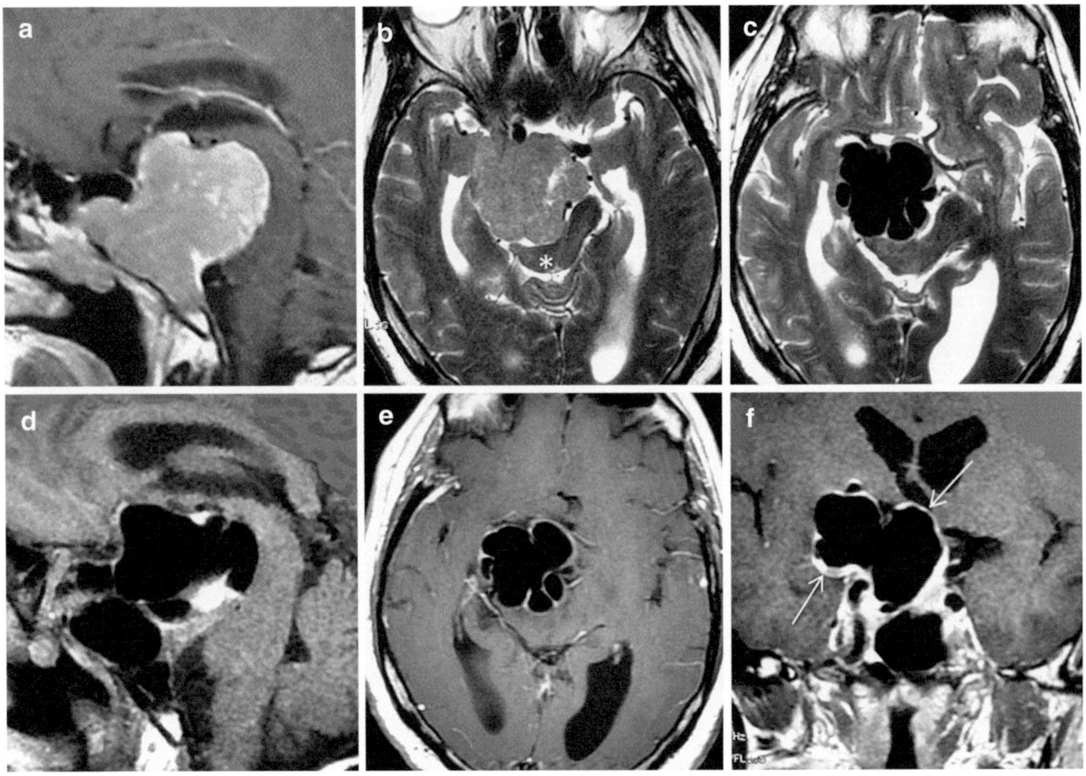

Fig. 9.7 60-year-old man with hemiparesis and headaches caused by a giant pneumatocyst. The patient has been treated by dopamine agonist for the last 6 months for a giant macroprolactinoma. (**a**) Sagittal CE T1WI at diagnosis, before the introduction of oral therapy. Huge invasive pituitary adenoma with supra- and infrasellar extension. (**b**) Axial T2WI reveals a compressive mass impinging the right cerebral peduncle (asterisk). (**c–f**) Axial T2, sagittal, axial, and coronal CE T1WIs demonstrate a polylobulated mass with signal void corresponding to the air trapped within the adenoma capsule that enhances after gadolinium injection (*arrows*)

Further Reading

Colao A, Sarno AD, Cappabianca P et al (2003) Gender differences in the prevalence, clinical features and response to cabergoline in hyperprolactinemia. Eur J Endocrinol 148(3):325–331

Iglesias P, Bernal C, Villabona C et al (2012) Prolactinomas in men: a multicentre and retrospective analysis of treatment outcome. Clin Endocrinol (Oxf) 77(2):281–287

Kreutz J, Vroonen L, Cattin F et al (2015) Intensity of prolactinoma on T2-weighted magnetic resonance imaging: towards another gender difference. Neuroradiology 57(7):679–684

10 Aggressive Pituitary Adenoma

Jean-François Bonneville

The definition of "aggressive" pituitary adenomas varies with the different specialties in charge of pituitary gland tumors. For the pathologist, for instance, "aggressivity" means that the dura of the sellar region is invaded, even if this is not recognized by the neurosurgeon, or if proliferation markers such as Ki-67 or P53 are detected. Radiologists may have their own definition.

"Aggressive" pituitary tumors grow rapidly: detecting a small change in volume in a short time commands perfect reproducibility of MRI images. Thus, it is strongly recommended to obtain MRI coronal projections strictly with the same angulation in daily practice, for instance as we proposed perpendicularly to a line tangential to the genu and the splenium of the corpus callosum, which is easily drawn on a sagittal view (Fig. 1.1). Other options are 3D MRI or tumoral volume calculation by manual segmentation (Fig. 10.1).

Tumors extending beyond a natural barrier such as the dura are considered invasive. Invasiveness can manifest itself by focal rupture of tumoral contours, clival invasion, or cavernous sinus invasion (Fig. 10.2). Abrupt/acute rupture of the sellar floor evokes more certainly bony invasion than a smooth change, meaning that the sellar floor is simply pushed away (Fig. 10.3).

Clival invasion has been recently individualized and has been recognized in 8 % of macroadenomas. Risk factors are female, large-volume tumor, and null-cell adenoma. CT in this case is superior to MRI in demonstrating a focal or widespread defect of the basisphenoid bone with decreased attenuation in underlying trabecular bone (Fig. 10.4). If not recognized, clival invasion can lead to severe operative complications.

Round lobulated exophytic nodules distorting tumoral contours may represent another feature of invasiveness.

Cavernous sinus invasion remains difficult to assess if limited. It generally starts posteriorly and is best demonstrated on axial T2W sequences. Evidence of invasion is through the presence of a breach in the medial dural wall of the cavernous sinus (Fig. 10.5). More invasive tumors are able to enlarge the dural pocket of the oculomotor nerve and pass into the subarachnoid space of the temporal lobe. A detailed description and illustrations of cavernous sinus invasion are given in Chap. 11. Pituitary adenomas with T2-hyperintense signal, which could correspond to sparsely granulated tumors, are usually considered more prone than tumors with T2 hypointensity to invade surrounded structures. This has been particularly demonstrated with GH-secreting pituitary adenomas (Figs. 14.7 and 14.8).

Microcystic tumoral pattern on T2WI could indicate some tendency to invasiveness, and has been reported more frequently in corticosilent pituitary adenomas (Fig. 10.6).

Carcinomas are very rare and can be distinguished only by the presence of metastases. They do not present with specific patterns. Chapter 17 is devoted to this condition.

J.-F. Bonneville et al., *MRI of the Pituitary Gland*, DOI 10.1007/978-3-319-29043-0_10

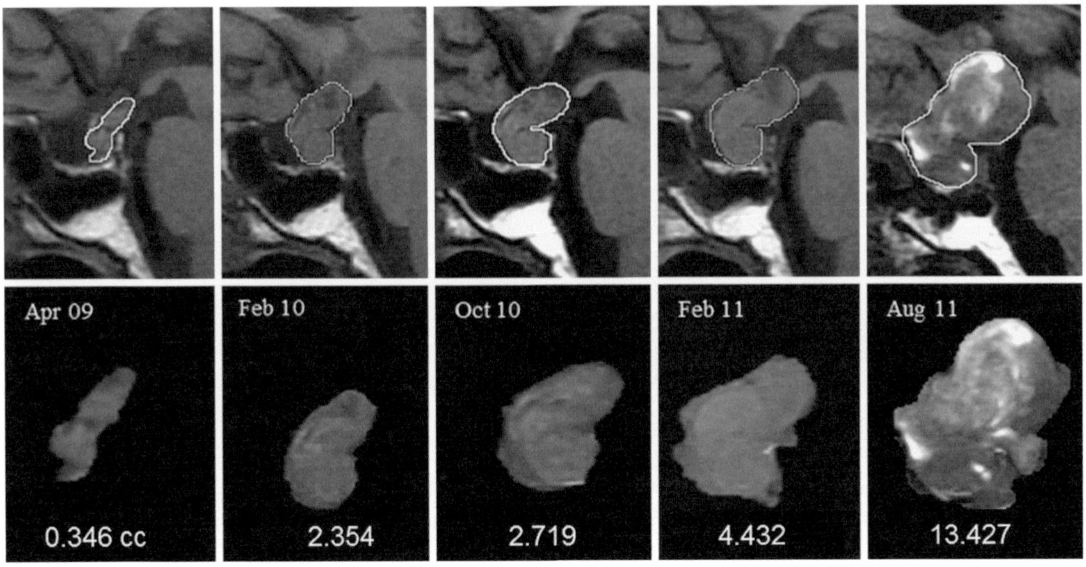

Fig. 10.1 Aggressive recurrent-resistant prolactinoma in a 43-year-old man. *Upper row*: serial sagittal T1WIs. Increased tumoral volume with time despite medical treatment. *Lower row*: volumetric assessment

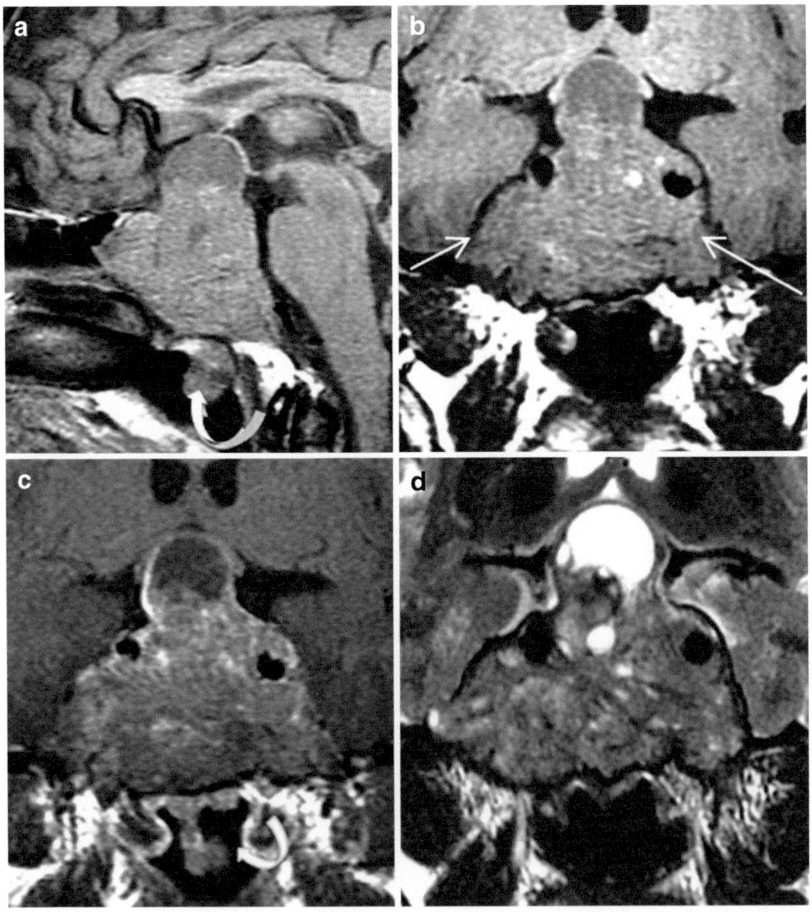

Fig. 10.2 Aggressive pituitary adenoma in a 47-year-old woman. Bitemporal hemianopia. (**a**, **b**) Sagittal and coronal T1WIs. (**c**) Coronal CE T1WI. (**d**) Coronal T2WI. The tumor invades both cavernous sinuses (*straight arrows*) and extends toward the nasopharyngeal space (*curved arrow*)

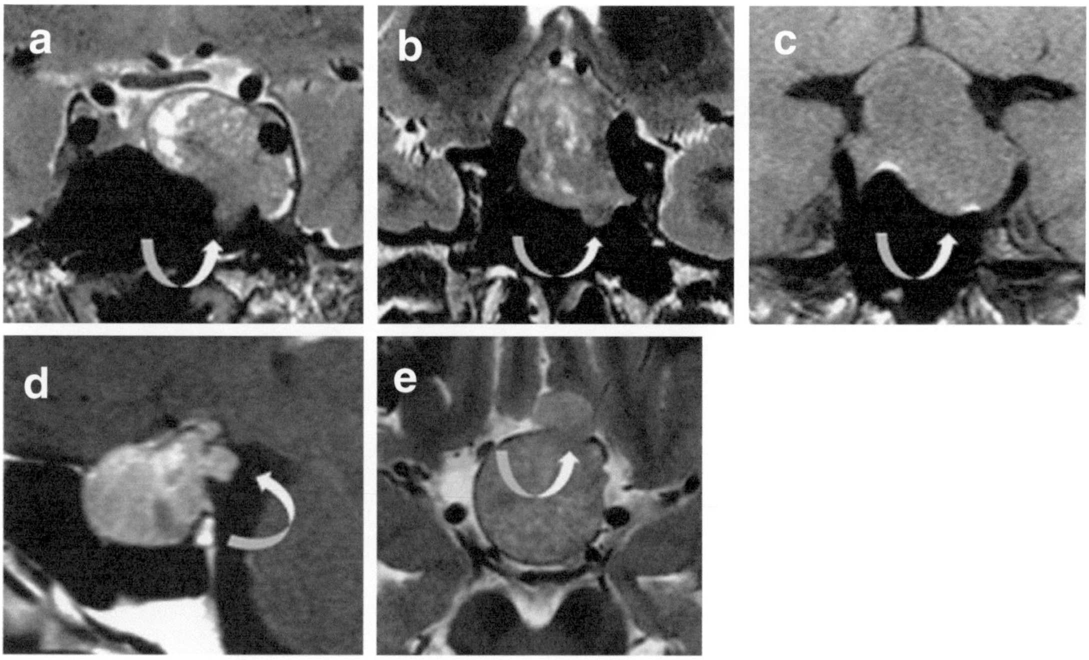

Fig. 10.3 Aggressive pituitary adenomas (except in **c**). (**a**, **b**) T2WIs. Acute changes of the sellar floor. (**c**) Coronal T1WI. Smooth change of the sellar floor, which is displaced downward but not invaded. (**d**, **e**) Sagittal CE T1 and axial T2WIs. Exophytic tumoral nodules

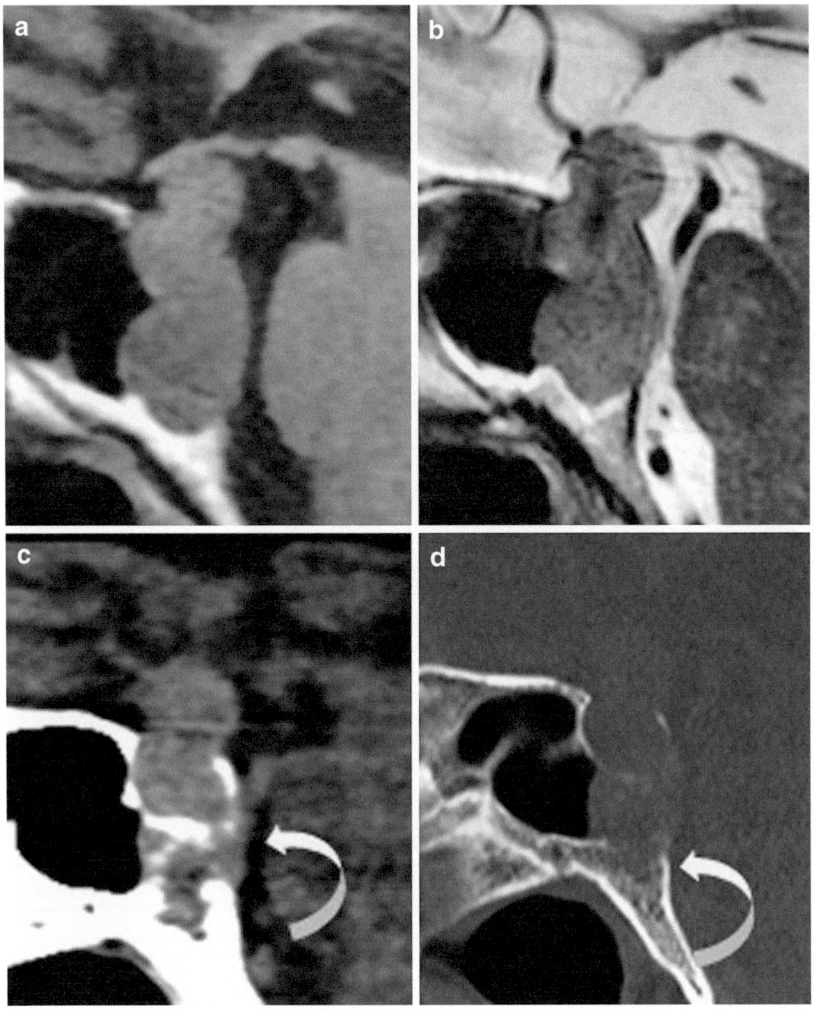

Fig. 10.4 Clival invasion. (**a**, **b**) Sagittal T1 and T2WIs. Large pituitary adenoma with limited suprasellar extension and extensive inferior extension. (**c**, **d**) Midsagittal CT, soft and bone window: osteolysis of the clivus (*arrows*)

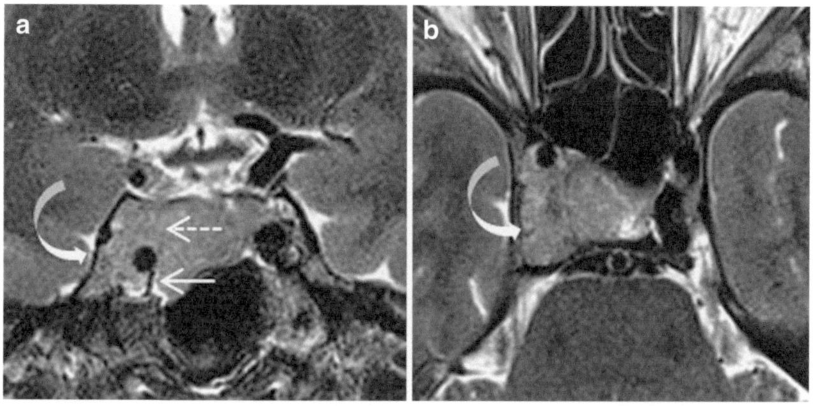

Fig. 10.5 T2 hyperintense GH-secreting adenoma with cavernous sinus invasion (*curved arrow*). (**a**, **b**) Coronal and axial T2WIs. The internal medial wall of cavernous sinus (*straight arrow*) is missing superiorly (*dotted line*)

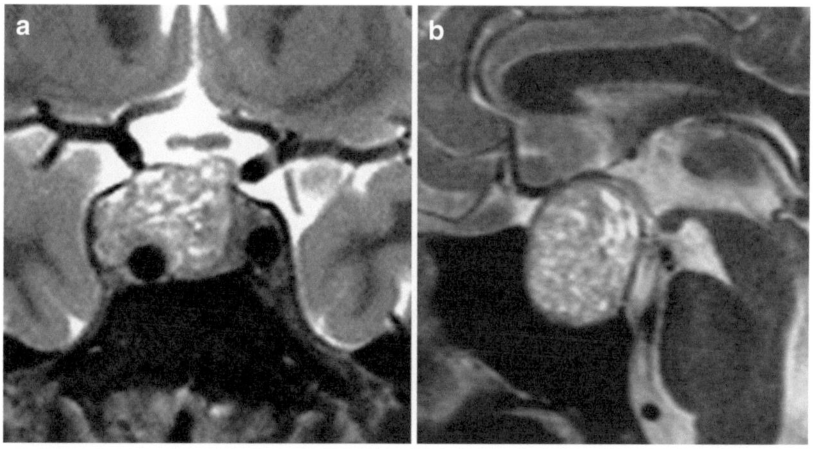

Fig. 10.6 Corticosilent pituitary adenomas in two patients. (**a**) Coronal T2WI: right-sided tumor invading right cavernous sinus with a microcystic pattern. (**b**) Sagittal T2WI: same microcystic appearance of a pituitary adenoma with suprasellar extension

Further Reading

Chen X, Dai J, Ai L et al (2011) Clival invasion on multi-detector CT in 390 pituitary macroadenomas: correlation with sex, subtype and rates of operative complication. AJNR Am Neuroradiol 32(4): 785–789

Potorac I, Petrossians P, Daly AF et al (2015) Pituitary MRI characteristics in 297 acromegaly patients based on T2-weighted sequences. Endocrinol Relat Cancer 22(2):169–177

Scheithauer BV, Kovacs KT, Laws ER Jr et al (1986) Pathology of invasive pituitary tumors with special reference to functional classification. J Neurosurg 65:733–744

11 Cavernous Sinus Invasion

Jean-François Bonneville

The diagnosis of cavernous sinus invasion by pituitary adenomas is of paramount importance, particularly for secreting pituitary adenomas: it is accepted that surgery alone is usually unable to cure the disease in these cases. Clinically, cavernous sinus invasion is most of the time silent. The radiological diagnosis of subtle cavernous sinus invasion remains difficult and can remain uncertain even with the highest quality MRI and the highest experience of the neuroradiologist. For these reasons, frequency of cavernous sinus invasion is differently appreciated in the literature.

Nevertheless, huge invasion of cavernous sinus is usually obvious: a tissue of an identical MR signal and an identical enhancement as those of the intrasellar component of the tumor completely encircles the intracavernous internal carotid artery. The lateral wall of the cavernous sinus is bulging. The normal enhancement of the venous extrasellar spaces is missing. Cavernous sinus invasion by pituitary adenomas is mostly unilateral, the laterally displaced normal pituitary gland "protecting" the contralateral cavernous sinus (Fig. 11.1). The lumen of the intracavernous internal carotid artery is usually unchanged, different to what is observed in cavernous sinus meningioma. When cavernous sinus invasion is massive, the pituitary adenoma can pass into the subarachnoid spaces of the temporal lobe. It was initially believed that this severe extension was through a rupture of the thick lateral dural wall of the cavernous sinus. In fact, the tumoral growth follows and enlarges the dural pocket accompanying the oculomotor nerve (Fig. 11.2).

In some cases, a simple displacement and a compression of the cavernous sinus structures by a lateral extension of the pituitary adenoma can mimic a true invasion; but here there is no perforation of the dural medial wall of the cavernous sinus. Asymmetrical tentorial enhancement has also been described with invasion, as in severe compression of the cavernous sinus by sellar tumor, and is then not specific. It may represent venous congestion in the tentorium caused by obstructed flow in the medial venous compartment of the cavernous sinus.

Historical classifications based on anatomical landmarks, such as those of Knosp or Cottier, are of no absolute value (Fig. 11.3). For Knosp, cavernous sinus invasion is "very likely" if the tumor extends laterally and passes a line drawn between the cross-sectional centers of the supra- and intracavernous segments of the internal carotid artery. Cottier suggests that a percentage of encasement of the internal carotid artery by tumoral tissue of more than 67 % makes invasion certain. Another criterion, the nonvisualization of the carotid sulcus venous compartment, as described by Bonneville with dynamic CT, is scarcely reproducible with MRI. Nevertheless, an intracavernous internal carotid artery remote from the sphenoid carotid sulcus is highly suggestive of cavernous sinus invasion (Fig. 11.4).

J.-F. Bonneville et al., *MRI of the Pituitary Gland*, DOI 10.1007/978-3-319-29043-0_11

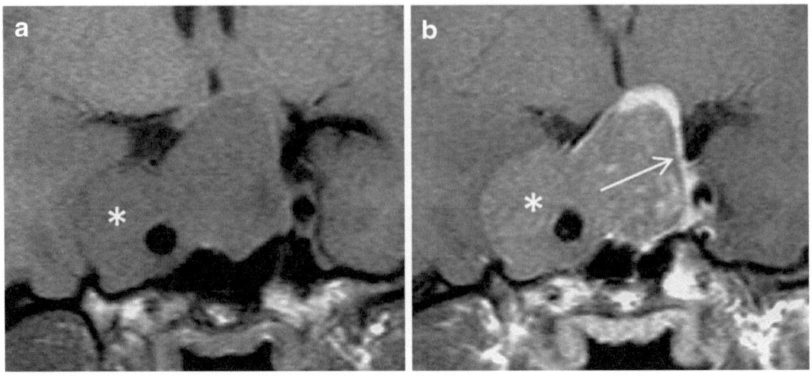

Fig. 11.1 Pituitary macroadenoma invading right cavernous sinus (*asterisk*). (**a**, **b**) Coronal T1 and CE T1 WIs. The internal carotid artery is totally encased by the tumor. The normal pituitary tissue (*arrow*) is displaced laterally and superiorly

Limited tumoral extensions within the cavernous sinus need to be detected, given that their presence can radically change the medical strategy. Their diagnosis needs high-quality, high-resolution MRI and special sequences, ideally with demonstration of the thin internal dural membrane separating the sellar content from the cavernous sinus. Such a demonstration is more frequently obtained with 3.0 T than with 1.5 T MR scanners. Early cavernous sinus extensions are located initially posteriorly, i.e., where the internal dural wall is the thinnest: high-resolution axial T2WIs are the most informative to detect these extensions and must be added to the usual sequences (Fig. 11.5). If not completely torn, the internal medial wall appears as an incomplete thin, T2-hypointense line floating as a curtain between cavernous sinus and pituitary fossa (Fig. 11.6). The second most frequent site of invasion is located in the concavity of the internal carotid artery siphon, with a tongue-like appearance best demonstrated on axial views. A shoulder-like tumoral expansion above the internal carotid artery seen on coronal view is also suggestive of cavernous sinus invasion (Fig. 11.7). Finally it is noticeable that, in pituitary adenomas treated medically, shrinkage of the intracavernous part of the tumor, if any, occurs in the same way as for the intrasellar component.

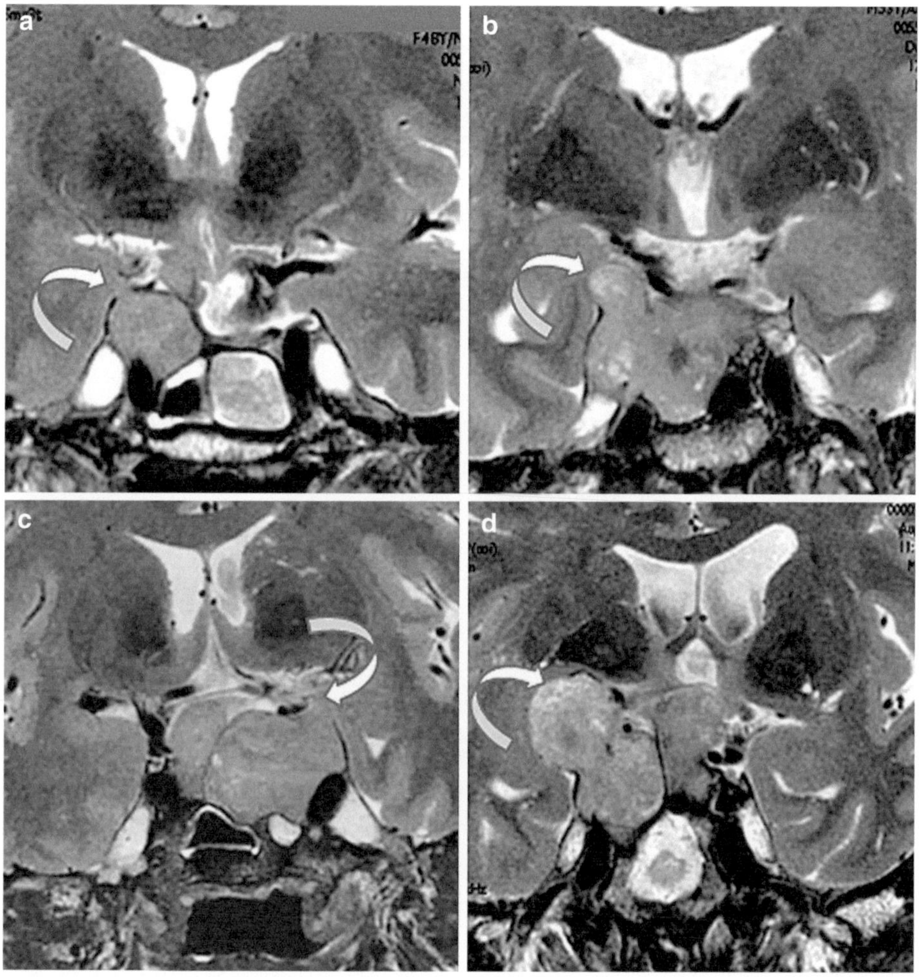

Fig. 11.2 Cavernous sinus invasion extended into the subarachnoid space of the temporal lobe in four patients with recurrence of pituitary adenoma. (**a**–**d**) Coronal T2WIs. Limited (**a**–**c**) and huge (**d**) tumoral extension, presumably through the dural pocket of the oculomotor nerve (*arrows*)

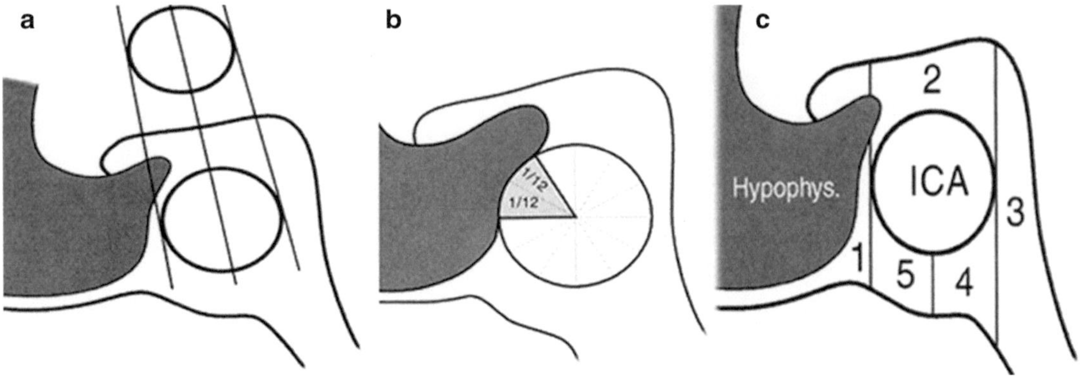

Fig. 11.3 (**a**) Knosp landmark. Cavernous sinus invasion is said to be very likely if the tumor passes the line joining the centers of intracavernous and supracavernous internal carotid artery sections. (**b**) Cottier landmark. Encasement of the internal carotid artery of more than 67 % is said to indicate cavernous sinus invasion, as is obliteration of the carotid sulcus venous compartment (5 in **c**)

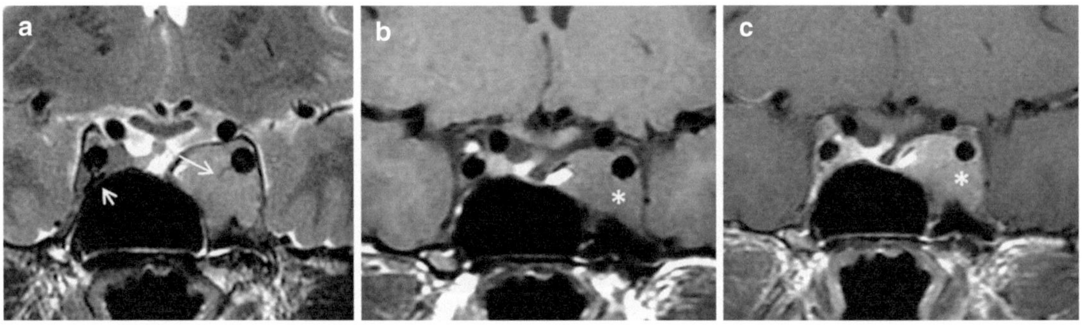

Fig. 11.4 Recurrent pituitary adenoma invading left cavernous sinus. (**a**–**c**) Coronal T2, T1, and CE T1 WIs. Normally, as seen in the right cavernous sinus, the intracavernous internal carotid artery is separated from the sphenoid carotid sulcus by a vein (*small arrow*) or is in close contact with the carotid sulcus. On the left, there is no visible vein of the carotid sulcus and the left internal carotid artery is distant from the sphenoid bone: invasion of the cavernous sinus is clear (*asterisk*). Note that the torn medial wall of cavernous sinus (*arrow*) is partially demonstrated only on T2WI (**a**)

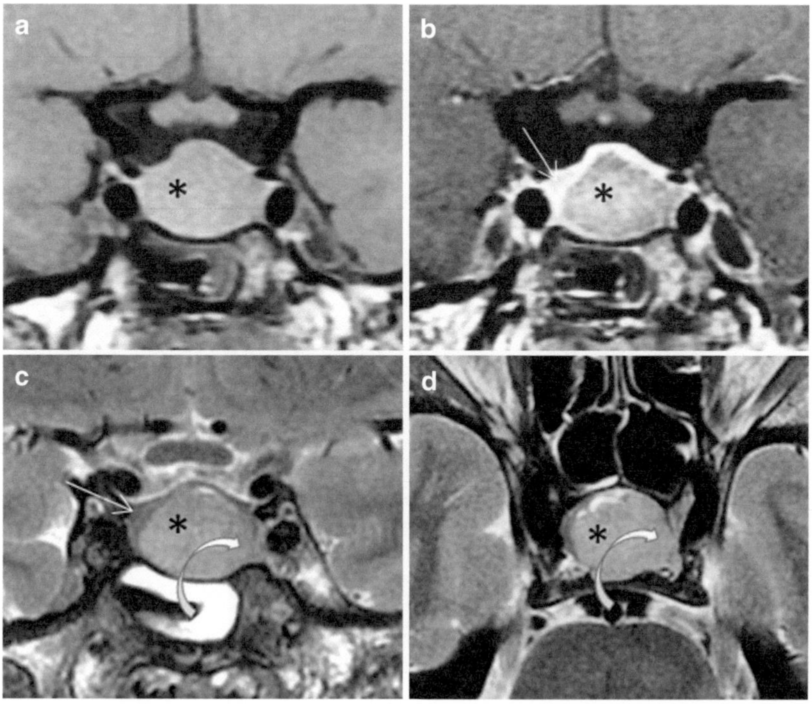

Fig. 11.5 T2-hyperintense GH-secreting pituitary adenoma with cavernous sinus invasion (*asterisk*). (**a–c**) Coronal T1, CE T1, and T2 WIs, and (**d**) axial T2WI. Compressed anterior pituitary gland (*straight arrow*). Limited left cavernous sinus invasion. Demonstration of the incomplete medial wall of the cavernous sinus (*curved arrow*) is only visible on T2WI

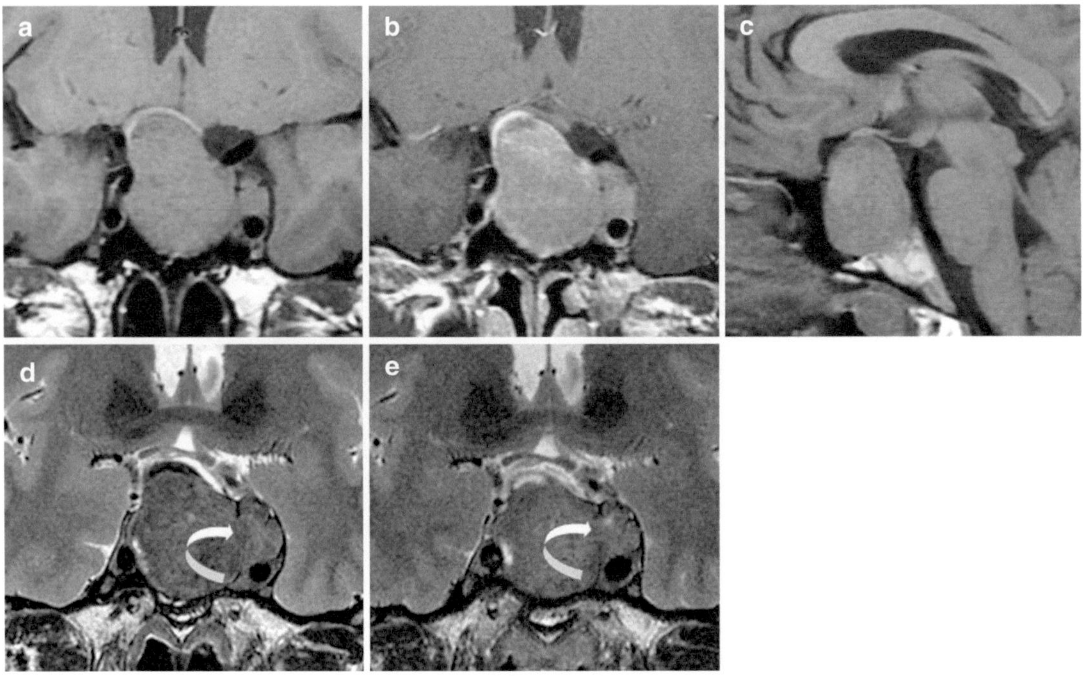

Fig. 11.6 Nonfunctioning macroadenoma invading left cavernous sinus. (**a**, **b**, **d**) Coronal T1, CE T1, and T2 WIs. (**c**) Sagittal T1WI. (**e**) Coronal T2WI after tumoral debulking. The torn medial wall of the cavernous sinus (*arrow* in **d**) is pushed laterally and less displaced after debulking in (**e**)

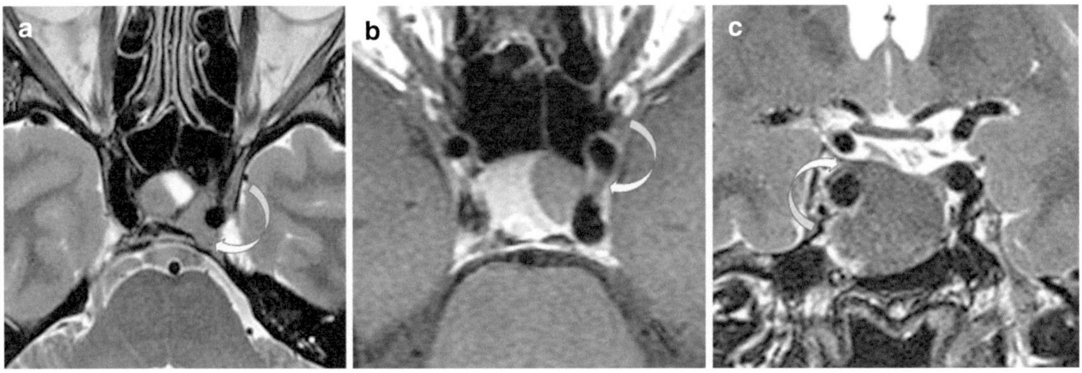

Fig. 11.7 Limited tumoral extensions to cavernous sinus (*arrows*). (**a**) Posterior extension on axial T2WI. (**b**) Between two segments of intracavernous internal carotid artery on axial CE T1WI. (**c**) Above the internal carotid artery on coronal T2WI

Further Reading

Cao L, Chen H, Hong J et al (2013) Magnetic resonance imaging appearance of the medial wall of the cavernous sinus. J Neuroradiol 40:245–251

Knosp E, Steiner E, Kitz K et al (1993) Pituitary adenomas with invasion of the cavernous sinus space: a magnetic resonance imaging classification compared with surgical findings. Neurosurgery 33(4):610–616

Yilmazlar S, Kocaeli H, Aydiner F et al (2005) Medial portion of the cavernous sinus. Clin Anat 18:416–422

12 Hemorrhagic Pituitary Adenoma

Jean-François Bonneville

Unlike pituitary apoplexia, pituitary adenoma hemorrhage is mostly a nonsymptomatic radiological finding, and is frequently called "subacute hemorrhage" in the literature. Most cases have no identifiable cause. Hemorrhage is quite frequent, mainly in nonfunctioning adenomas and in macro- and microprolactinomas treated with dopamine agonists or not. This condition is generally benign and seems in some cases to favor the cure of the disease. Pituitary adenoma hemorrhage is also common in childhood and adolescence.

Hemorrhage MR signal varies with many conditions and principally with time. As benign pituitary hemorrhage is asymptomatic, only subacute and chronic phases are usually observed.

In the subacute phase, hemorrhage appears as a hyperintense area on T1WI and mostly hyperintense on T2WI (Fig. 12.1). In the chronic phase, the hematoma may appear as T1 hypointense, and a T2-hypointense peripheral ring of hemosiderin may represent the only marker of an old hemorrhage. Nevertheless, this sign is inconstant, the absence of a blood-brain barrier in the pituitary gland allowing an efficient turnover, thus preventing hemosiderin from deposit. T2W gradient-echo sequences are more sensitive for the demonstration of such an old hemorrhage (Fig. 12.2). So-called intratumoral "cysts" presenting with T1 hypointensity and T2 hyperintensity likely represent old hemorrhagic cavities or infarction (Fig. 12.3).

In a significant number of macroprolactinomas, a fluid-fluid level is present in old hemorrhage, the supernatant corresponding to extracellular methemoglobin and the subnatant to erythrocyte membranes and intracellular deoxyhemoglobin. The supernatant is hyperintense in both T1WI and T2WI; the subnatant is of low signal on T2WI (Fig. 12.4). However, signal intensities of blood products depend on the age of the hemorrhage and may vary. The fluid-fluid level may be demonstrated on T2WI only. It permits differentiation of sellar lesions liable to present with T1 hyperintensity, i.e., hemorrhagic pituitary adenomas, craniopharyngiomas, and Rathke cleft cysts. While pituitary adenomas have a strong tendency to bleed, this phenomenon is much rarer in craniopharyngiomas or Rathke cleft cysts. Thus, a T1-hyperintense sellar tumor harboring a fluid-fluid level has to be diagnosed as a pituitary adenoma until proven otherwise.

Hemorrhage can also concern microadenomas and primarily microprolactinomas, but fluid-fluid level is rarer in such cases. Hemorrhagic microadenomas may be mistaken for intrasellar T1-hyperintense protein-rich Rathke cleft cysts. It must be borne in mind that most pituitary adenomas, even tiny, produce a mass effect—on the sellar floor, the pituitary stalk, the upper surface of the gland, and/or the posterior lobe (Fig. 12.5)—in contrast to Rathke cleft cysts. Rathke cleft cysts show few or no mass effects and their wall can be depressed, for instance by a coexisting pituitary adenoma (Fig. 21.3).

J.-F. Bonneville et al., *MRI of the Pituitary Gland*, DOI 10.1007/978-3-319-29043-0_12

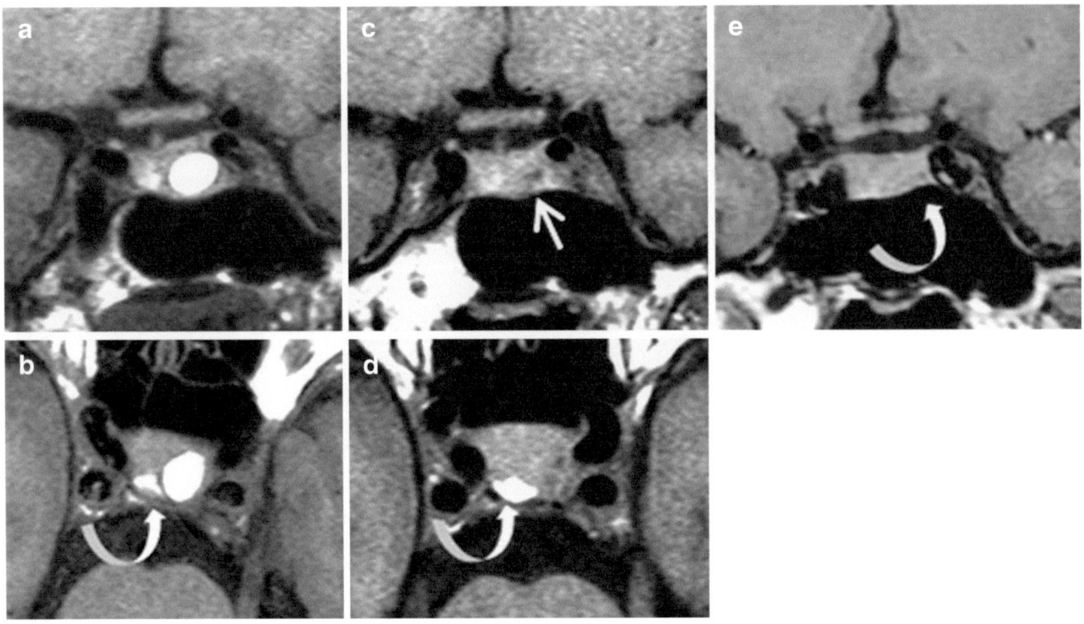

Fig. 12.1 Hemorrhagic prolactinoma. Amenorrhea/galactorrhea. Prolactin is 65 ng/ml. (**a**, **b**) Coronal and axial T1WIs: rounded T1-hyperintense left-sided mass; depression of the sellar floor, bulging of the sellar diaphragm, tilting of the infundibulum, and compression of the posterior lobe (*arrow*). (**c**, **d**) Coronal and axial T1WIs after 1 year of cabergoline treatment. Prolactin level is normal. Tiny residual T1-hypointense image (*straight arrow*) without mass effect; the posterior lobe is no longer distorted (*arrow*). (**e**) Coronal T1WI 1 year later, still on cabergoline treatment. The height of the anterior lobe is slightly decreased on the left and the microadenoma image has vanished. Note the remodeling of the sellar floor (*arrow*)

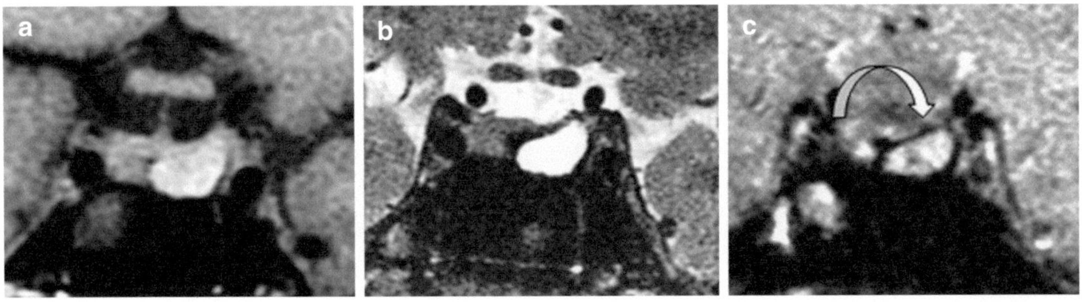

Fig. 12.2 Pituitary adenoma with old hemorrhage. (**a**–**c**) Coronal T1, coronal T2, and T2W gradient-echo sequences. The left-sided adenoma is T1 hyperintense and T2 hyperintense. Peripheral dark rim of hemosiderin in (**c**) (*arrow*)

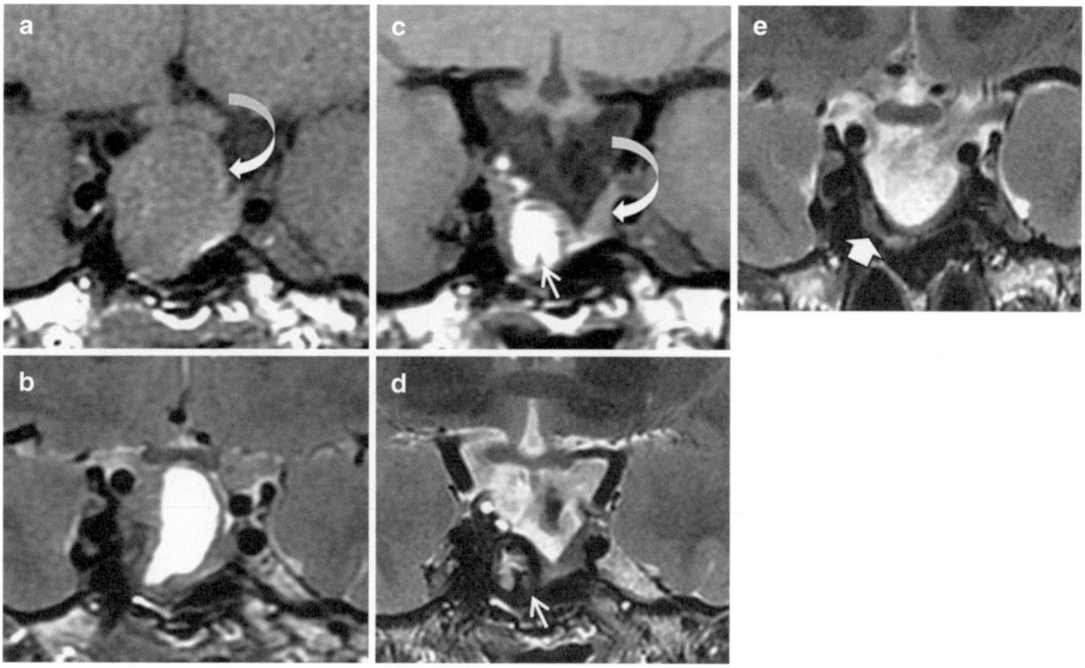

Fig. 12.3 Macroprolactinoma in a 27-year-old man. Prolactin is 1800 ng/ml. (**a**, **b**) Coronal T1 and T2 WIs at diagnosis. The lesion is slightly T1 hypointense and markedly T2 hyperintense, evoking necrotic or old hemorrhagic changes of the left part of the tumor. Normal anterior pituitary tissue (*curved arrow*). (**c**, **d**) Coronal T1 and T2 WIs 3 months later, with cabergoline 2 mg per week. Dramatic shrinkage of the tumor and asymptomatic recent hemorrhage of the right part of the adenoma (*straight arrows*). Remodeling of normal anterior pituitary tissue (*curved arrow*). (**e**) Coronal T2WI at 1 year. "Empty sella." Thin residual T2-hyperintense abnormal tissue on the right (*thick arrow*). Prolactin level is 8 ng/ml

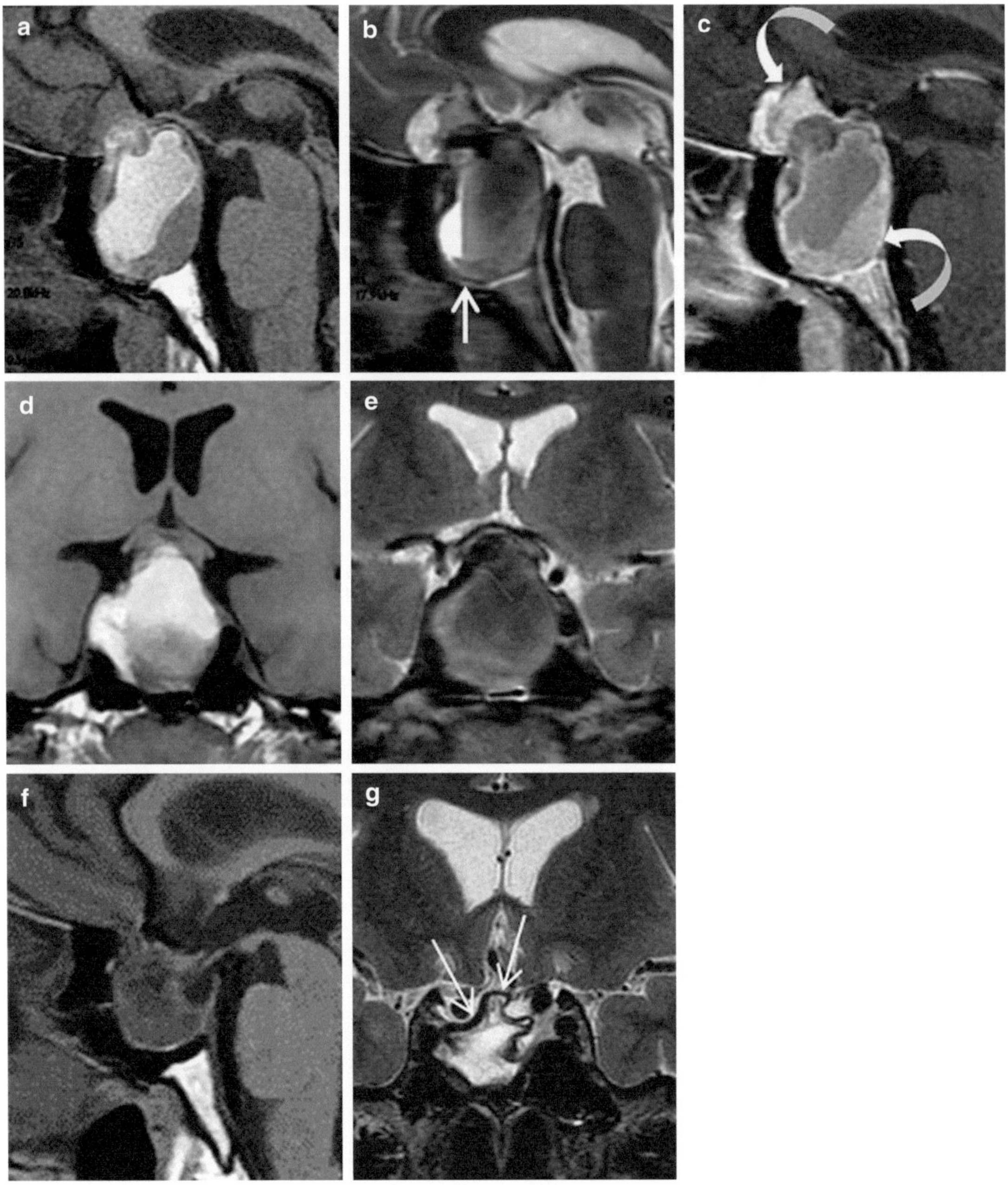

Fig. 12.4 Hemorrhagic macroprolactinoma revealed by a visual field defect in a 28-year-old woman. Prolactin is 118,000 mIU/l. (**a**–**c**) Sagittal T1, T2, and CE T1 WIs. (**d**, **e**) Coronal T1 and T2 WIs. Heterogeneous intra- and suprasellar mass threatening the optic chiasm with predominant T1 hyperintensity. Fluid-fluid level with T2 hypointensity of the infranatant in (**b**) (*straight arrow*). Enhancement of the solid part of the tumor after gadolinium injection (*curved arrows*). (**f**, **g**) Sagittal T1 and coronal T2 WIs after 8 years of irregular treatment with cabergoline. Prolactin is still 25,000 mIU/l. Dramatic shrinkage of the mass, which appears hypointense on T1WI and hyperintense on T2WI. Peripheral T2-hypointense rim corresponding to the margins of the residual adenoma impregnated with hemosiderin (*thin arrows*)

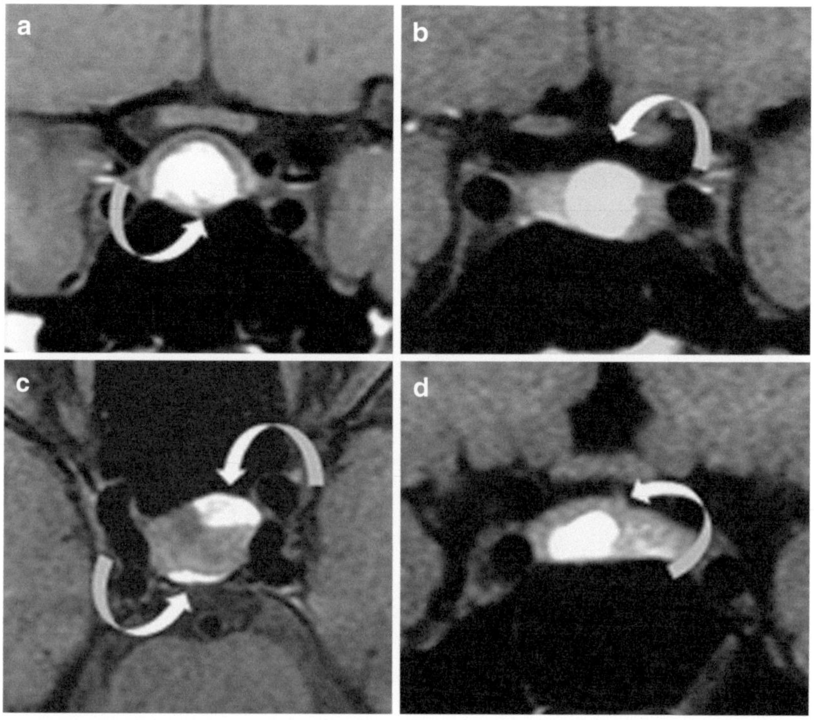

Fig. 12.5 Hemorrhagic pituitary adenomas demonstrating mass effect. (**a**, **b**) On the sellar floor and sellar diaphragm on coronal T1WIs. (**c**) On the anterior wall of the sella and the posterior lobe on axial T1WI. (**d**) On the pituitary stalk on coronal T1WI

Further Reading

Kinoshita Y, Tominaga A et al (2014a) Pituitary adenomas in childhood and adolescence with a focus on intratumoral hemorrhage. Pituitary 17(1):1–6

Kinoshita Y, Tominaga A, Usui S et al (2014b) Impact of subclinical hemorrhage on the pituitary gland in patients with pituitary adenomas. Clin Endocrinol (Oxf) 80(5):720–725

Sarwar KN, Huda MS, Van de Velde V et al (2013) The prevalence and natural history of pituitary hemorrhage in prolactinoma. Clin Endocrinol Metab 98(6):2362–2367

13 Pituitary Apoplexy

Jean-François Bonneville and Fabrice Bonneville

Pituitary apoplexy is a relatively frequent serious complication of pituitary adenoma, most of the time nonsecreting, and usually reveals the tumor. Pituitary apoplexy is sometimes mistaken for a pituitary hemorrhage, which is a much less severe condition or is even asymptomatic, and whose MRI features are different: for instance, demonstration of a fluid-fluid level at the early stage of the disease rules out the diagnosis of pituitary apoplexy.

It is striking that most pituitary apoplexies complicate pituitary macroadenomas with a suprasellar extension threatening the optic chiasm, but rarely giant adenomas, as if hemorrhagic infarction preferentially occurs when the responsible pituitary adenoma is still contained by the sellar diaphragm (Fig. 13.1). Pituitary apoplexy can be spontaneous or can follow trauma, surgery, pregnancy, anticoagulation, or estrogen therapy. A multitude of rare precipitating events has been reported, such as a case of pituitary apoplexy following sphenoid mucocele rupture (Fig. 39.5).

Pituitary apoplexy is an emergency. Symptoms (sudden onset of headache, frequently oculomotor nerve palsy, or decreased visual acuity and asthenia) can simulate subarachnoid hemorrhage, meningitis, or stroke. Diagnosis must be made as soon as possible to initiate treatment, i.e., surgical decompression in cases of severe visual symptoms or, more usually, endocrine replacement therapy.

Radiological diagnosis may be difficult in the early stage, the classical predominant hyperintensity on T1WI being frequently absent, either because infarction or because hemorrhage is still in the form of deoxyhemoglobin (Figs. 13.2 and 13.3). A "brushed" specific pattern (Figs. 13.2 and 13.6) of alternating subtle T1-hyperintense and -hypointense areas within the sellar mass may suggest apoplexy before the more characteristic T1-hyperintense signal of blood becomes visible. T2WI is more sensitive by demonstrating heterogeneous low signal intensity.

DWI can show an increased signal intensity in comparison with the normal gray and white matter and a low apparent diffusion coefficient, consistent with restricted diffusion (Fig. 13.4). This sequence has great value in the rare cases of ischemic pituitary necrosis without hemorrhage.

Reactional thickening of the sphenoidal sinus mucosa constitutes an excellent sign that is present from the early stage (Figs. 13.2, 13.4, 13.5, and 13.6). This thickening corresponds to a swelling of the subepithelial layer of the sphenoid sinus mucosa; it does not indicate infectious sinusitis and thus does not rule out the choice of the transsphenoidal route if surgery is scheduled.

Sequential MRI will demonstrate a gradual increase in the T1-hyperintense signal, from the periphery toward the center of the mass, corresponding to the transformation of deoxyhemoglobin to methemoglobin. In parallel, T2WIs demonstrate irregular hypointense areas in the more central part of the mass. T2*W gradient-echo MRI can be helpful in detecting pituitary hemorrhage as a "dark mass."

J.-F. Bonneville et al., *MRI of the Pituitary Gland*, DOI 10.1007/978-3-319-29043-0_13

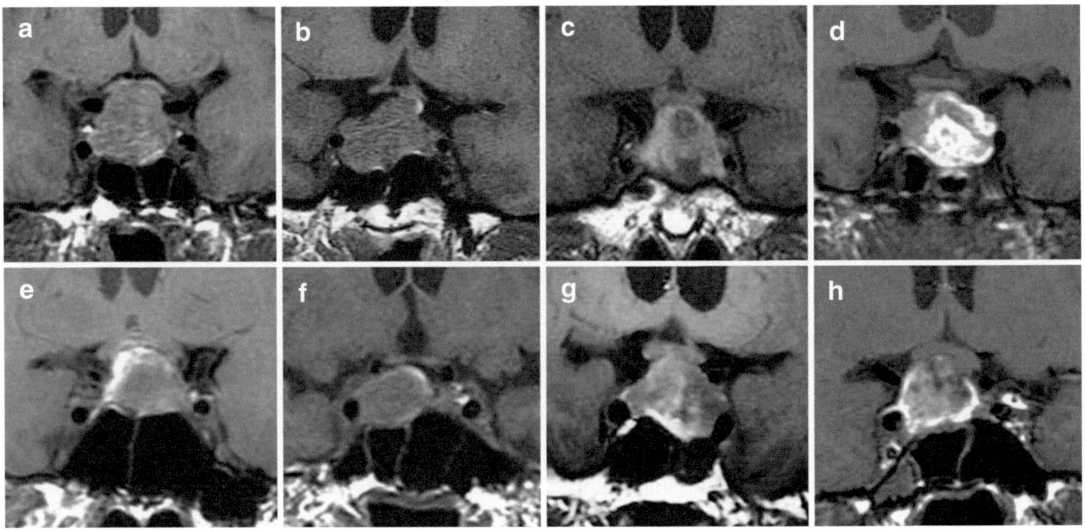

Fig. 13.1 A series of pituitary apoplexies. (**a–h**) Coronal T1WIs. Note the very similar size of the responsible macroadenomas just abutting the optic chiasm. There were no giant adenomas in this series

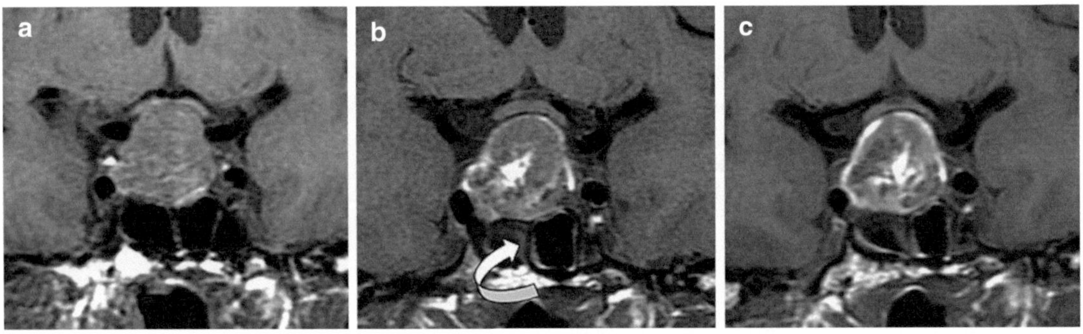

Fig. 13.2 Serial T1WIs of a patient with pituitary apoplexy. (**a**) 12 h after the onset of symptoms (sudden headache, fatigue, and right third oculomotor nerve palsy). Pituitary mass abutting the optic chiasm and yielding a heterogeneous signal with linear alternating areas of T1 hyper- and hypointensities, showing a general striated or "brushed" pattern. (**b**) At 24 h: peripheral and central areas of spontaneous T1-hyperintense signal. Thickening of the sphenoid sinus mucosa (*arrow*). (**c**) At 36 h: increased hyperintense areas and further thickening of the sphenoid sinus mucosa

After gadolinium injection peripheral enhancement is noted, with no or minimal enhancement of the necrosed central part of the mass (Fig. 13.6).

Pituitary apoplexy more rarely can be purely ischemic, theoretically without blood evidence even after a few days (Fig. 13.7), although secondary hemorrhagic transformation may occur.

A retroclival infiltrate (Figs. 13.6 and 13.8) associated with pituitary apoplexy has been recently described and interpreted as a hematoma. However, enhancement of retroclival mass thickening after gadolinium administration may be observed, and raises the question of its exact nature; the hypothesis of engorgement of the basilar venous sinus and retroclival dura has also to be evoked. Acute hemorrhage beyond the sellar region has also been described in the subarachnoid spaces and even in the ventricular system. Ischemic stroke may also occur following pituitary apoplexy. Two mechanisms have been described: early stroke by direct compression of the internal carotid artery (Fig. 13.9), or

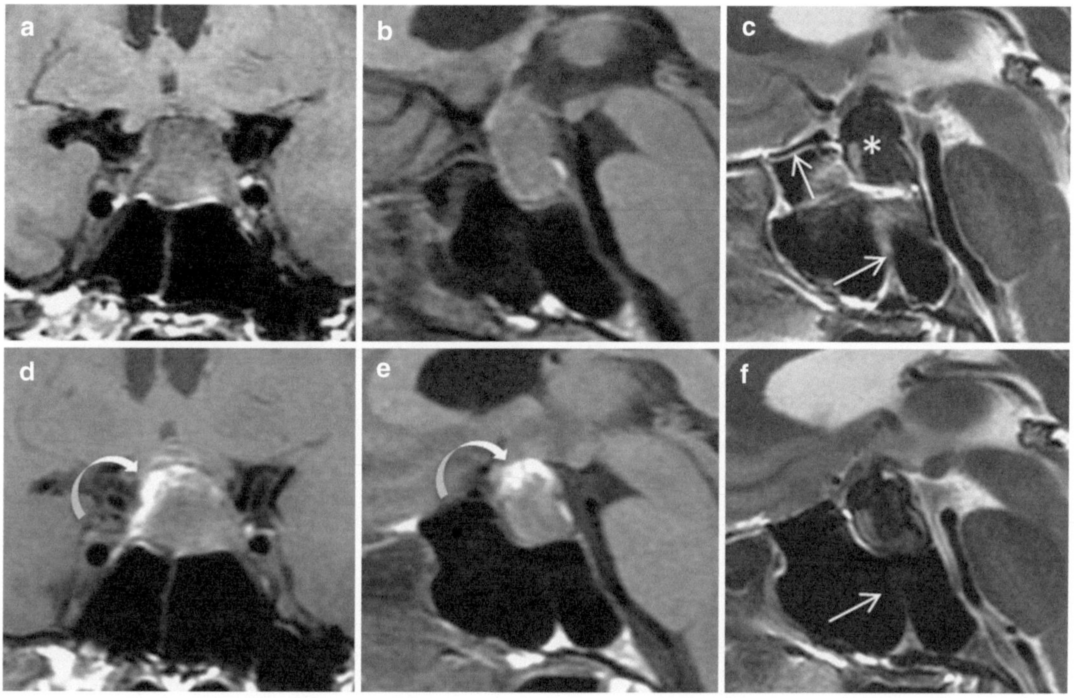

Fig. 13.3 Pituitary apoplexy in a patient presenting with sudden onset of an isolated headache. MRI at day 1. (**a**, **b**) Coronal and sagittal TIWIs; (**c**) sagittal T2WI. Intra-suprasellar tumor without evidence of hemorrhage on T1WI; on T2WI, marked hypointense mass (*asterisk*) and thickening of the sphenoid sinus mucosa (*arrows*). (**d–f**) Same sequences at day 4. Faint peripheral T1 hyperintensity signaling the presence of methemoglobin (*curved arrows*). Thickening of the sphenoid sinus mucosa has vanished

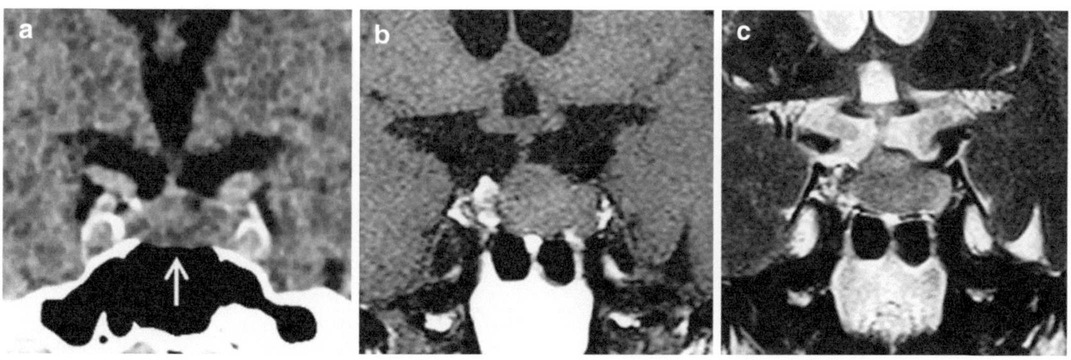

Fig. 13.4 Apoplexy, ischemic form, in a 73-year-old man presenting with sudden onset of severe headache and nausea. (**a**) Coronal CT scan. Discrete hypodensity of a pituitary mass and thinning of the sellar floor (*arrow*). (**b–d**) T1, T2, and CE T1 WIs. The mass is T1 isointense and T2 hyperintense; there is rim enhancement after contrast, but the central part of the mass does not enhance (*asterisk*). (**e**) Axial DWI shows marked hyperintensity of the lesion (*curved arrow*), thus confirming the ischemic origin of the apoplexy (Courtesy of Ch. Magnin, MD)

Fig. 13.4 (continued)

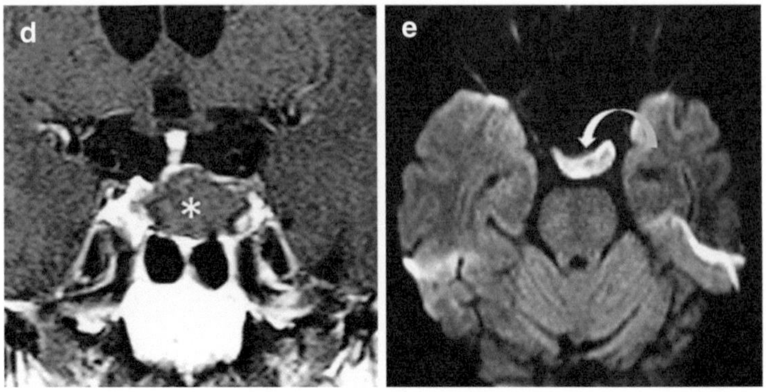

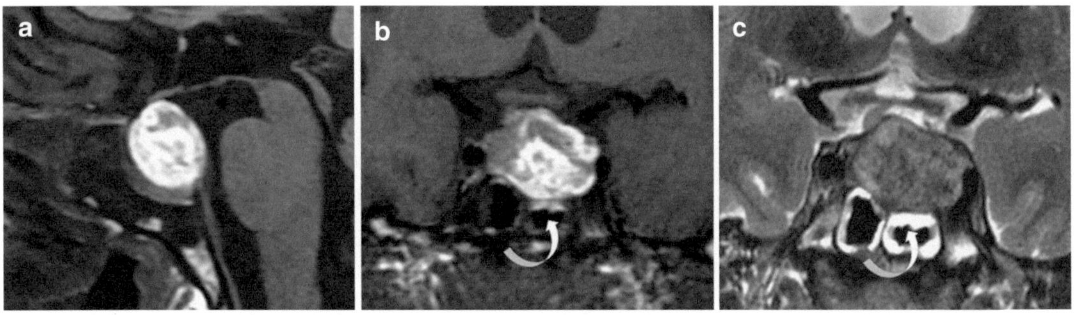

Fig. 13.5 Pituitary apoplexy seen at 1 week. (**a**, **b**) Sagittal and coronal noncontrast T1WIs. (**c**) Coronal T2WI. Frank T1 hyperintense heterogeneous signal in (**a**) and faint hypointensities on T2. Thickened sphenoid sinus mucosa (*curved arrows*)

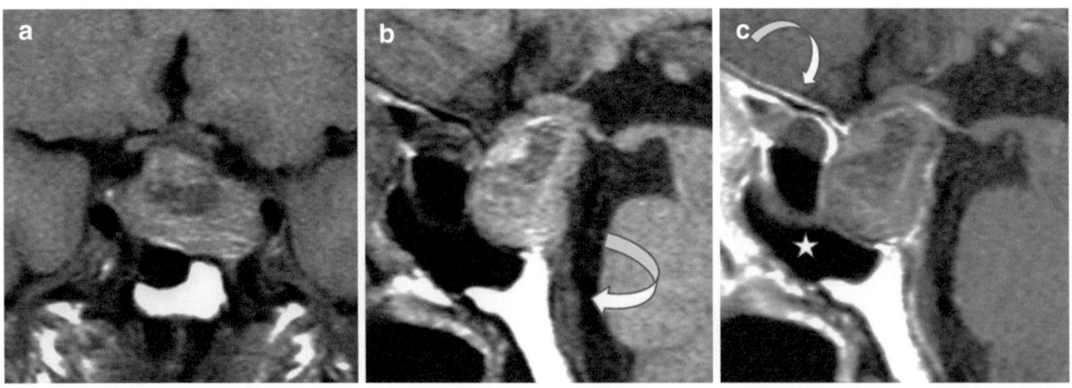

Fig. 13.6 Pituitary apoplexy at 2 days. (**a**) Coronal T1WI. (**b**, **c**) Sagittal T1 and CE T1 WIs. Characteristic "brushed" pattern of a lesion abutting the optic chiasm. Retroclival hematoma (*large arrow*). Thickened sphenoid sinus mucosa (*asterisk*). Intense enhancement of the pre-sellar dura (*small curved arrow*)

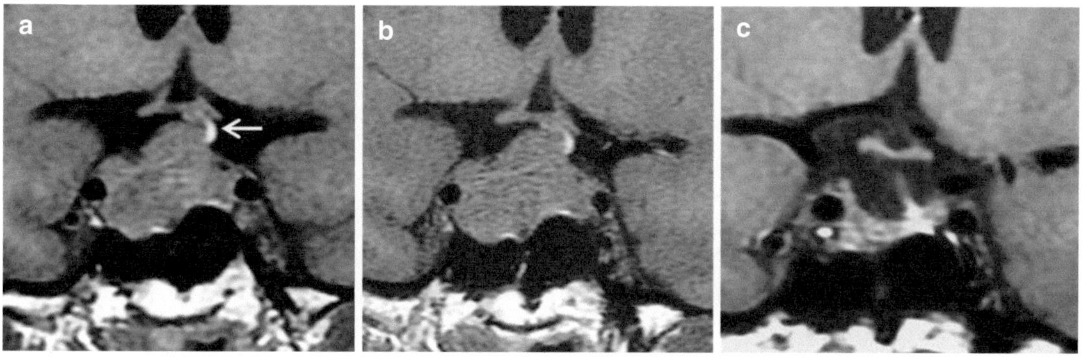

Fig. 13.7 Pituitary apoplexy, ischemic form. Coronal T1WI. (**a**) At admission, typical "striated-brushed" pattern of the mass. Ectopic antidiuretic hormone storage at the dome of the lesion (*arrow*). (**b**) Three days later, no change and no evidence of hemorrhage: apoplexy-infarction? (**c**) Spontaneous shrinkage of the mass 2 months later

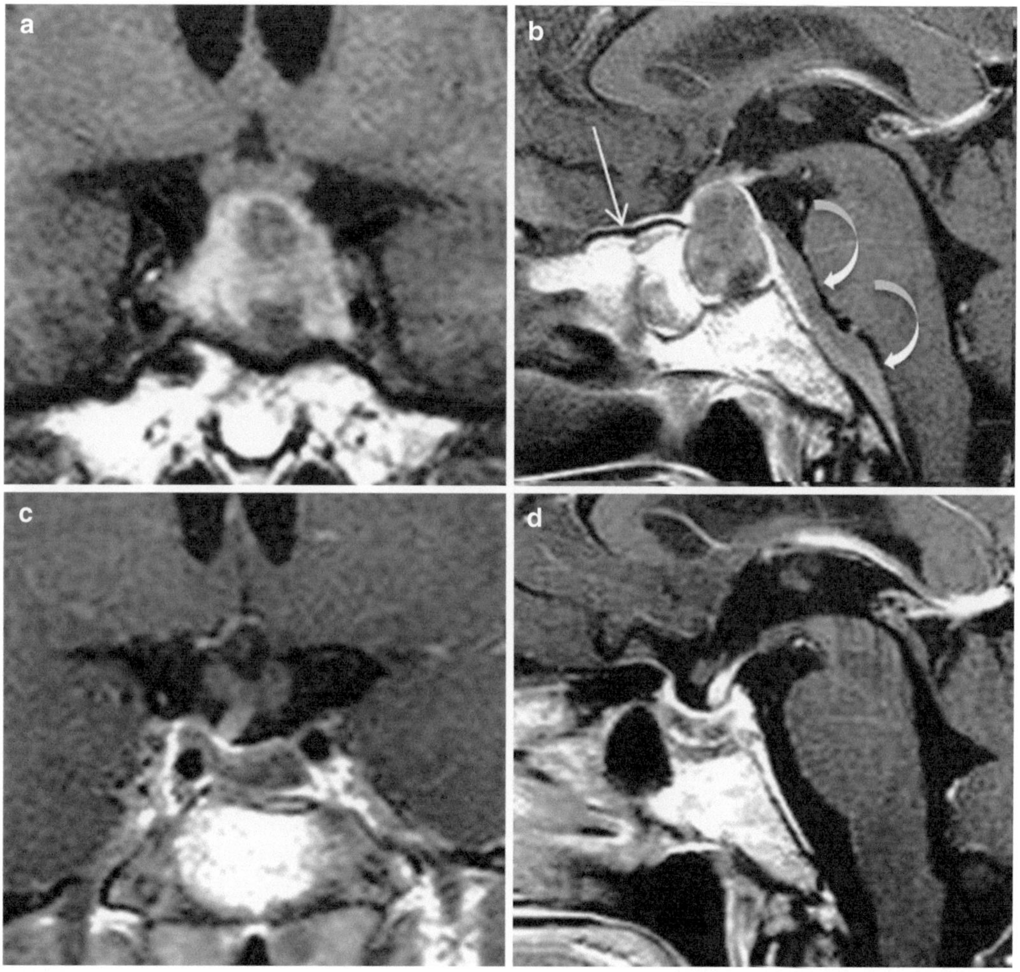

Fig. 13.8 Retroclival hematoma in pituitary apoplexy. (**a**, **b**) Coronal T1 and sagittal CE T1 WIs 5 days after the onset of symptoms. Spontaneous T1-hyperintense heterogeneous mass abutting the optic chiasm. After gadolinium injection thick retroclival hematoma (*curved arrows*) and thickened presellar dura (*straight arrow*) are apparent, but the pituitary mass itself is not enhancing. (**c**, **d**) Coronal and sagittal CE T1WIs at 6 months. Spontaneous shrinkage with hardly any enhancement of the sellar content. Disappearance of the retroclival hematoma and of the enhancement of the dura

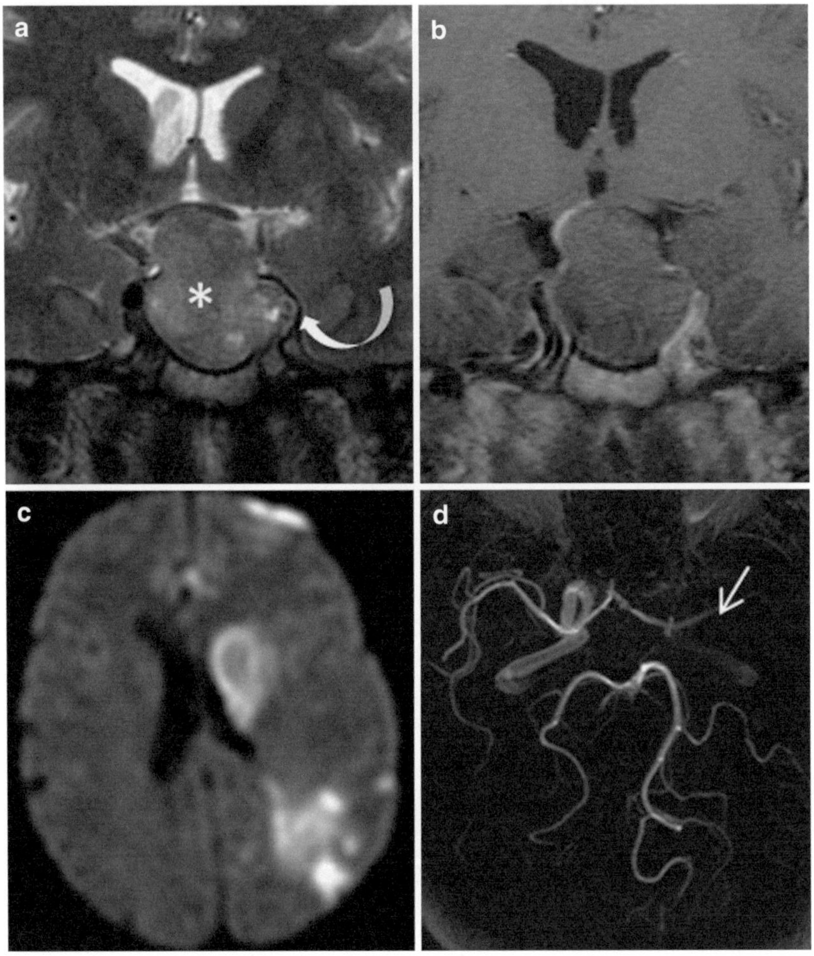

Fig. 13.9 62-year-old man with pituitary apoplexy and right hemiplegia caused by stroke. Coronal (**a**) T2WI and (**b**) CE T1WI show in a clinical setting of acute apoplexy a large intra-suprasellar nonenhancing necrosed adenoma (*asterisk*) compressing the left intracavernous internal carotid artery (*curved arrow*). (**c**) DWI demonstrates multiple foci of hyperintensity scattered in the left cerebral hemisphere, evocative of acute stroke, owing to low flow in the left middle cerebral artery (*arrow*), as demonstrated by (**d**) MRA

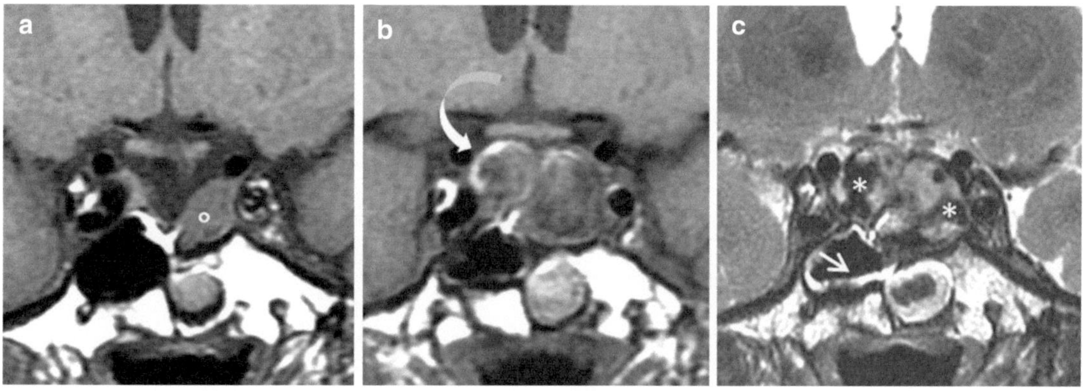

Fig. 13.10 Posttraumatic apoplexy of a nonsecreting pituitary adenoma remnant in a 68-year-old woman operated on twice, 30 and 20 years ago. (**a**) Coronal noncontrast T1WI. Left pituitary adenoma remnant (*circle*) 2 years after last surgery. No follow-up. 18 years after last MRI control, severe high-velocity head trauma with occurrence of headache and left abducens nerve palsy. (**b**, **c**) Coronal T1 and T2 WIs. Characteristic picture of pituitary apoplexy at the early phase with limited peripheral T1 hyperintensity (*curved arrow*) and more diffuse areas of T2 hypointensities (*asterisks*). Typical thickening of the sphenoid sinus mucosa (*small arrow*)

delayed stroke attributable to vasospasm subsequent to subarachnoid hemorrhage. Therefore, an overview of intracranial arteries may be advisable in cases of pituitary apoplexy.

If surgery is postponed or not indicated, shrinkage of the mass occurs in some weeks or months (Figs. 13.7 and 13.8). Regrowth of pituitary adenoma may occur at some distance from the apoplexy episode. Apoplexy of a pituitary remnant can be observed as late as 15 years after surgery (Fig. 13.10). Lastly, complications of pituitary apoplexy can be observed, such as subarachnoid or intraventricular hemorrhage and stroke resulting from internal carotid artery compression.

Further Reading

Bi WL, Dunn IF, Laws ER Jr (2015) Pituitary apoplexy. Endocrine 48(1):69–75

Briet C, Salenave S, Chanson P (2015) Pituitary apoplexy. Endocrinol Metab Clin North Am 44(1):199–209

Capatina C, Inder W, Karavitaki N et al (2015) Management of endocrine disease: pituitary tumour apoplexy. Eur J Endocrinol 172(5):R179–R190

14 Acromegaly

Iulia Potorac and Jean-François Bonneville

One of the most evocative clinical presentations is that of acromegaly. The facial coarsening with frontal skull bossing, enlargement of nose, lips, and tongue, mandibular prognathism, and acral enlargement are the main features that support the diagnosis. Moreover, acromegalic patients also describe paresthesias, headaches, hyperhidrosis, and menstrual or sexual function complaints. There is deepening of the voice resulting from modifications of the vocal cords and hyperpneumatization of sinuses, all of which are consequences of the excessive GH secretion. Untreated, acromegaly leads to increased mortality and impaired quality of life. Acromegalic patients are prone to cardiovascular complications, arterial hypertension, type 2 diabetes mellitus, colon polyps, and thyroid nodules. They also often develop sleep apnea syndrome and arthropathies.

Biologically, the diagnosis of acromegaly is established when IGF1 levels are higher than the normal sex- and age-adjusted ranges and when GH secretion during an OGTT (oral glucose tolerance test) fails to suppress. Control of the disease is considered to be attained when IGF1 is normalized and random GH measurement is inferior to 1 ng/ml.

The incidence of acromegaly is of approximately four to five cases per million individuals per year. Usually, men are diagnosed at younger ages and their IGF1 levels are generally higher in comparison with female patients. In the large majority of cases, acromegaly is caused by a GH-secreting pituitary adenoma. In two-thirds of cases these are macroadenomas, but giant lesions (>4 cm) are rare. However, thanks to the recent advances of the MRI technique and especially of 3.0-T scanners and high-resolution images obtained in T2W sequences, microadenomas are now more frequently diagnosed than previously, when small lesions could have passed unnoticed.

Furthermore, microadenomas associated with an empty sella or necrotic adenomas are not infrequently encountered (Fig. 14.1). Moreover, enlarged intracavernous internal carotid arteries can press on the pituitary gland, thus possibly masking a pituitary microadenoma (Figs. 14.2 and 14.3). The presence of such vascular anomalies prompts the preoperative realization of an angio-MRI, which will in some cases detect associated arterial aneurysms (Fig. 59.1).

There seems to be a negative correlation between adenoma size and patient age. Larger adenomas are usually diagnosed in younger patients and are responsible for higher levels of GH secretion, whereas older patients are often diagnosed with smaller adenomas that respond well to medical treatment. This age–size correlation is also supported by the observations of the recently discovered syndrome termed X-linked acro-gigantism. This is an early-onset form of gigantism with growth acceleration occurring as early as the first year of life, caused by an important GH hypersecretion. MRI finds either diffuse hyperplasia or large macroadenomas, often with an important suprasellar extension at diagnosis (Fig. 14.4).

J.-F. Bonneville et al., *MRI of the Pituitary Gland*, DOI 10.1007/978-3-319-29043-0_14

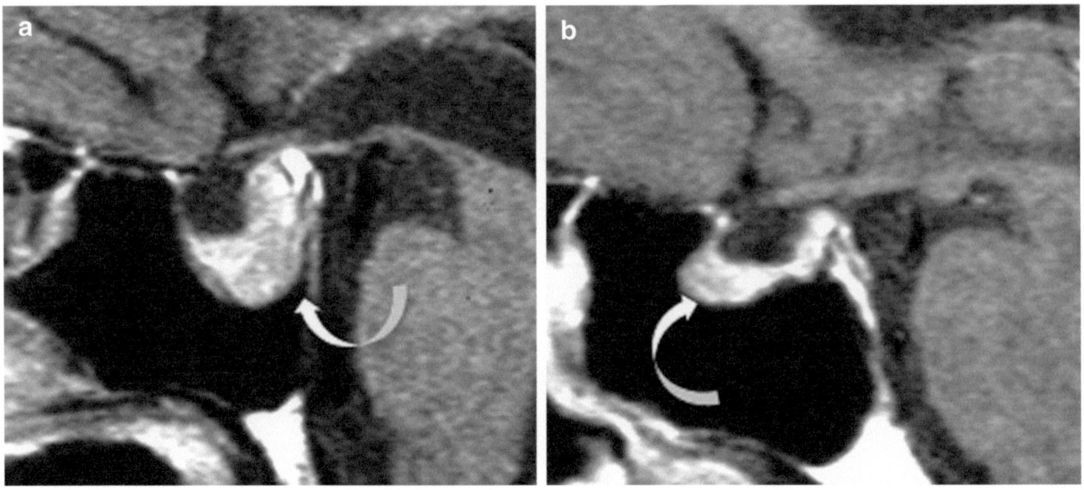

Fig. 14.1 GH-secreting pituitary adenoma and partial empty sella in elderly. (**a**, **b**) CE T1WIs. Microadenomas (*arrows*)

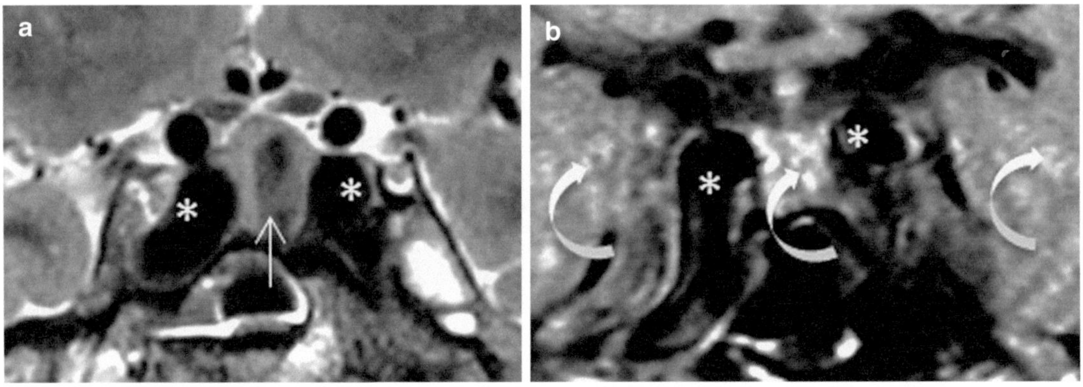

Fig. 14.2 GH-secreting pituitary adenomas and ectasic internal carotid arteries in two acromegalic patients. (**a**) Coronal T2WI. (**b**) Coronal T1WI. Enlarged internal carotid arteries (*asterisks*) narrow the frontal diameter of the sellar content, increase flow artifacts (*curved arrows*), and may mask a pituitary microadenoma. In (**a**) the intrasellar adenoma (*arrow*) is T2 hypointense

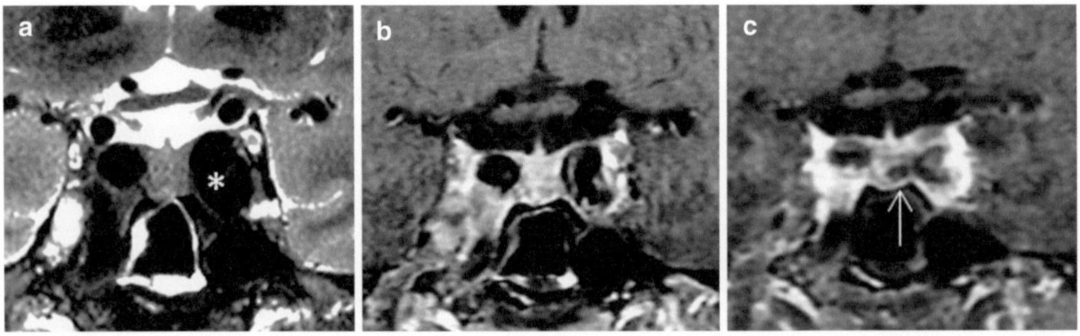

Fig. 14.3 Acromegaly in a 52-year-old man (**a**, **b**) Coronal T2 and CET1WIs. IGF1 is 2× upper limit of normal (ULN). Dolichoectasic internal carotid arteries (*asterisk*) and narrow sella. The GH-secreting microadenoma is only demonstrated on dynamic MRI (**c**) (*arrow*)

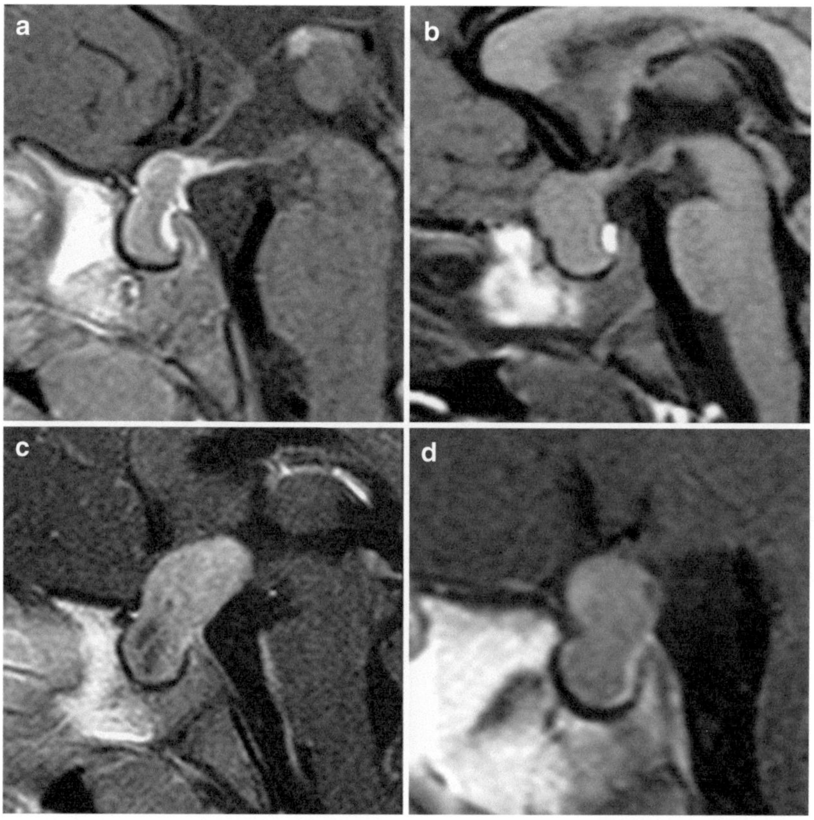

Fig. 14.4 GH-secreting pituitary adenomas with suprasellar extension in four children younger than 3 years with X-linked acro-gigantism. (**a**, **c**, **d**) Sagittal CE T1WIs. (**b**) Sagittal T1WI. Note that the sphenoid sinus is not yet aerated, thus potentially explaining the upward extension of these adenomas (Courtesy of A. Daly, MD)

Curiously, GH-secreting adenomas have a tendency to expand toward the sphenoid sinus and more rarely cranially, toward the optic chiasm (Fig. 14.5). They can even have an isolated inferior extension (cranially, the adenoma does not surpass the sellar diaphragm) in nearly one-quarter of cases (Fig. 14.6). Because of this particular pattern of extension, optic chiasm compression symptoms rarely manifest at presentation in acromegaly, and this is possibly one of the reasons why the disease evolution is so long before diagnosis. There are several theories attempting to explain this pattern of extension, although the reason that seems most likely is the GH-induced hyperpneumatization of the sphenoid sinus with bone apposition on the outer surface and internal resorption, rendering the sellar outline frail.

GH-secreting adenomas have a particular feature in terms of T2W signal intensity. In more than 50 % of cases, they are T2 hypointense when compared with the signal of the normal pituitary gland or that of the gray matter. These T2-hypointense adenomas are usually smaller, less invasive into the cavernous sinus, and more rarely compressive of the optic chiasm than T2-hyper- or isointense GH-secreting adenomas (Fig. 14.7). The T2-hypointense adenomas are also associated to higher IGF1 levels, a testament to their higher GH-secretory potential. Invasion of the cavernous sinus is an important predictive factor for surgical cure. Very subtle invasions can be present, and their detection prior to surgery is important as this will influence the chances of surgical cure. One key for the diagnosis of limited intracavernous sinus invasion is to obtain

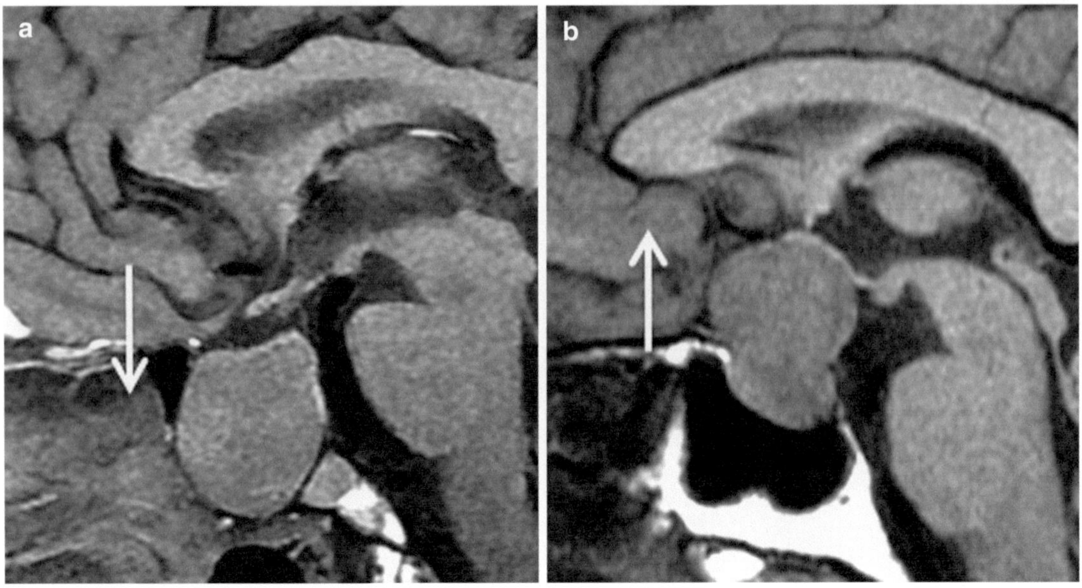

Fig. 14.5 GH-secreting pituitary macroadenoma. (**a**, **b**) Sagittal T1WIs. Most GH-secreting pituitary adenomas (as in **a**) have a tendency to extend downward while most nonsecreting adenomas (as in **b**) extend upward and frequently threaten the optic chiasm

high-resolution coronal and axial T2WIs (Fig. 14.8). These images could capture the torn aspect or the absence of the thin dural medial wall of the cavernous sinus (see Chap. 11).

The gold standard in the treatment of GH-secreting pituitary adenomas is transsphenoidal surgery. Unfortunately, surgical results depend on several factors (among which adenoma features, cavernous sinus invasion, and the experience of the neurosurgeon are the most important), and cure is not always obtained, especially in the case of macroadenomas. Therefore, in many cases adjunctive medical treatment is necessary. Somatostatin analogs have been used in the management of acromegaly for several decades, and have an established antisecretory and antitumoral effects whether they are administered pre- or postsurgically. The benefit of somatostatin analogs as presurgical treatment have been analyzed in multiple studies, but currently the opinions are still divided. It seems, however, that macroadenomas are more likely to benefit from a presurgical somatostatin analog treatment. The response to somatostatin analogs seems to be better in the case of T2-hypointense adenomas. After only 6 months of treatment, T2-hypointense adenomas are associated with a greater reduction of IGF1 levels and GH secretion and a more important tumor shrinkage (Fig. 14.9). In some cases, a change of signal, from T2 hypointense to T2 hyperintense, may accompany adenoma shrinkage (Fig. 14.10). A new medical treatment option is the GH-receptor antagonist, pegvisomant, which is efficient at normalizing IGF1 values but usually has no effect on tumor volume. In the rare cases where surgery and medical treatment cannot control GH hypersecretion or tumor growth, radiotherapy can be employed. With the recent advances, radiotherapy ensures tumoral control with fewer side effects than occurred previously.

Histologically, GH-secreting adenomas are separated into densely granulated and sparsely granulated. Densely granulated adenomas have been shown to have a more intense GH secretion and a better response to somatostatin analog treatment. These adenomas could correspond to the T2-hypointense ones on MRI, but so far few studies on a small number of patients have properly addressed this matter. Ongoing studies are investigating this issue to assess whether MRI would be able to predict the granulation pattern

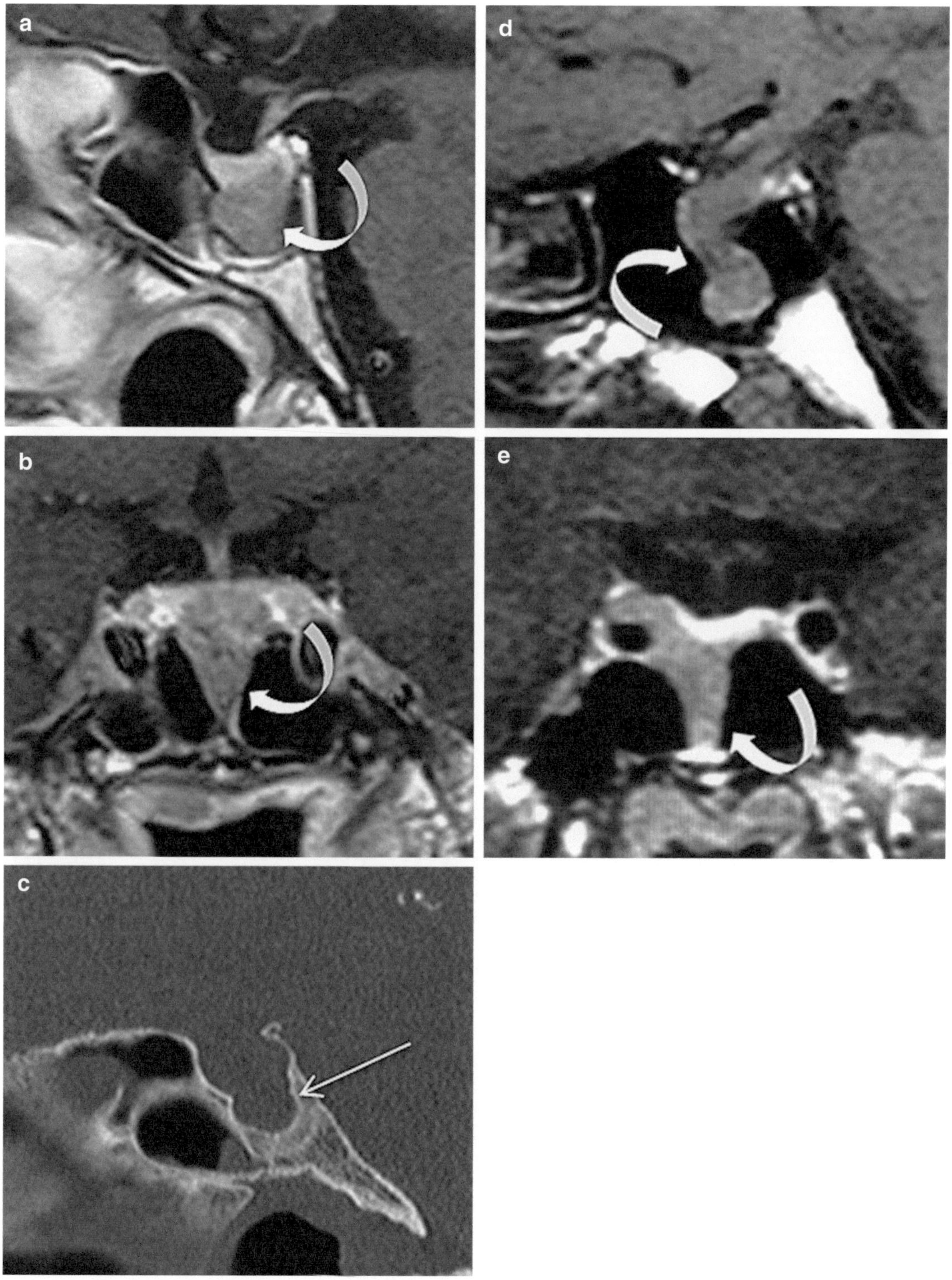

Fig. 14.6 GH-secreting pituitary adenomas with isolated inferior extension in two acromegalic patients. (**a**, **b**) Sagittal and coronal CE TIWIs. (**c**) Sagittal CT. (**d**, **e**) Sagittal T1 and CE T1 WIs. Such inferior tumoral extensions, which are rarely seen in nonacromegalic patients, seem limited by the sphenoid septa. Note the peculiar pattern of the sella turcica change in (**c**). Patient in (**a**–**c**) has an IGF1 3× UNL, and prolactin was 60 ng/ml

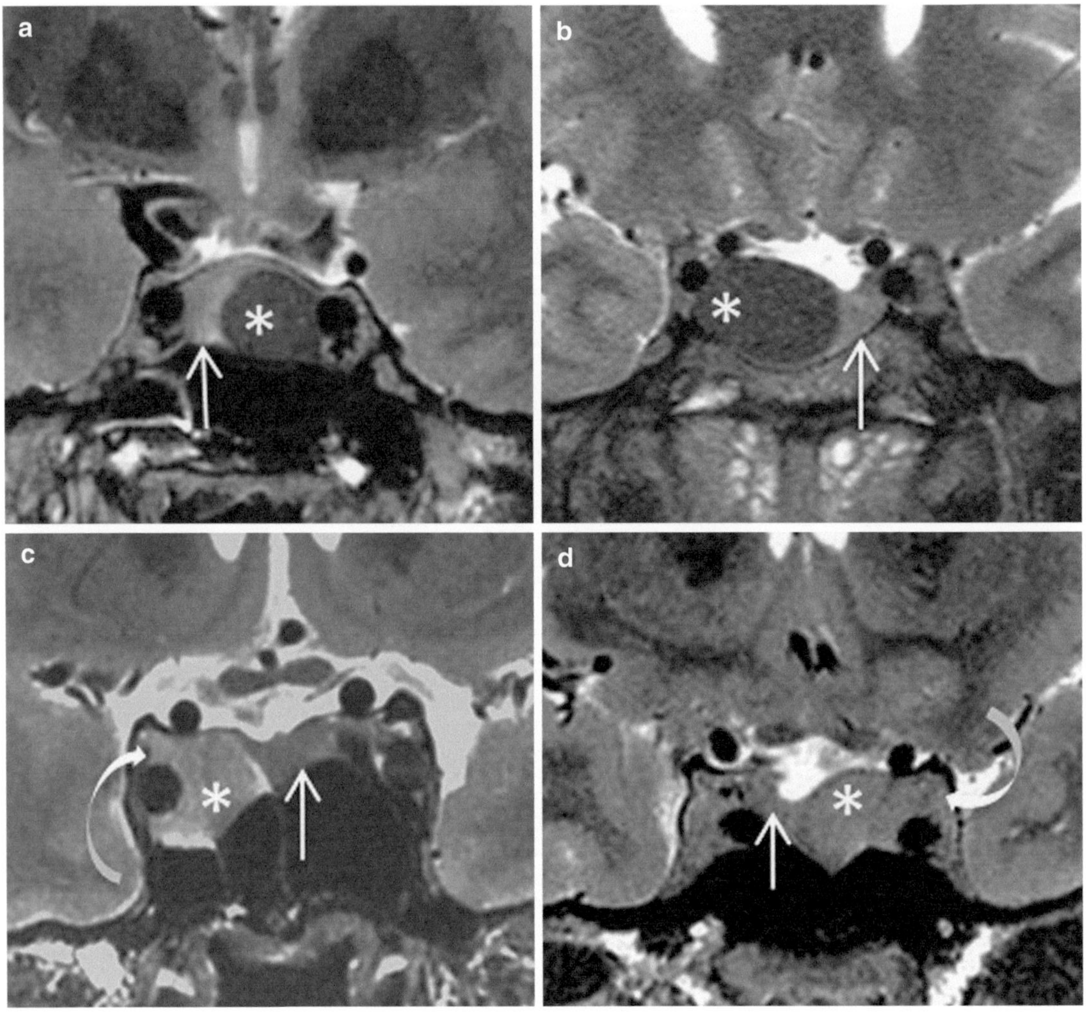

Fig. 14.7 GH-secreting pituitary adenomas. (**a**–**d**) Coronal T2WIs. If compared with the normal pituitary gland (*arrows*), the adenomas (*asterisks*) are T2 hypointense (**a**, **b**) or T2 hyperintense (**c**, **d**). Both T2-hyperintense adenomas invade the cavernous sinus (*curved arrows*)

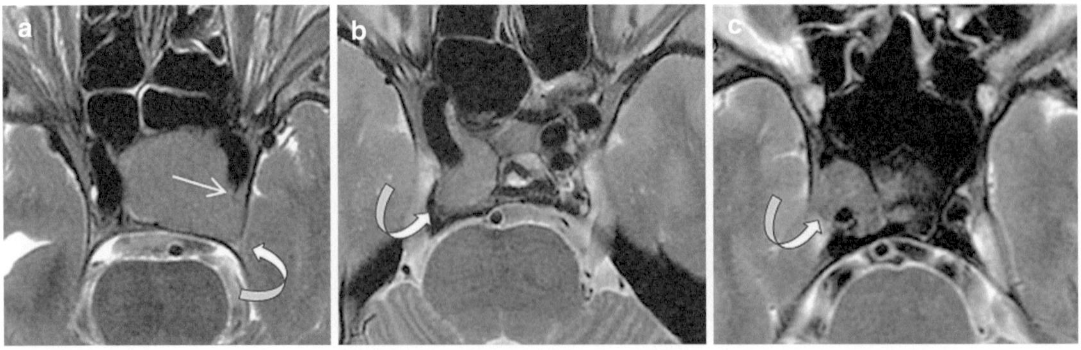

Fig. 14.8 Cavernous sinus invasion in three different patients with predominant posterior extension (*curved arrows*). (**a**–**c**) Axial T2WIs. In (**a**) there is a small residual flap of the medial wall of cavernous sinus (*straight arrow*)

of GH-secreting pituitary adenomas before surgery.

Acromegaly is usually a sporadic disease, but can also be a manifestation of a syndromic or familial disease. The McCune–Albright syndrome classically reunites the triad polyostotic fibrous dysplasia, café-au-lait skin spots, and peripheral precocious puberty. Biologically, excess GH secretion can be found in some patients, but pituitary anomalies on MRI are only present in one-third of these cases (Fig. 14.11). As a familial disease, acromegaly can manifest as part of multiple endocrine neoplasia type 1 (MEN1), Carney complex (CC), or familial isolated pituitary adenoma syndrome (FIPA). MEN1 is defined by the familial association of primary

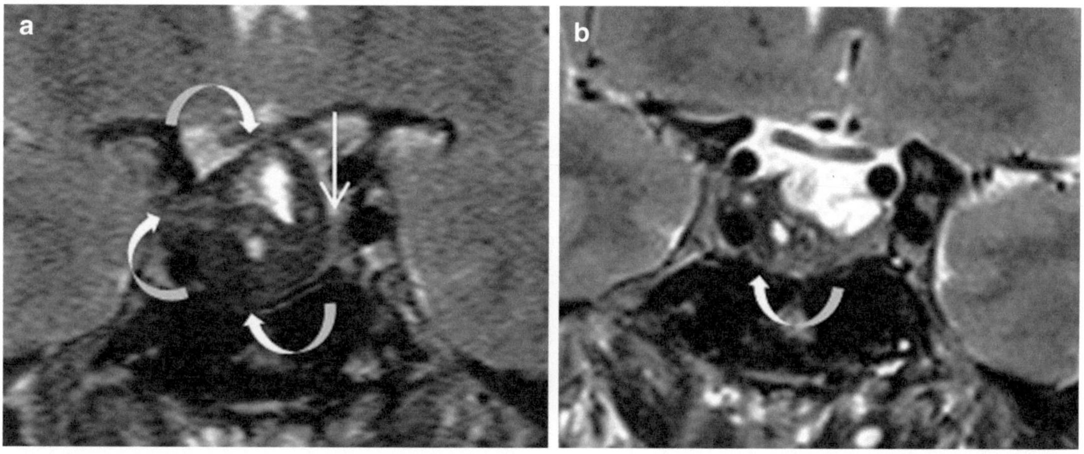

Fig. 14.9 Large GH-secreting pituitary adenoma in a 52-year-old man. IGF1 is 3.5× UNL. (**a**, **b**) Coronal T2WIs before and 6 months after somatostatin analog treatment. The adenoma is T2 hypointense with hyperintense areas of degenerative changes, and well circumscribed (*arrow*). Normal pituitary gland (*straight arrow*). Impressive adenoma shrinkage after treatment

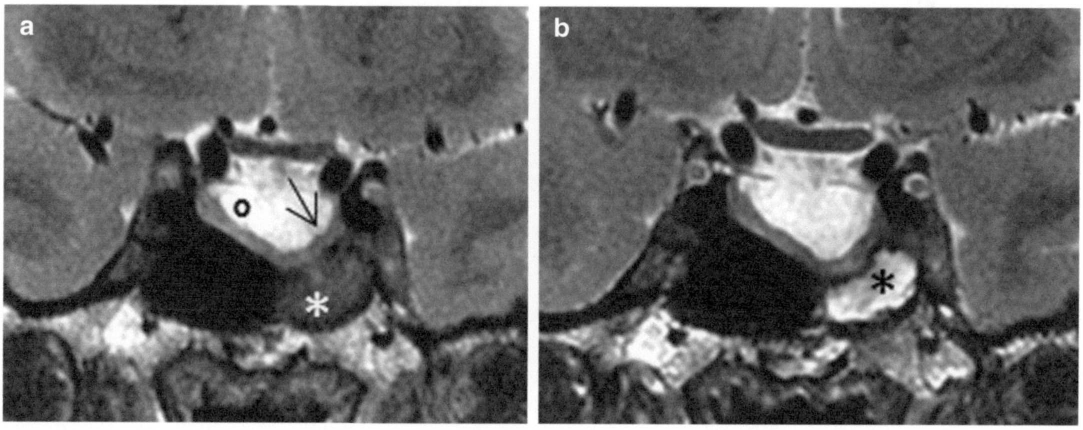

Fig. 14.10 GH-secreting pituitary adenomas before and after 6 months of treatment with somatostatin analogs. (**a**, **b**) Coronal T2WIs in a 52-year-old woman. Acromegalic symptoms for 2 years only. IGF1 is 3.5× UNL. The adenoma (*asterisk*), associated with an empty sella (*circle*), is located in the sphenoid sinus. Its T2 signal is less intense than that of the pituitary gland (*arrow*) and becomes frankly hyperintense after medical treatment (**b**). (**c**, **d**) Coronal T2WIs in a 72-year-old woman. Acromegalic symptoms for 10 years. IGF1 is 4× UNL. The pituitary adenoma (*asterisk*) has destroyed the sellar floor and is inside the sphenoid sinus. Its T2 signal is nearly identical to that of the pituitary gland (*arrow*) and turns hyperintense after treatment

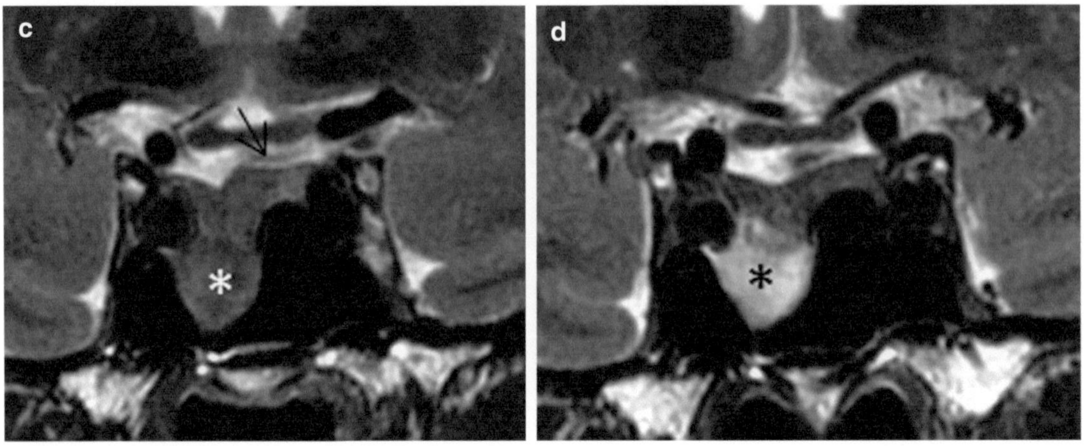

Fig. 14.10 (continued)

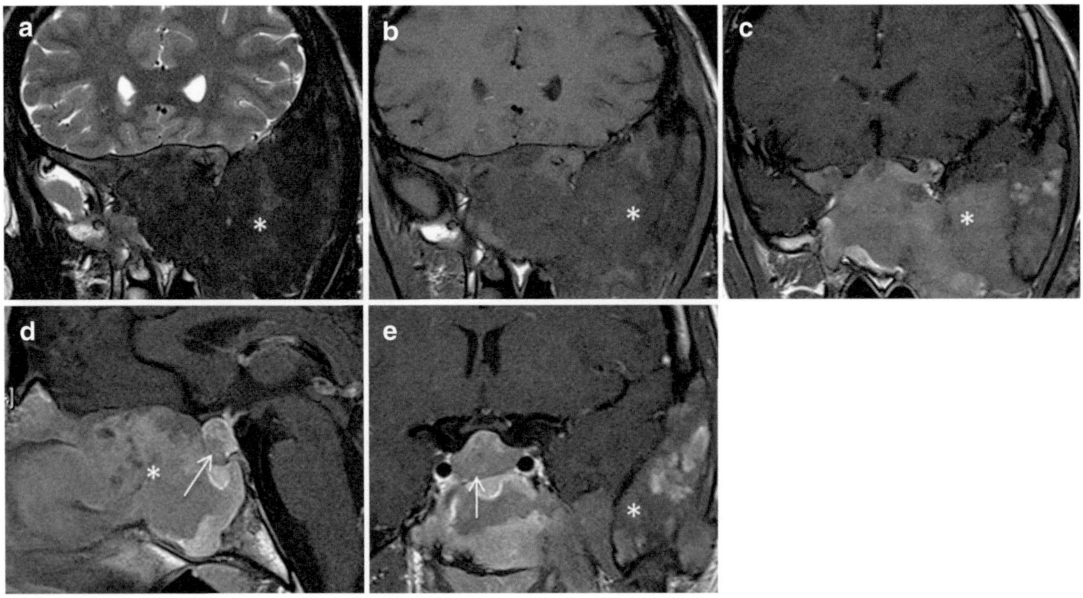

Fig. 14.11 GH-secreting pituitary adenoma and McCune–Albright syndrome (**a**-**c**) coronal T2, T1 and CET1WIs; (**d**, **e**) sagittal and coronal CET1WIs. Characteristic pattern of polyostotic fibrous dysplasia (*asterisks*) and pituitary adenoma (*arrow*) (Courtesy of G. Raverot MD, PhD)

hyperparathyroidism, pancreatic, gastrointestinal, and thoracic neuroendocrine tumors, pituitary adenomas (most frequently, prolactinomas), and adrenal adenomas. CC is a syndrome that associates endocrine anomalies (primary pigmented nodular adrenocortical disease, GH- and prolactin-secreting pituitary adenomas, thyroid and gonadal tumors) and non-endocrine manifestations (lentiginosis, blue nevi, schwannomas, cardiac, skin, and breast myxomas). FIPA was identified by Beckers as the familial occurrence of pituitary adenomas without other manifestations of the syndromic diseases known to associate with pituitary adenomas at the time, i.e., MEN1 or CC. GH-secreting adenomas are well represented in the FIPA families, especially the cases with AIP gene mutations. These AIP mutation-positive acromegalic patients have larger and more invasive pituitary adenomas that often require complex management, as disease control is obtained only with difficulty.

Further Reading

Hagiwara A, Inoue Y, Wakasa K et al (2003) Comparison of growth hormone–producing and non–growth hormone–producing pituitary adenomas: imaging characteristics and pathologic correlation. Radiology 228: 533–538

Heck A, Ringstad G, Fougner SL et al (2012) Intensity of pituitary adenoma on T2-weighted magnetic resonance imaging predicts the response to octreotide treatment in newly diagnosed acromegaly. Clin Endocrinol (Oxf) 77:72–77

Potorac I, Petrossians P, Daly AF et al (2015) Pituitary MRI characteristics in 297 acromegaly patients based on T2-weighted sequences. Endocr Relat Cancer 22(2):169–177

15 Cushing Disease

Jean-François Bonneville

Cushing disease represents a difficult challenge for the neuroradiologist involved in pituitary diseases. A definite demonstration of the frequently tiny responsible pituitary microadenoma is of major importance for defining the medical strategy.

Classic features of chronic cortisol excess include asthenia, weight gain, diabetes mellitus, hypertension, thromboembolism, proximal myopathy, osteoporosis, acne, alopecia, and purple striae. Biological diagnosis of Cushing disease is based on certification of hypercortisolism (by measurement of urine free cortisol, late night cortisol, and 1 mg dexamethasone suppression test), which is ACTH dependent. However, biochemical confirmation of the pituitary origin of the disease is uncertain in many cases.

A nonpituitary source of ACTH, such as lung neuroendocrine tumors, may be responsible, more frequently in men: this diagnosis may be evoked in patients presenting with a relatively short history of symptoms after elimination of a causative corticotropic pituitary adenoma.

The radiological patterns of corticotropic pituitary macroadenomas do not differ from those of other pituitary adenomas, although some aspects can be disturbing (Fig. 15.1). However, microadenomas represent 50 % of the whole and many are very small and yet symptomatic. Corticotropic pituitary adenomas are located centrally or laterally in the sella and have the same MRI characteristics as other pituitary adenomas, except somatotropinomas; i.e., they demonstrate a more or less T2-hyperintense signal and a T1-hypointense signal, (Fig. 15.2) but may also be isointense. There is faint or no enhancement after gadolinium injection. Dural invasion is considered frequent but not always identifiable on the most sophisticated MRI studies. Half-dose gadolinium (0.05 mmol/kg) is recommended to avoid a too strong enhancement, which could mask a picoadenoma (less than 2–3 mm). High-resolution MRI and long acquisition times are the main factors. The superiority of 3.0-T machines is without question. Optimized sequences are regularly proposed, each new one giving theoretically better results than the previous ones, but increases the risk of false-positive findings. Recently, it has been suggested that enhancement parameters in dynamic MRI can help to distinguish ACTH-producing adenomas from nonfunctioning pituitary adenomas, the time–intensity curve featuring a rapidly enhancing and slow washout pattern in the first ones. Administration of corticotropin-releasing hormone during 3-T MRI has also been proposed to improve their detection.

When Cushing disease is strongly suspected and biologically confirmed, our policy is as follows (Fig. 15.3): in a first session, high-resolution, long-acquisition time sagittal 3-mm T1, 2-mm coronal T2, 3-mm coronal T1, and 2.5-mm coronal CE T1WIs are obtained. If necessary, an axial T1W sequence is frequently added, looking for an imprint on the posterior lobe or for the presence of an incidentaloma, for example an incidental intrasellar Rathke cleft cyst. If a doubtful

J.-F. Bonneville et al., *MRI of the Pituitary Gland*, DOI 10.1007/978-3-319-29043-0_15

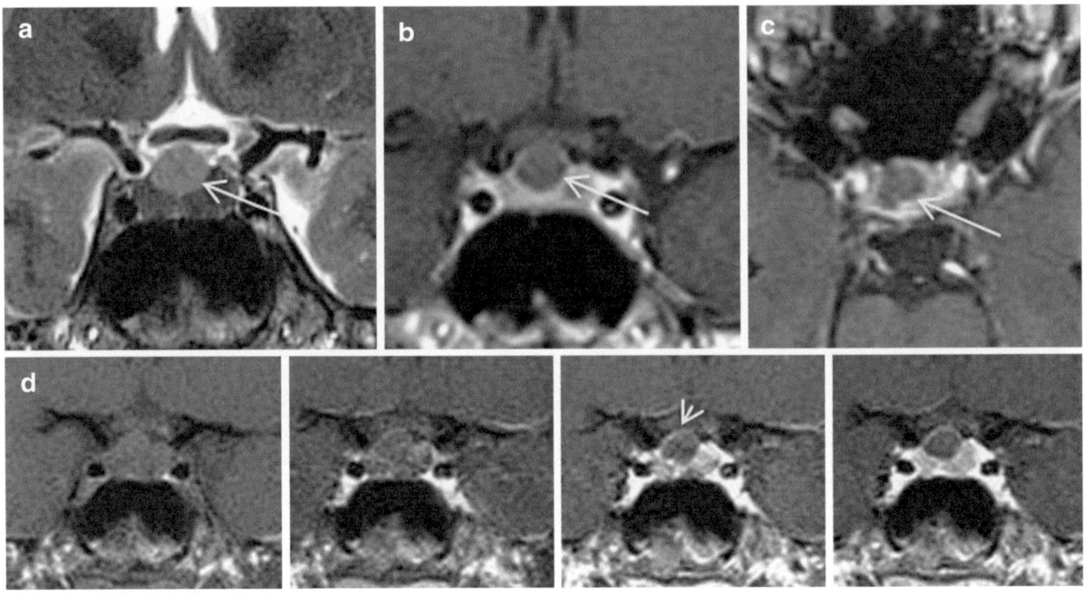

Fig. 15.1 Corticotropic adenoma mimicking a Rathke cleft cyst in a 27-year-old woman. (**a**, **b**) Coronal T2 and CE T1 WIs. T2 hyperintense, unenhanced rounded lesion very similar to a Rathke cleft cyst lying on the anterior pituitary with appearance of an egg in an egg-cup. (**c**) Axial CE T1WI. The lesion is off-midline and presents with irregular contours (*arrows*). (**d**) Dynamic imaging. Delayed enhancement of the pituitary gland. The "cyst" wall enhances with the pituitary (*short arrow*). Inferior venous sampling has confirmed the pituitary origin of ACTH hypersecretion

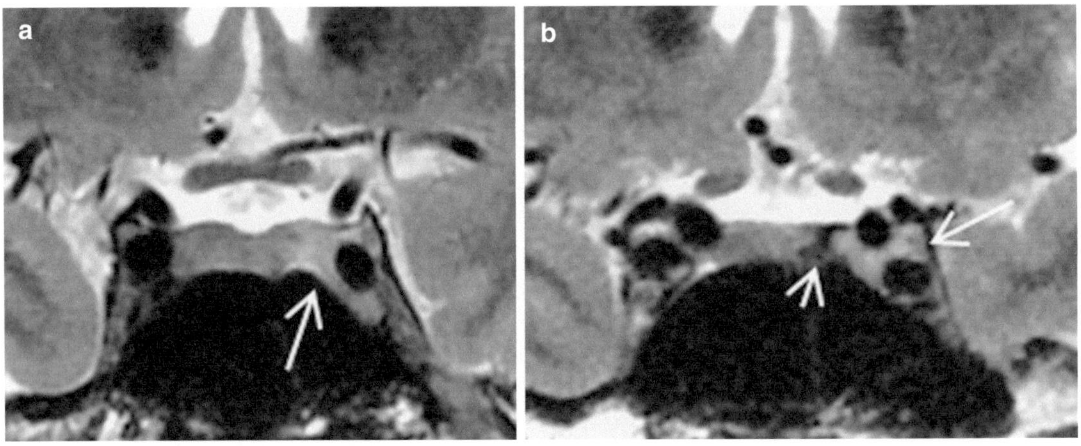

Fig. 15.2 Left-sided corticotropic microadenoma invading cavernous sinus in a 38-year-old woman. Coronal T2WIs before (**a**) and 3 months after surgery (**b**). In (**b**), a T2-hyperintense tumoral remnant (*long arrow*) encircles the intracavernous internal carotid artery; a T2-hypointense area indicates a small hemorrhagic postoperative area (*short arrow*). The patient was not cured

tiny T2-hyperintense or T1-hypointense image is shown, an additional half-dose of gadolinium is intravenously injected and a coronal T1W sequence is repeated 30 min later (Fig. 15.4). Delayed enhancement of such a suspicious area eliminates an artifact but cannot differentiate the diagnosis between pituitary microadenoma and unidentified incidentaloma.

When a pituitary microadenoma is not identified or remains questionable at this point, a

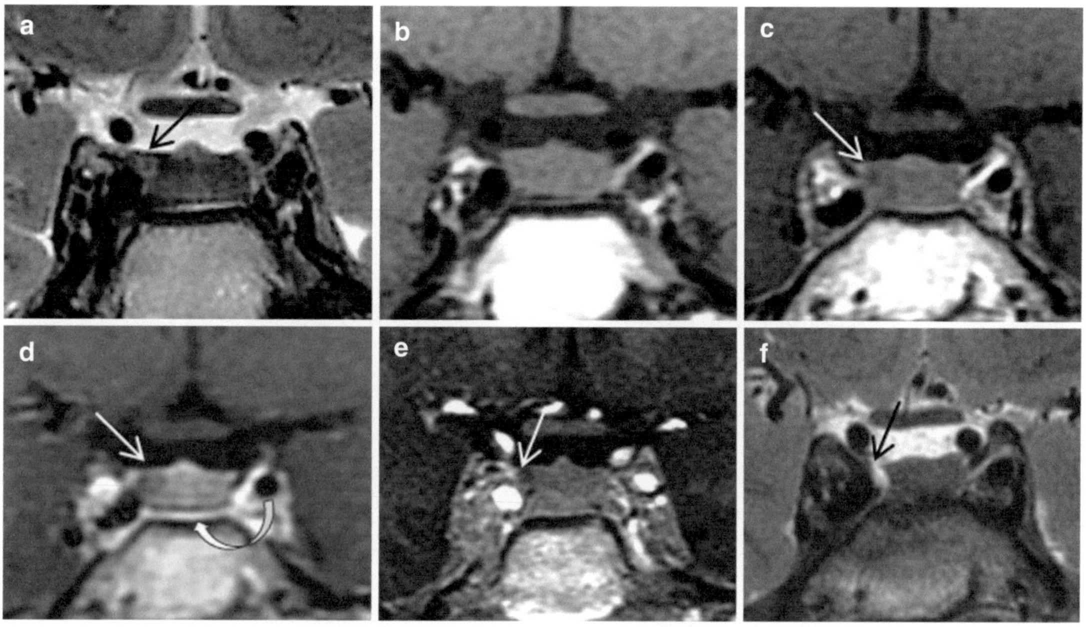

Fig. 15.3 Cushing disease in a 26-year-old woman. (**a–c**) Coronal T2, T1, and CE T1 WIs. A right-sided microadenoma is suspected in (**a**) and (**c**) (*arrows*). A second MRI session was scheduled 3 weeks later. (**d**) Dynamic MRI and (**e**) Coronal 3D fast gradient-echo CE T1WI reinforced the suspicion. Presence of an inferior coronary sinus (*curved arrow*) is considered here an anatomical variant. After selective removal of the microadenoma, the patient was totally cured. (**f**) Coronal T2WI. Defect of the anterior pituitary representing the surgical bed (*black arrow*)

second MRI session is scheduled a few weeks later and a different technical protocol is implemented. Dynamic imaging is obtained (Fig. 15.5), followed by inframillimetric gradient-echo sequences with 3D reformatting images. Interpretation of dynamic images must be very cautious and can lead to serious mistakes: it is essential to localize precisely the posterior lobe whose enhancement occurs physiologically before that of the anterior lobe. An intrasellar area of early delayed enhancement may correspond to an yet unenhanced normal anterior lobe and not to a pituitary microadenoma. Such a mistake is not infrequent in radiological reports and can lead to a false-positive diagnosis.

In a patient with an ACTH-dependent hypercortisolemia, demonstrating an "image" within the pituitary gland does not solve the issue. Artifacts, particularly partial volume artifacts (Fig. 15.6), remain a difficulty: in this instance, combined coronal and axial projections and 3D reformatting images are useful. Insidiously, an artifact can coexist with a microadenoma. The number of detected incidentalomas increases with MRI resolution, thus with 3-T MR scans; those located on midline can be quite easily diagnosed as Rathke cleft cysts, their signal being mostly T1 hyperintense; their specific location just in front of the posterior lobe is better appreciated on axial T1W fat-saturated images. Intrasellar lesions located off-midline can correspond to a corticotropic microadenoma, a nonfunctioning microadenoma, or an unidentified incidentaloma. Nevertheless, if a rigorous imaging protocol is undertaken under the supervision of an experienced neuroradiologist, the responsible corticotropic microadenoma is identified in a large proportion of patients with Cushing disease.

It is our opinion that patients suspected of Cushing disease must be supported in specialized neuroradiological centers, and should be managed by specialized endocrinologists and neurosurgeons. This strategy will avoid in many cases the recourse to inferior petrous sinus sampling to confirm the pituitary origin of the disease.

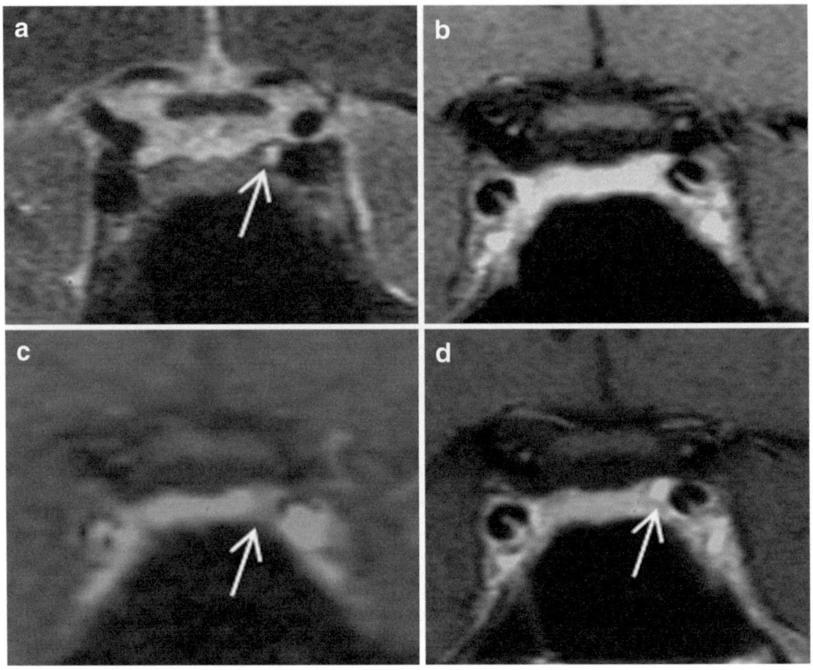

Fig. 15.4 Cushing disease in a 44-year-old woman. (**a**) Coronal T2WI. Localized bulging of the sellar diaphragm above a 2-mm hyperintense area (*arrow*). (**b**) CE T1WI. The lesion is masked. (**c**) Dynamic sequence. Defect in enhancement on the left (*arrow*). (**d**) Delayed CE T1WI. Late enhancement of the pituitary adenoma

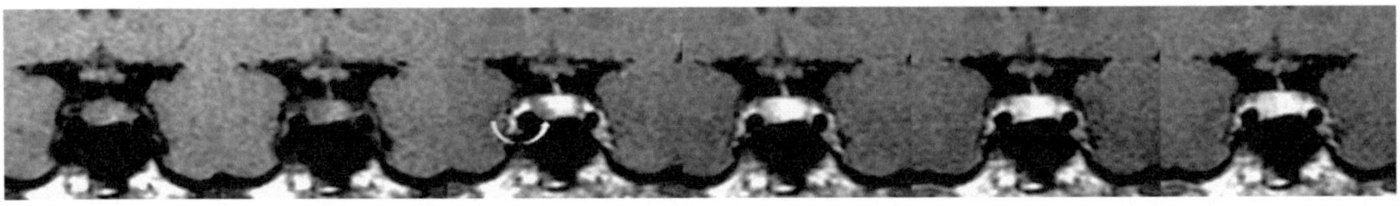

Fig. 15.5 Pitfall with dynamic imaging in a patient with suspected Cushing disease. Normal dynamic sequence with gadolinium injection. Each image is separated by 30 s. On image 3, there is normal early enhancement of the posterior pituitary (which is located off-midline in 50 % of normal individuals). On the right, the anterior pituitary is not enhanced, simulating a pituitary adenoma (*curved arrow*). On the next images, a normal enhancement of the pituitary content is observed

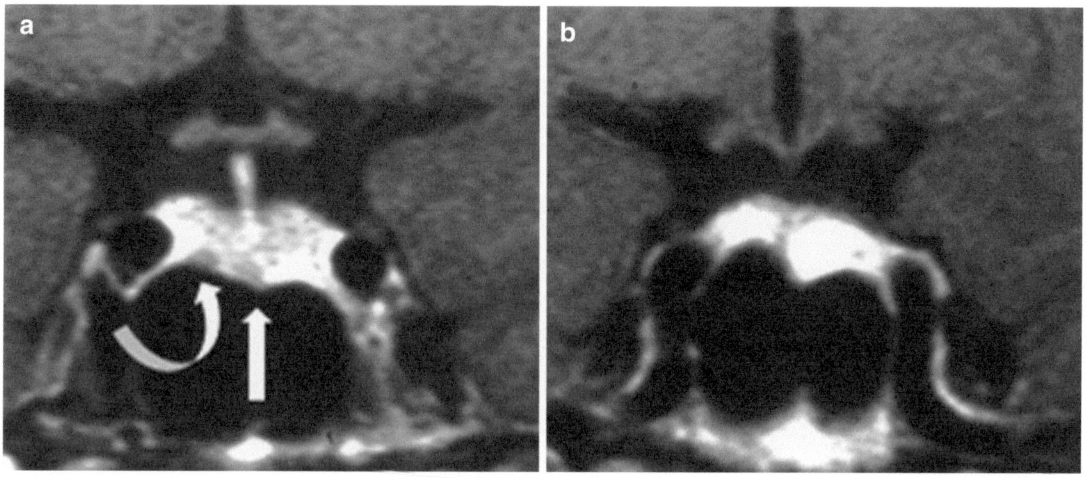

Fig. 15.6 Partial volume artifact and microcorticotropic adenoma. (**a**, **b**) Contiguous coronal CE TIWIs. Partial volume artifact (*curved arrow*) related to an asymmetrical sphenoid sinus as shown in (**b**). A corticotropic microadenoma located on the midline (*straight arrow*) was missed on previous studies

Further Reading

Bonneville JF, Cattin F, Bonneville F et al (2002) Pituitary gland imaging in Cushing disease. Neurochirurgie 48(2–3 Pt 2):173–178

Erickson D, Erickson B, Watson R et al (2010) 3Tesla MRI with and without corticotropin releasing hormone stimulation for the detection of microadenomas in Cushing syndrome. Clin Endocrinol (Oxf) 72: 793–799

Ntali G, Grossman A, Karavitaki N (2015) Clinical and biochemical manifestations of Cushing's. Pituitary 18(2):181–187

16 Silent Corticotroph Pituitary Adenoma

Fabrice Bonneville

Silent corticotroph pituitary adenomas are pituitary adenomas that require special attention. They are clinically and biologically silent but harbor ACTH-secreting cells at pathology. They may convert into active adenoma responsible for Cushing disease. Because they are endocrinologically silent, silent corticotroph adenomas are usually diagnosed when large and behave like nonfunctioning macroadenomas, being responsible for headaches, visual impairment, or pituitary deficiency (Fig. 16.1). Hemorrhage and apoplexy may be more prevalent that in nonfunctioning adenomas and ACTH-secreting adenomas (Fig. 16.2). Silent corticotroph adenomas can recur easily (Fig. 16.3), and present as aggressive tumors with frequent invasion of the cavernous sinus. Surgical treatment may fail, thus leading to different trials of multimodal therapy, including stereotactic radiosurgery, somatostatin analogs, and chemotherapy such as temozolomide.

Interestingly, a recent paper reported suggestive MRI features of silent corticotroph adenomas. Indeed, when compared with ACTH-secreting or nonfunctioning macroadenomas, silent corticotroph adenomas appeared significantly more frequently with a multimicrocystic pattern, best demonstrated on T2WI (Figs. 16.1, 16.3, and 16.4). In our experience there is a trend for silent corticotroph pituitary macroadenomas to harbor a multimicrocystic component, but this pattern is not pathognomonic, and may be observed in ACTH-secreting and gonadotropic adenomas as well. In general, corticotroph adenomas, when large, have a high chance of developing cysts, either macrocysts, microcysts, or a combination of both (Fig. 16.5). Apoplexy is another way to discover silent corticotroph adenoma. MRI is then nonspecific and the nature of the underlying adenoma remains unspecified, except if a non-necrosed area of the adenoma appears with the suggestive multimicrocystic pattern.

J.-F. Bonneville et al., *MRI of the Pituitary Gland*, DOI 10.1007/978-3-319-29043-0_16

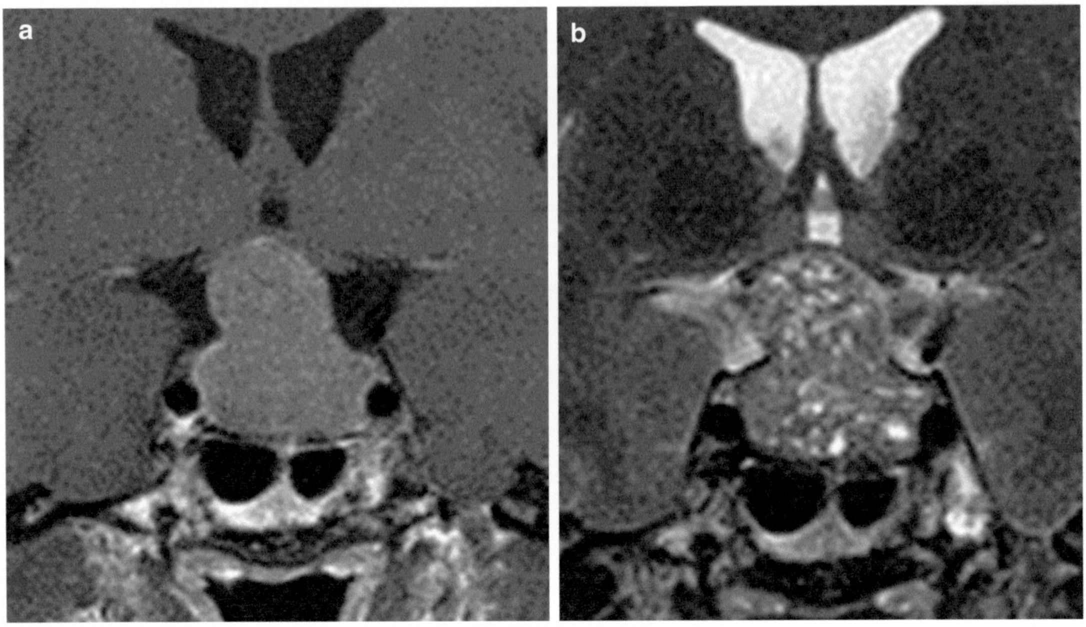

Fig. 16.1 Silent corticotroph pituitary macroadenoma in a 35-year-old woman with headaches, vertigo, and tinnitus. Laboratory studies revealed mild hyperprolactinemia and hypothyroidism. Surgery was performed and the diagnosis of silent corticotroph adenoma confirmed by pathology. (**a**) Coronal CE T1WI demonstrates a typical figure-of-8 shaped intra-suprasellar homogeneous adenoma. (**b**) Coronal T2WI depictes a unique multimicrocystic pattern, a feature frequently observed in silent corticotroph adenomas

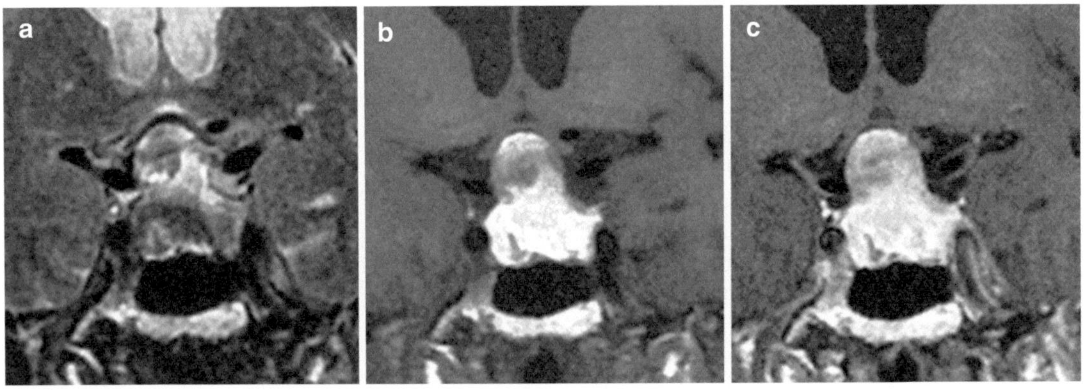

Fig. 16.2 Apoplexy of a silent corticotroph pituitary macroadenoma in a 71-year-old woman with visual impairment and headaches lasting for a few weeks. Coronal T2, T1, and CE (**a**–**c**) T1 WIs reveal heterogeneous signal intensity with predominant T1 hyperintensity and T2 hypointensity of an intra-suprasellar adenoma impinging on the optic chiasma. Pathological examination of the resected tissue demonstrated positive ACTH expression

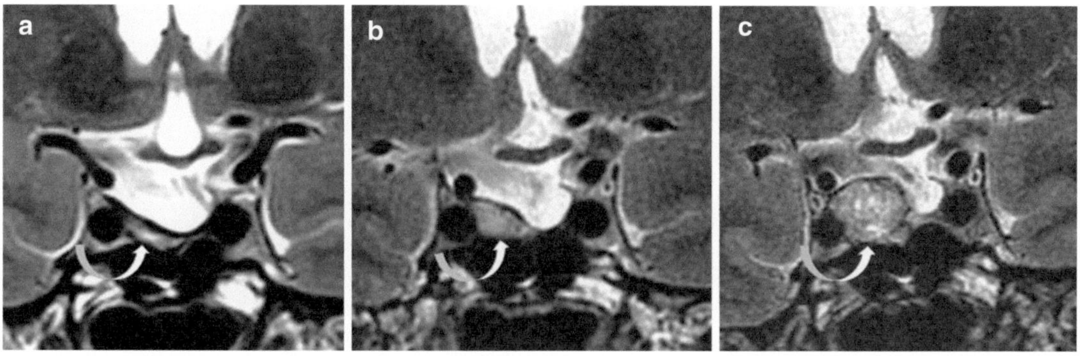

Fig. 16.3 Recurrent silent corticotroph pituitary adenoma in a 52-year-old man. (**a–c**) Coronal T2WIs. Episode of severe headache evoking a pituitary apoplexy 4 months previously with subsequent pituitary deficiency. (**a**) Small right T2-hyperintense tumoral remnant (*arrow*). (**b**) Two years later, increased size of the remnant (*arrow*). (**c**) Frank recurrence with obvious increased of tumoral volume 8 months later (*arrow*). Microcystic MRI pattern. Adenomectomy was performed and the diagnosis of corticotroph adenoma obtained by pathological examination

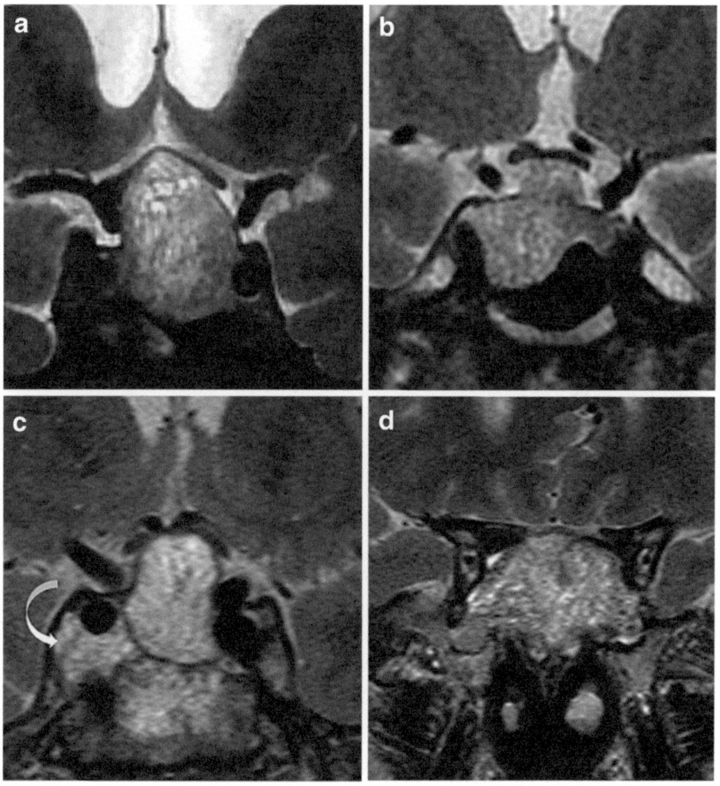

Fig. 16.4 Coronal T2WIs (**a–d**) in different patients with pathologically proven silent corticotroph pituitary adenomas. All adenomas harbor a multimicrocystic pattern, a feature suggestive of this entity. Cavernous sinus invasion is obvious in (**c**) (*arrow*)

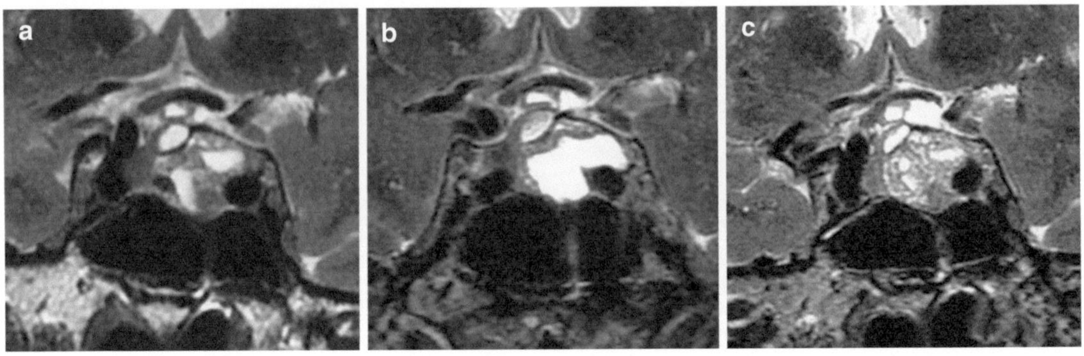

Fig. 16.5 Recurrent silent corticotroph pituitary adenoma in a 67-year-old woman. Visual field defect. (**a**–**c**) Coronal T2WIs. Rapid changes of the cystic MR pattern. (**a**) Four years after surgery. (**b**) Six months and (**c**) 12 months later

Further Reading

Cazabat L, Dupuy M, Boulin A et al (2014) Silent, but not unseen: multimicrocystic aspect on T2-weighted MRI in silent corticotroph adenomas. Clin Endocrinol 81:566–572

Cooper O (2015) Silent corticotroph adenomas. Pituitary 18:225–231

Nishioka H, Inoshita N, Sano T, Fukuhara N, Yamada S (2012) Correlation between histological subtypes and MRI findings in clinically nonfunctioning pituitary adenomas. Endocr Pathol 23:151–156

17 Pituitary Carcinoma

Jean-François Bonneville

Pituitary carcinomas are defined as pituitary adenomas with documented craniospinal and/or systemic metastases. The requirements to establish the diagnosis of pituitary carcinoma are today well specified: the primary tumor must be identified by histology; metastases, subarachnoid or systemic, must not be contiguous with the primary sellar tumor itself; and the structural features of the metastases should be similar to those of the primary tumor. Thus defined, pituitary carcinomas are extremely rare: only approximately 140 cases have been reported in the literature. The majority of pituitary carcinomas are hormonally active, principally ACTH- and prolactin-producing tumors. The prognosis is very poor despite the use of various regimens of cytotoxic chemotherapy such as temozolomide. The median survival is 12 months, and slightly longer for those patients with metastases confined to the CNS. The pathogenesis of malignant transformation is unclear. Pituitary carcinomas arise after a long patency period of time, up to 20 years, mostly from pituitary macroadenomas treated by surgery or irradiation. It does not appear that radiotherapy has a major carcinogenic role. The pathways metastases can take from pituitary adenoma include blood-borne, drop, and CNS dissemination, the latter possibly occurring after surgery. It has been said that the primary pituitary adenoma is frequently aggressive with cavernous sinus invasion, but these features are inconstant. Descriptions of pituitary carcinomas on MRI are scarce in the literature. It does not seem that any specific aspect has been reported, apart from aggressiveness and rapid growth (Fig. 17.1). Sites of metastases include the spinal cord, lung, pancreas, liver, kidney, and bone (Fig. 17.2).

J.-F. Bonneville et al., *MRI of the Pituitary Gland*, DOI 10.1007/978-3-319-29043-0_17

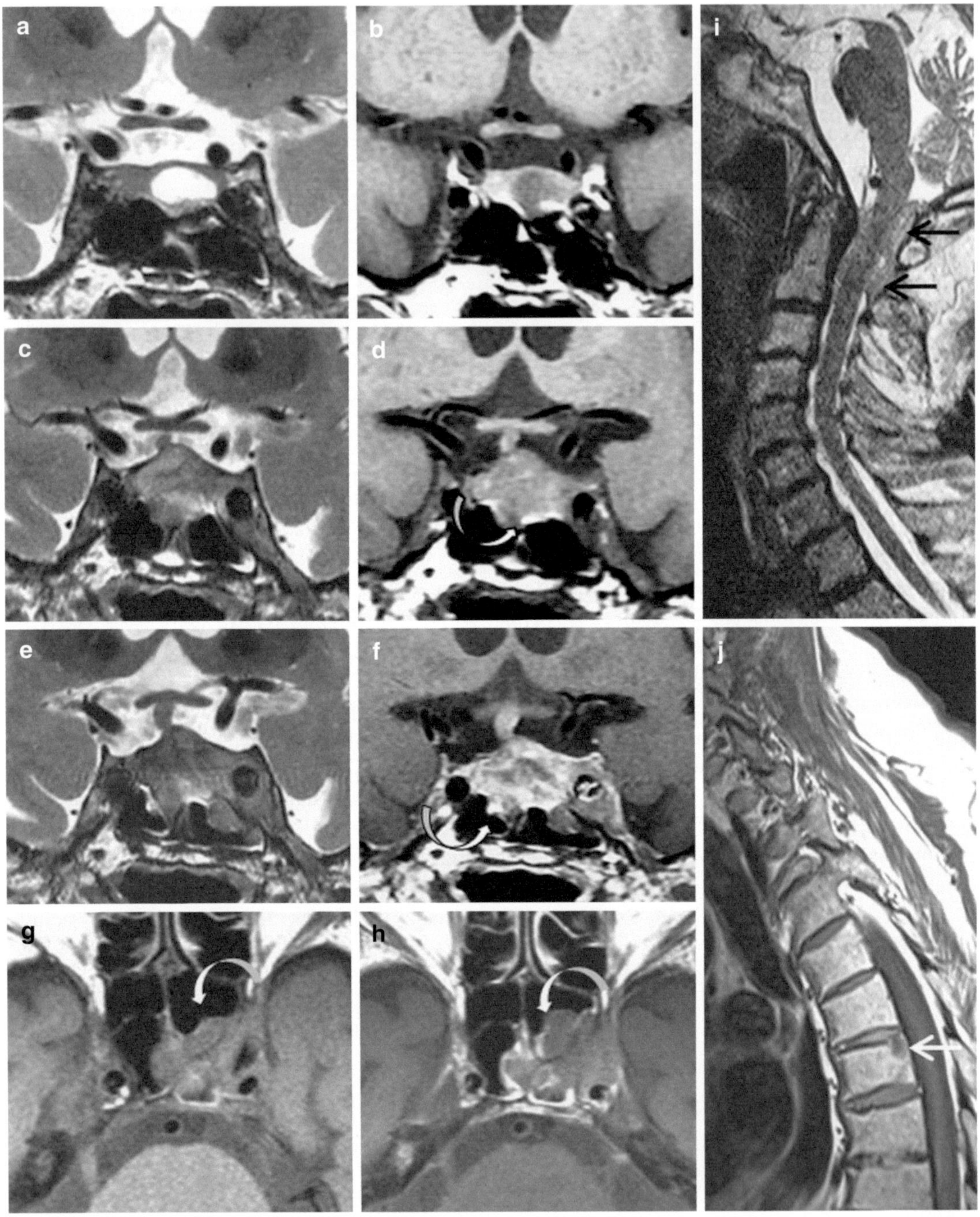

Fig. 17.1 Pituitary carcinoma. (**a**, **b**) Coronal T2 and T1 WIs. Pituitary microadenoma discovered by chance in a 69-year-old man. No follow-up. (**c**, **d**) Seven years later. Severe headache, rhinorrhea, and left oculomotor nerve paresis. Coronal T2 and T1 WIs show enlarged sellar mass with erosion of the sellar floor (*arrow*) and extension to left cavernous sinus. (**e**, **f**) Two weeks later. Aggravation of the medical status. Coronal T2 and CE T1WIs show further very rapid tumoral extension to the sphenoid sinus (*arrow*). (**g**, **h**) Comparative axial T1 and CE T1 WIs demonstrating rapid tumoral extension to sphenoid sinus in 2 weeks (*arrows*). (**i**, **j**) Sagittal T1 and T2 WIs of the spinal cord. Epidural metastases (*black arrows*) and bone metastases (*white arrow*)

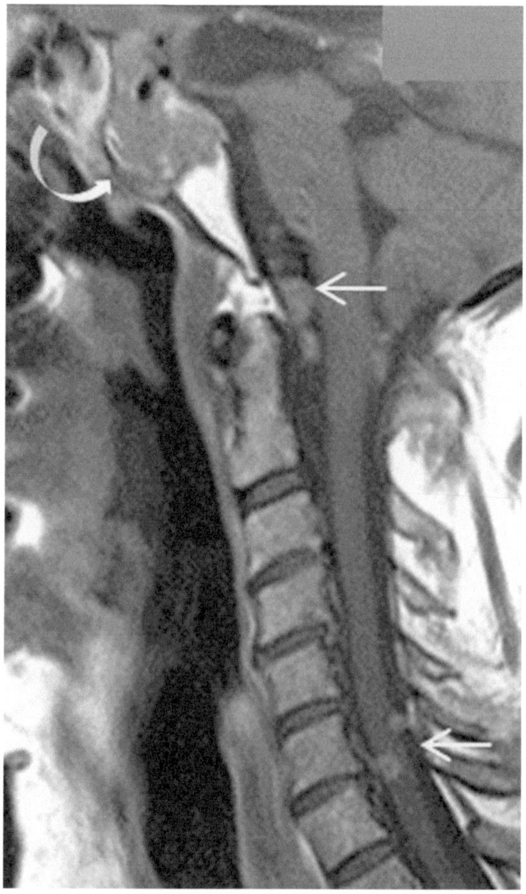

Fig. 17.2 Pituitary carcinoma in a 45-year-old man. Tumoral recurrence 1 year after removal of a silent ACTH pituitary adenoma. Sagittal CE T1WI. Pituitary mass invading sphenoid sinus (*curved arrow*). Subarachnoid metastases (*straight arrows*) (Courtesy of G. Raverot, MD, PhD)

Further Reading

Balili I, Sullivan S, Mckeever P et al (2014) Pituitary carcinoma with endolymphatic sac metastasis. Pituitary 17(3):210–213

Heaney A (2014) Management of aggressive pituitary adenomas and pituitary carcinomas. J Neurooncol 117(3):459–468

Park KS, Hwang JH, Hwang SK et al (2014) Pituitary carcinoma with fourth ventricle metastasis: treatment by excision and Gamma-knife radiosurgery. Pituitary 17(6):514–518

18 Ectopic Pituitary Adenoma

Jean-François Bonneville

Ectopic pituitary adenomas are defined by the presence of adenomatous pituitary tissue outside the sella and are distinctly separate from the pituitary gland. They are believed to originate from remaining pituitary cells resting along the path of the embryological formation of the pituitary gland. Ectopic pituitary adenomas can be nonfunctioning or secreting, particularly ACTH, GH, and prolactin secreting. The most common site is by far the sphenoid sinus, followed by the cavernous sinus, clivus, nasal cavity, nasopharynx, suprasellar region, and third ventricle. Sphenoid sinus ectopic pituitary adenomas can manifest themselves through a mass effect such as headache and nasal obstruction if large enough, or with symptoms of hormonal excess. Most case reports deal with Cushing disease, and it is accepted today that the sphenoid sinus must be carefully screened if pituitary MRI is negative in the setting of hypercortisolism (Fig. 18.1). Ectopic pituitary adenomas are generally heterogeneous with areas of T1 hypointensity and T2 hyperintensity, and moderate enhancement after contrast administration. Dynamic MRI can help to differentiate ectopic ACTH-secreting from nonfunctioning ectopic adenomas, the time–intensity curve featuring a rapidly enhancing and slow washout pattern in ACTH adenomas. Involvement of adjacent bone is frequent with large ectopic pituitary adenomas. Pituitary adenomas arising from the pituitary stalk are not stricto sensu ectopic adenomas, since the stalk is normally enfolded by an extension of normal anterior pituitary tissue (Fig. 18.2). An empty sella can coexist with an ectopic adenoma (Fig. 18.3). Ectopic pituitary adenomas must be distinguished from pituitary adenomas invading the sphenoid sinus, sometimes through a tiny hole pierced in the sellar floor best detected by CT (Fig. 18.4). Distinction sometimes can be almost impossible before surgery. Careful analysis of case reports of so-called ectopic pituitary adenomas have revealed that some are in fact intrasellar adenomas invading the sphenoid sinus.

J.-F. Bonneville et al., *MRI of the Pituitary Gland*, DOI 10.1007/978-3-319-29043-0_18

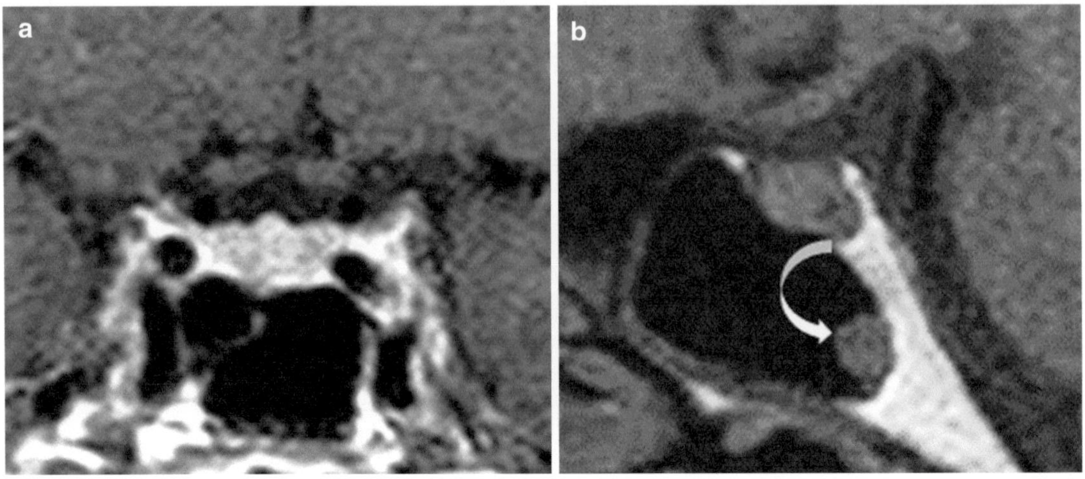

Fig. 18.1 Sphenoid sinus ectopic corticotropic adenoma in a 50- year-old woman. (**a**) Coronal CE T1WI. Normal anterior pituitary. (**b**) Sagittal T1WI demonstrates a "polyp" at the posterior part of the sinus (*arrow*) corresponding to a corticotropic adenoma at histological examination (With permission of Springer Science and Flitsch J et al, *Pituitary* (2015) 18:279–282)

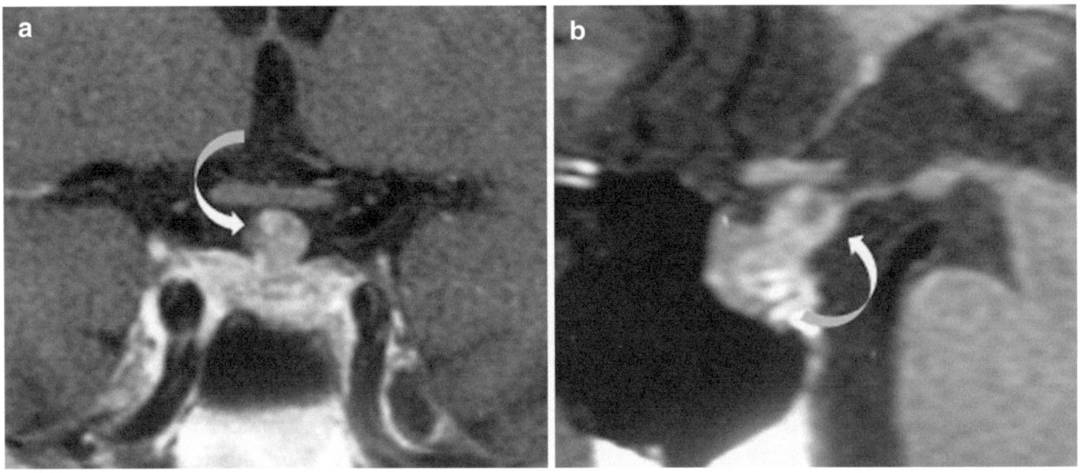

Fig. 18.2 Pituitary stalk corticotropic "ectopic" adenoma in a 50-year-old-woman with Cushing disease. (**a**, **b**) Coronal and sagittal CE T1WI. Note that pituitary stalk ectopic adenomas are not considered as true ectopic adenomas by some authors (Courtesy of Ph. Chanson, MD, PhD)

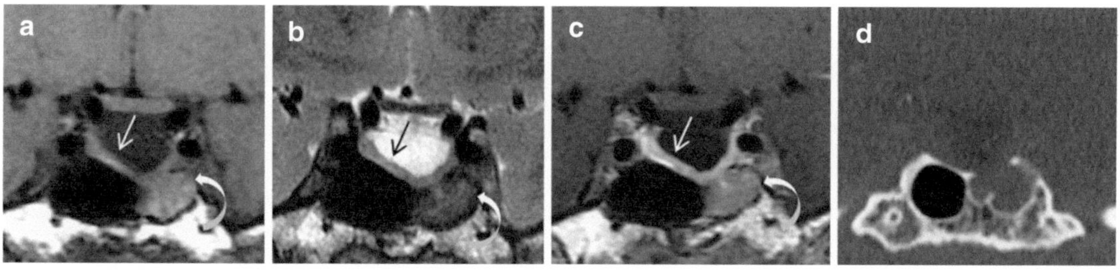

Fig. 18.3 GH-secreting "ectopic" pituitary adenoma and empty sella in a 42-year-old-woman. (**a–c**) Coronal T1, T2, and CE T1 WI. (**d**) Coronal CT. The signal of the anterior pituitary gland (*straight arrow*) is normal at the bottom of the empty sella. The pituitary adenoma (*curved arrow*) appears to have no connection with the pituitary gland, but sellar floor erosion is demonstrated in (**d**). True ectopic adenoma with secondary erosion of the sella, or the opposite?

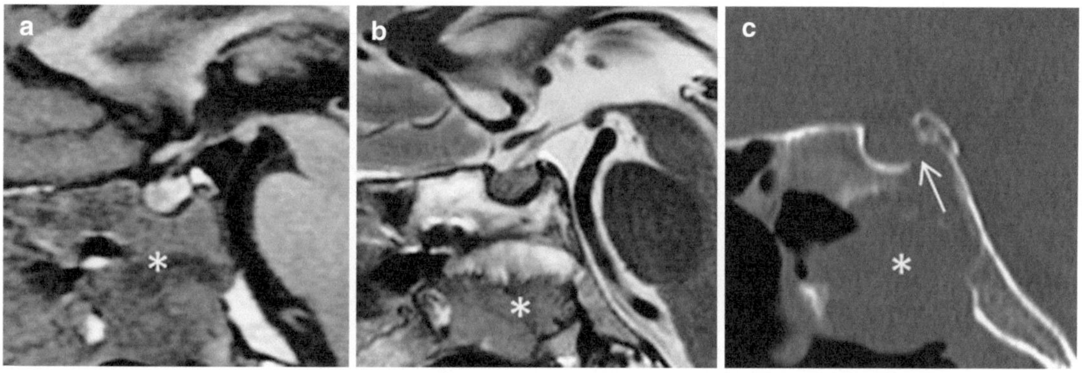

Fig. 18.4 Sphenoid sinus prolactinoma in a 47-year-old-man with nasal obstruction and a sphenoid mass on CT. Surgery is in favor of a mucocele, but histological examination finds prolactin cells. Prolactin level obtained after surgery was 1275 ng/ml. (**a**, **b**) Sagittal T1 and T2 WI. Heterogeneous mass occupying the sphenoid sinus (*asterisk*); the pituitary gland appears normal. (**c**) Sagittal CT reveals a localized erosion of the sellar floor (*arrow*)

Further Reading

Flitsch J et al (2015) A pitfall in diagnosing Cushing's disease: ectopic ACTH-producing pituitary adenoma in the sphenoid sinus. Pituitary 18:279–282

Johnston PC, Kennedy L, Weil RJ et al (2014) Ectopic ACTH-secreting pituitary adenomas within the sphenoid sinus. Endocrine 47(3):717–724

Thompson LD, Seethala RR, Müller S (2012) Ectopic sphenoid sinus pituitary adenoma (ESSPA) with normal anterior pituitary gland: a clinicopathologic and immunophenotypic study of 32 cases with a comprehensive review of the English literature. Head Neck Pathol 6(1):75–100

Yang BT, Chong VFH, Wang ZC et al (2010) Sphenoid sinus ectopic pituitary adenomas: CT and MRI findings. Br J Radiol 83(987):218–224

19 Rathke Cleft Cyst: Asymptomatic

Jean-François Bonneville and Fabrice Bonneville

Rathke cleft cysts (RCC) are the most frequent pituitary lesions revealed on MRI. They are intra-/suprasellar lesions believed to derivate from remnants of the Rathke pouch; therefore, one major characteristic is their strict and quite constant location on the midline. Nevertheless, RCC located off-midline may be encountered. They can originate either intra- or suprasellarly and their precise origin is best recognized if small, i.e., less than 10 mm in size. The displacement of the normal pituitary gland depends on the precise origin of the cyst. If initially intrasellar, RCCs are located on the midline, just in front and in close contact with the posterior lobe. Axial T1WI is in this case the most informative (Figs. 19.1 and 19.2), while a small hyperproteinic RCC may be mistaken for a large posterior lobe on sagittal view (Fig. 19.3). If initially suprasellar, RCCs originate from the pars tuberalis of the Rathke pouch. They are depicted on the upper surface of the pituitary gland or embedded in the pituitary with the appearance of an egg in an egg-cup, on the midline (Figs. 19.4 and 19.5). Asymptomatic RCCs involving the pituitary stalk (Fig. 19.6a–f) probably share the same origin; they must be differentiated from a deep infundibular recess of the third ventricle or from a pathological enlargement of the infundibulum. Rare RCCs can be encountered off-midline in the suprasellar cistern (Fig. 19.6g–i). Double RCCs may coexist. Concomitant pituitary adenomas are not exceptional (see Chap. 21). RCCs are classically described as pituitary cystic lesions with smooth contours, without calcification and no rim enhancement. "MicroRCCs," one to a few millimeters in diameter, are seen with increasing frequency with high-field MR scanners, either intrasellarly or at the distal end of the pituitary stalk; they have to be considered as anatomic variants (Fig. 19.5), since such microRCCs are present in routine autopsies in up to 33 % of normal pituitary glands. Larger RCCs, around 5–10 mm in size, are also frequent and nearly always asymptomatic (Fig. 19.7). In contrast to what is observed with pituitary adenomas, the sella turcica is unchanged. This is particularly remarkable on axial sequences where it can be observed that the anterior wall of the sella is not or scarcely distorted in front of RCCs even as large as 10 mm in diameter. RCCs larger than 12 mm may be symptomatic (for a fuller description see Chap. 20). RCCs can be stable, enlarge slowly or more rapidly, or shrink or even disappear, and can recur. Some changes have been depicted during pregnancy (see Chap. 8). From a general point of view, evolution of RCC is unpredictable. For this reason, serial imaging and visual field examination seem reasonable for those RCCs around 1 cm in diameter or less if the RCC is suprasellar in location. The cyst content is composed either of a thick mucus rich in protein and mucopolysaccharide or, much less frequently, of a CSF-like transparent fluid with low viscosity. The former is present in the vast majority of intrasellar cysts and is responsible for a more or less T1-hyperintense signal, depending

J.-F. Bonneville et al., *MRI of the Pituitary Gland*, DOI 10.1007/978-3-319-29043-0_19

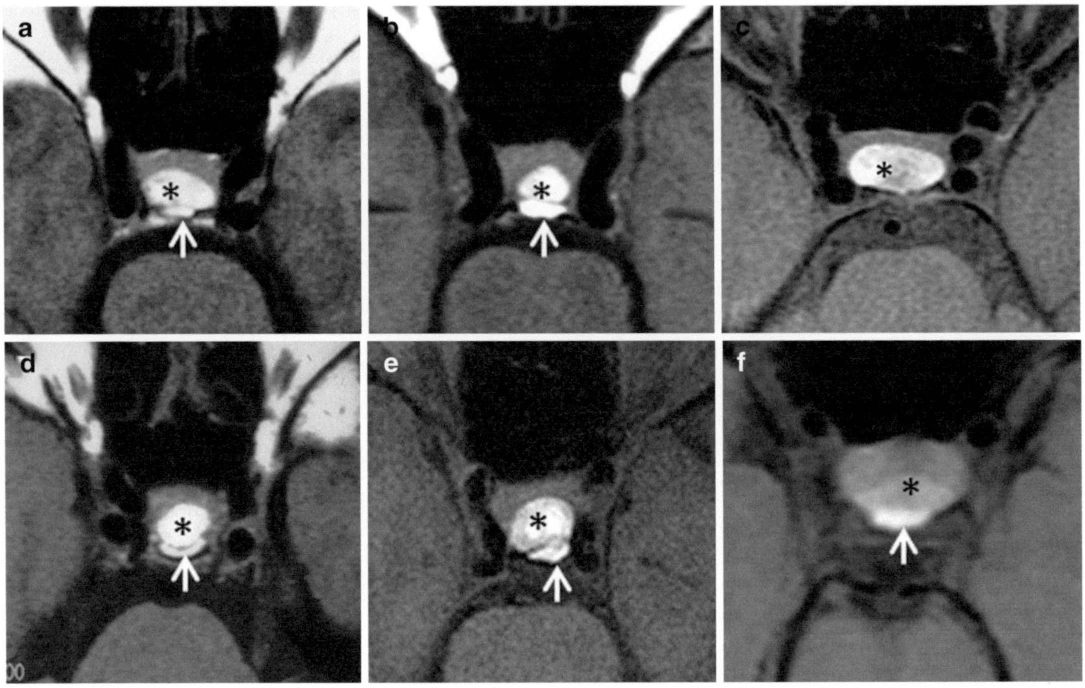

Fig. 19.1 RCCs on axial T1 (**a**, **b**, **d**) and axial T1 fat-saturated WI (**c**, **e**, **f**). RCCs (*asterisks*) are located between anterior and posterior lobes and are in close contact with the posterior lobe. The posterior lobe itself (*white arrows*) is in close contact with the dorsum sellae excepted in **c**

on the protein concentration and degree of dehydration of the cyst content. The usual absence of mass effect observed with RCC, together with their midline location, easily permits their differentiation from hemorrhagic pituitary adenomas. The less frequent CSF-like RCCs are T1 hypointense (Fig. 19.8) and are seen more frequently in suprasellar than in intrasellar locations. Spontaneous changes in signal can occur with time. Intracystic waxy nodules are observed in 75 % of the cases in T1-hyperintense RCC. The main components of these nodules are protein and cholesterol. Most are floating freely within the cyst and their position can change with time; a few are adherent to the cyst wall. The signal of these hyperproteinic nodules is isointense or slightly hyperintense on T1, and frankly hypointense on T2WI. They do not enhance or faintly enhance after contrast administration and are unique or, more rarely, multiple. They can be large, occupying almost the whole cyst, or extremely tiny (Fig. 19.9). In all cases, their recognition warrants the diagnosis of RCC. The activity of mucus-producing cells is variable, and responsible for variations of the cyst size together with absorption of cystic fluid. Factors influencing mucus secretion and, therefore, RCC size increase, are unknown. The cyst wall is very thin, lined usually by a single-cell respiratory-type epithelium often with goblet cells. Thus, the wall of asymptomatic RCC is not visible after gadolinium injection. A potential cause of errors is the enhancement of the normal pituitary gland surrounding the RCC, thus mimicking wall enhancement (Fig. 19.10). Rapid enhancement of the normal pituitary tissue early after contrast injection may help to avoid confusion with cyst wall enhancement that may be seen in symptomatic RCC. Nonenhancement of the cyst wall is essential to differentiate RCC from craniopharyngioma, in which the wall is thicker and stratified, and from complicated RCC.

MRI characteristics of most asymptomatic RCC, namely, no or faint sellar change, unique intrasellar midline location, close contact with the posterior lobe for intrasellar RCC, T1 hyper-

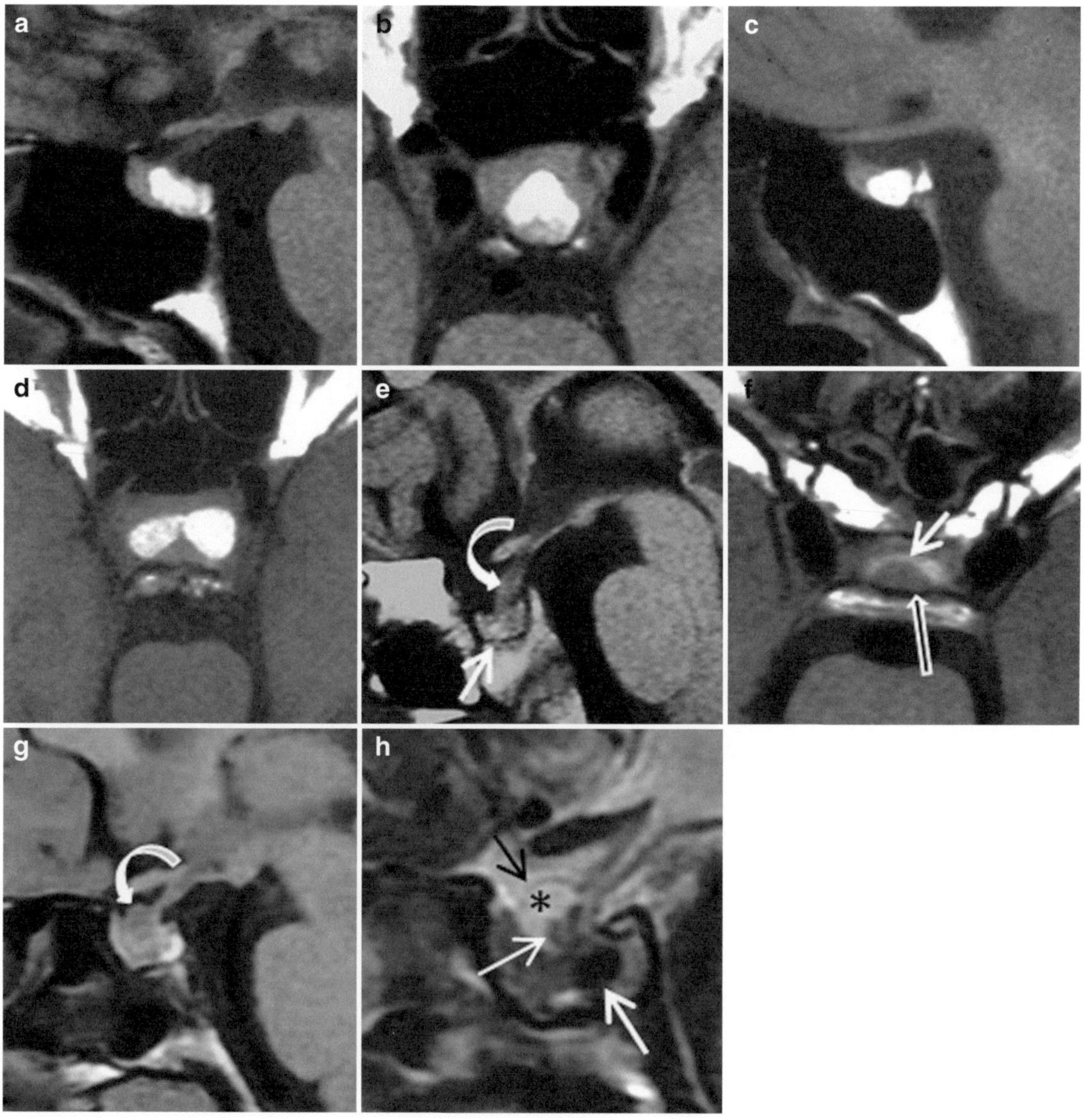

Fig. 19.2 RCCs on sagittal (**a**, **c**, **e**, **g**) and axial (**b**, **d**, **f**) T1WIs. (**h**) Sagittal T2WI. Particular features: (**a**, **b**) Elongated RCC in an elongated sella. (**c**, **d**) Bilobulated RCC. (**e**, **f**) Asymptomatic RCC and infundibuloneurohypophysitis in a 5-year-old boy; thickened pituitary stalk (*curved arrow*); enlarged T1 isointense posterior lobe (*black* and *white arrow*) outlined by an arch-like RCC (*white arrow*) compressed by the abnormal posterior lobe. (**g**, **h**) Double RCC on sagittal T1 and T2 WIs. An anterior T2-hyperintense RCC (*asterisk*) presents a hyperproteinic nodule (*thin white arrow*); the posterior RCC is T2 hypointense (*thick white arrow*). Both are almost invisible on T1WI

intensity without fluid level, T2-hypointense hyperproteinic nodules, and no cyst wall enhancement, usually make the diagnosis of most RCCs easy. These characteristic features should permit one to dramatically restrict the use of the vague term “incidentaloma” too frequently used in radiological reports. Although the vast majority of RCCs remain asymptomatic, some give rise to clinical manifestations. Rapid increase in cyst volume, change of signal, and post-gadolinium rim enhancement can be predictive markers of complications (see Chap. 20).

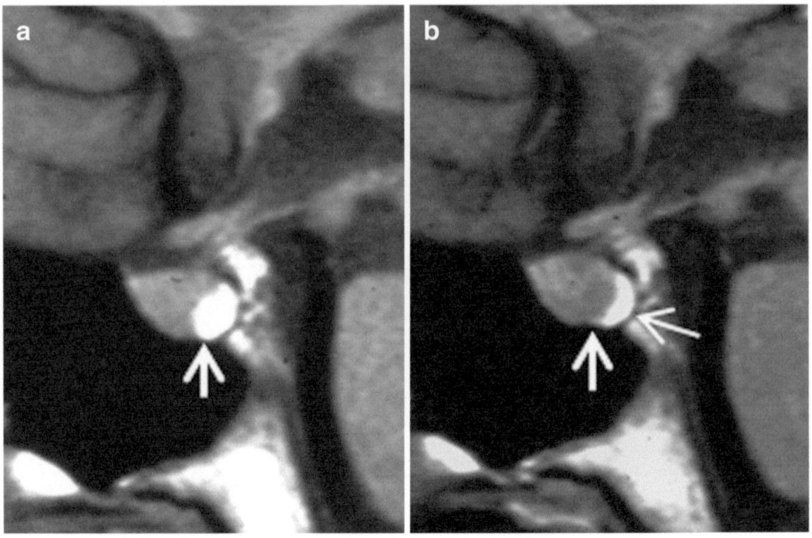

Fig. 19.3 (**a**, **b**) Sagittal T1WIs. RCC (*thick arrow*): spontaneous T1 signal change in a few months (from T1 hyperintense to T1 hypointense). The posterior lobe (*thin arrow*) cannot be distinguished from RCC in (**a**)

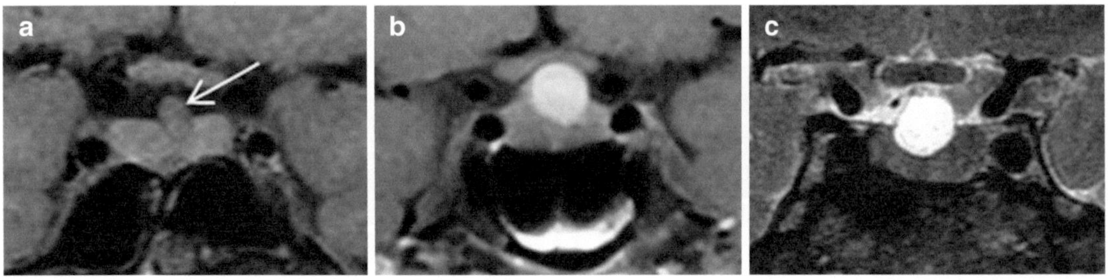

Fig. 19.4 Coronal T1 (**a**, **b**) and T2 WIs (**c**) in three patients with RCC. Egg in an egg-cup pattern. RCC is slightly T1 hypointense in (**a**) if compared with the normal anterior pituitary, markedly hyperintense in (**b**), and T2 hyperintense in (**c**)

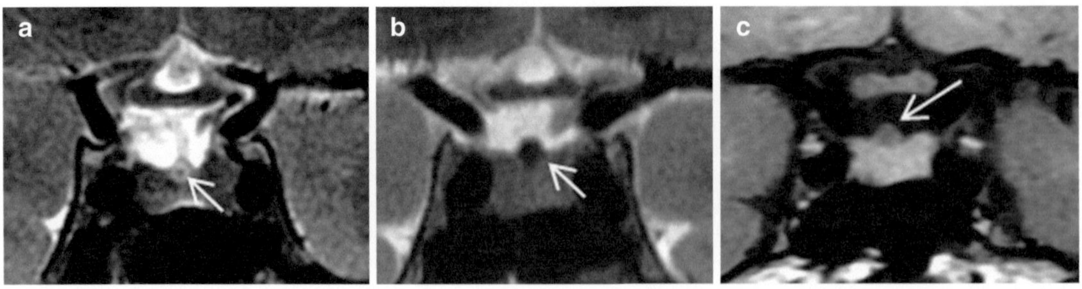

Fig. 19.5 MicroRCCs at the sellar diaphragm level. (**a**, **b**) Coronal T2WI and (**c**) T1WI. RCC is T2 hyperintense with a central hypointense hyperproteinic micronodule (*arrow*) in (**a**), T2 hypointense in (**b**), T1 hypointense in (**c**)

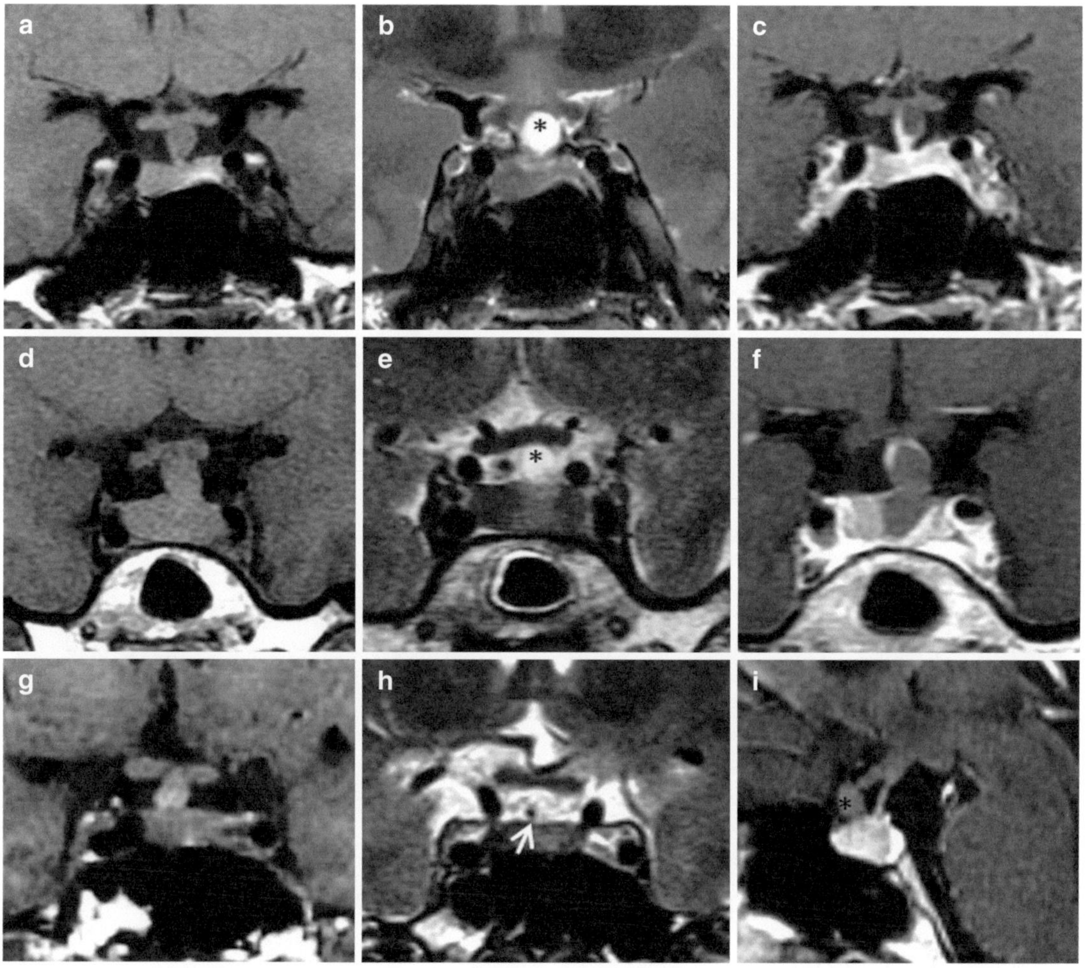

Fig. 19.6 (**a–c**) Coronal T1 (**a**, **d**, **g**), coronal T2 (**b**, **e**, **h**) and sagittal CE TI WIs (**c**, **f**, **i**). RCC of the pituitary stalk (**a–c**), intrasellar RCC extended to the pituitary stalk (**d–f**), and off-midline RCC of the suprasellar cistern (**g–i**). All RCCs are T2 hyperintense (*asterisk*) with a tiny T2-hypointense nodule in (**h**) (*arrow*). Postcontrast enhancement of a distorted pituitary stalk in (**c**) and (**f**) with incomplete and thin enhancement of RCC wall. In (**i**), the T1 nonenhanced RCC (*asterisk*) is located in front of the pituitary stalk

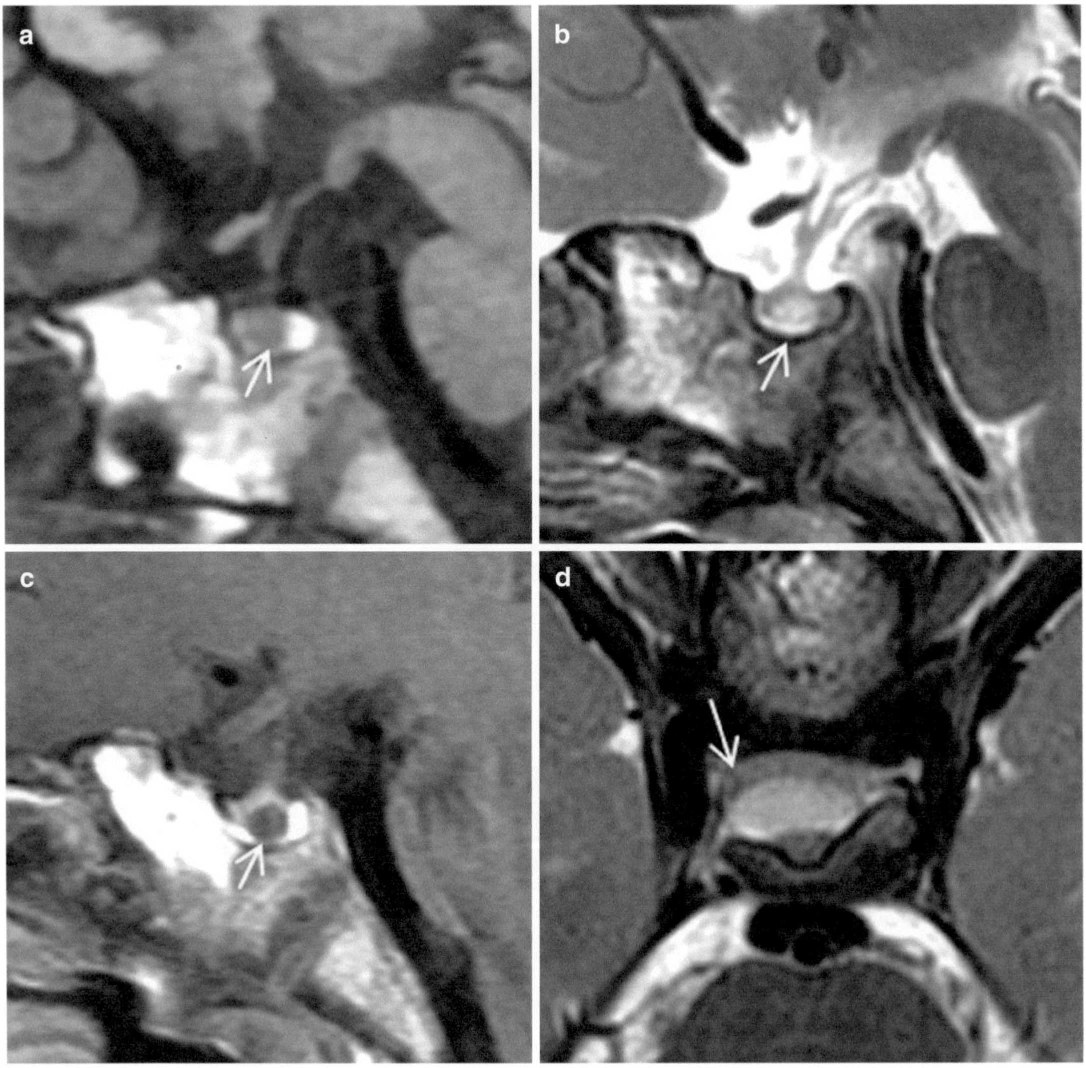

Fig. 19.7 Asymptomatic RCC in a 4-year-old boy. (**a**–**c**) Sagittal T1, T2, and CE T1 WIs. (**d**) Axial T2WI. Characteristic shape and location of an RCC with a CSF-like signal on sagittal and axial images (*arrow*)

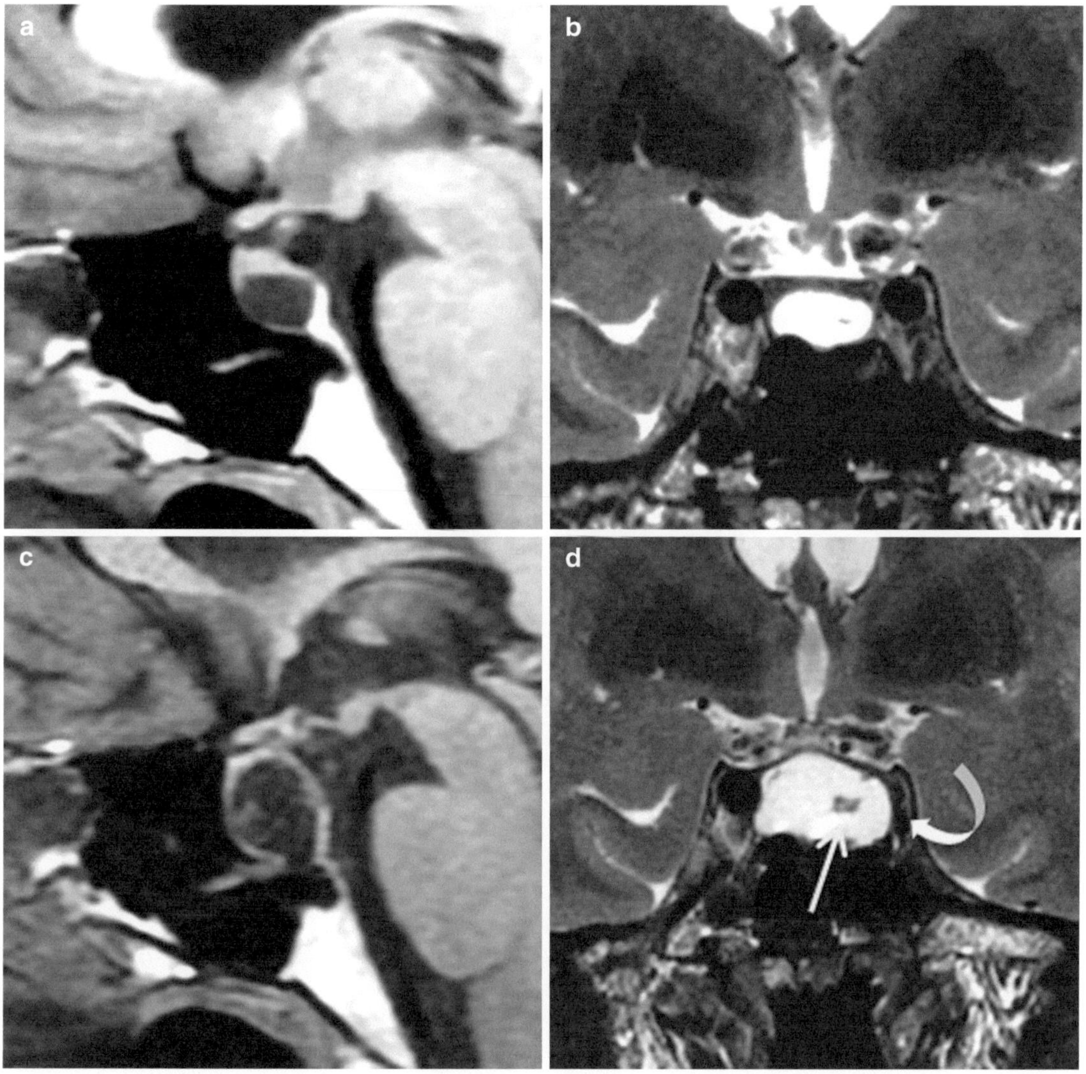

Fig. 19.8 Asymptomatic RCC in a 32-year-old woman followed yearly for 8 years. (**a**, **c**) Sagittal T1WI and (**b**, **d**) Coronal T2WI. RCC is markedly T1 hypointense and T2 hyperintense. Hyperproteinic nodule (*arrow*). Low-speed cyst volume increase in 8 years. The patient remains asymptomatic but a follow-up is necessary. Note the incidental finding of an asymptomatic thrombosis of left internal carotid artery in (**d**) (*curved arrow*)

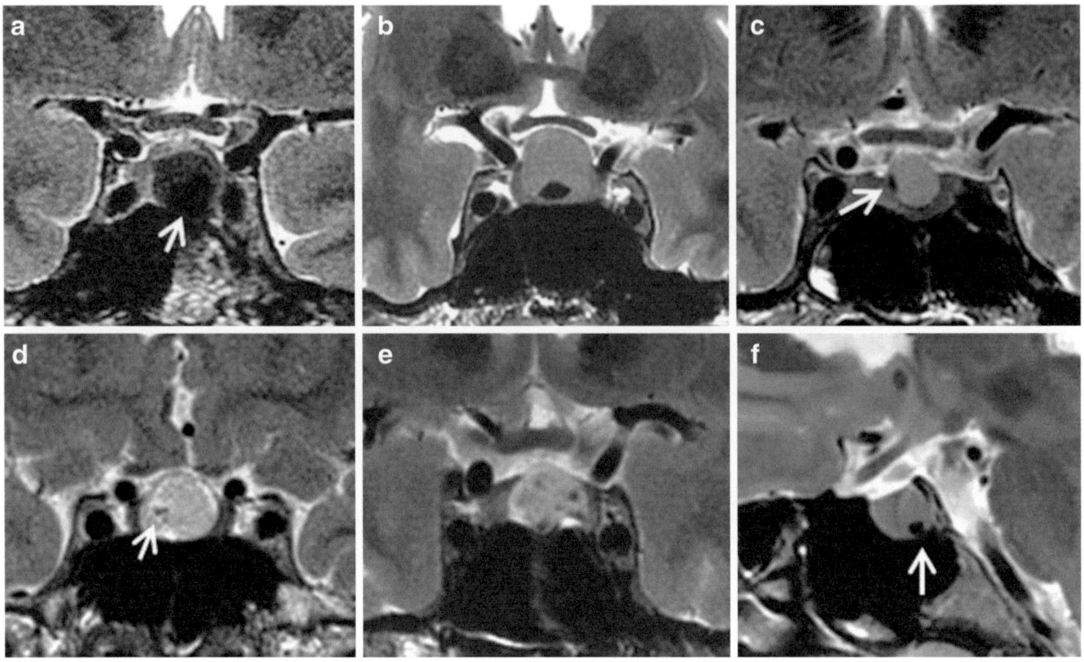

Fig. 19.9 RCCs with T2-hypointense hyperproteinic nodules. (**a–e**) Coronal T2WIs. (**f**) Sagittal T2WI. The nodules can be massive (**a**), small (**b**, **f**), tiny (**c**, **d**), or, more rarely, multiple (**e**)

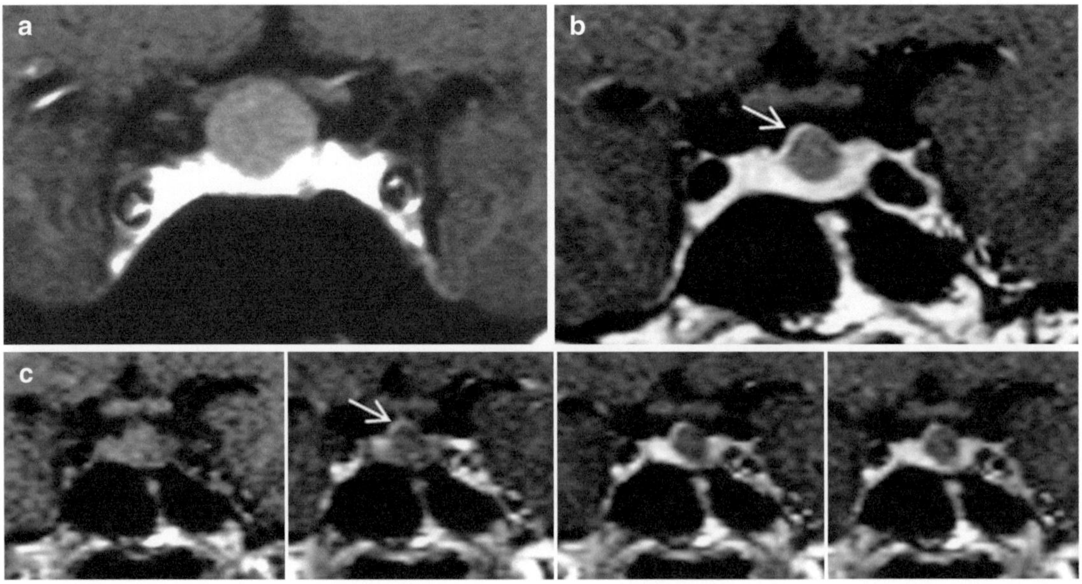

Fig. 19.10 RCCs after gadolinium injection on coronal CE T1WIs (**a**, **b**). Characteristic pattern with no rim enhancement in (**a**). Thin enhancement (*arrow*) of the displaced pituitary gland simulating RCC partial wall enhancement in (**b**). In (**c**), dynamic sequence confirms that the enhancement occurs early and involves the displaced anterior pituitary (*arrow*) and not the RCC wall which, if at all, should occur later

Further Reading

Bonneville F, Cattin F, Marsot-Dupuch K et al (2006) T1 signal hyperintensity in the sellar region: spectrum of findings. Radiographics 26(1):93–113

Byun WM, Kim OL, Kim D (2000) MR imaging findings of Rathke cleft cysts: significance of intracystic nodules. AJNR Am J Neuroradiol 21(3):485–488

Trifanescu R, Ansorge O, Wass JA et al (2012) Rathke cleft cysts. Clin Endocrinol (Oxf) 76(2):151–160

20 Rathke Cleft Cyst: Symptomatic and Complicated

Jean-François Bonneville

Rathke cleft cysts (RCCs) are a very common incidental finding: with the improvement in MRI techniques, their frequency in living patients is now approaching that seen at autopsy. Most are millimetric and located either intrasellarly on the midline, between anterior and posterior pituitaries, or lying on the upper surface of the gland at the level of the distal end of the pituitary stalk (Fig. 19.1). They have to be considered as anatomical variants and do not warrant any follow-up. RCC may become symptomatic either by mass effect or through complications. Mass effect (chronic headache, visual field defect, pituitary deficiency) may appear with an increase in cyst size when mucus production exceeds absorption. Complications may include inflammation, infection, hemorrhage, apoplexy, or rupture. RCCs 5–10 mm in diameter are frequent and cannot be usually held responsible for symptoms unless it can be demonstrated that a cyst has shrunk, as can be observed in some patients with pituitary insufficiency seen late after the onset of symptoms (Fig. 20.1). In these cases, the exact nature of the "complication" can remain unknown. Nevertheless, the natural history of these 4–8-mm asymptomatic cysts is unpredictable (Fig. 20.2), and the obvious fact that a symptomatic RCC one day was asymptomatic must be kept in mind. Our policy, in the setting of such an incidental finding, is to monitor these cysts at 1 year with strictly the same MRI projections. Serial MRI are then spaced out, but only if there is no change of size or signal of the cyst and if there is no postgadolinium enhancement of the cyst wall. Of course the nearer is the cyst to the optic chiasm, the more careful will be the monitoring. RCCs 1 cm and larger can be symptomatic or asymptomatic (Figs. 20.3 and 20.4), so their responsibility in the setting of chronic or repeated episodic headaches can be difficult to assert unless inflammation is demonstrated. Cyst wall inflammation appears on MRI as rim enhancement after gadolinium injection (Fig. 20.5). Such an inflammation could be related to an intermittent foreign-body reaction caused by mucinous contents, and therefore is more frequently observed with T1-hyperintense RCC. Inflammation of the cyst wall may increase mucus secretion and, therefore, cyst volume. It can extend to the surrounding anterior pituitary tissue, giving rise to a secondary hypophysitis with gonadotropin, ACTH, TSH, and/or GH deficiencies and hyperprolactinemia (Fig. 20.6). Diabetes insipidus is also frequent and can be isolated. In patients with repeated episodic headaches and demonstration of cyst wall enhancement, i.e., inflammation, some authors have proposed surgical treatment of RCC to avoid hypophysitis and its hormonal consequences. Partial or even complete cyst shrinkage can occur spontaneously with time, leading to an erroneously termed "empty sella." In our experience, a complicated RCC represents a not infrequent cause of pituitary insufficiency or diabetes insipidus of "unknown origin." Cyst infection and bacterial meningitis occur principally in mucinous

J.-F. Bonneville et al., *MRI of the Pituitary Gland*, DOI 10.1007/978-3-319-29043-0_20

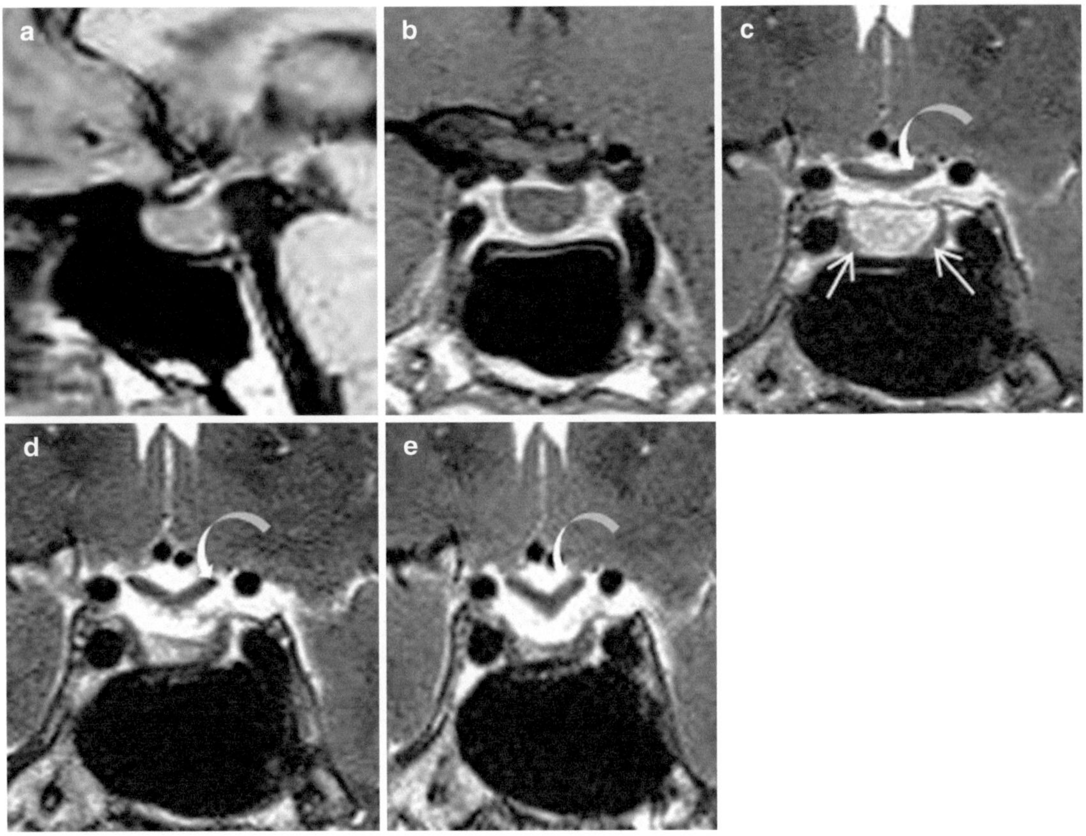

Fig. 20.1 Pituitary insufficiency for 2 months in a 43-year-old man. "Complicated" RCC. (**a–c**) Sagittal T1, coronal CE T1, and coronal T2 WIs at diagnosis. T1 isointense "egg in an egg-cup" nonenhanced intrasellar cyst displacing the normal pituitary gland on the periphery (*straight arrow*). The optic chiasm is not strictly horizontal, but mildly lowered (*curved arrow*), meaning that the cyst was previously larger. (**d**, **e**) Coronal T2WIs 4 and 10 months later. Progressive shrinkage of the cyst and optic chiasm ptosis in parallel (*curved arrow*)

RCC (Fig. 20.7). The shared venous drainage of the sellar content and the sphenoid sinus has been proposed as a mechanism of secondary infection. Intracystic hemorrhage is rare except in patients with coagulation disorders. It is represented by a fluid-fluid level better seen on sagittal and axial sequences. Depending of the RCC protein concentration and, therefore, of the T1 signal intensity, the hemorrhagic compartment can appear more or less intense than the rest of the cyst. In some cases, diagnosis of cyst hemorrhage can be difficult on T1WI, but the presence of a fluid level on T2WI is characteristic of a hemorrhagic event. Sudden hemorrhage can lead to rapid extension of cyst or even cyst rupture, possibly responsible for chemical meningitis (Fig. 20.8). The term "RCC apoplexy" (hemorrhagic or nonhemorrhagic) is used in the literature for different pathologies: symptomatic RCC hemorrhage or pituitary apoplexy in contact with an RCC or true RCC apoplexy. Hemorrhagic RCC apoplexy (Fig. 20.9) is very rare; its mechanism is presumed to be the repeated bleeding from the thin blood vessels in the cyst wall or from the hypophyseal blood vessels by compression or shearing stress. The mechanism of nonhemorrhagic RCC apoplexy is not clearly understood. In fact, the term "RCC apoplexy" refers to a symptomatology of acute severe headache and possibly meningismus, visual disturbance,

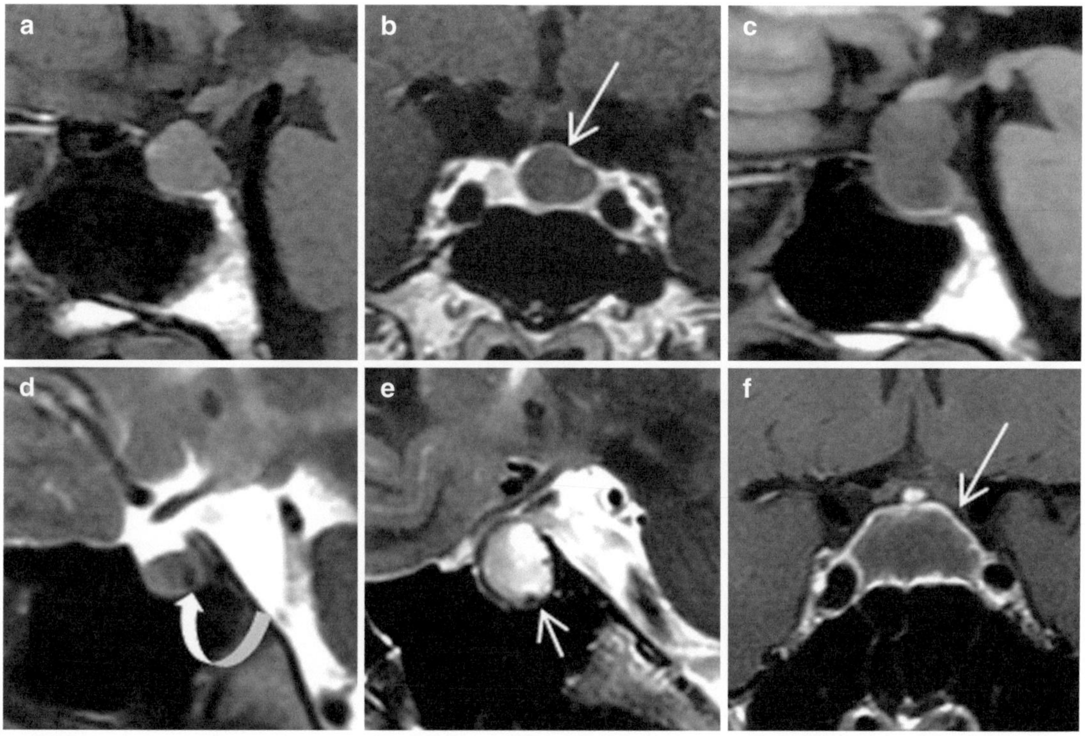

Fig. 20.2 Complicated RCC in two patients. *Upper row*. Diabetes insipidus for 2 months in a 55-year-old woman. (**a**, **b**) Sagittal T1 and coronal CE T1WIs. Intrasellar mass isointense to the brainstem with rim enhancement after contrast injection (*arrow*), thus signifying that the RCC is (or was) symptomatic. (**c**) Sagittal T1WI 6 months later. Rapid cyst enlargement with T1 signal becoming hypointense. *Lower row*. Headache and blurred vision in an 18-year-old woman. (**e**, **f**) Sagittal T2 and coronal CE T1 WIs. Characteristic features of a complicated RCC: T2-hyperintense sellar mass with suprasellar extension and T2-hypointense nodule (*short arrow*). Ring enhancement (*arrow*). (**d**) Sagittal T2 brain MRI performed 2 years previously in the assessment of paresthesias. T2-hypointense image (*curved arrow*), the location of which evokes a small, very common RCC. This case raises the issue of the management of RCC discovered by chance

oculomotor nerve palsies, and impairment of pituitary function. Clinical and imaging features can be very similar to those observed with pituitary apoplexy. Sphenoidal mucosal thickening is often present in both pituitary and RCC apoplexy. But intracystic nodules are found only in RCC. The largest RCCs, up to 30–40 mm in diameter, are mostly T1 hypointense (Fig. 20.10). Symptoms are related to mass effect and include frontal headache (though not always) and visual field defect and/or optic nerve impairment. Oculomotor nerves palsies are more commonly observed in case of acute cyst enlargement. Cyst recurrences are frequent after cyst puncture, and MR follow-up is mandatory in all cases (Fig. 20.11).

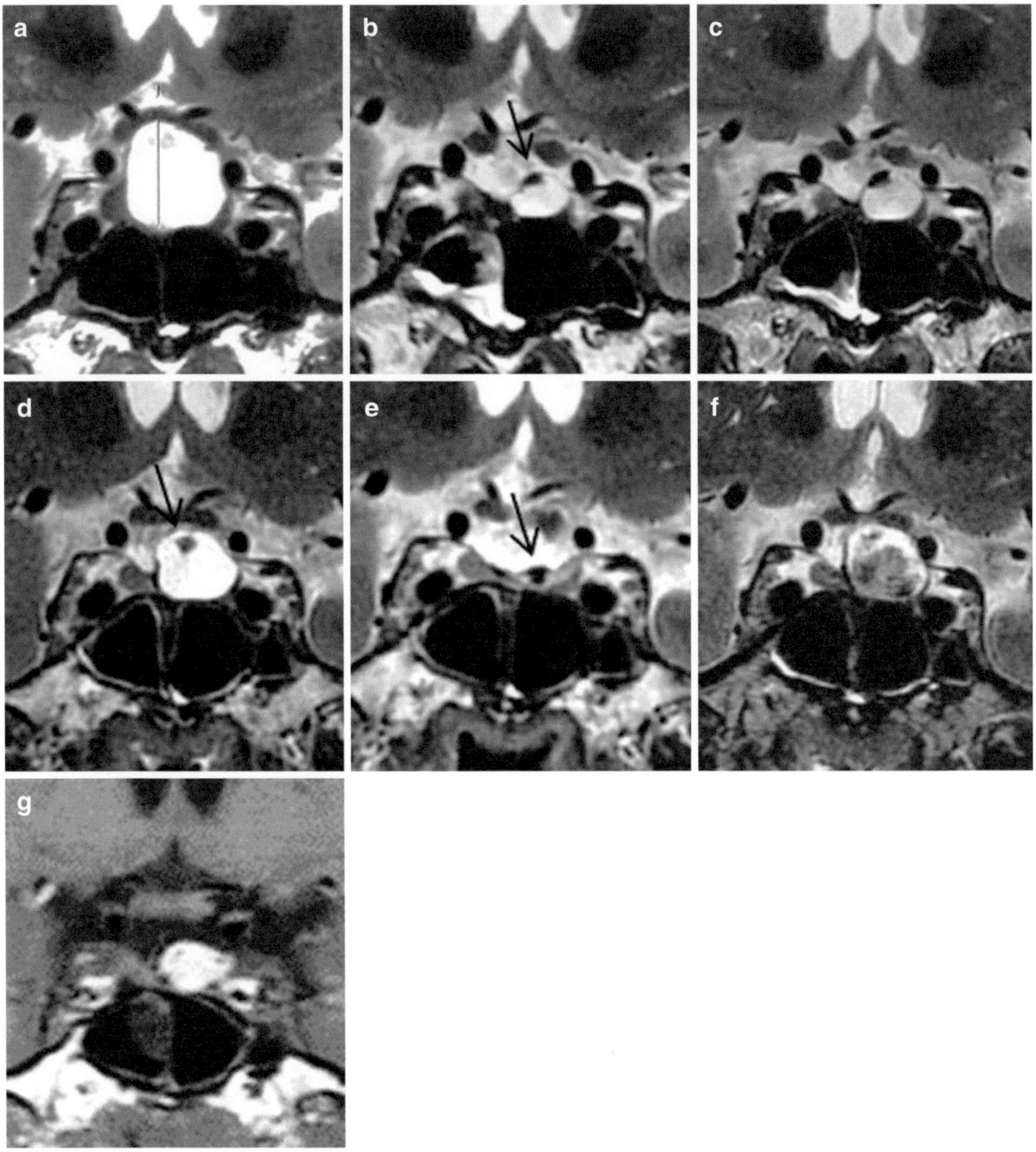

Fig. 20.3 Same patient as in Fig. 20.2 upper row. (**a**–**f**) Coronal T2WIs and (**g**) coronal T1WI. (**a**) corresponds to Fig. 20.2(**d**). The optic chiasm is raised (**a**). The cyst is punctured and remains asymptomatic for 5 years. MRI pattern 2 months postoperatively (**b**), then yearly (**c**–**g**). Variable cyst volume changes. Unchanged small hyperproteinic nodule (*arrows*)

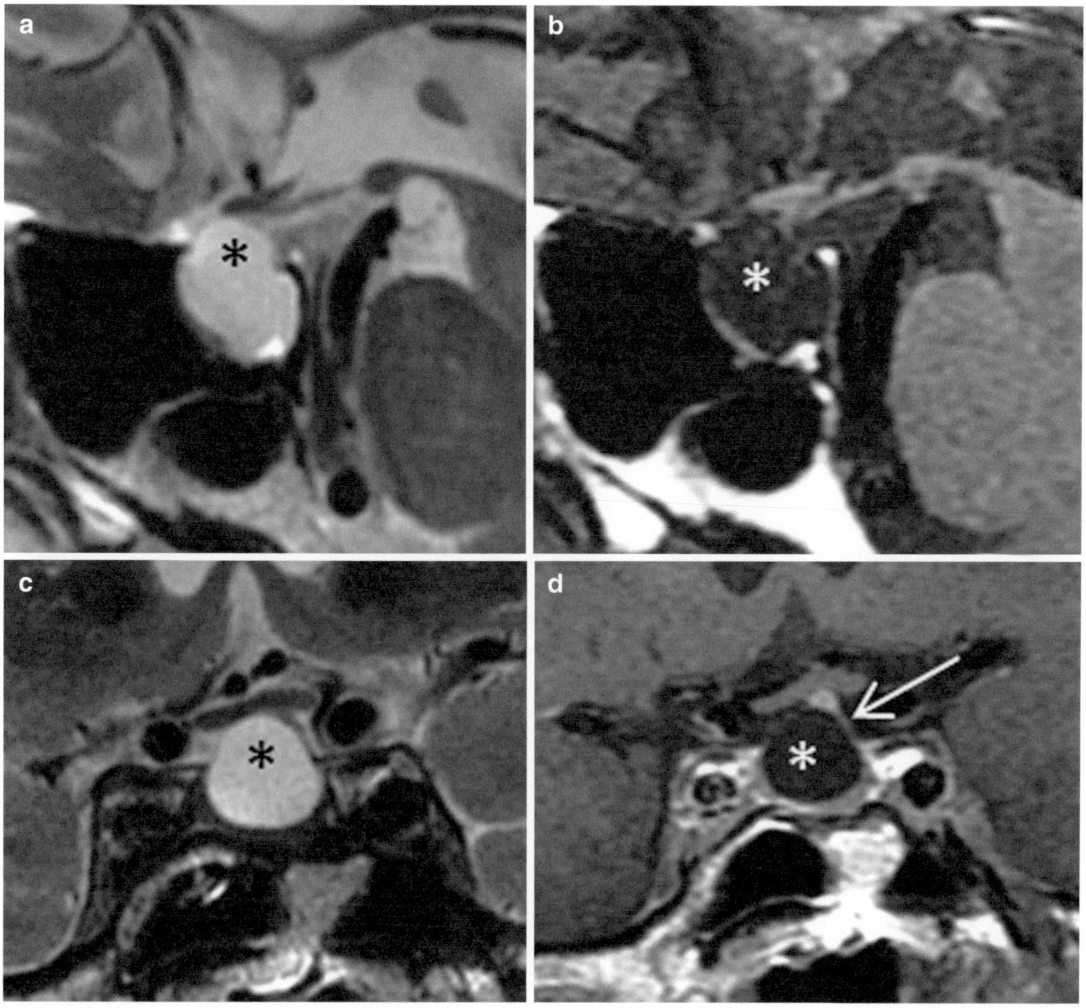

Fig. 20.4 Pituitary insufficiency and hyponatremia in an 82-year-old woman. (**a**, **b**) Sagittal T2 and T1 WIs. (**c**, **d**) Coronal T2 and CE T1 WIs. The RCC (*asterisk*) is T2 hyperintense and T1 hypointense. Slight tilting of optic chiasm. Band-like enhancement (*arrow*) is the pituitary stalk and not a cyst rim. The symptomatology is probably from a chronic compression of the anterior pituitary gland

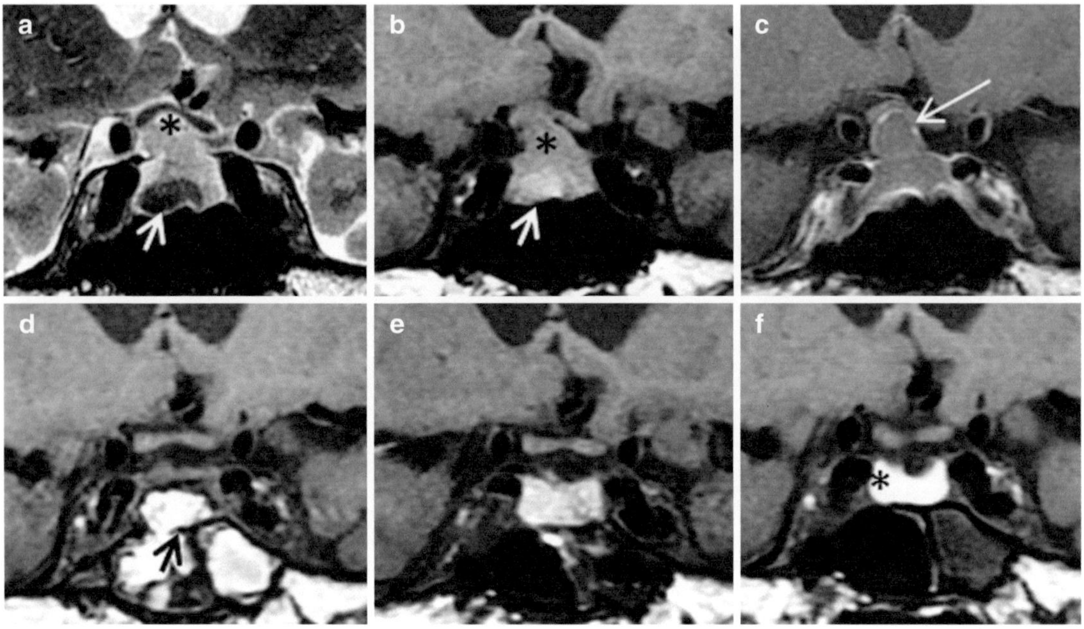

Fig. 20.5 Pituitary insufficiency and visual field defect in a 68-year-old man. (**a–c**) Coronal T2, T1, and CE T1 WIs. T2-hyperintense RCC (*asterisk*) with T2-hypointense and slightly T1-hyperintense characteristic hyperproteinic nodule (*thick short arrow*). The optic chiasm is distorted. Postgadolinium thin-rim enhancement (*long arrow*). (**d–f**) Postoperative coronal T1WIs respectively 4 days, 3 months, and 1 year after cyst puncture. Fat packing (*black arrow*) with chemical shift artifact in (**d**). Cyst recurrence in (**e**). In (**f**), persistent T1-hyperintense cyst related to higher proteinic concentration and dehydration

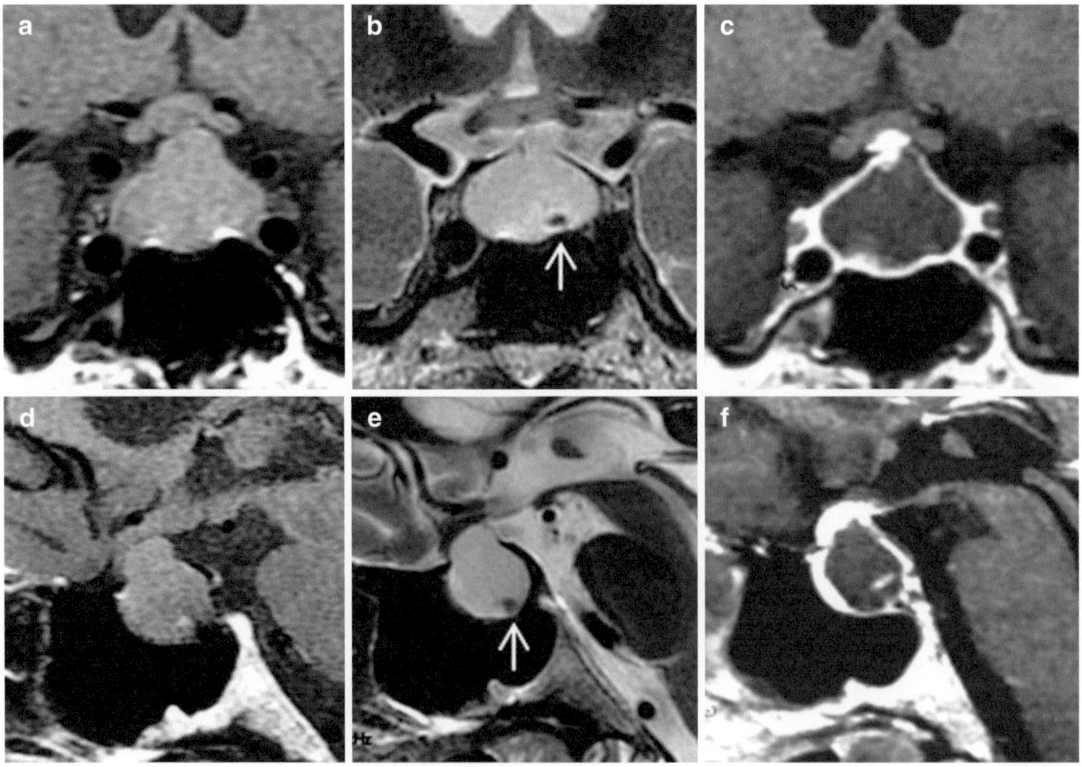

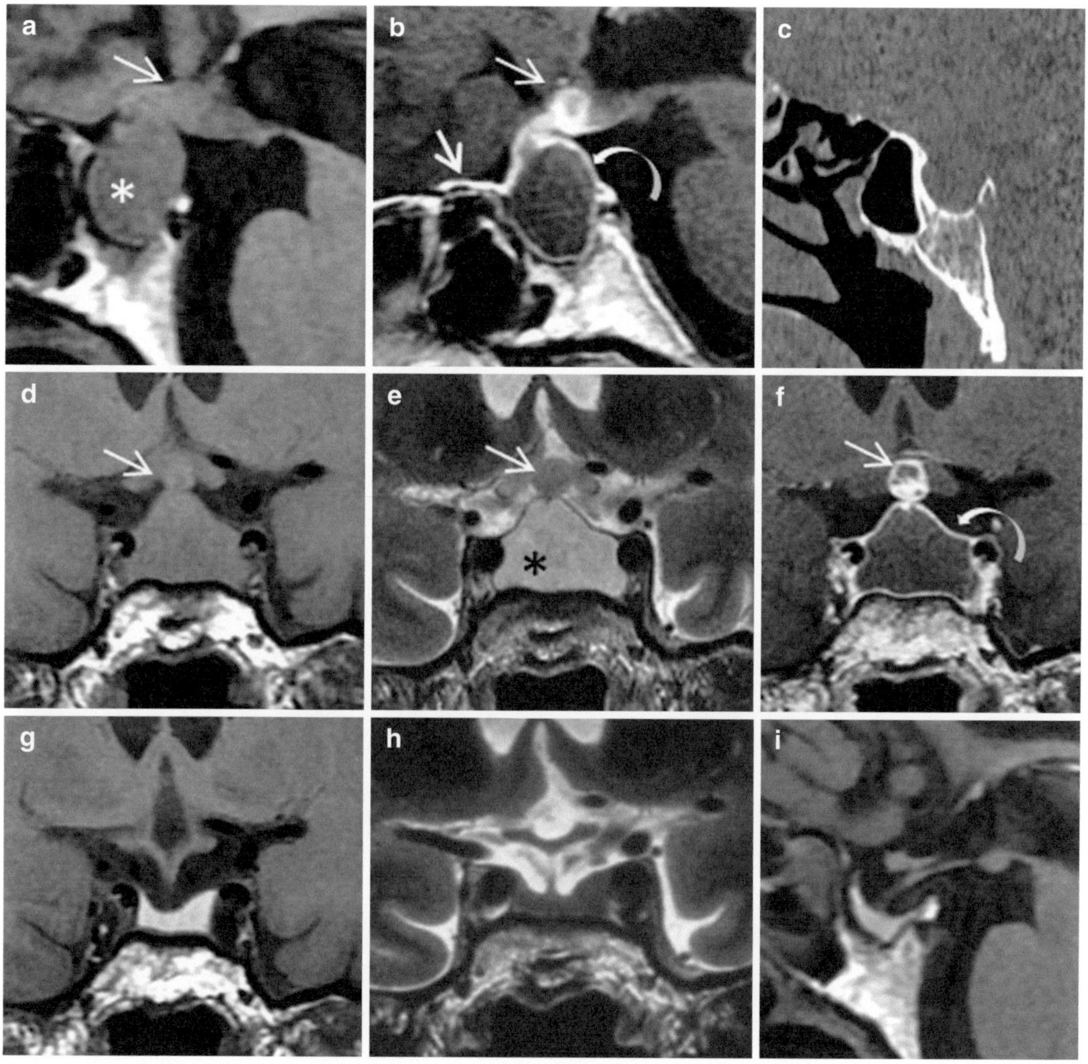

Fig. 20.7 Infected RCC in a 61-year-old man. Sudden onset of severe frontal headache rapidly followed by asthenia, shiver, and right third oculomotor nerve palsy. Lumbar puncture in favor of bacterial meningitis. (**a**, **b**) Sagittal T1 and CE T1 WIs. (**c**) Reformatted CT. (**d–f**) Coronal T1, T2, and CE T1 WIs. Thickened infundibulum (*thin arrow*) and intra-suprasellar mass (*asterisk*) slightly T1 hypointense relative to the brainstem and T2 hyperintense. Marked enhancement of the presellar dura (*thick arrow*) and the cyst wall (*curved arrow*). Infected RCC confirmed at surgery. (**g–i**) Coronal T1, T2, and sagittal T1 WIs 2 months later. Persistent pituitary insufficiency. Residual frankly T1-hyperintense intrasellar content confirming positively the diagnosis of RCC

Fig. 20.6 Complicated RCC in a 47-year-old man. Sudden onset of panhypopituitarism 3 months previously. No headache. (**a–c**) Coronal T1, T2, and CE T1 WIs. (**d–f**) Sagittal T1, T2, and CE T1 WIs. Intra- and suprasellar mass mildly T1 hyperintense and T2 hyperintense. Intracystic nodule (*arrow*). Marked postcontrast rim enhancement. At surgery, yellow-brown viscous liquid

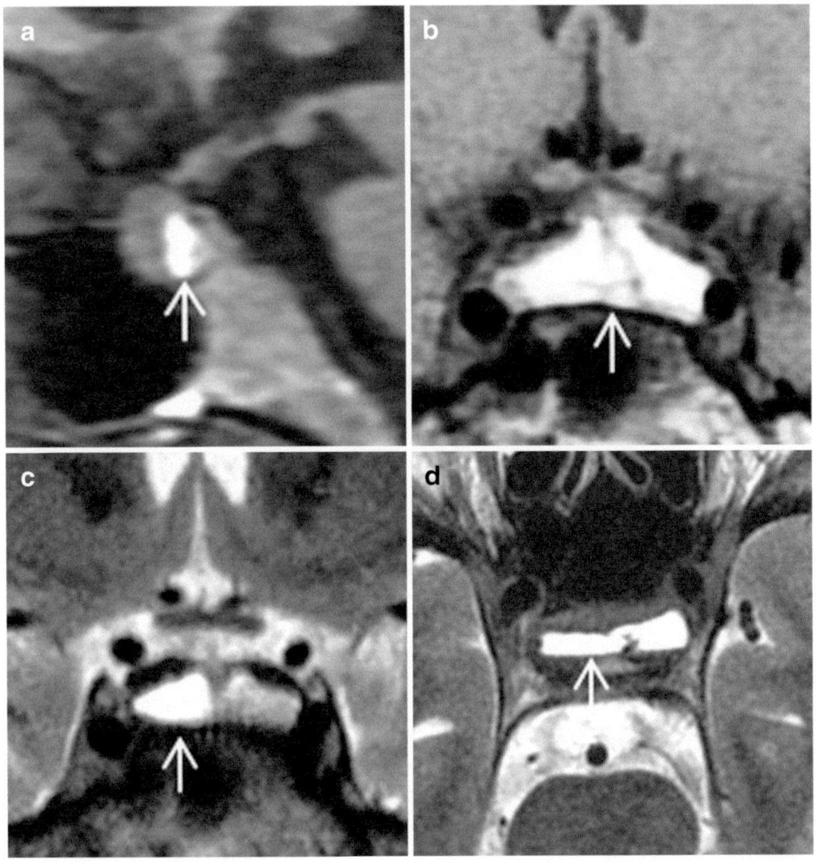

Fig. 20.8 Presumed ruptured RCC in a 31-year-old pregnant woman 3 weeks before delivery. Acute headache. Aseptic meningitis confirmed by lumbar puncture. (**a**) Sagittal T1. (**b**, **c**) Coronal T1 and T2 WIs. (**d**) Axial T2WI. T1- and T2-hyperintense mass located between anterior pituitary and posterior pituitary with a cracked pattern evoking a ruptured RCC (*arrow*)

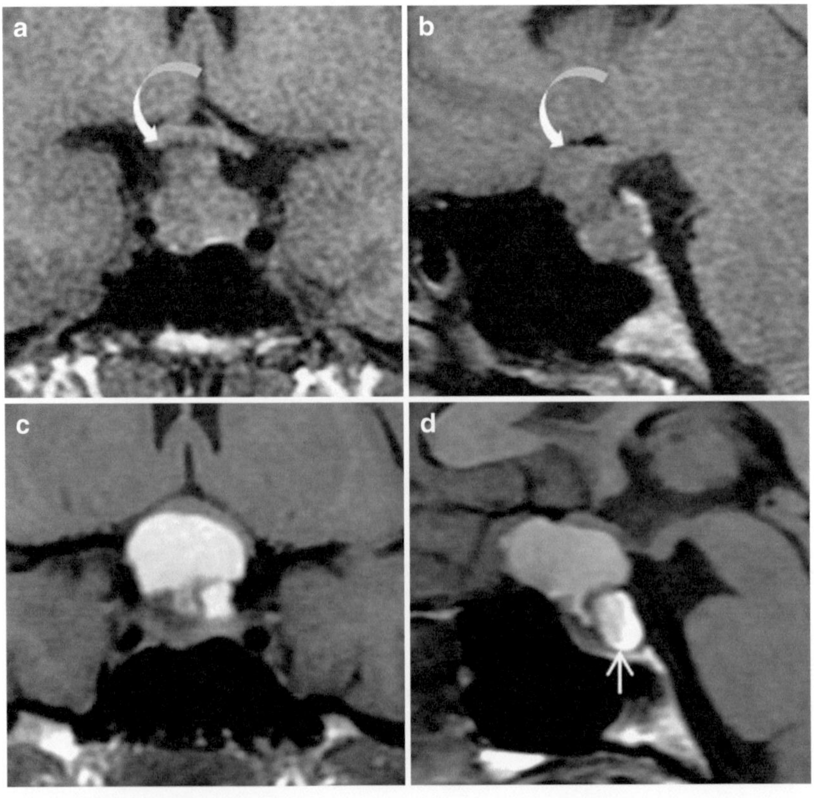

Fig. 20.9 RCC hemorrhagic apoplexy in a 37-year-old woman. Amenorrhea for 1 year, increased weight, altered vision. (**a**, **b**) Coronal and sagittal T1WIs at diagnosis. T1-isointense intra-suprasellar mass abutting the optic chiasm (*arrow*). (**c**, **d**) Sudden severe headache 2 months later. Coronal and sagittal T1WIs without contrast. Dramatic size increase and T1 hyperintensity of the cyst with a fluid-fluid level (*arrow*) indicating intracystic hemorrhage

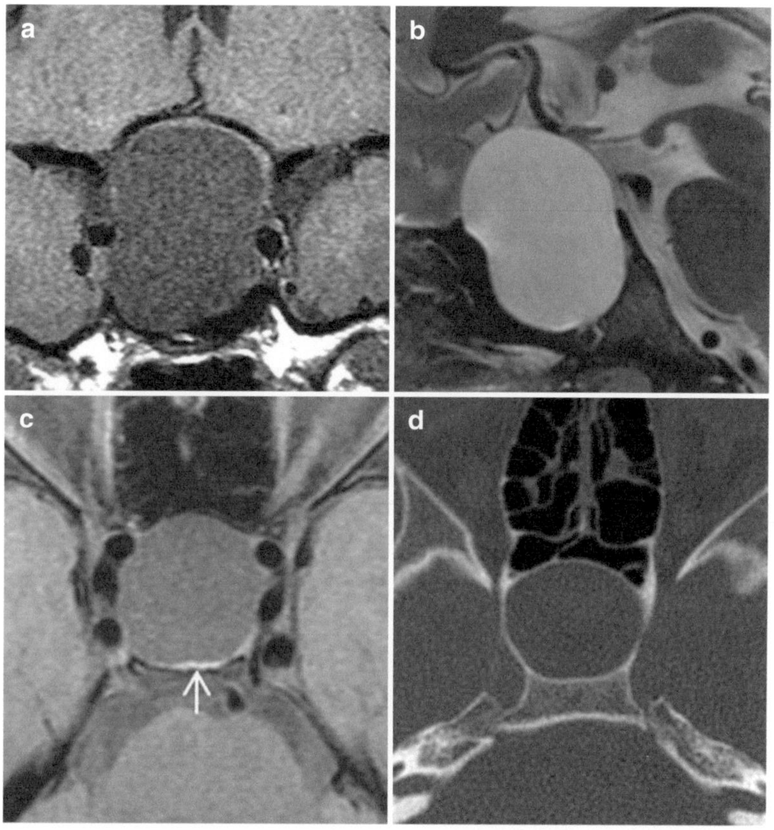

Fig. 20.10 RCC with suprasellar extension in an 18-year-old man with hypogonadism, bilateral visual field defect, and mild headache. (**a**) Coronal T1WI, (**b**) sagittal T2WI, (**c**) axial T2WI, (**d**) axial CT. Large intra-suprasellar cystic mass, hypointense on T1 and hyperintense on T2, compressing the optic chiasm. Compression of the posterior pituitary (*arrow*). Regular enlargement of the sella

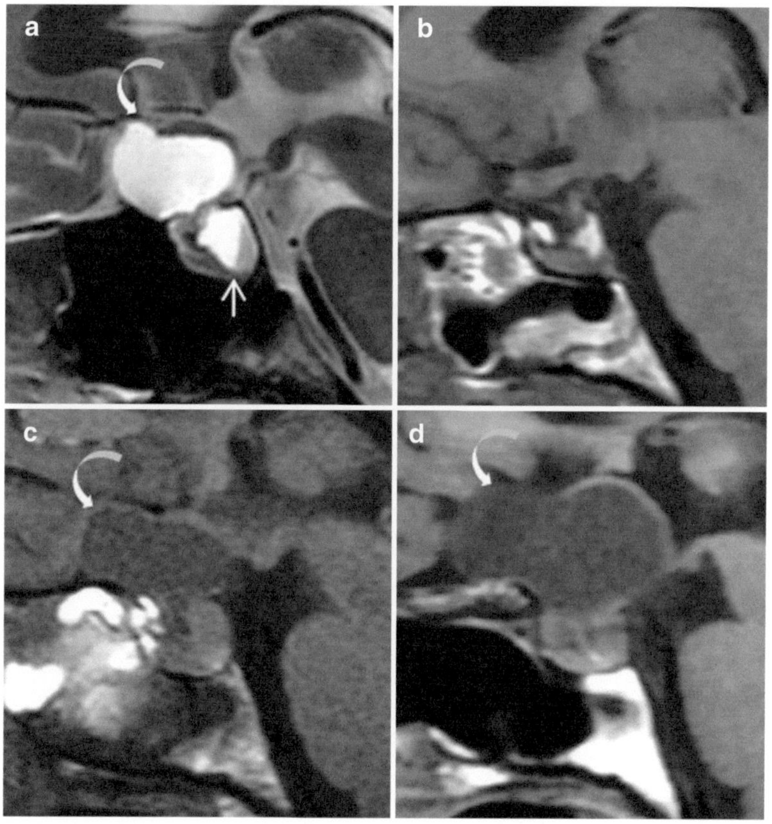

Fig. 20.11 Same patient as Fig. 20.9. RCC evolution. (**a**) Sagittal T2WI before surgery. (**b**) Sagittal T1WI 4 days after surgery. The cyst has disappeared. (**c**, **d**) Sagittal T1WIs. Rapid cyst recurrences (*arrows*) after cyst puncture

Further Reading

Binning MJ, Liu JK, Gannon J et al (2008) Hemorrhagic and nonhemorrhagic Rathke cleft cysts mimicking pituitary apoplexy. J Neurosurg 108(1):3–8

Han SJ, Rolston JD, Jahangiri A et al (2014) Rathke cleft cysts: review of natural history and surgical outcomes. J Neurooncol 117(2):197–203

Trifanescu R, Ansorge O, Wass JA et al (2012) Rathke cleft cysts. Clin Endocrinol (Oxf) 76(2):151–160

21 Pituitary Adenoma and Concomitant Sellar Lesions

Jean-François Bonneville

The concomitance of two different pathologies within the sella is considered very rare in the clinical setting but not in autopsy studies. From a radiological point of view and since the advent of high-field MRI scanners, particularly 3.0 T, pituitary adenomas and Rathke cleft cysts (RCC) coexist not infrequently, particularly if tiny intrasellar RCC are considered: millimetric T1-hyperintense cysts in contact with the anterior surface of the posterior lobe are frequently missed if axial T1W images are not obtained. Small (2–3 mm in diameter) RCC located at the junction of the pituitary stalk and the anterior pituitary are also frequent (Fig. 21.1)

Diagnosis of coexisting pituitary adenomas and RCC can be difficult without a careful analysis of the MR images. Isolated intrasellar RCC have a characteristic pattern. Most are mucoid and then hyperintense on T1W images, and present a precise shape and constant position on axial T1W images: they are located strictly on the midline, just in front of the posterior lobe, with a regularly convex anterior surface. In current practice, these characteristics permit one to optimize the frequently made diagnosis of "incidentaloma" in that of "Rathke cleft cyst discovered by chance," and then to propose a medical strategy and follow-up precisely appropriate to the lesion. These immutable characteristics of RCC are modified in the case of a concomitant second pituitary lesion (Fig. 21.2). In these circumstances, the exact diagnosis can become uncertain on conventional sagittal and coronal images, but not on axial T1W images, preferentially T1W fat-saturated images, to avoid the chemical shift artifact made by the often fatty dorsum sellae (Fig. 21.3). T1-hyperintense RCC can sometimes be confused with T1-hyperintense hemorrhagic microadenomas. The images can be very disturbing in cases of pregnancy after medical treatment of a prolactinoma with concomitant RCC (Fig. 21.4). The key is that, if compared with pituitary adenomas, intrasellar RCC are not responsible for a mass effect (Fig. 21.5). Thus in the case of concomitant intrasellar RCC and pituitary microadenoma, it is observed that the adenoma imprints on the cyst—even if the cyst is larger—and never the opposite (Fig. 21.6). This observation indicates low pressure inside the cyst. These features make the diagnosis of concomitant intrasellar pituitary adenoma and RCC simple provided that axial T1W images are obtained. Coexistence of pituitary adenomas with other sellar or parasellar lesions can complicate the diagnosis, for instance, aneurysms (Fig. 59.1) and meningiomas of the sellar diaphragm (Fig. 21.7), cavernous sinus, or tuberculum sellae. Lastly, case reports of double or even triple secreting pituitary adenomas, multihormonal or not, are more frequently being reported alongside the improvement in MRI scanners.

J.-F. Bonneville et al., *MRI of the Pituitary Gland*, DOI 10.1007/978-3-319-29043-0_21

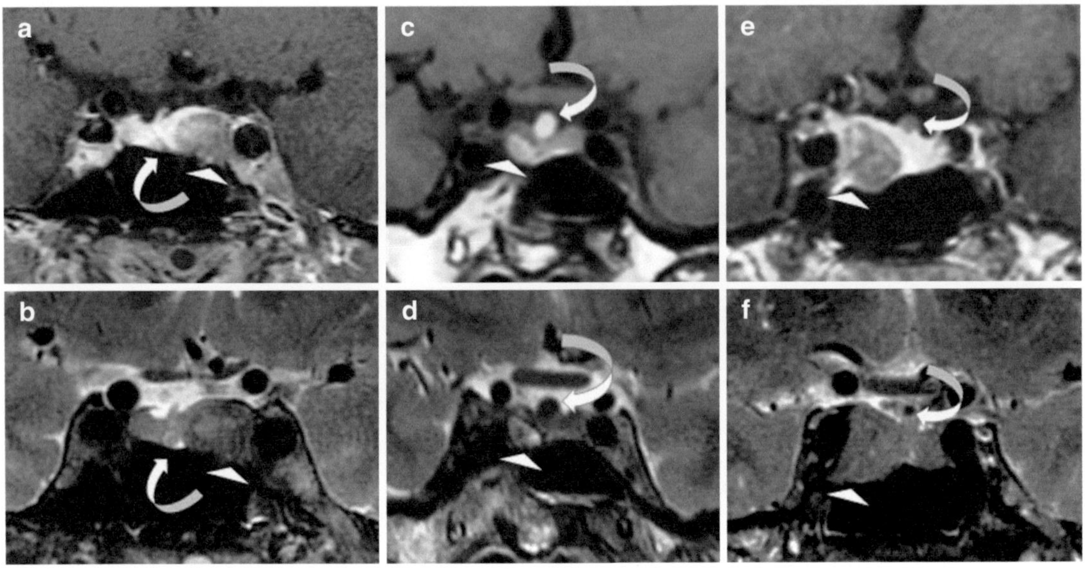

Fig. 21.1 Coexisting microadenomas (*arrowheads*) and RCC (*curved arrows*). (**a**, **b**) Coronal CE T1 and T2 WI. Left-sided pituitary adenoma and RCC on the midline. (**c**, **d**) Coronal T1 and T2 WI. Right-sided pituitary adenoma and RCC at the sellar diaphragm level. The cyst is T1 hyperintense and T2 hypointense. (**e**, **f**) Coronal CE T1 and coronal T2 WI. Right-sided pituitary adenoma and RCC at the sellar diaphragm level. The cyst is not enhanced in (**e**) and presents in (**f**) a characteristic punctiform T2 hypointensity corresponding to a hyperproteinic micronodule

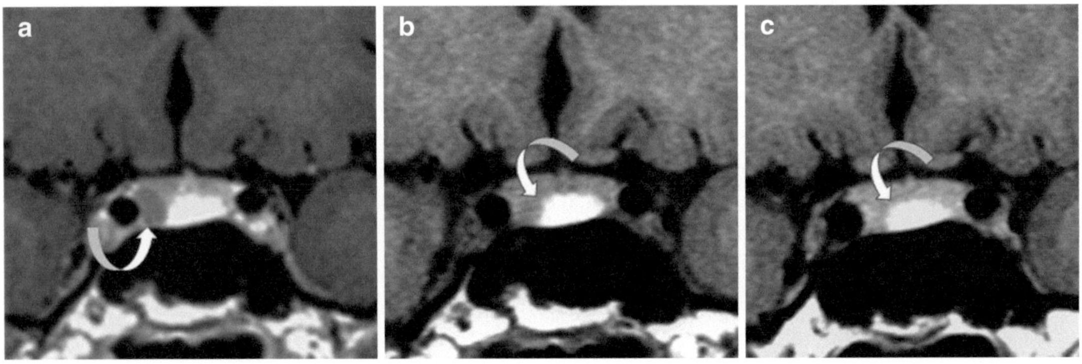

Fig. 21.2 Spaniomenorrhea-galactorrhea in a 26-year-old-woman. RCC and prolactinoma. Prolactin is 68 ng/ml. (**a**, **b**) Coronal CE T1 and T1 WI without contrast: right-sided microprolactinoma (*arrow*) in contact with a large T1-hyperintense RCC. In (**b**), better demonstration of the mass effect caused by the adenoma: unilateral bulging of the sellar diaphragm, displacement of the pituitary stalk, lowering of the sellar floor, and imprint of the adenoma onto the right margin of an RCC. (**c**) After 2 months of treatment with cabergoline, prolactin is 4 ng/ml; partial shrinkage of the adenoma and disappearance of its imprint onto the cyst

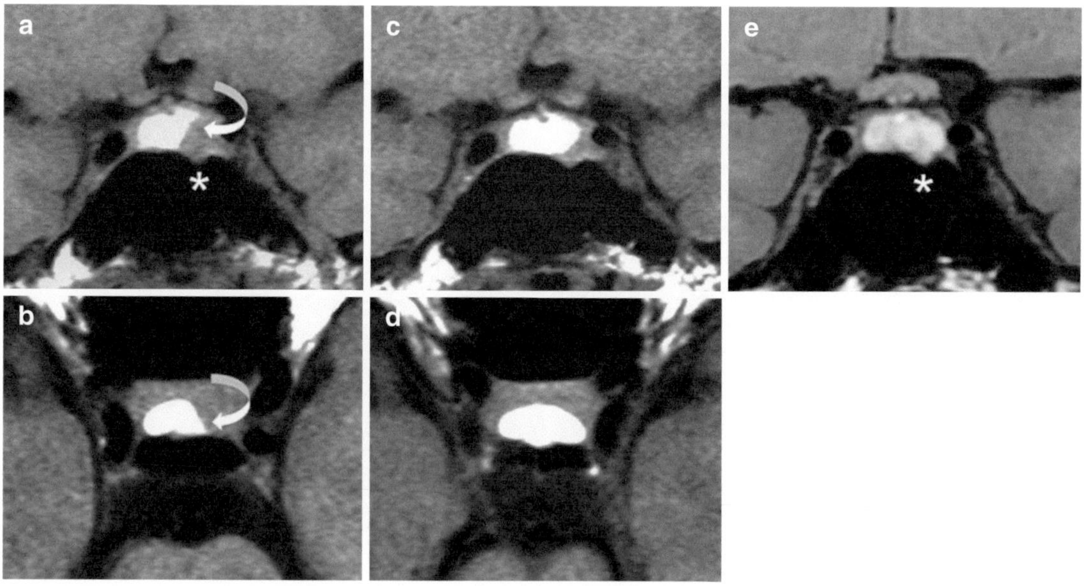

Fig. 21.3 Secondary amenorrhea in a 22-year-old woman. Prolactin is 81 ng/ml. (**a**, **b**) Coronal and axial T1WI. A left-sided T1-isointense prolactinoma (*curved arrow*) is responsible for a mass effect onto the sellar diaphragm, the pituitary stalk, and the sellar floor (*asterisk*); it imprints markedly onto the left margin of an RCC. The diagnosis is easier on the axial image. (**c**, **d**) Same sequences after 6 months of treatment with cabergoline. Shrinkage of the adenoma; the RCC now has its usual perfectly symmetrical shape on axial view. (**e**) Coronal T1WI 5 years later. The patient is always on cabergoline; the cyst occupies the whole sella and evens fills a small depression of the sellar floor originally created by the microprolactinoma (*asterisk*)

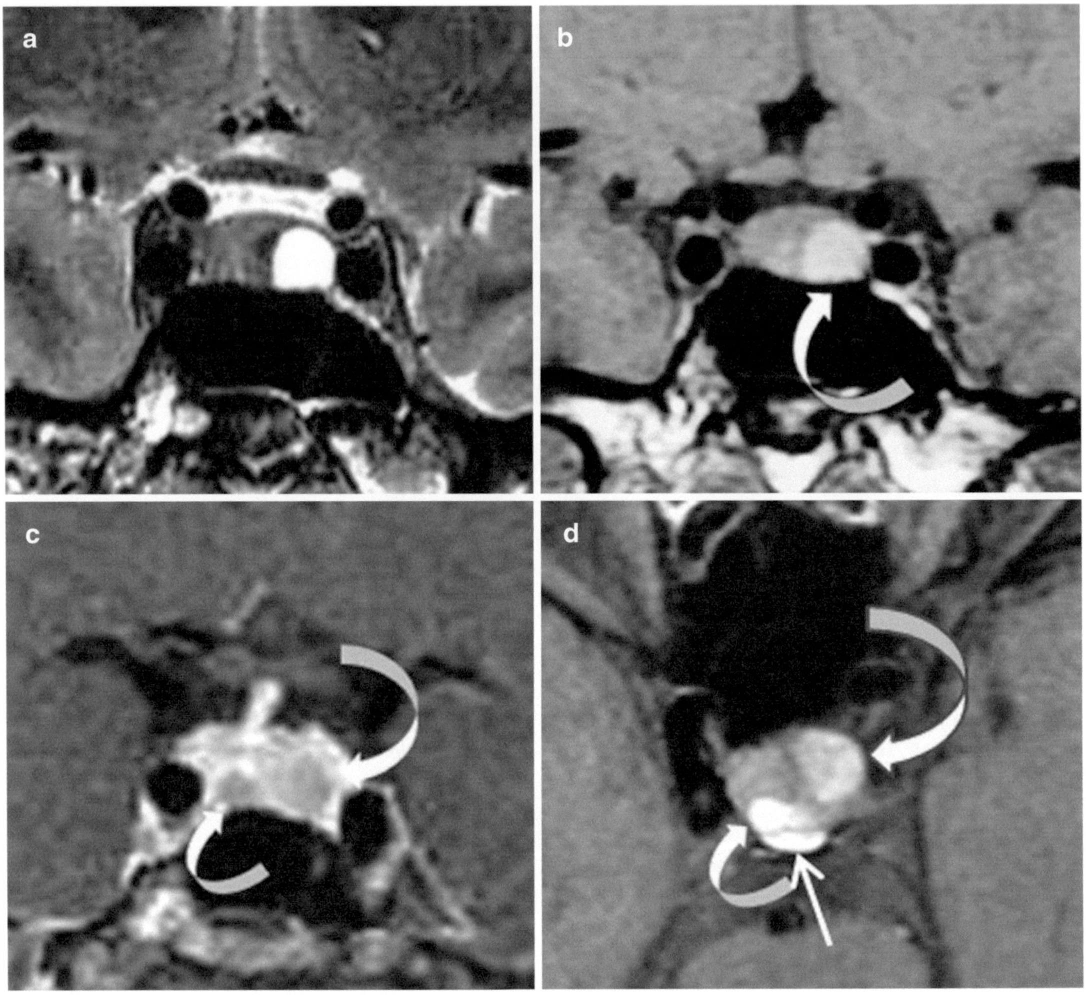

Fig. 21.4 Post-pill amenorrhea. Prolactin is 60 ng/ml. Coronal T2 (**a**), unenhanced T1 (**b**), and CE T1 WI (**c**) reveal a left-sided microprolactinoma (*large curved arrow*). Hyperintensity on T1WI is in favor of an hemorrhagic transformation. After gadolinium injection (**c**), a 4-mm right-sided lesion is demonstrated slightly posterior to the adenoma (*small curved arrow*). The diagnosis is obtained on axial T1WI without contrast injection (**d**): in front of the posterior lobe (*straight arrow*), a hyperintense RCC (*small curved arrow*) is deformed by the hemorrhagic pituitary adenoma, which imprints on the anterior wall of the sella (*large curved arrow*)

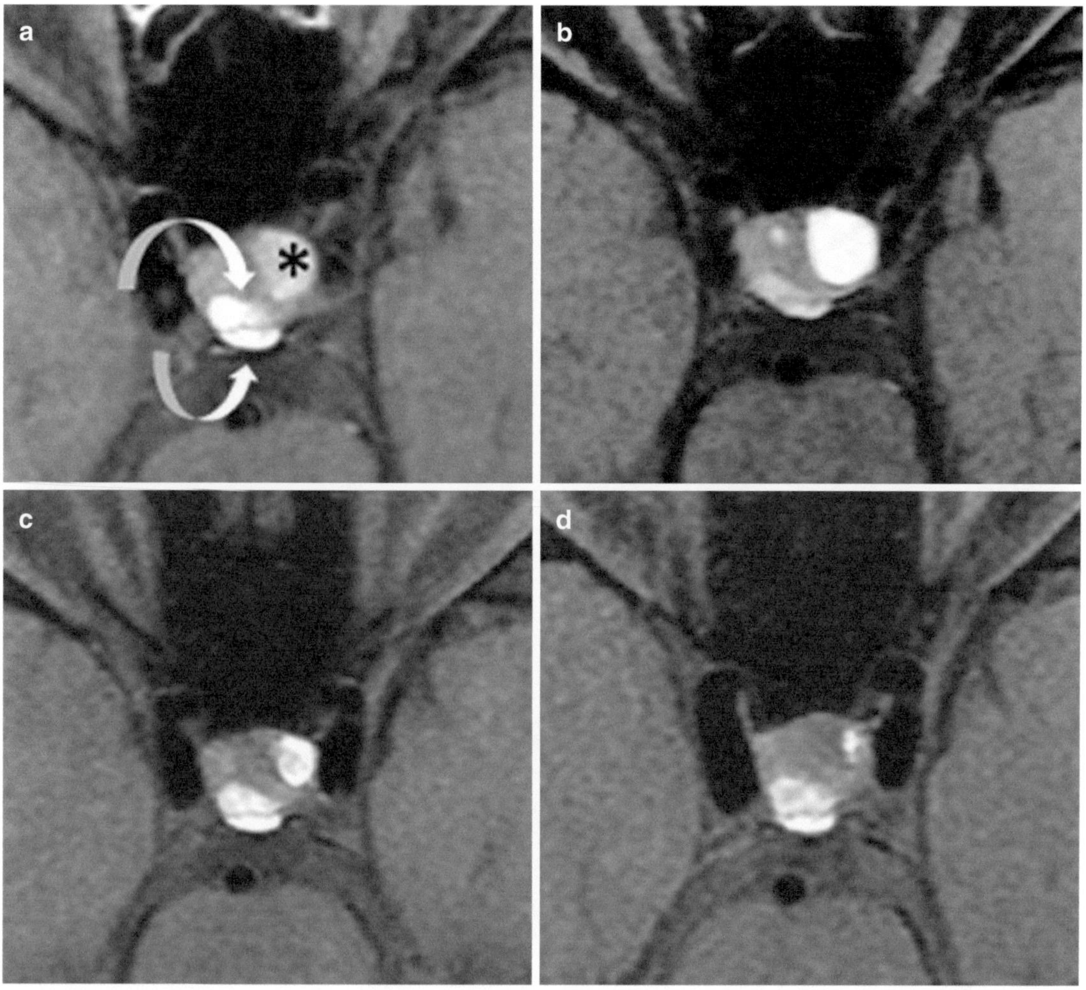

Fig. 21.5 Same patient as Fig. 21.4. Nonenhanced axial T1WIs. (**a**) At presentation. Posterior lobe (*lower arrow*); RCC (*upper arrow*); hemorrhagic prolactinoma (*asterisk*). A pregnancy occurs after cabergoline treatment; cabergoline is withdrawn. Axial T1WI (**b**) is obtained at the 7th month of pregnancy. The hemorrhagic microprolactinoma is slightly enlarged, resulting in an increased compression of the RCC; the posterior lobe is slightly flattened. Three months after normal delivery (**c**), the prolactinoma is decreased in size and the RCC has re-expanded. (**d**) Two years later, normal prolactin level with cabergoline: further expansion of the cyst together with shrinkage of the adenoma

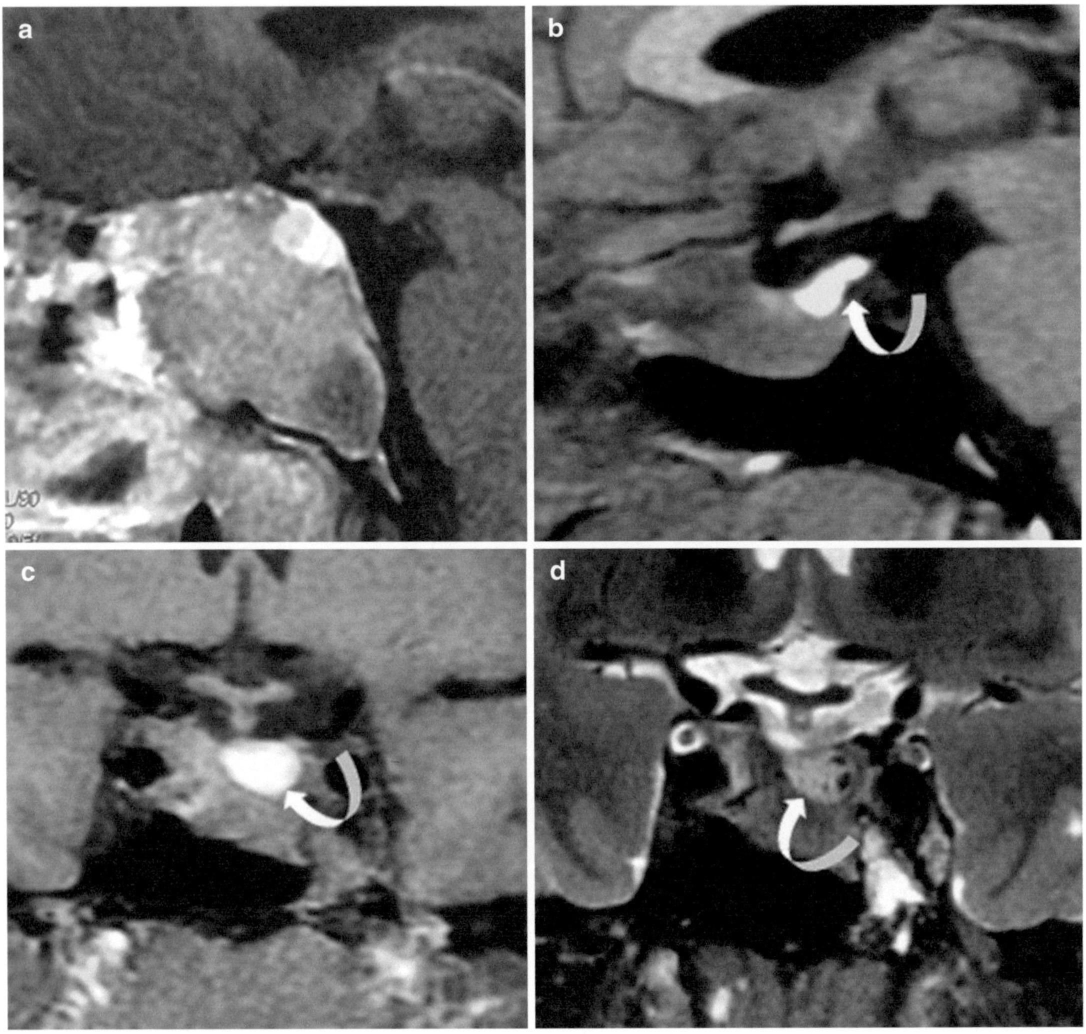

Fig. 21.6 Mixed GH-prolactin pituitary adenoma in a 31-year-old man with gynecomastia. IGF1 is 1,269 ng/ml and prolactin 260 ng/ml. (**a**) Sagittal CE T1WI (erroneously, nonenhanced sequences were not obtained) evoked first a "tumor" of the sphenoid sinus before laboratory tests were known. One year later, after treatment with somatostatin analogs and cabergoline: (**b**, **c**) Sagittal and coronal T1WIs and (**d**) coronal T2WI. Shrinkage of the adenoma; a bright spot identified at the posterior part of the sella (*arrow*) is too large to represent vasopressin storage location. Pathognomonic pattern of an RCC with intracystic T2-hypointense hyperproteinic micronodules

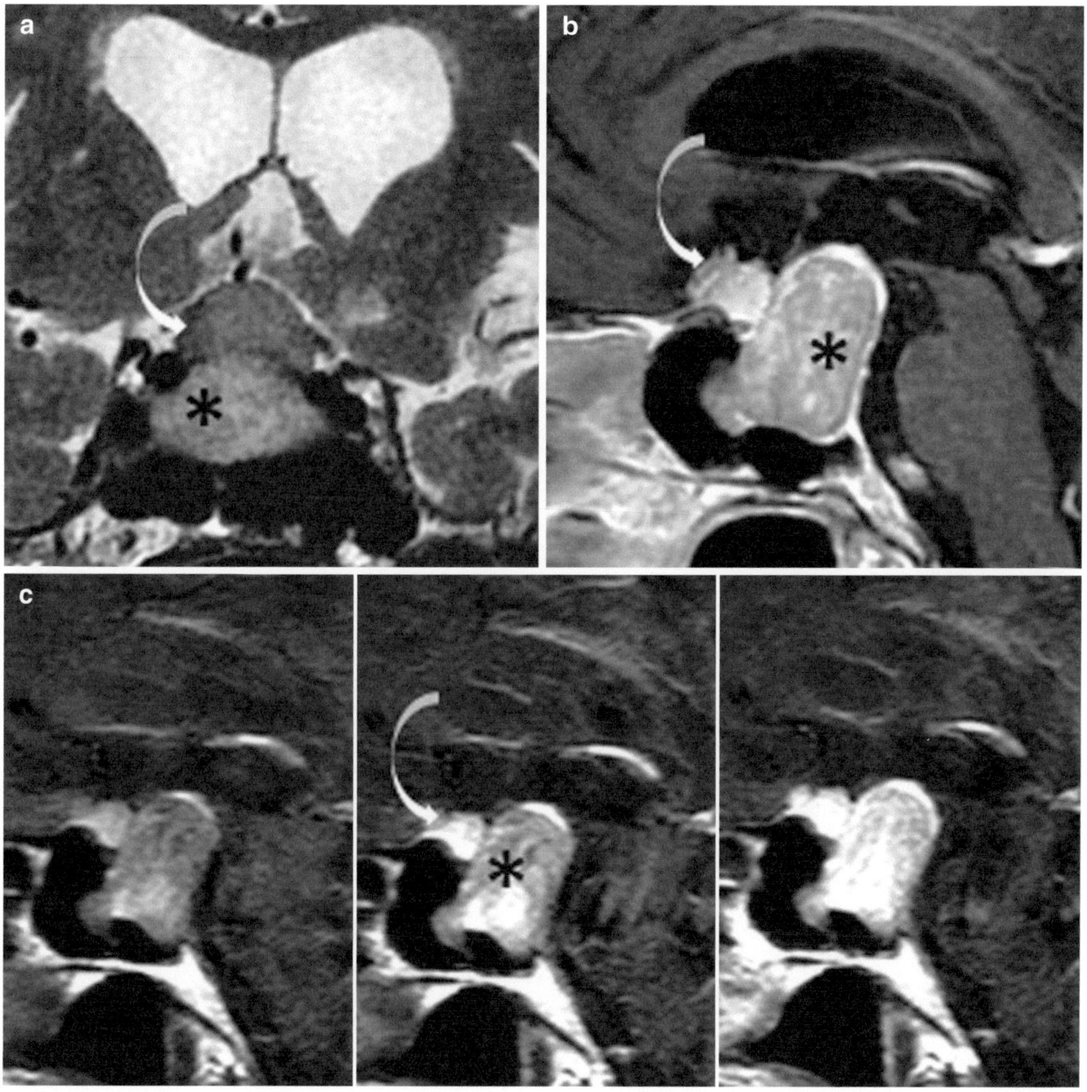

Fig. 21.7 Concomitant pituitary macroadenoma and tuberculum sellae meningioma. (**a**) Coronal T2WI, (**b**) sagittal CE T1WI, (**c**) dynamic images. The meningioma (*arrow*) appears less T2 hyperintense than the adenoma (*asterisk*) in (**a**) and more enhanced after gadolinium injection in (**b**). On dynamic imaging (**c**), meningioma enhancement appears first

Further Reading

Jin G, Hao S, Xie J et al (2013) Collision tumors of the sella: coexistence of pituitary adenoma and craniopharyngioma in the sellar region. World J Surg Oncol 11:178

Meij BP, Lopes MB, Vance ML et al (2000) Double pituitary lesions in three patients with Cushing's disease. Pituitary 3(3):159–168

Noh SJ, Ahn JY, Lee KS, Kim SH (2007) Pituitary adenoma and concomitant Rathke's cleft cyst. Acta Neurochir (Wien) 149:1223–1228

22 Craniopharyngioma

Sonia Nagi

Craniopharyngioma is an epithelial tumor, classified as WHO grade 1. Although histologically benign, craniopharyngiomas are aggressive neoplasms, and recurrences are common because complete surgical resection is difficult. They represent approximately 5 % of all intracranial tumors. Craniopharyngiomas are derived from remnants of the Rathke pouch and can occur anywhere along the course of the craniopharyngeal duct, from the nasopharynx to the third ventricle. They are usually sporadic. Rare cases of adamantinous craniopharyngiomas have been associated with Gardner syndrome, a variant of familial adenomatous polyposis. Craniopharyngiomas are characterized by a bimodal age distribution, with a main peak in children (5–14 years) and a second peak in adults (fifth to seventh decade). They most commonly involve the suprasellar and sellar area (75 %), where they are either anterior or posterior to the optic chiasm. In fewer cases, their location is purely suprasellar (20 %) or entirely intrasellar (5 %). There are two histologic subtypes: the adamantinous type, most common form, typically seen in children and adolescents; and the papillary type, seen almost exclusively in adults. Adamantinous craniopharyngiomas are usually lobulated and cystic tumors, containing a dark greenish brown fluid. These cysts contain variable amounts of cholesterol, keratin, protein, methemoglobin, and necrotic debris, which account for their variable appearance on MRI. They are usually associated with calcification and often demonstrate local brain invasion, being adherent to adjacent vessels and nerves. Papillary craniopharyngiomas are generally well-circumscribed, predominantly solid tumors. The solid component may rarely contain small cystic areas or calcifications. The third ventricle is a common location of this subtype. Clinical symptoms are variable, on account of the variable location. Headache, visual field defects, decreased visual acuity, and hormone disturbance are the common clinical symptoms in the suprasellar location. The most common endocrine dysfunctions encountered in children are growth retardation and delayed or precocious puberty. Global hypopituitarism, hyperprolactinemia, and diabetes insipidus are the other endocrine disorders encountered. Less commonly, patients may present with cognitive impairment or personality change.

Adamantinous craniopharyngiomas classically occur in childhood or adolescence and typically present with three components: solid, cystic, and calcified portions, which occupy the suprasellar cistern (Figs. 22.1, 22.2, 22.3, and 22.4). The cystic component is single or multiple, and usually hyperintense on T1, T2, and FLAIR weighted images because of the presence of proteinaceous liquid. Less commonly, a CSF-like signal pattern can be seen in huge craniopharyngiomas with a thick wall enhancement. The solid component has variable signal intensities and shows contrast enhancement. Small necrotic areas account for its inhomogeneous signal before and after contrast administration. Calcifications

J.-F. Bonneville et al., *MRI of the Pituitary Gland*, DOI 10.1007/978-3-319-29043-0_22

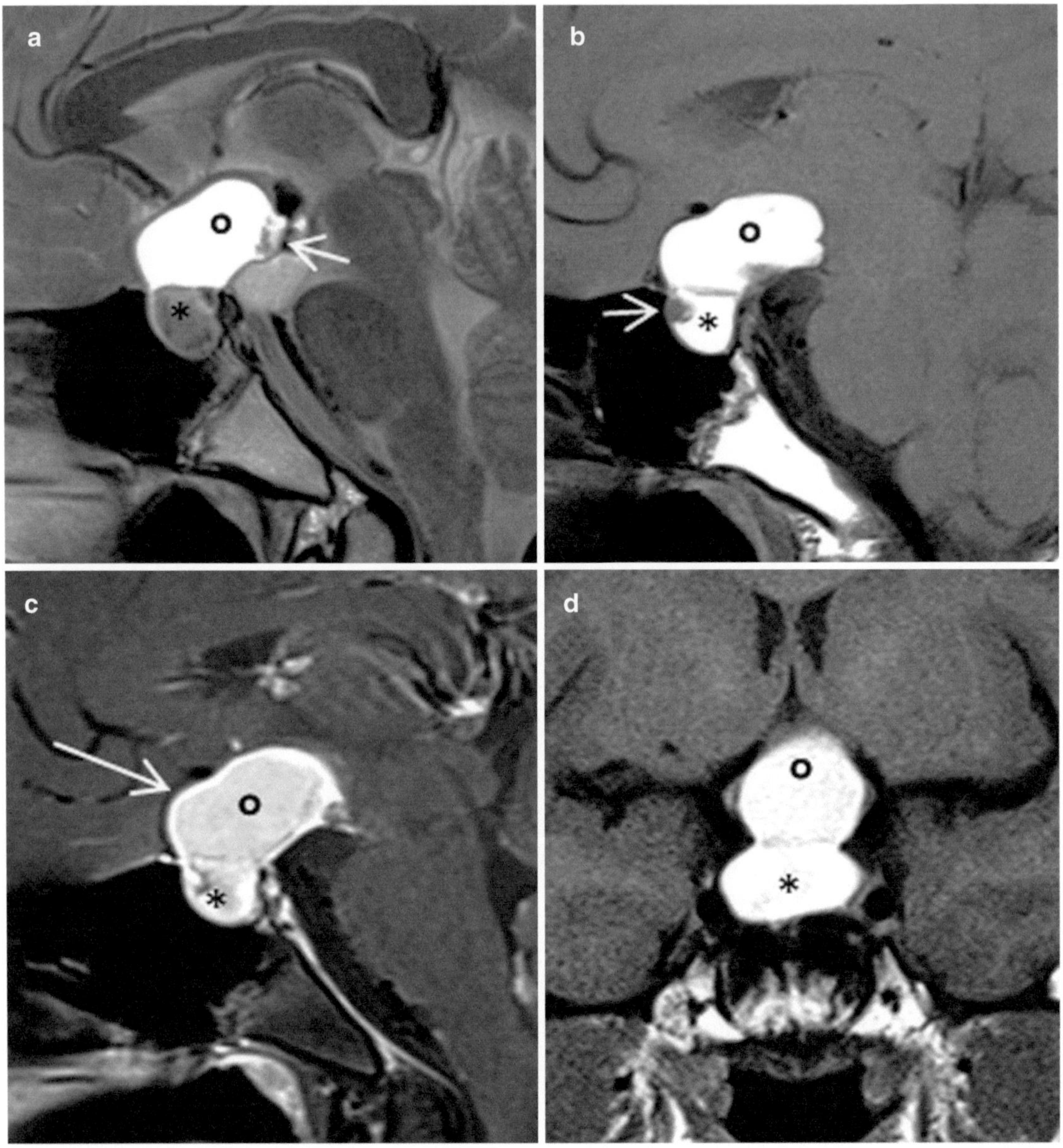

Fig. 22.1 A 16-year-old girl with headaches, secondary amenorrhea, and left hemianopsia. Intra- and suprasellar cystic adamantinous craniopharyngioma. (**a–c**) Sagittal T2, T1 and CE T1 fat-saturated WIs. Intrasellar heterogeneous cyst without sellar change (*asterisk*). Suprasellar hyperintense cyst (*circle*) with thin peripheral enhancement (*long arrow*). Nodular calcifications in both portions (*short arrows*). (**d**) Coronal T1WI. Superior extension with optic chiasm compression

Fig. 22.2 A 7-year-old boy with headaches and vomiting. Suprasellar adamantinomatous craniopharyngioma. (**a**, **b**) Sagittal heavily T2 and CE T1 WIs. (**c**, **d**) Coronal T2 and axial FLAIR WIs. Suprasellar multiloculated mixed mass with varying mainly bright signal intensities (*asterisk*) and solid calcified component heterogeneously enhanced (*thick arrow*). Cyst wall enhancement (*thin arrows*). Note posterior fossa extension with brainstem and cerebellar compression (*curved arrow*). Hydrocephalus by interventricular foramen obstruction. (**e**, **f**) Axial T1 and T2*WIs. Spontaneous hyperintense cyst signal due to proteinaceous content (*asterisk*). Markedly hypointense calcifications (*thick arrow*)

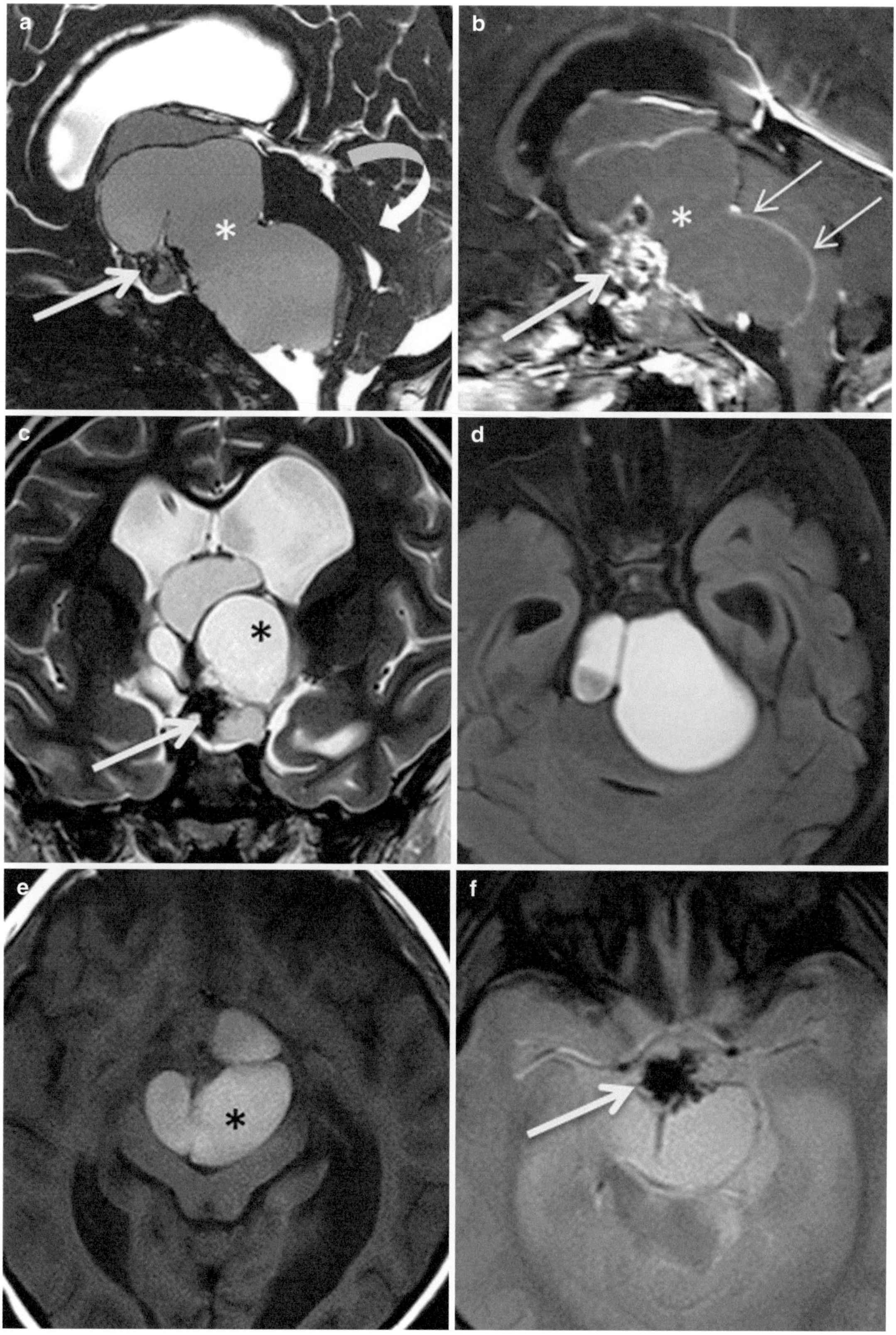
a
b
c
d
e
f

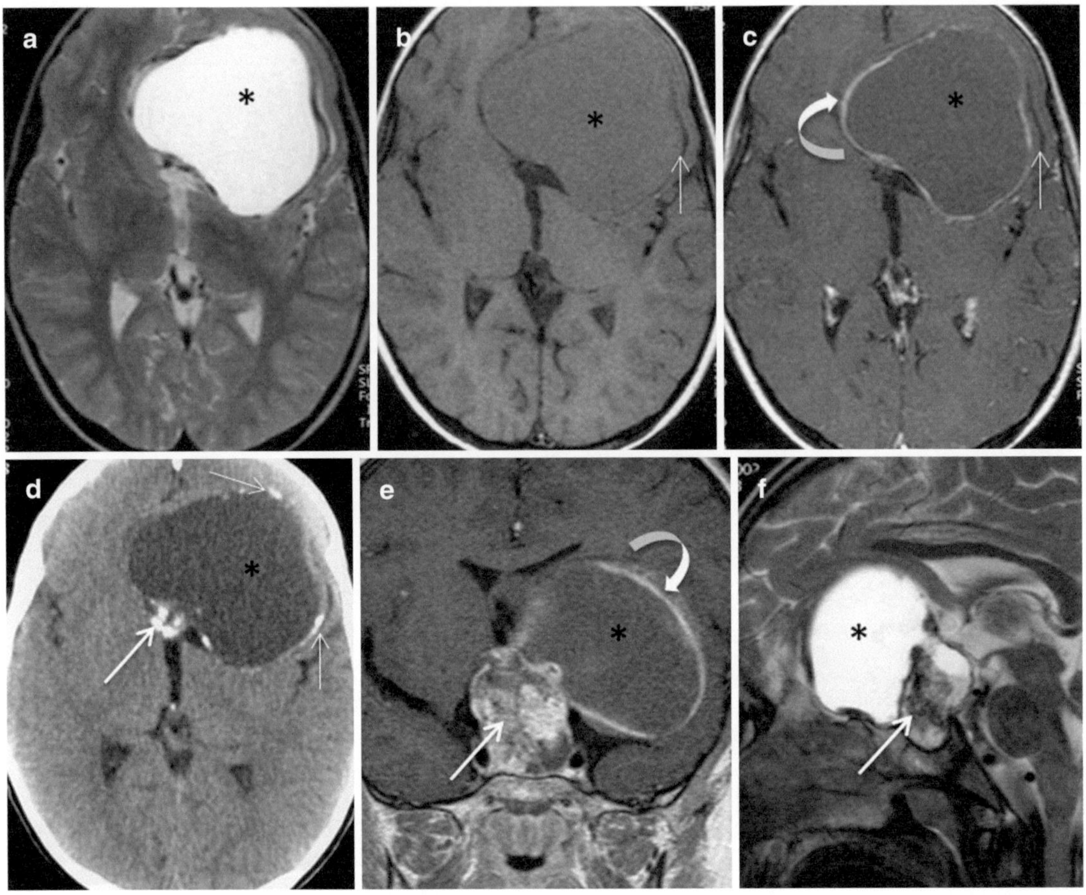

Fig. 22.3 An 8-year-old boy with afebrile seizures, bilateral optic atrophy, reduced visual acuity, and left temporal hemianopia. Intra- and suprasellar adamantinomatous craniopharyngioma. (**a–d**) Axial T2, T1, CE T1 WIs and CT scan. (**e**) Coronal CE T1WI. (**f**) Sagittal T2WI. Intra- and suprasellar mixed mass with cystic (*asterisk*) and calcified tissular component (*arrow*). The cyst wall is T1 hypointense and hyperdense with discontinuous calcifications (*thin arrows*). Heterogeneous enhancement of the solid component (*arrows*). Cyst wall enhancement (*curved arrows*)

are common (90 % of cases) and are better demonstrated by T2* sequence. However, their confirmation by a CT scan is sometimes necessary. Lipid resonances are usually detected in proton MR spectroscopy. Huge craniopharyngiomas can extend in all directions. The sella is often enlarged and may be eroded.

Papillary craniopharyngiomas usually appear as a solid or mixed, predominantly solid and cystic, spherical tumor in the suprasellar region (Fig. 22.4). They are characterized by a more upward growth toward the third ventricle. The solid parts classically show isointense signal intensity on T1 and T2 WI, with a hypointense signal on DWI with increased apparent diffusion coefficient reflecting the low-grade character. They present homogeneous or reticular enhancement because of their small necrotic areas. They less frequently contain calcifications. Nevertheless, their imaging features are nonspecific, and differential diagnosis is based on the age of the patient and the location of the tumor. Surgical removal is easier in this subtype than in the adamantinous type. Peritumoral edema spreading along the optic tracts was initially considered to be specific to craniopharyngiomas. Similar optic tract edema has been described since then in other parasellar tumors such as ade-

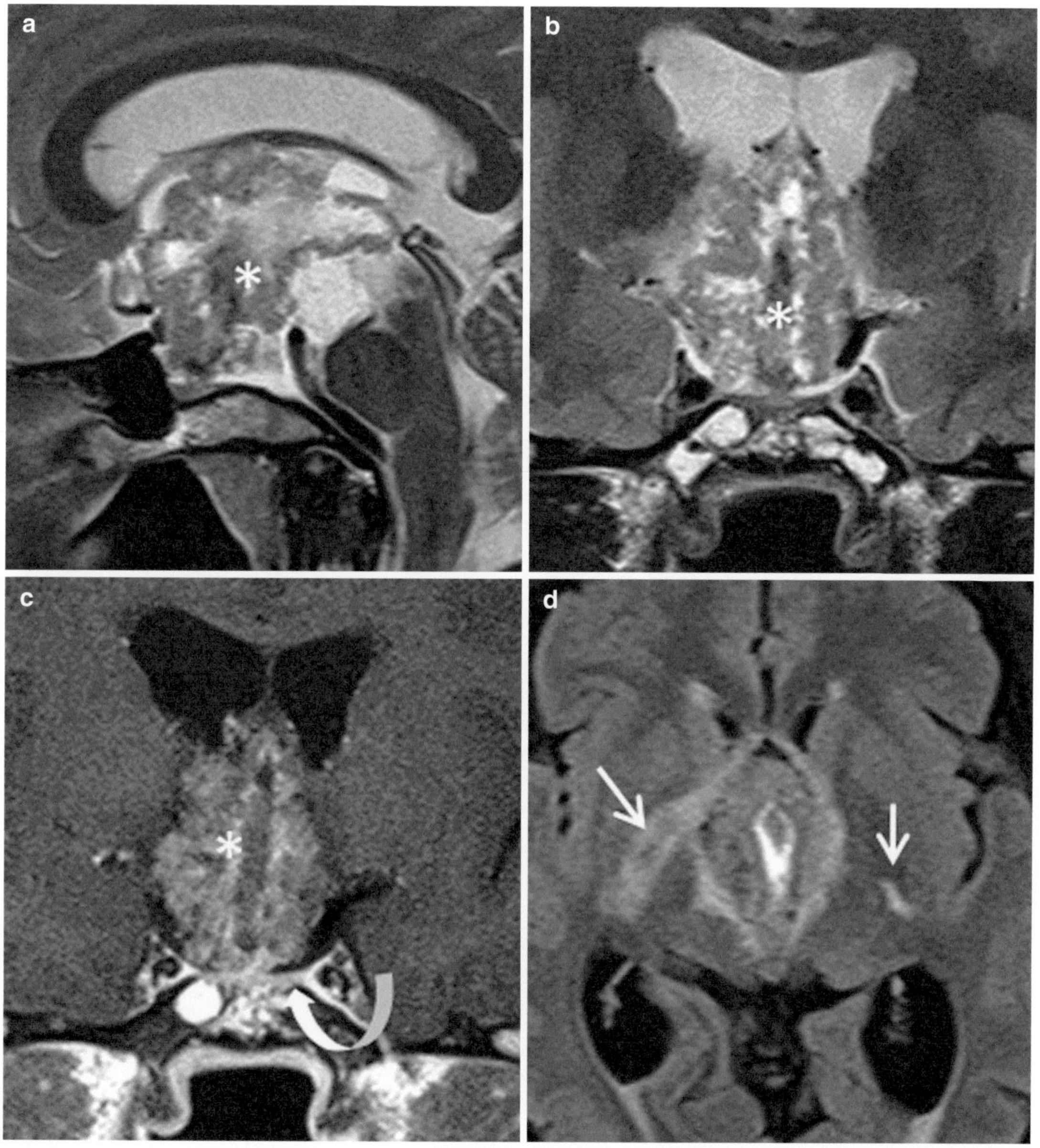

Fig. 22.4 A 28-year-old man with hypogonadotropic hypogonadism and diabetes insipidus. Suprasellar papillary craniopharyngioma. (**a**, **b**) Sagittal and coronal T2WIs. Mixed predominantly solid and cystic suprasellar mass with iso- to hyperintense signal (*asterisk*). (**c**) Coronal CE T1WI. Heterogeneous enhancement (*asterisk*), flattened pituitary gland (*curved arrow*). (**d**) Axial FLAIR WI. Bilateral edema along optic tracts (*arrows*)

nomas, germ cell tumors, gliomas, meningiomas, and lymphomas. This could be related to distension of perivascular spaces, which represent a drainage route of interstitial fluid into the subarachnoid space, their outflow pathway into the subarachnoid spaces being blocked by suprasellar tumor (Figs. 22.4 and 22.5). Occasionally, craniopharyngiomas are located in the third ventricle (Fig. 22.6). Rare locations include posterior fossa, sphenoid bone, and nasopharynx. Distant spread of craniopharyngioma is a rare complication that occurs independently of the subtype. Locations include cerebral hemispheres, posterior fossa, brainstem, basal ganglia, and lumbar

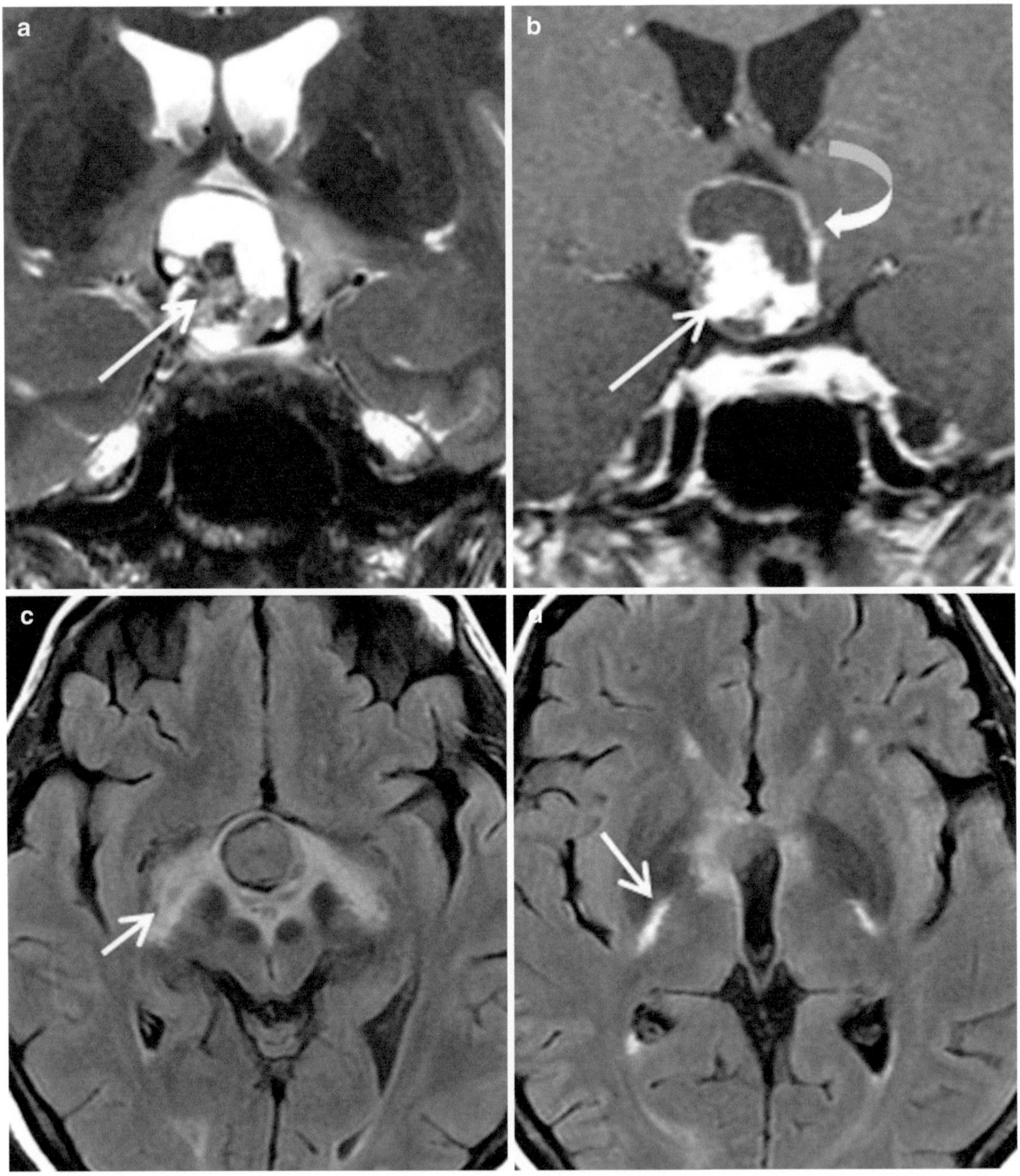

Fig. 22.5 A 22-year-old woman with reduced visual acuity. Suprasellar adamantinous craniopharyngioma. (**a**, **b**) Coronal T2 and CE T1WIs. Suprasellar mass with cystic component enhancing peripherally (*curved arrow*) and solid component enhancing heterogeneously (*long arrow*). (**c**, **d**) Axial FLAIR WI. Bilateral marked edema along the optic tracts (*short arrows*)

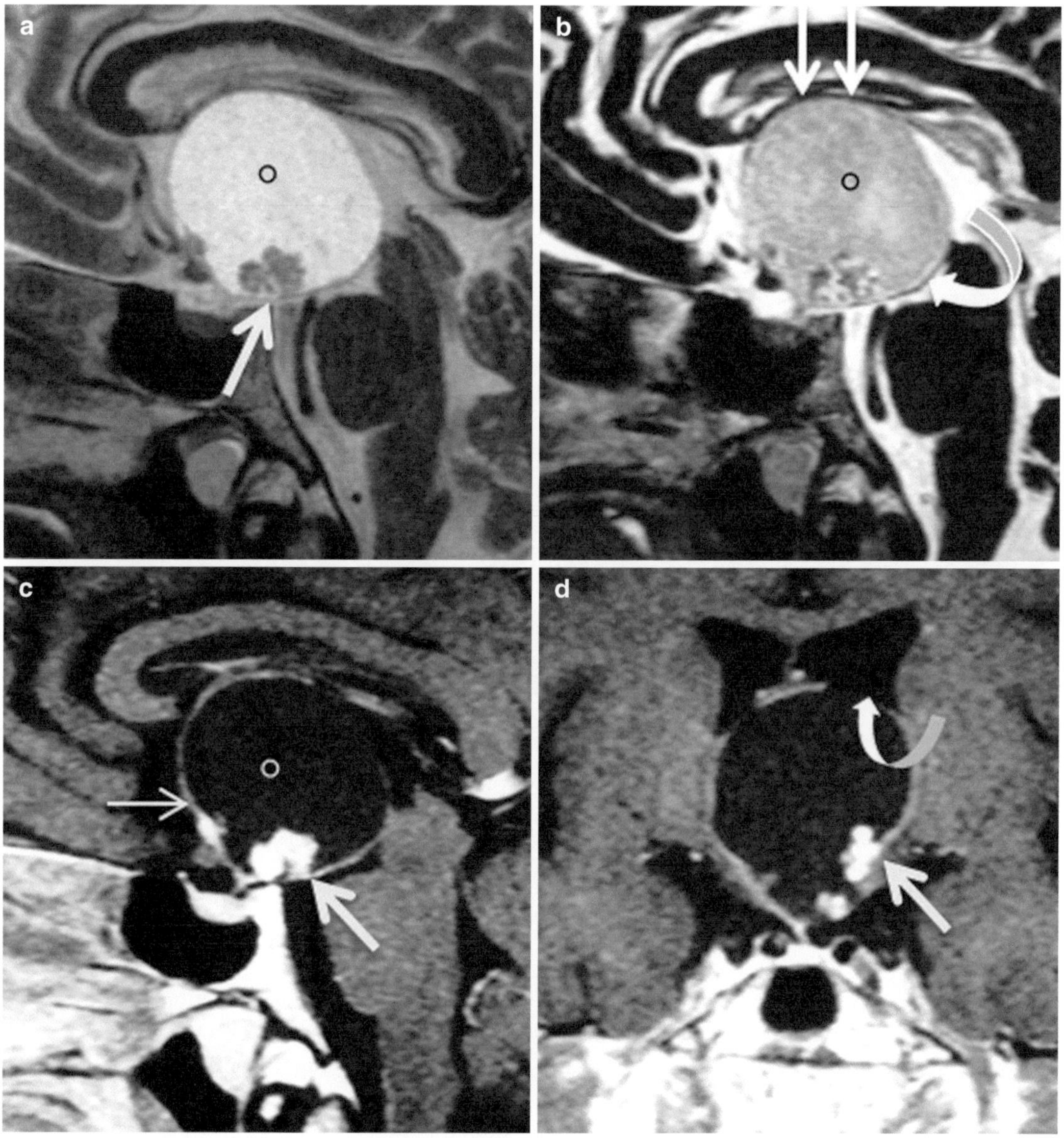

Fig. 22.6 A 54-year-old man with headaches, visual disturbance, difficulty in walking, and memory disorder. Third ventricular craniopharyngioma. (**a–c**) Sagittal T2, heavily T2, and CE T1 WIs. Mixed cystic (*circle*) and tissular (*thick arrow*) mass within the third ventricle. Tissular portion (*thick arrow*) and thin wall cyst (*thin arrow*) enhancement. Note the downward bowing of the floor of the third ventricle by the mass (*curved arrow*) and fornix displacement (*double thick arrow*). (**d**) Coronal CE T1WI. Interventricular foramen obstruction (*curved arrow*). Note normal pituitary gland

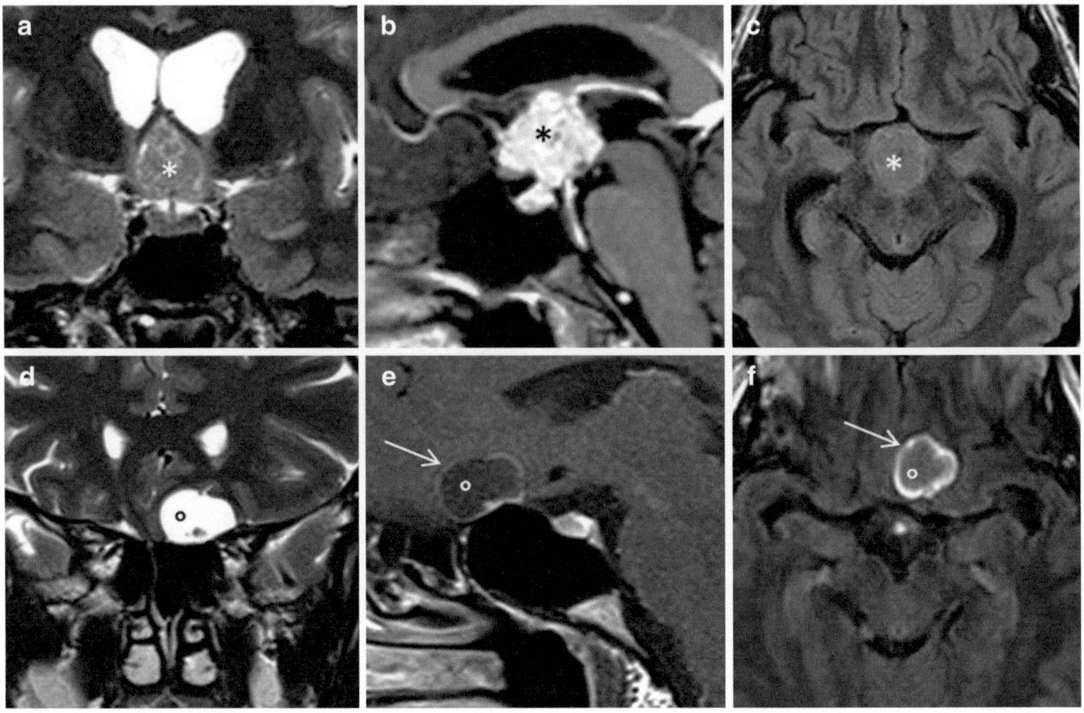

Fig. 22.7 A 43-year-old woman with headaches. Suprasellar papillary craniopharyngioma with recurrence 1 year after surgery away from suprasellar region, along the surgery path. (**a**) Coronal T2WI. Isointense suprasellar mass (*asterisk*). (**b**) Sagittal CE T1WI. Reticular diffuse enhancement (*asterisk*). (**c**) Axial FLAIR WI. Homogeneous isointense signal (*asterisk*). One year after complete surgical resection: (**d**) Coronal T2WI. Extra-axial left parasagittal and presellar hyperintense cystic mass (*circle*). (**e**) Sagittal CE T1WI. Peripheral enhancement (*thin arrow*) sparing the central area (*circle*). No suprasellar tumor relapse. (**f**) Axial FLAIR WI. Hyperintense cyst wall (*thin arrow*) and hypointense central area (*circle*)

spine. The mechanism is poorly understood, but most cases are thought to result from spread along the surgical path (Fig. 22.7). Metastatic leptomeningeal craniopharyngiomas have been reported, as a result of dissemination along CSF pathways (Fig. 22.8). Craniopharyngiomas with multiple recurrences and malignant transformations have been reported. The key factor associated with craniopharyngioma recurrence is the quality of surgical resection. Adhesion or encasement of adjacent cranial nerves or vessels (Fig. 22.7) significantly increases surgical morbidity. Differential diagnosis includes Rathke cleft cyst (Fig. 22.9), pituitary adenoma (Fig. 22.10), dermoid cyst, epidermoid cyst, teratoma, and pilomyxoid astrocytoma. Treatment usually consists of surgical resection with or without adjuvant radiation therapy.

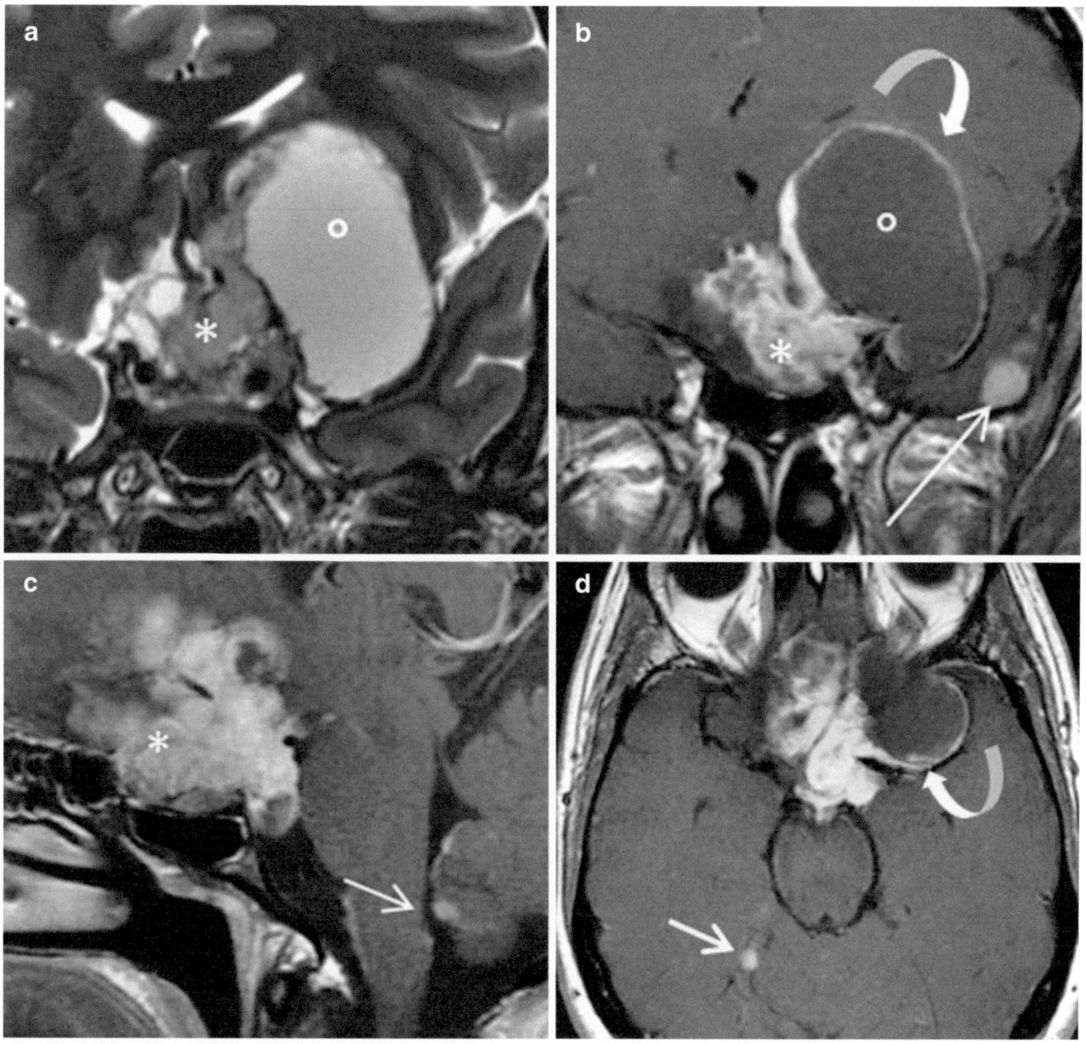

Fig. 22.8 A 32-year-old woman with headaches. Intra- and suprasellar adamantinous craniopharyngioma with concomitant leptomeningeal metastasis. (**a**, **b**) Coronal T2 and CE T1 WIs. Solid heterogeneous enhanced portion (*asterisk*), cystic portion (*circle*) with ring enhancement (*curved arrow*). Extra-axial left temporal nodular enhancement (*long arrow*). (**c**, **d**) Sagittal and axial CE T1WIs. Leptomeningeal enhancement in posterior fossa involving medulla and inferior roof of fourth ventricle (*short arrow*). Nodular enhancement in tentorium cerebelli (*thick arrow*). Note the encasement of the left middle cerebral artery

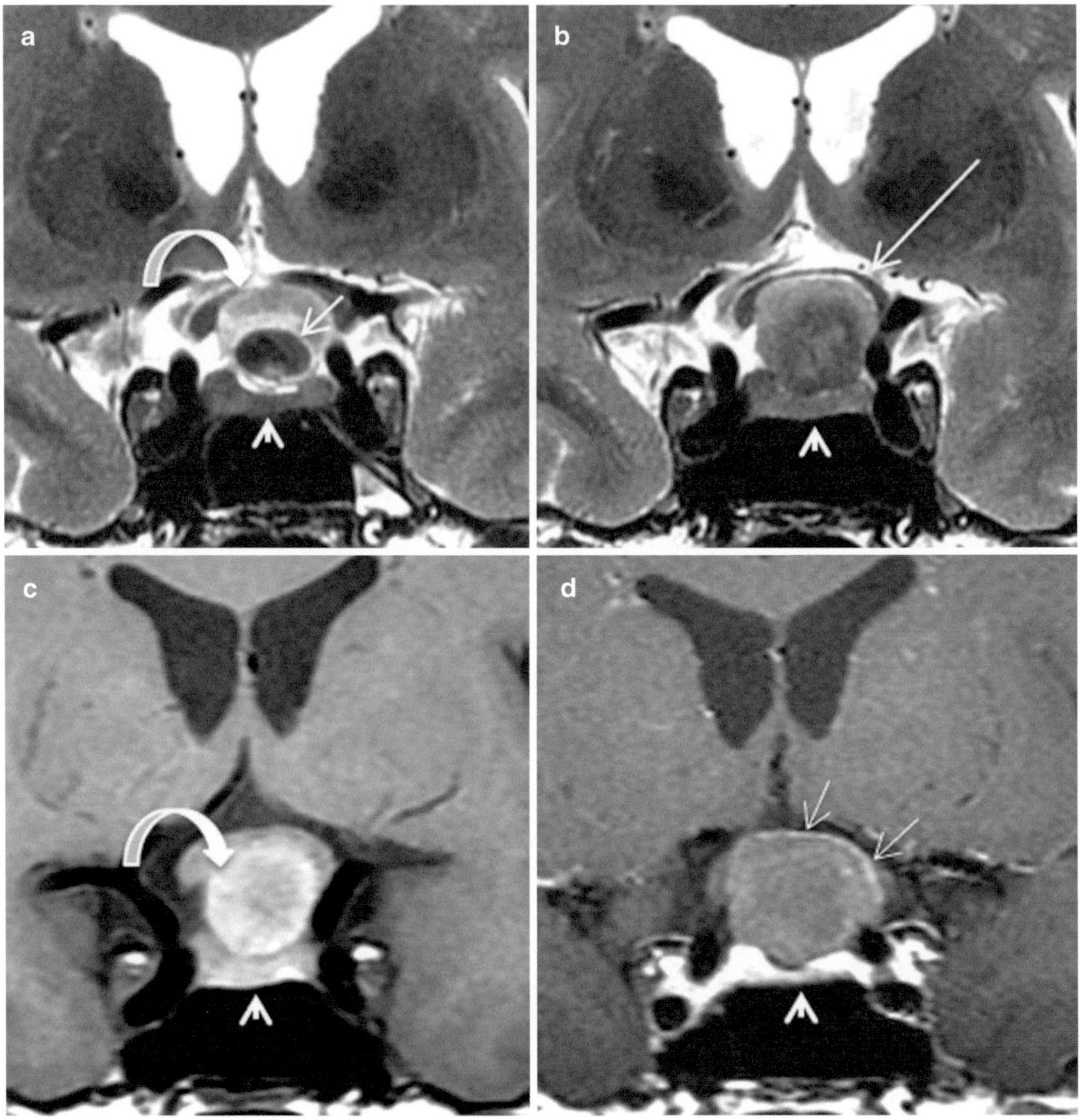

Fig. 22.9 A 57-year-old woman with decreased visual acuity. Suprasellar adamantinous craniopharyngioma mimicking a Rathke cleft cyst. (**a**, **b**) Coronal T2WIs. (**c**, **d**) Coronal T1 and CE T1 WIs. Round suprasellar mass with heterogeneous slightly T2 and T1 hyperintense content (*curved arrow*) and central T2 hypointense nodule (*thin arrow*). The mass is located above the pituitary gland (*short arrow*). Upward displacement and thinning of the optic chiasm (*long arrow*). Peripheral enhancement (*double arrow*) spearing the central area. Homogeneous enhancement of the pituitary gland (*short arrow*)

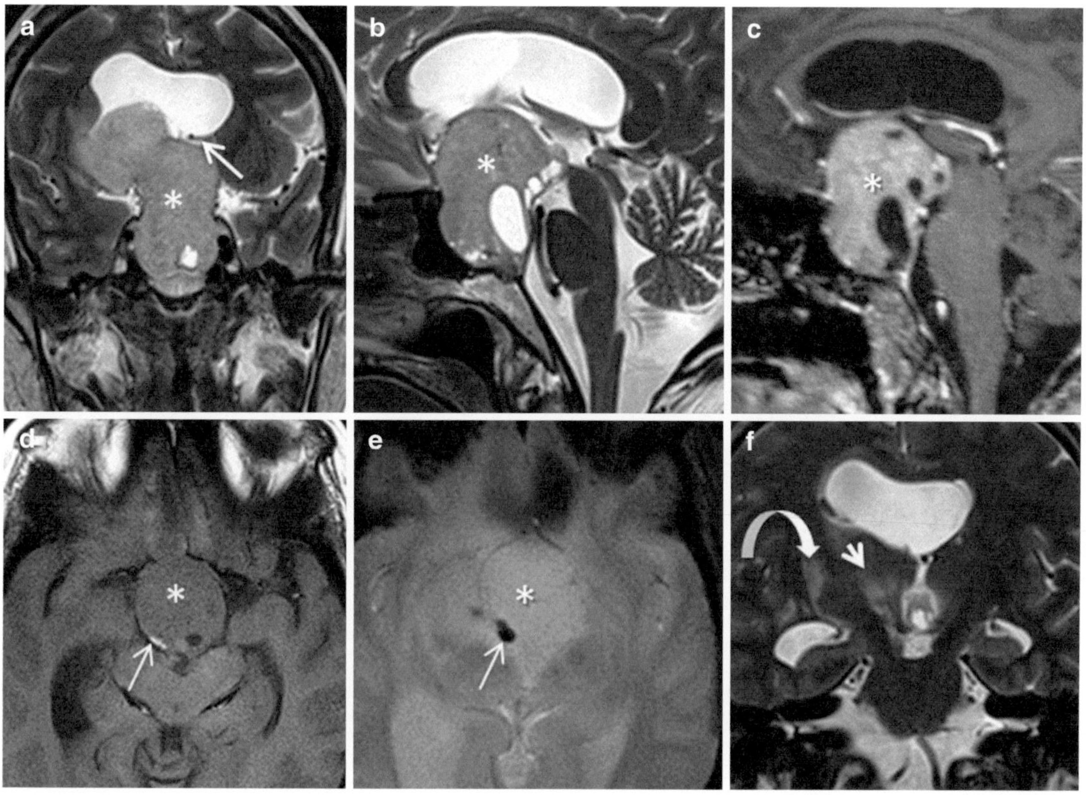

Fig. 22.10 A 54-year-old woman with headaches, visual disturbance, and left hemiparesis gradually increasing for 2 years. Intra- and suprasellar papillary craniopharyngioma mimicking a pituitary macroadenoma. (**a**, **b**) Coronal and sagittal T2WIs. Solid heterogeneous mass (*asterisk*) with hyperintense cystic areas and superior extension giving a figure-of-eight configuration. Hydrocephalus by obstruction of interventricular foramen (*thick arrow*). (**c**) Sagittal CE T1WI. Enhancement of the mass sparing intralesional cyst components (*asterisk*). (**d**, **e**) Axial T1 and T2* WIs. The mass is isointense on T1 with peripheral calcification (*thin arrow*). (**f**) Coronal T2WI. transependymal edema extending to right internal capsule (*curved arrow*). Edema along the optic tracts (*short arrow*)

Further Reading

Choi SH, Kwon BJ, Na DG et al (2007) Pituitary adenoma, craniopharyngioma, and Rathke cleft cyst involving both intrasellar and suprasellar regions: differentiation using MRI. Clin Radiol 62:453–462

Lee HJ, Wu CC, Wu HM et al (2015) Pretreatment diagnosis of suprasellar papillary craniopharyngioma and germ cell tumors of adult patients. Am J Neuroradiol 36:508–517

Saeki N, Nagai Y, Matsuura I et al (2004) Histologic characteristics of normal perivascular spaces along the optic tract: new pathogenetic mechanism for edema in tumors in the pituitary region. Am J Neuroradiol 25:1218–1222

23 Pre- and Suprasellar Meningiomas

Françoise Cattin

The meningioma is the most common intracranial tumor in adults, with 20 % occurring at the skull base. This benign tumor arises from arachnoidal cells of the meninges. The common sites of origin are the planum sphenoidale, the tuberculum sellae, the clinoid processes, the sellar diaphragm, and the cavernous sinus. Pre- and suprasellar meningiomas can be revealed by anosmia, frontal syndrome, and visual disturbance when the optic chiasm or optic nerves are compressed. Meningioma appears iso to hyperintense on T2WI and is hypo- to isointense on T1WI. Postcontrast scan shows marked homogeneous enhancement of the mass on both CT and MRI (Fig. 23.1). The presence of a ring of CSF delineating the tumor contours is frequent. Hyperostosis is commonly associated with meningiomas of the planum sphenoidale, tuberculum sellae, and clinoid processes (Fig. 23.2). Upward convexity of the jugum sphenoidale in front of the insertion of the meningioma, termed blistering, is a fundamental but not pathognomonic sign of meningioma. It may result in the extension of the underlying sinus, a phenomenon named pneumosinus dilatans. Extensive edema can be observed around the large presellar meningioma: the vasogenic edema associated with meningioma is thought to be related to tumor secretion of vascular endothelial growth factor (Fig. 23.3). Heterogeneous enhancement can be related to intratumoral calcifications or cysts. In the largest hypervascularized tumors, tortuous and enlarged peritumoral vessels and intratumoral vasculature can be visualized (Fig. 23.4). Extension of the presellar meningioma along the dural sheath of the optic nerve may occur (Fig. 23.5). Posterior extension of the large meningioma arising from the planum sphenoidale or tuberculum sellae can completely recover the sellar diaphragm, making difficult the identification of the site of tumoral insertion. Meningiomas of the sellar diaphragm are the most tricky. The normal pituitary gland is usually easily identifiable below the tumor on high-resolution T1 and T2 WI (Fig. 23.6). Dynamic MR sequence shows the more intense and earlier enhancement of the meningioma when compared with the normal pituitary gland (Fig. 23.7). Moreover, dynamic imaging can be helpful in the rare cases of association of meningioma and pituitary adenoma (Fig. 21.7). It is important to remember that meningiomas are often multiple; complete MR examination of the brain is needed in all cases. On DWI, the ADC is often low in meningioma (Fig. 23.8). However, this sequence does not have a major role in the differential diagnosis. On perfusion imaging, sellar meningiomas show high values of rCBV and signal intensity curves with little or no return to the baseline levels, similarly to adenomas. Bladowska has proposed the use of fixed cutoff values to differentiate meningioma from pituitary adenoma: maximum rCBV exceeding 7.14 and mean rCBV above 5.74 with a time–intensity curve not returning to the baseline level are suggestive of the diagnosis of meningioma. Perfusion imaging is not a reliable

J.-F. Bonneville et al., *MRI of the Pituitary Gland*, DOI 10.1007/978-3-319-29043-0_23

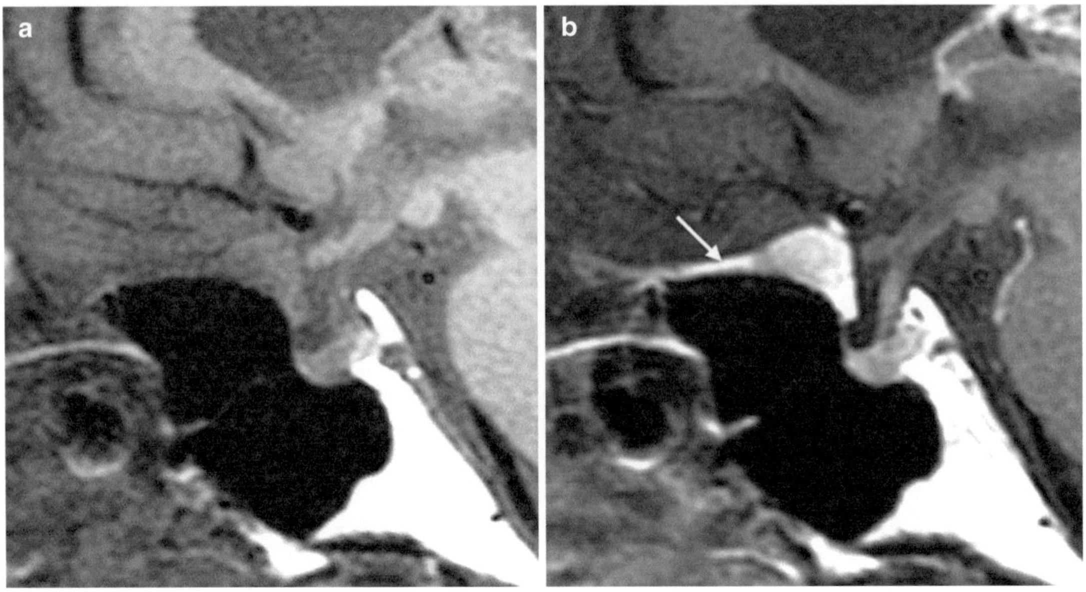

Fig. 23.1 Meningioma of the tuberculum sellae. (**a**, **b**) Sagittal T1 and CE T1 WIs. Before contrast, the lesion is isointense to the gray matter and strongly and homogeneously enhances. The adjacent presellar dura is thickened (*arrows*). The pituitary gland is normal

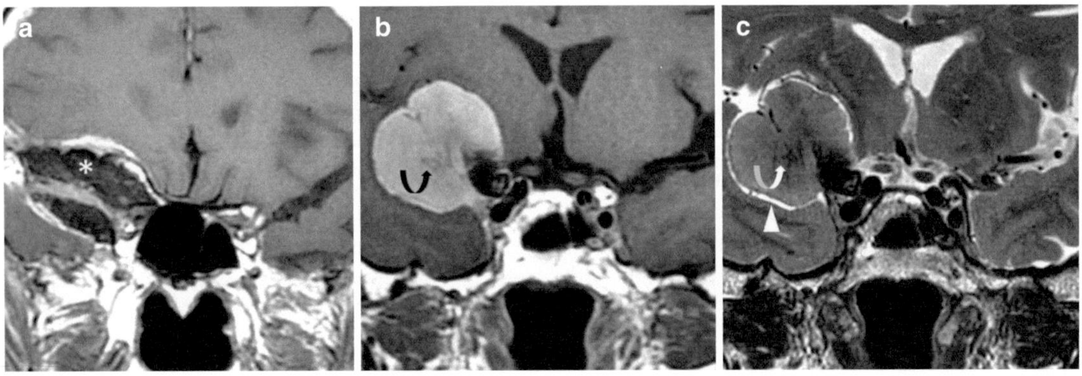

Fig. 23.2 Large meningioma of the lesser sphenoid wing. (**a**–**c**) Coronal CE T1WIs and coronal T2WI. Huge osteoma of the right lesser sphenoid wing (*asterisk*). The intratumoral vasculature is faintly visible (*curved arrows*). The tumor is surrounded by a thin layer of CSF (*arrowhead*)

technique to differentiate the different histological types of meningioma; however, the CBV is markedly increased in angiomatous meningioma. MR spectroscopy, which demonstrates increased choline peak, no N-acetylaspartate, and alanine peak at 1.46 ppm (inconstant), is not particularly useful in the differential diagnosis. Moreover, the bony structures of the skull base and pneumatization of the sphenoid sinus are frequently the source of artifacts degrading the spectrum.

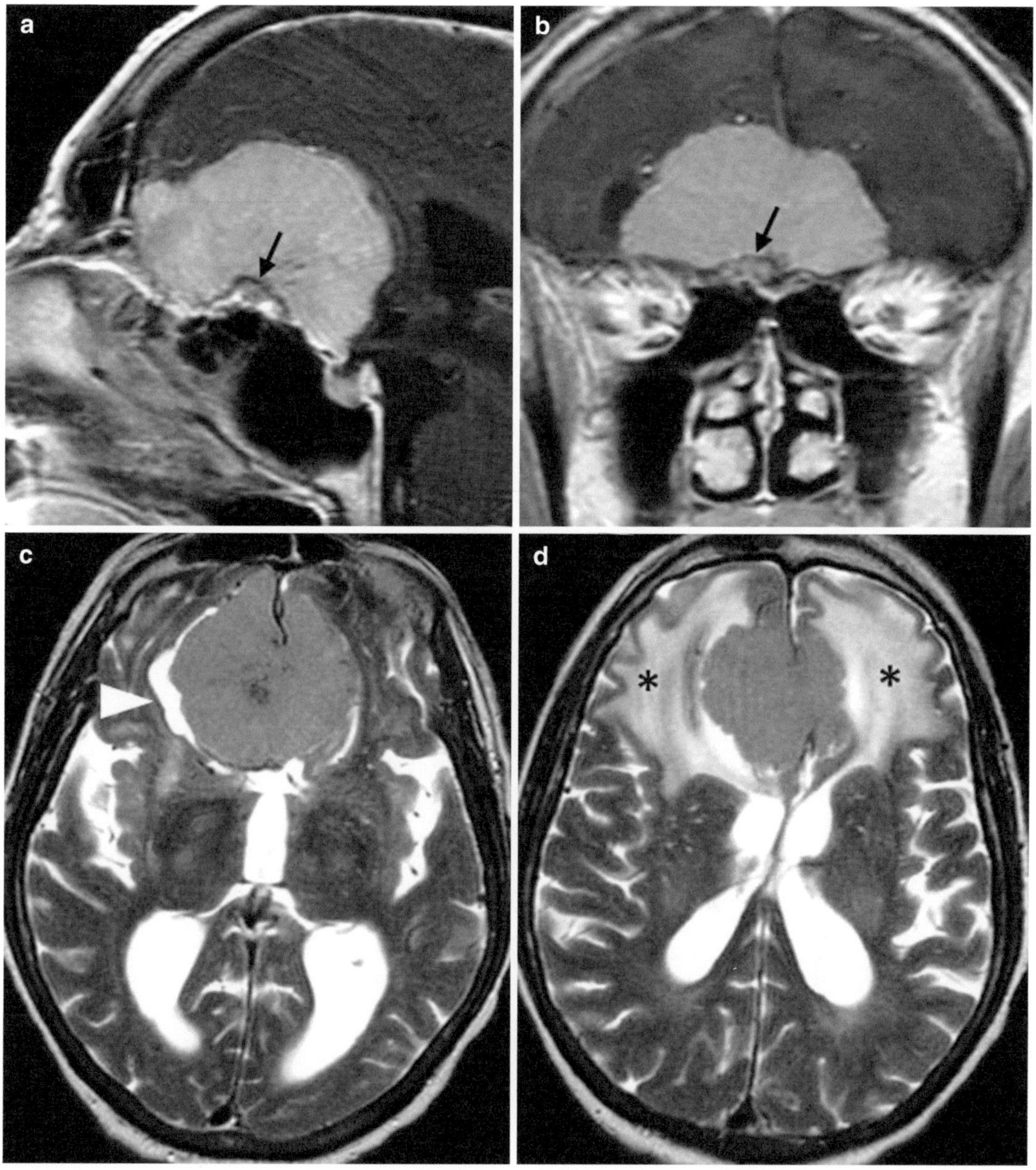

Fig. 23.3 Huge presellar meningioma. (**a**, **b**) Sagittal and coronal CE T1WIs. Thick osteoma (*arrow*) of the jugum sphenoidale. (**c**, **d**) Axial T2WIs. Demonstration of a CSF cleft between the meningioma and the brain parenchyma on the right side (*arrowhead*) and extensive edema in the adjacent white matter (*asterisks*)

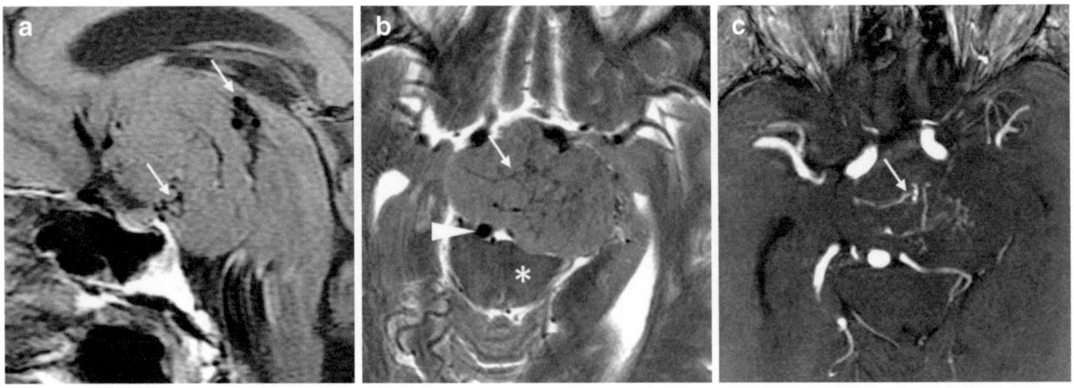

Fig. 23.4 Supra- and retrosellar angiomatous meningioma arising from the dorsum sellae. (**a**–**c**) Sagittal T1WI, axial T2WI, and 3D time-of-flight MRA. The pons is compressed and posteriorly displaced (*asterisk*) and the basilar artery is pushed to the right (*arrowhead*). Visualization of high-flow vessels in the tumor (*arrows*)

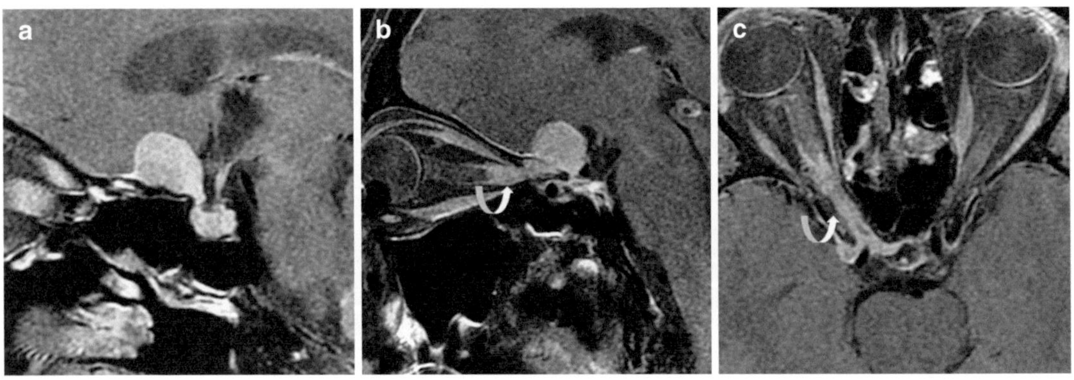

Fig. 23.5 Meningioma of the jugum sphenoidale. (**a**–**c**) Sagittal, oblique parasagittal, and axial CE T1WIs with saturation of the fat signal. The meningioma is extending along the dural sheath of the right optic nerve (*curved arrows*)

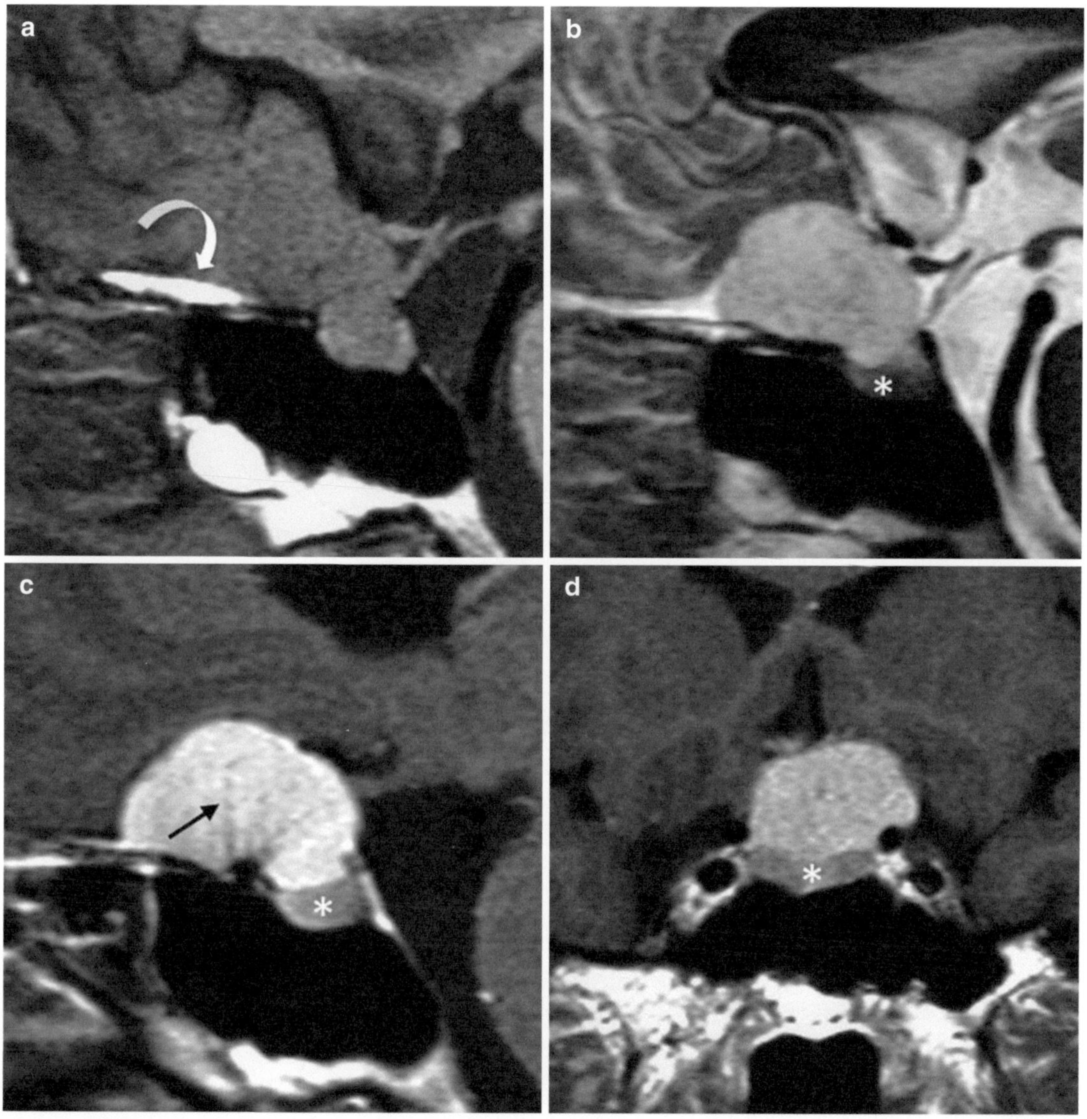

Fig. 23.6 Presellar meningioma with posterior extension in the suprasellar cistern. (**a**) Sagittal T1WI. Differentiation between the tumor and the pituitary gland is not possible. The diagnosis of meningioma of the planum sphenoidale can be evoked in the presence of a thick linear hyperintense image in the presellar region (*curved arrow*) corresponding to the insertion osteoma. (**b**) Sagittal T2WI. Marked hypersignal of the meningioma allows easy delineation of the underlying normal pituitary gland (*asterisk*). (**c**, **d**) Sagittal and coronal CE T1WIs. The enhancement of the meningioma is much more intense than that of the normal pituitary gland (*asterisk*). In (**c**) note the visualization of intratumoral vasculature (*arrow*)

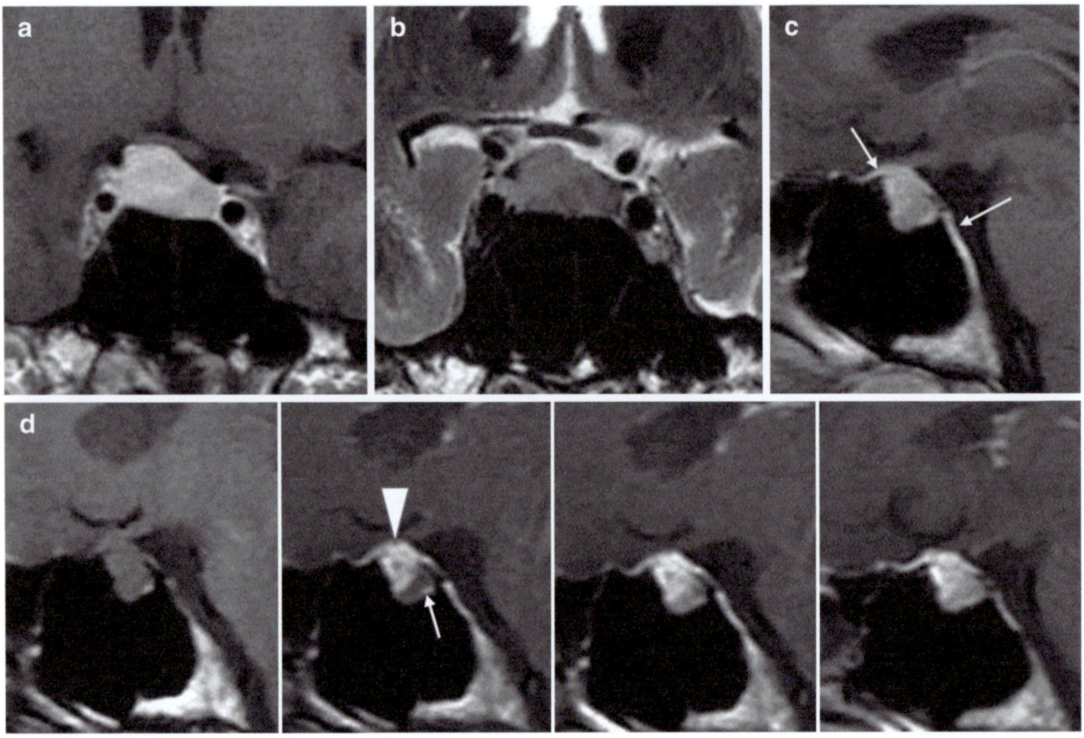

Fig. 23.7 Meningioma of the sellar diaphragm. (**a**) Coronal CE T1WI. Asymmetrical enlargement and bulging of the sellar content. The optic chiasm is raised on the right side. The enhancement is more intense in the upper part of the sellar content. (**b**) Coronal T2WI. The signal is discretely more intense on the right side. (**c**) Sagittal CE T1WI. The sella turcica is not enlarged. Visualization of a small anterior and posterior dural tail (arrows). (**d**) Dynamic MRI. Early and intense enhancement of the anterior and superior part of the sellar content, suggestive of the presence of sellar diaphragm meningioma (*arrowhead*). The normal pituitary gland is pushed inferiorly and posteriorly (*arrow*); its enhancement appears later. At the end of the dynamic scanning, the sellar content is fairly homogeneous

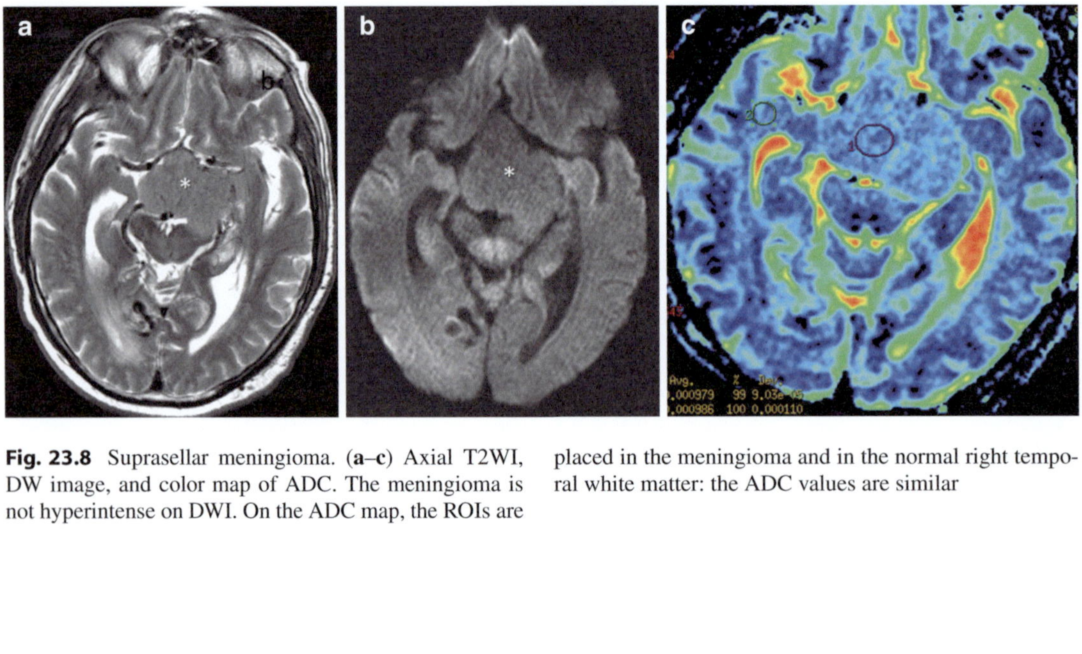

Fig. 23.8 Suprasellar meningioma. (**a**–**c**) Axial T2WI, DW image, and color map of ADC. The meningioma is not hyperintense on DWI. On the ADC map, the ROIs are placed in the meningioma and in the normal right temporal white matter: the ADC values are similar

Further Reading

Bladowska J, Zimny A, Guzinski (2013) Usefulness of perfusion-weighted magnetic resonance imaging with signal-intensity curves analysis in the differential diagnosis of sellar and parasellar tumors: preliminary report. Eur J Radiol 82(8):1292–1298

Nagar VA, Ye JR, Ng WH et al (2008) Diffusion-weighted MRI: diagnosing atypical or malignant meningiomas and detecting tumor differentiation. AJNR Am J Neuroradiol 29:1147–1152

Saloner D, Uzelac A, Hetts S, Martin A, Dillon W (2010) Modern meningioma imaging techniques. J Neurooncol 99:333–340

Cavernous Sinus Meningioma

24

Françoise Cattin

Cavernous sinus tumors most frequently are revealed by oculomotor deficit, ptosis, diplopia, anisocoria, or complete ophthalmoplegia. Involvement of the trigeminal nerve with facial numbness or facial pain can occur. Compression of the internal carotid artery with reduction of the arterial lumen has been held responsible for ischemic events. Two types of cavernous sinus meningiomas have to be distinguished: some meningiomas arise from the lateral dural wall (Fig. 24.1) while others are developed exclusively inside the cavernous sinus. The main features are enlargement of the cavernous sinus and thickening of its lateral wall, which is markedly hypointense on T2WI (Fig. 24.2). A dural tail, linear meningeal thickening, and enhancement extending from the edge of the tumor to the ipsilateral tentorium are almost always present but not specific. It can be observed in other extra-axial lesions, such as schwannoma, metastasis, lymphoma, pituitary diseases, and granulomatous disorders. The dural tail reflects the neoplastic dural infiltration or reactive vascularity, or both, draining in the adjacent dura. The tumor can extend anteriorly toward the optic canal, the superior orbital fissure, the great wing of the sphenoid, and posteriorly toward the Meckel cave and the prepontine cistern. Encasement of the internal carotid artery and constriction of its lumen is common (Fig. 24.3). 3D TOF MRA can help to visualize the internal carotid artery stenosis and assess the intracranial collateral vascularization. Cavernous sinus meningiomas frequently extend into the sella turcica, pushing the pituitary gland toward the opposite side. The medial limit of the tumor is usually well defined on T2WI, owing to the hypersignal of the meningioma in comparison with normal pituitary gland, while CE T1WI usually demonstrates similar homogeneous enhancement of meningioma and pituitary gland. Dynamic MRI can help to distinguish the meningioma from the compressed normal pituitary gland. A cavernous meningioma with intrasellar extension may be responsible for an enlargement of the inferior intercavernous sinus (Fig. 24.4). Multiple meningiomas of the sellar region can occur (Fig. 24.5). MRI appearance of cavernous sinus meningioma is usually typical. The main differential diagnosis is pituitary adenoma with cavernous sinus invasion. In some cases, cavernous hemangioma, metastasis, lymphoma, trigeminal schwannoma, or thrombosed intracavernous internal carotid artery aneurysm can simulate a meningioma. Looking at the sphenoid sinus itself may be of precious help, as intracavernous meningiomas may invade it by passing through its bony walls after thickening them instead of destroying them, a feature not encountered in other lesions (Fig. 24.6).

J.-F. Bonneville et al., *MRI of the Pituitary Gland*, DOI 10.1007/978-3-319-29043-0_24

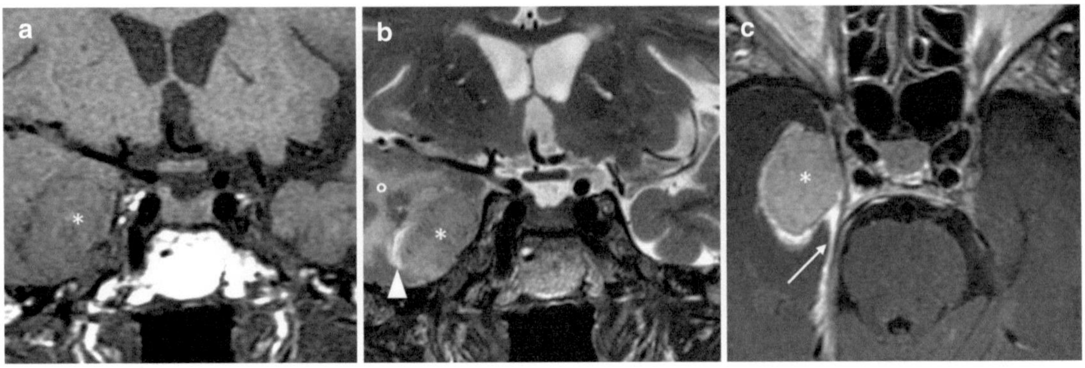

Fig. 24.1 Large parasellar meningioma inserted on the lateral wall of the right cavernous sinus (*asterisk*). (**a**) Coronal T1WI. The lesion is isointense to the surrounding brain tissue. (**b**) Coronal T2WI. Demonstration of peritumoral white matter edema (*circle*). Note a small cleft of CSF (*arrowhead*). (**c**) Axial CE T1WI. Homogeneous enhancement of the meningioma and dural tail along the free edge of the tentorium (*arrow*)

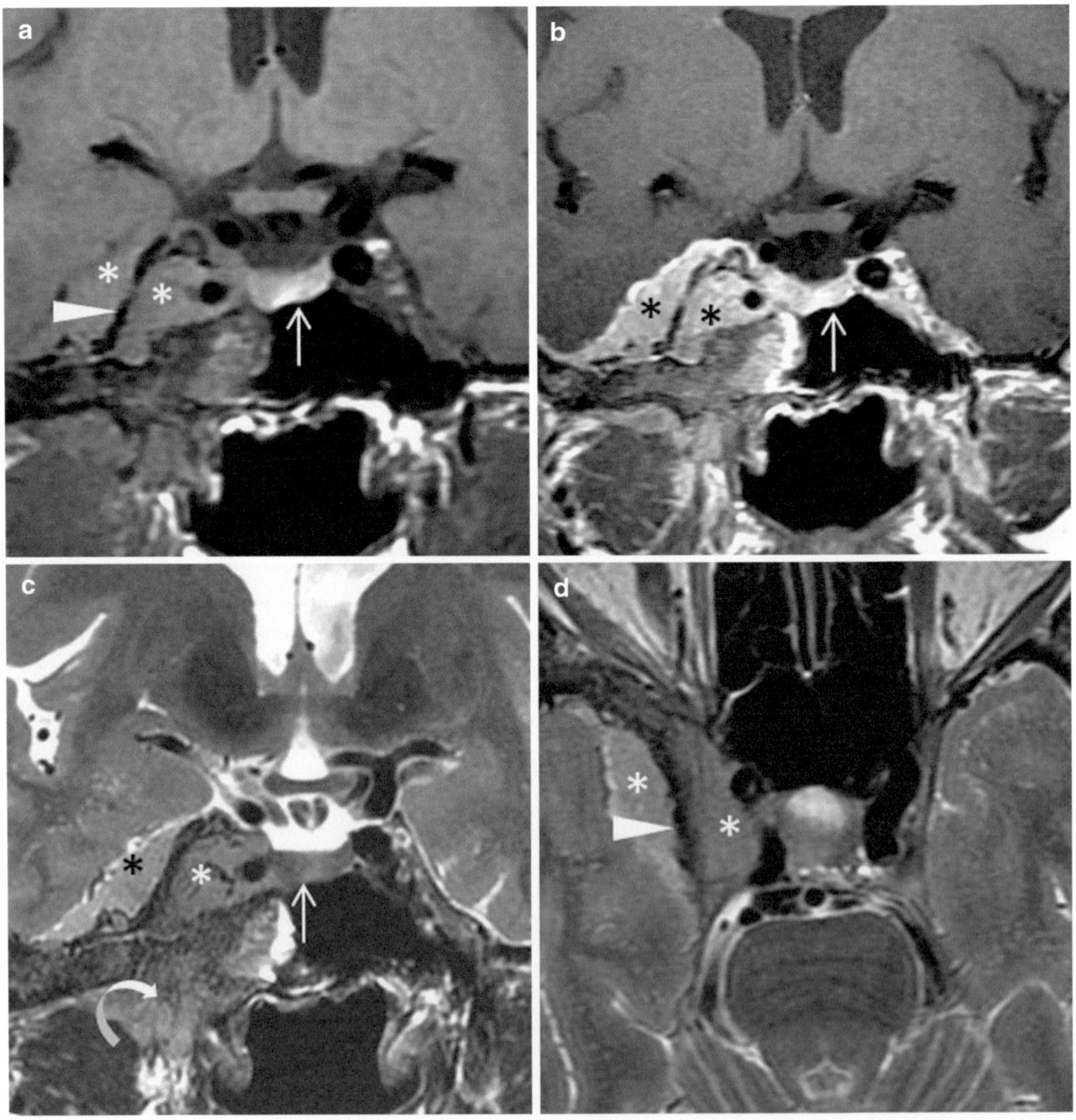

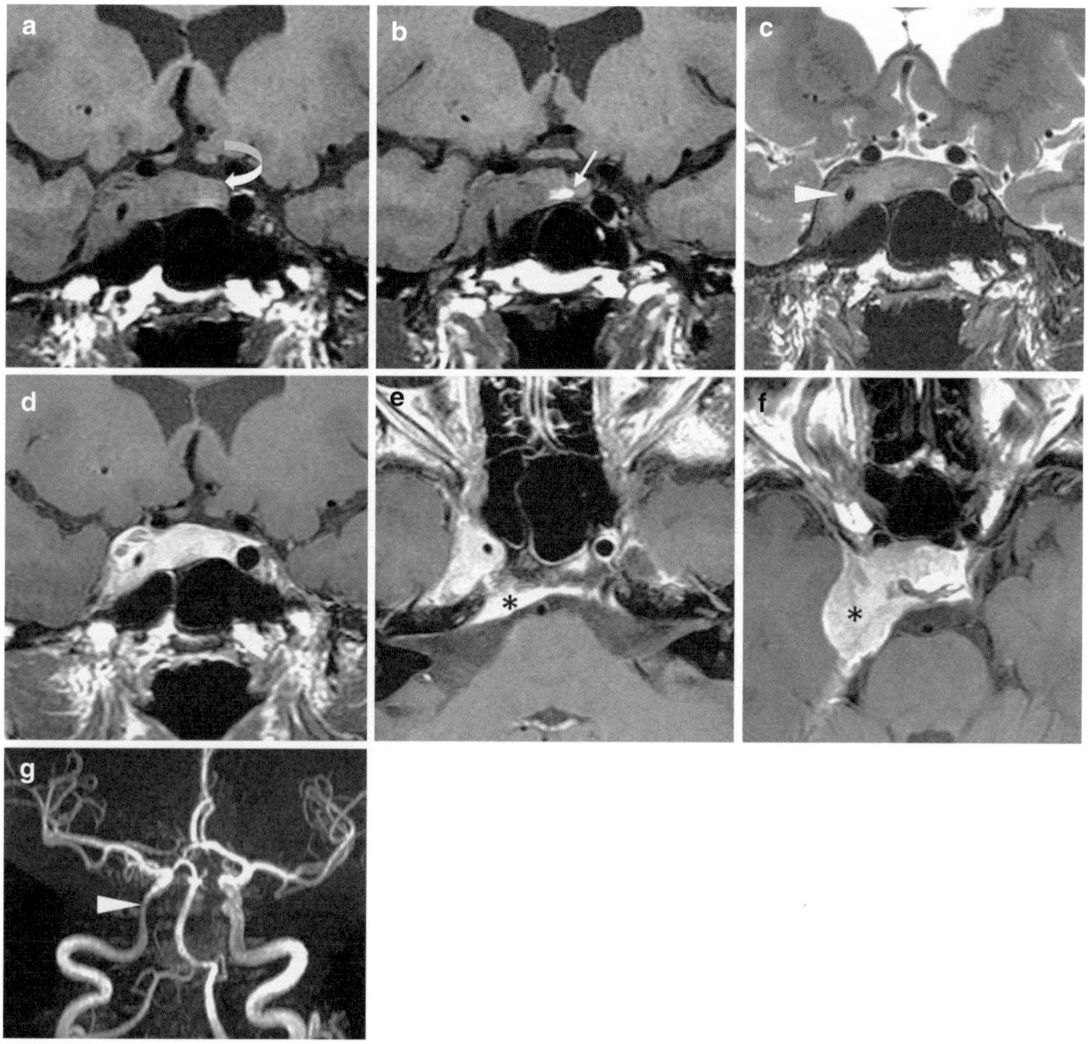

Fig. 24.3 Meningioma of right cavernous sinus with intrasellar extension. (**a**, **b**) Coronal T1WIs. Bulging of the lateral wall of the right cavernous sinus and convexity of the upper pole of the sellar content. The tumoral tissue is isointense to the gray matter and hypointense to the normal anterior lobe (*curved arrow*) pushed to the left side and to the posterior lobe (*straight arrow*). (**c**) Coronal T2WI. The meningioma is discretely hyperintense. There is a severe reduction of the right intracavernous internal carotid artery lumen (arrowhead). (**d**) Coronal CE T1WI. This sequence is less informative than T1WI before contrast. Meningioma and normal pituitary gland are not differentiated. (**e**, **f**) Axial CE T1WIs. Demonstration of the posterior extension in the prepontine cistern and along the free edge of the tentorium (*asterisks*). (**g**) 3D TOF MRA confirms the stenosis of right intracavernous internal carotid artery (*arrowhead*)

Fig. 24.2 Meningioma of the right cavernous sinus growing on both sides of the lateral wall of the cavernous sinus (*asterisks*), into the cavernous sinus and toward the temporal fossa (*curved arrow*). (**a–c**) Coronal T1, CE T1 and T2 WIs. (**d**) Axial T2WI. T2 signal of the meningioma is more intense than that of the pituitary gland (*thin arrow*), but enhancement is nearly similar. There is a marked thickening of the lateral wall of the right cavernous sinus (*arrowhead*)

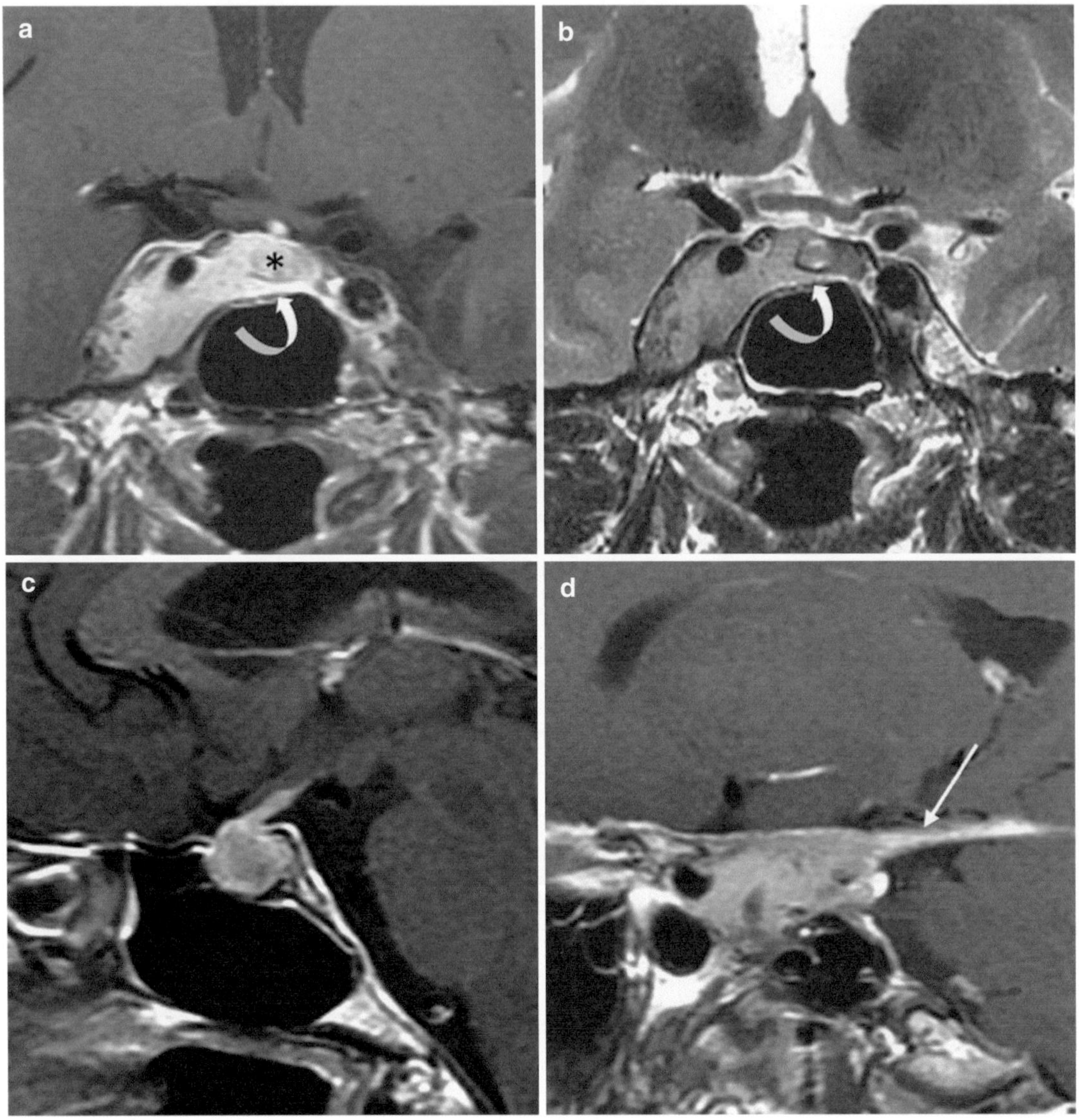

Fig. 24.4 Meningioma of right cavernous sinus with intrasellar extension. (**a**) Coronal CE T1WI and (**b**) T2WI. The normal pituitary gland is pushed to the left (*asterisk*). The inferior intercavernous sinus is prominent (*curved arrow*). (**c**) Midline sagittal CE T1WI. Intrasellar extension of the right cavernous sinus meningioma associated with a thick inferior intercavernous sinus is responsible for the upper bulging of the pituitary gland. (**d**) Right parasagittal CE T1WI shows the posterior extension of the meningioma along the free edge of the tentorium (*arrow*)

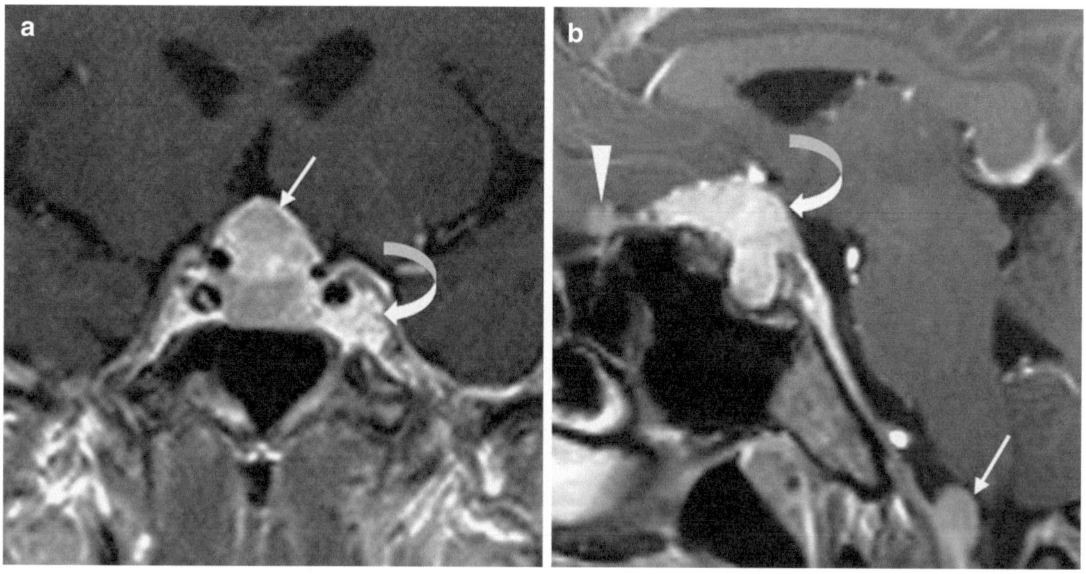

Fig. 24.5 Multiple meningiomas. Two different patients. (**a**) Coronal CE T1WI. Association of a meningioma of the jugum sphenoidale (*arrow*) and a meningioma of the left cavernous sinus (*curved arrow*). (**b**) Sagittal CE T1WI. Association of a meningioma of the cribriform plate (*arrowhead*), a meningioma of the jugum sphenoidale (*curved arrow*), and a meningioma of the foramen magnum (*arrow*)

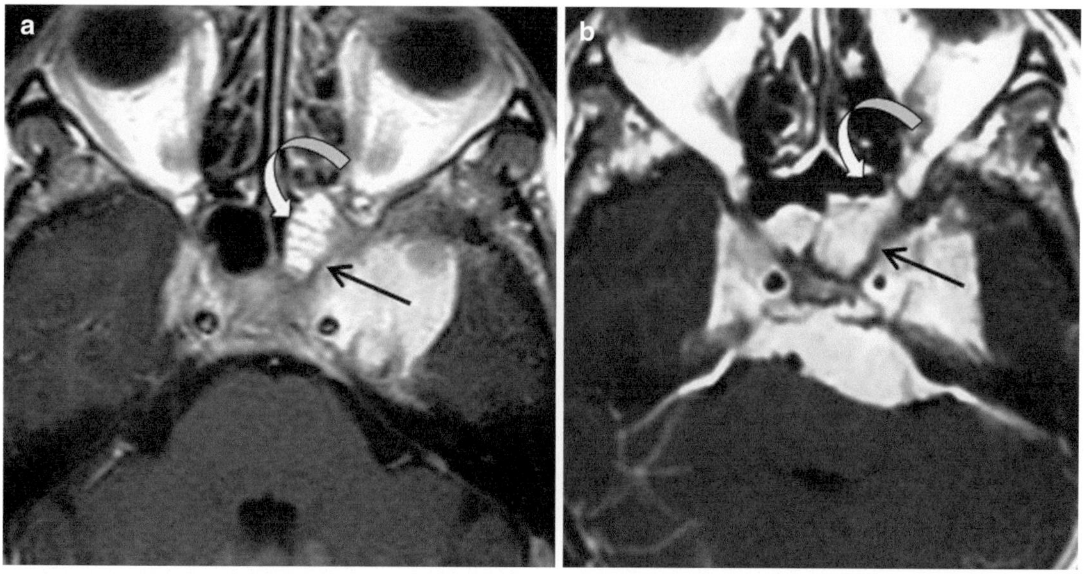

Fig. 24.6 Typical cavernous sinus meningiomas with intrasphenoidal extension. (**a**, **b**) Axial CE T1WIs of two different cases of meningiomas, one being unilateral, the other bilateral. Note that the meningiomas have grown through the bony walls of the sphenoid sinus (*curved arrows*) without any osteolysis, but contrastingly with thickening of them (*straight arrows*)

Further Reading

Abdel Razek AAK, Castillo M (2009) Imaging lesions of the cavernous sinus. AJNR Am J Neuroradiol 30: 444–452

Lee JH, Lee HK, Park JK et al (2003) Cavernous sinus syndrome: clinical features and differential diagnosis with MR imaging. AJR Am J Roentgenol 181:583–590

Ruscalleda J (2005) Imaging of parasellar lesions. Eur Radiol 15:549–559

25 Intraoperative MRI

Michael Buchfelder and Sven-Martin Schlaffer

Since MRI today is the standard procedure for depicting pituitary adenomas with the best possible resolution, it seems reasonable that attempts have been made to integrate MR scanners into operative suites for intraoperative imaging. There are many variants of such dedicated systems available, with 0.15 T (low field) or 1.5 T and 3.0 T (high field) magnets. Usually, the surgical procedure is interrupted for imaging. In any situation, for generating intraoperative images either the patient or the magnet has to move. Depending on the field strength of the system, the acquisition times and the quality of the images vary considerably.

In general, when the surgeon feels that he has achieved the best possible radicality of tumor resection, the surgical procedure is interrupted and an intraoperative MR image is generated. To be able to differentiate residual tumor and blood within the resection cavity, T2W sequences are preferable for intraoperative investigations (Figs. 25.1 and 25.2). The decompression of optic pathways and the resection of suprasellar tumor components can be reliably documented with either type of system.

Postoperative artifacts such as hemorrhage into the tumor cavity and surgical packing within the operative field, which frequently distort the appreciation of surgical radicality dramatically in the early postoperative period (Dina et al. 1993), are avoided if the imaging is done just a few minutes after tumor extraction. One major advantage of the direct depiction of residual tumor during the operative procedure is that, once such is depicted, it can be attacked in a very targeted fashion (Buchfelder and Schlaffer 2012). Thus, in many patients with residual tumor that has escaped the surgeon's eye, the resection can be successfully completed.

Numerous papers have reported that not only the percentage of patients with complete tumor resection is increased with the use of intraoperative imaging but also the total amount of adenoma tissue resected. This concerns all types of pituitary adenomas, with the exception of pituitary microadenomas. In these, to date the advantage of intraoperative MRI in pituitary surgery is less convincing, since the resection rates without intraoperative imaging already approach 90 % in many series, and small tumor residuals are more difficult to depict intraoperatively.

Intraoperative MRI is the most sensitive procedure to date to facilitate resection control, and has a much higher sensitivity than ultrasound or CT. However, the costs of installing dedicated MR scanners in operative suites are high, and thus financial aspects today prevent the more widespread availability of the technology.

J.-F. Bonneville et al., *MRI of the Pituitary Gland*, DOI 10.1007/978-3-319-29043-0_25

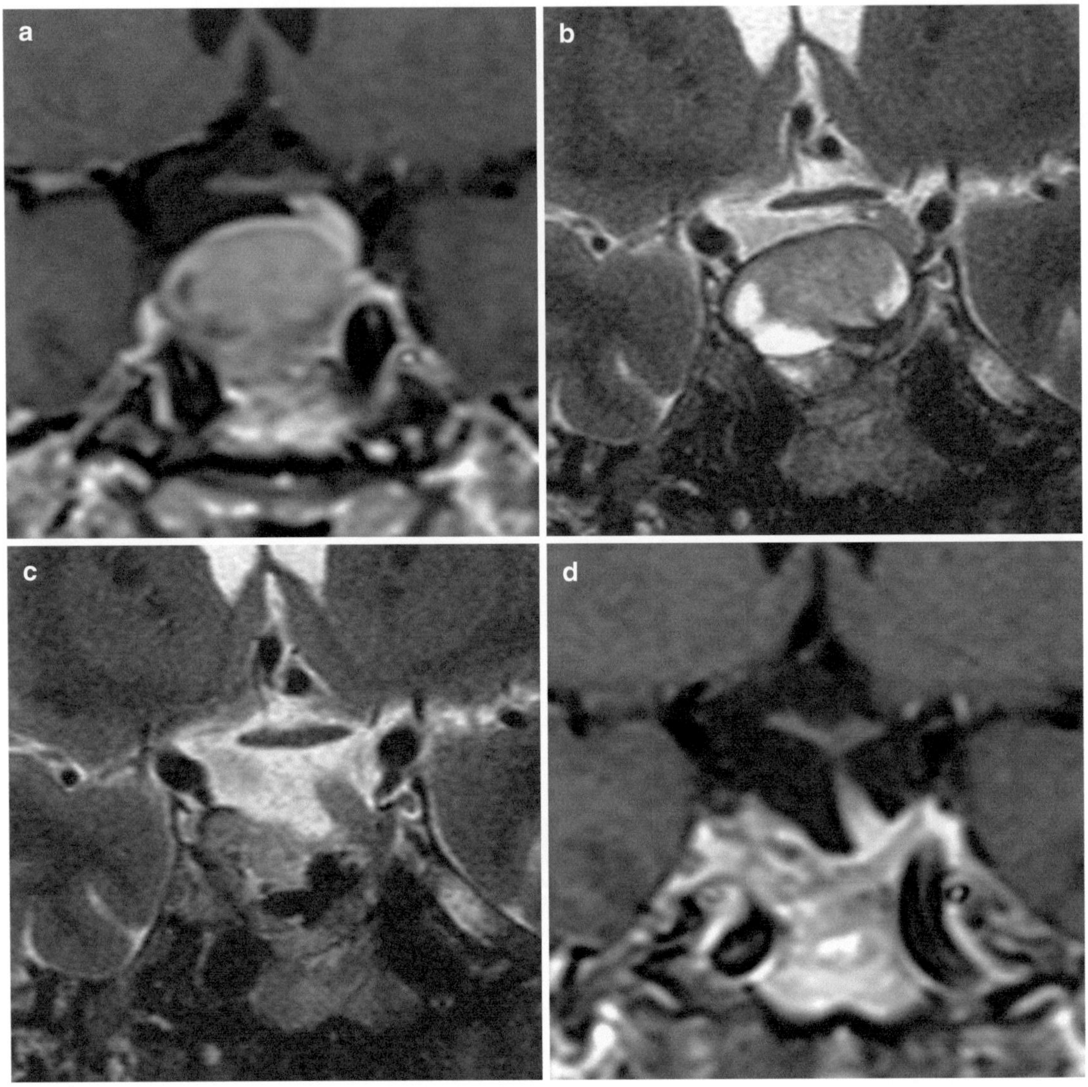

Fig. 25.1 Recurrent nonfunctioning pituitary adenoma in a 37-year-old patient. (**a**) Coronal CE T1WI before surgery. (**b**) Intraoperative coronal T2WI before resection. (**c**) Intraoperative coronal T2WI after resection. (**d**) Coronal CE T1WI 3 months later

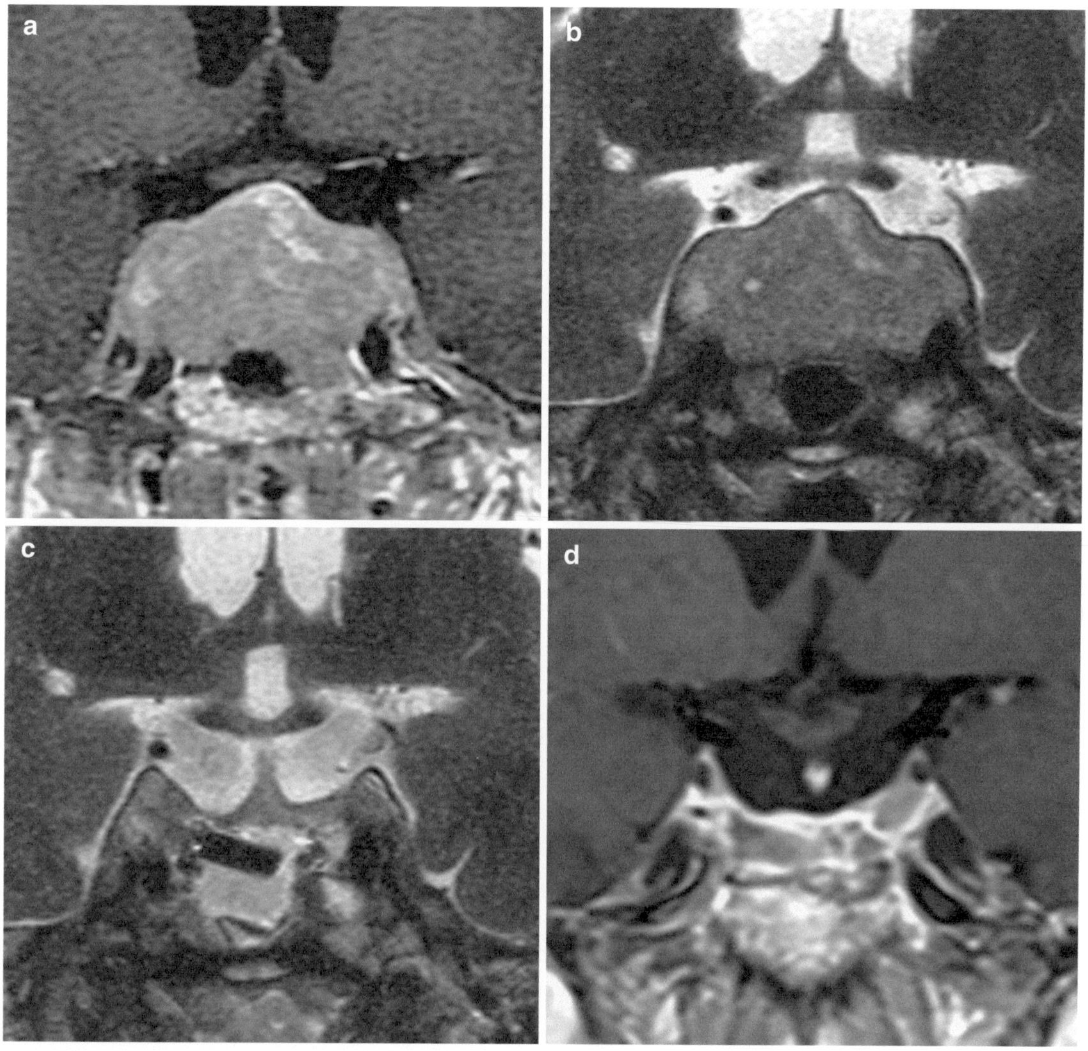

Fig. 25.2 Recurrent nonfunctioning pituitary adenoma in a 75-year-old patient after one transsphenoidal surgery. (**a**) Preoperative CE T1WI. (**b**) Intraoperative pre-resection coronal T2WI. (**c**) Intraoperative post-resection coronal T2WI. (**d**) Coronal CE T1WI 3 months postoperatively

References

Buchfelder M, Schlaffer SM (2012) Intraoperative magnetic resonance imaging during surgery for pituitary adenomas: pros and cons. Endocrine 42:483–495

Dina TS, Feaster SH, Laws ER, Davis DO (1993) MR of the pituitary gland postsurgery: serial MR studies following transsphenoidal resection. Am J Neuroradiol 14:763–769

The Early Postoperative Sella

26

Jean-François Bonneville

Reading a postoperative sellar MRI is generally considered as one of the most difficult challenges during imaging of the sellar region, particularly in the immediate postoperative period. Early postoperative MRI is usually not performed in most pituitary centers, and the corresponding literature is scarce. Presence of blood products and packing material have been accused of masking the sellar content and possible residual tumor in the first weeks after surgery. In our experience, this is true only with pituitary tumors with liquid (hemorrhagic or necrotic) content (Fig. 26.1). Early MRI, at day 3 or 4 after transsphenoidal surgery, is routinely obtained in our center and compared with the operative report. We do not perform immediate postoperative MRI, as proposed by some, the T1 signal of blood being still at day 1 isointense to the brain. At this stage, we strongly recommend noncontrast T1W sequences, which are the most informative. Conversely, we consider T2WI more prone to differentiate normal residual pituitary tissue from tumoral remnant beyond 3 months postoperatively. It is our opinion that gadolinium perfusion, at this stage, complicates the interpretation of MRI and must be avoided. Early postoperative MRI has numerous advantages: it can detect complications before the patient leaves the hospital, such as hemorrhage outside the tumoral limits (Fig. 26.2), overpacking of the sella (Fig. 26.3) or CSF fistula (Fig. 26.4). Some depletion of vasopressin storage can be observed on day 4 postoperative MRI, best appreciated on axial T1W fat-saturated noncontrast images. In case of postoperative diabetes insipidus, complete extinction of the bright spot will occur some days later, i.e., after complete depletion of vasopressin storage. MRI permits visualization of the surgical bed and mostly a tumoral remnant, if any, more easily if a hemostatic packing has been put in place. In any case, early postoperative MRI facilitates the reading of future examinations. MRI characteristics of hemostatic materials (Gelfoam, Surgicel) packed in the few days after surgery are as follows. It is a mass with regular contours, T1 isointense with the gray matter, with a peripheral rim of T1 hyperintensity corresponding to methemoglobin deposit (Fig. 26.5). Air bubbles caught in the fabric appear as inframillimetric rounded T1-hypointense images. The part of surgical bed free of hemostatic material corresponds to either tumoral remnant or normal residual pituitary tissue, the latter being usually smaller than the former. In the case of cavernous sinus invasion, the normal anterior pituitary gland is found contralaterally, but is frequently not clearly identified on early postoperative MRI. Of course, MR signal of tumoral remnant is identical to that of the tumor before surgery. Apart from cavernous sinus, location of the tumoral remnant is driven by the laws of ballistics, i.e., superiorly in the suprasellar cistern, and inferiorly and posteriorly within the sphenoid sinus (Fig. 26.6). Autogenous subcutaneous fat graft taken from the abdominal wall or from the lateral thigh is used in case of CSF leak; it is easily recognized in the form of a T1-hyperintense brilliant homogeneous polylobulated mass surrounded by a dark

J.-F. Bonneville et al., *MRI of the Pituitary Gland*, DOI 10.1007/978-3-319-29043-0_26

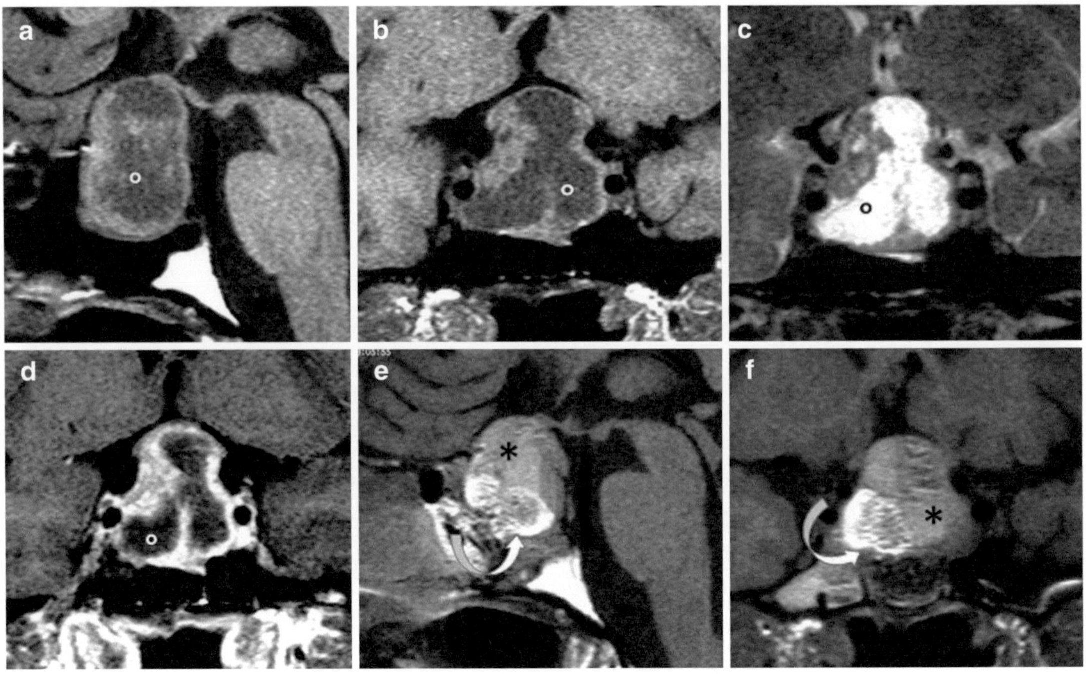

Fig. 26.1 Large necrotic pituitary nonfunctioning adenoma with suprasellar extension. (**a**, **b**) Sagittal and coronal T1WI. (**c**) Coronal T2 and (**d**) Coronal CE T1WI. Large amount of necrosis illustrated by T1-hypointense and T2-hyperintense areas with no enhancement after contrast injection (*circle*). (**e**, **f**) Sagittal and coronal T1W noncontrast images at day 4 after transsphenoidal surgery. There is no shrinkage of the mass. The surgical bed is occupied by blood (*asterisk*) and Surgicel impregnated with deoxyhemoglobin (*arrow*). The residual normal pituitary tissue is not distinguishable

T1-hypointense line oriented perpendicular to the frequency-encoded direction and corresponding to chemical shift artifact (Fig. 26.7). Fat signal is suppressed with the use of fat-saturated sequence. If necessary, surgeons can also use vaporized glue instead of Surgicel to assure hemostasis of the surgical area. In these cases, the sellar content appears homogeneously isointense to the brain, potentially making it difficult to differentiate serous collection from residual tumor. T2WI can help (Fig. 27.4). Muscle, fascia, cartilaginous matter, and bone collected from the nasal approach or silicone plate used to seal the sella are better identified on follow-up MRI.

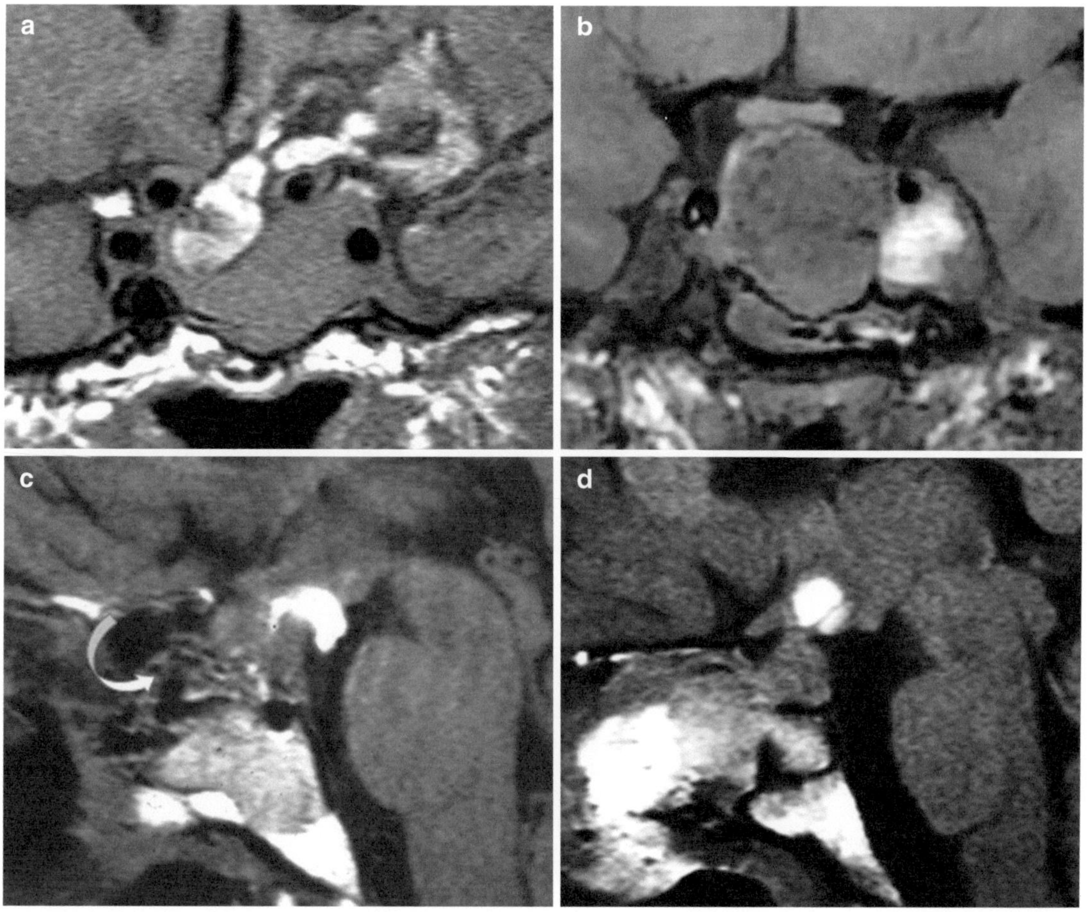

Fig. 26.2 Complications after pituitary surgery. Coronal (**a**, **b**) and sagittal (**c**, **d**) noncontrast T1WIs at day 4 after surgery. T1-hyperintense areas representative of hemorrhage in suprasellar cistern (**a**), cavernous sinus (**b**), interpeduncular subarachnoid space (**c**), and hypothalamus (**d**). Note in (**c**) the presence in the sphenoid sinus of multiple metallic artifacts resulting from surgical instrument microchips (*arrow*)

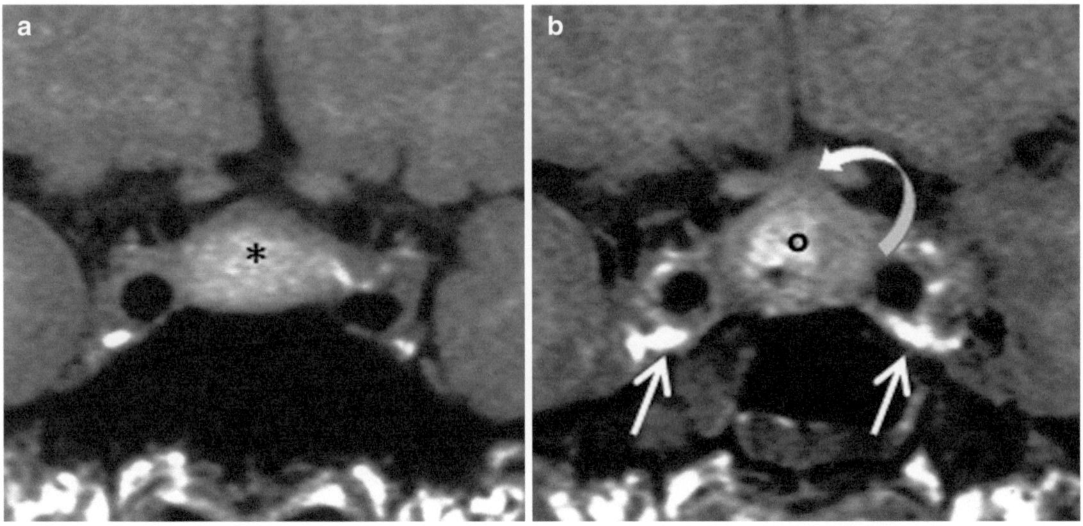

Fig. 26.3 Sella overpacking. (**a**, **b**) Noncontrast T1WIs before and 4 days after surgery. (**a**) Pituitary macroadenoma with limited suprasellar extension. T1 hyperintensity represents intra-adenomatous hemorrhage (*asterisk*). (**b**) Overpacking with Surgicel (*circle*) gives rise to an increased volume of the mass with abuts on the optic chiasm (*arrow*). T1 hyperintensity of the veins of the cavernous sinus (*straight arrows*) indicates slow flow caused by intrasellar hyperpressure

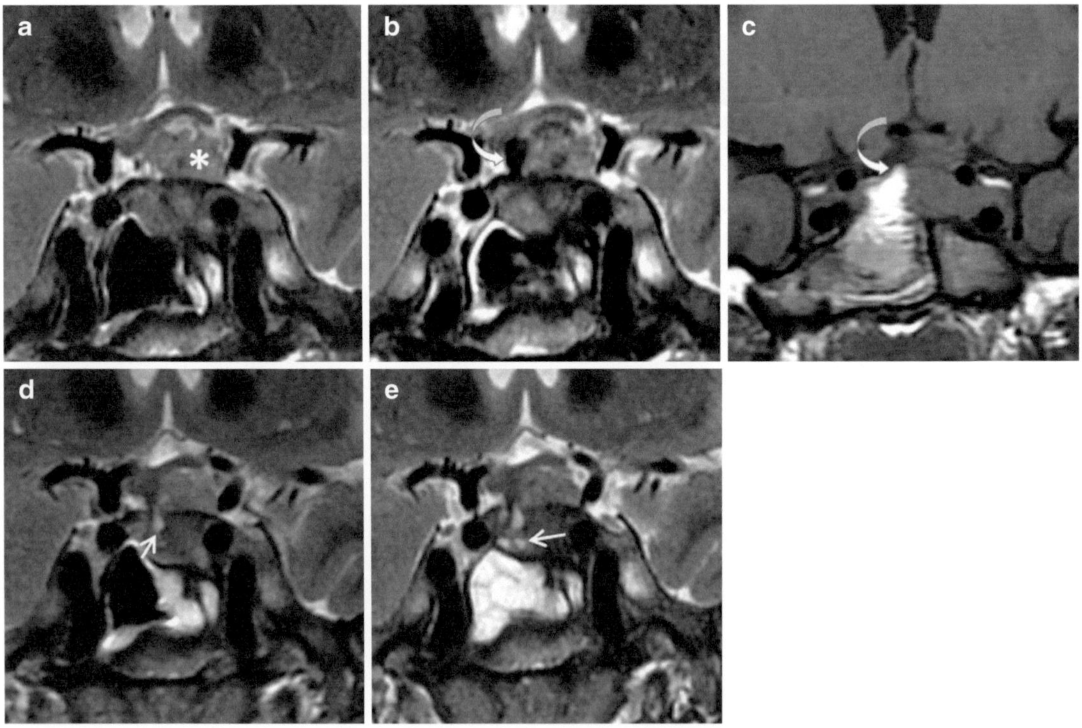

Fig. 26.4 CSF fistula. (**a**) Coronal T2WI. Pituitary adenoma with suprasellar extension (*asterisk*). (**b**) Coronal T2WI at day 4 after transsphenoidal surgery. Intracisternal T2 hypointense mass evoking the presence of blood (*arrow*). (**c**) Coronal T1WI on the same day demonstrates a piece of Surgicel impregnated with blood beyond the sellar diaphragm and constituting a fragile seal (*arrow*). (**d**, **e**) Coronal T2WIs at 12 and 13 weeks. Resorption of Surgicel packing leads to CSF fistula, materialized by CSF droplets (*straight arrows*) more numerous in (**e**)

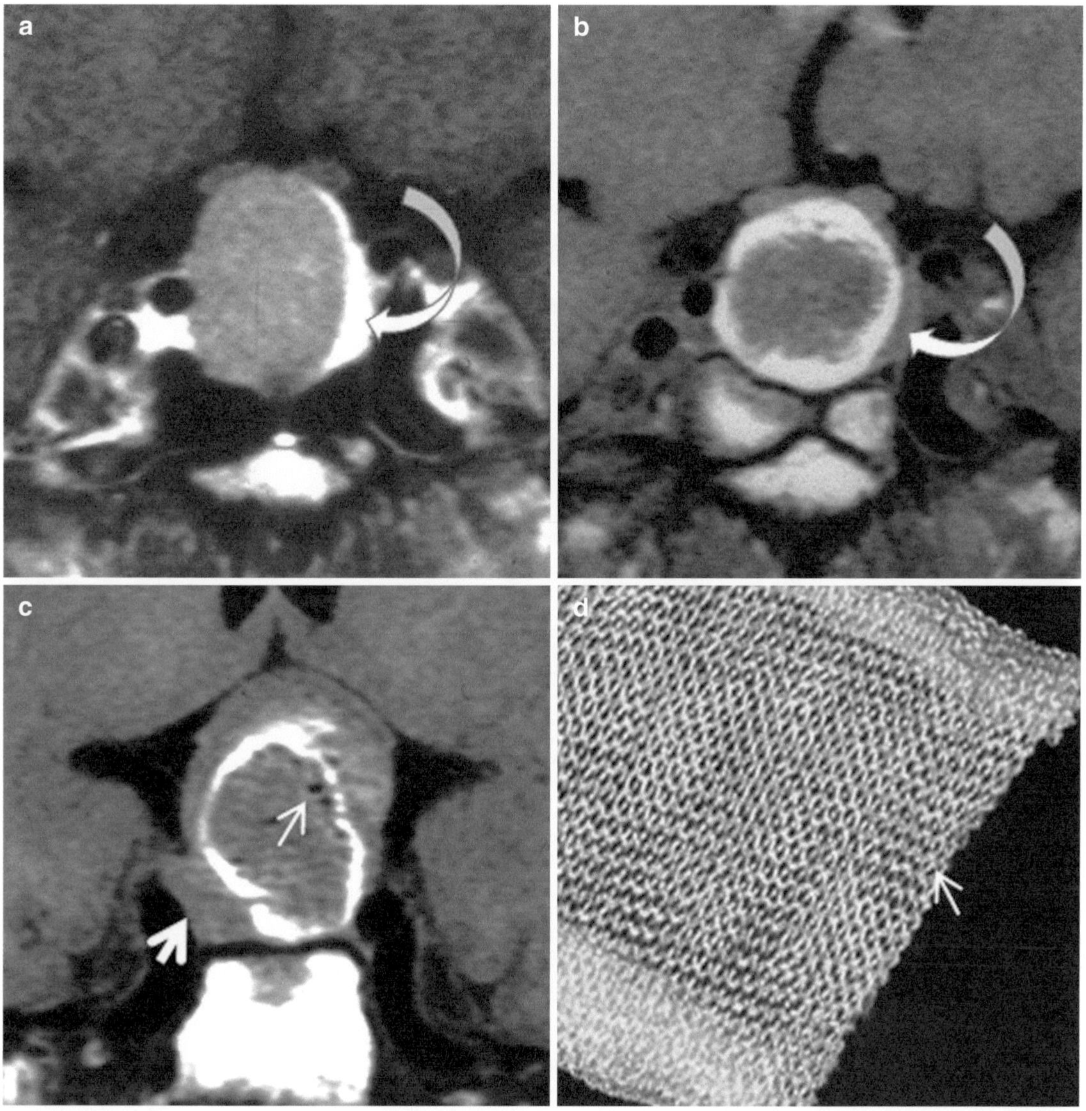

Fig. 26.5 MRI characteristics of Surgicel 4 days after surgery. (**a**, **b**) Coronal CE T1WI before (**a**) and coronal T1WI noncontrast at day 4 after surgery (**b**). Pituitary adenoma abutting the optic chiasm. The normal pituitary gland is compressed against the medial wall of left cavernous sinus in (**a**) and well distinguished in (**b**) (*arrows*). The sella is occupied by a T1-hypointense mass with a peripheral T1 hyperintense rim corresponding to Surgicel and methemoglobin in periphery. (**c**) Macroadenoma compressing the optic chiasm in another patient. Coronal T1W noncontrast image at day 4. Similar appearance of the surgical packing. Small air bubbles trapped in the tissue (*small arrow*). High suspicion of tumor remnant inferiorly (*thick arrow*). (**d**) Photograph of a piece of Surgicel

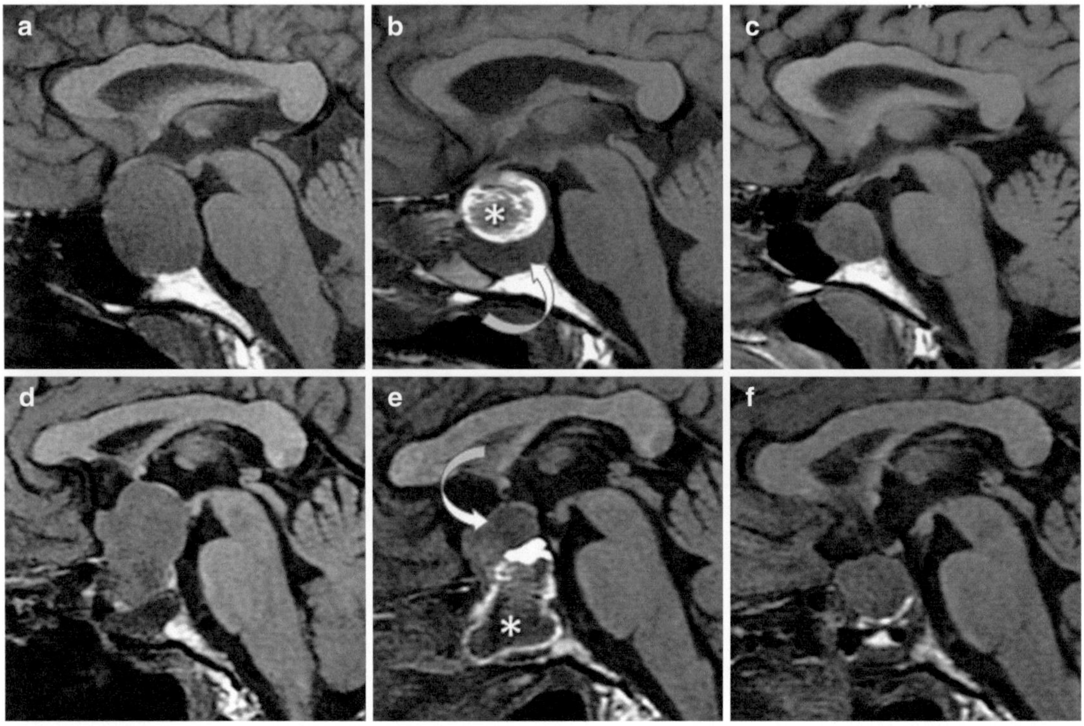

Fig. 26.6 Tumoral remnants at day 4 after surgery. (**a–f**) Noncontrast sagittal T1WI. Two different patients (*upper* and *lower rows*). (**a**, **d**) Initial MRI of pituitary macroadenomas. (**b**, **e**) Surgicel packing (*asterisk*) sharply delineates an inferior (**b**) and superior (**e**) remnant. (**c**, **f**) Remodeling of the tumoral remnant 6 months later

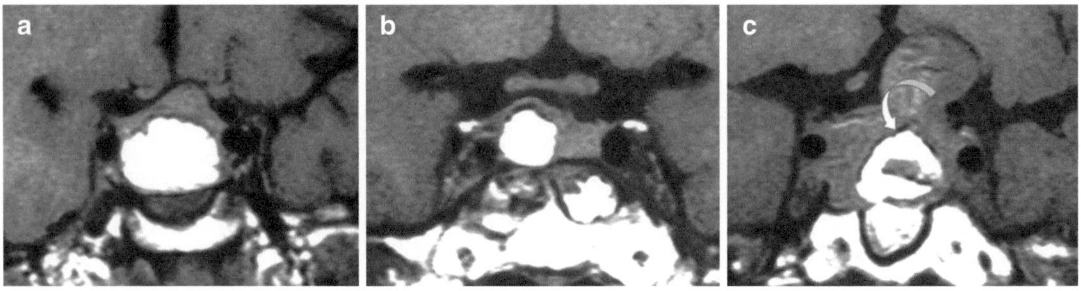

Fig. 26.7 Characteristic patterns of autologous fat grafting in three patients. (**a–c**) Coronal T1WIs. Highly T1-hyperintense mass with regular lobulated outline and chemical shift artifact (*arrow*)

Further Reading

Bonneville JF, Bonneville F, Schillo F et al (2003) Follow-up MRI after transsphenoidal surgery. J Neuroradiol 30:268–279

Stofko DL, Nickles T, Sun H, Dehdashti AR (2014) The value of immediate postoperative MR imaging following endoscopic endonasal pituitary surgery. Acta Neurochir (Wien) 156(1):133–140

Yoon PH, Kim DI, Jeon P, Lee SI, Lee SK, Kim SH (2001) Pituitary adenomas: early postoperative MR imaging after transsphenoidal resection. AJNR Am J Neuroradiol 22:1097–1104

27 The Late Postoperative Sella

Jean-François Bonneville

Pituitary centers which do not realize an immediate or 4-day postoperative MRI follow-up usually obtain an MRI at 3–6 months in search of a possible tumoral remnant. We recommend sagittal and coronal 3-mm thick T1WI and coronal 2-mm thick T2WI, ideally with a 3.0 T scanner. For easy comparison with the MRI follow-up to come, it is of uppermost importance to obtain coronal sequences with the same angulation, such as perpendicularly to the subcallosal plane (Fig. 27.1). In this way, recurrent tumors can be diagnosed and managed earlier (Fig. 27.2). An axial T2W 2-mm thick sequence is also useful if a small tumoral remnant is suspected at the posterior part of the cavernous sinus. If vasopressin storage has to be determined, an additional noncontrast axial T1W sequence is obtained. In our hands, contrast injection is frequently unnecessary and not routinely used. At 3 months postoperatively the Surgicel packing, if any, is not entirely resorbed; it will resorb later, by 6 months' follow-up (Fig. 27.3). If tissue glue has been used, complete shrinkage of postoperative sellar mass can be delayed (Fig. 27.4). Fat graft, if implanted in the sella in the case of CSF fistula, shrinks partially, but will persist long term, as long as 10–25 years (Fig. 27.3). Fat graft can also migrate into the sphenoid sinus if the sellar floor has not been reconstructed. The rate of resorption of autologous fat graft remains largely unpredictable. In some rare circumstances, particularly if the patient has gained weight, an increased volume of the sellar fat graft can be observed (Fig. 27.5), as it is elsewhere in the body when fat is used for correction of soft tissue volume loss or for cosmetic reasons such as breast augmentation. T1 hyperintensity of the normal pituitary tissue is sometimes transiently observed in the few months after surgery (Fig. 27.6). We have hypothesized that this phenomenon reflects a transient hormonal synthesis increase of the small-volume residual pituitary. Most of the packing other than fat being resorbed at 6 months is sellar content consisting of normal pituitary residual tissue and/or tumoral remnant. We suggest that coronal high-resolution, 2-mm thick T2W sequences coupled with 3-mm thick noncontrast T1W sequences are the most informative to differentiate both, and that contrast-enhanced MRI can be frequently spared. At 6 months, final remodeling of the normal pituitary gland has occurred; it appears frequently as a homogeneous triangular or oval small mass in contact with the sellar floor and the medial wall of the cavernous sinus. On T2WI, the T2 signal of the tumoral remnant, if any, is nearly always more or less hyperintense if compared with that of the residual normal pituitary tissue excepted in some somatotropinomas. The pituitary stalk is tilted towards the normal pituitary. In case of doubt, i.e., normal pituitary versus tumoral remnant, sequential MRI rigorously performed with the same parameters and the same inclination will frequently demonstrate a slight increase volume of the remnant and no change in the normal pituitary gland remnant (Fig. 27.7). Nevertheless, some remnants can stay unchanged for years, but perfect reproducibility of sequential MRIs permits one to

J.-F. Bonneville et al., *MRI of the Pituitary Gland*, DOI 10.1007/978-3-319-29043-0_27

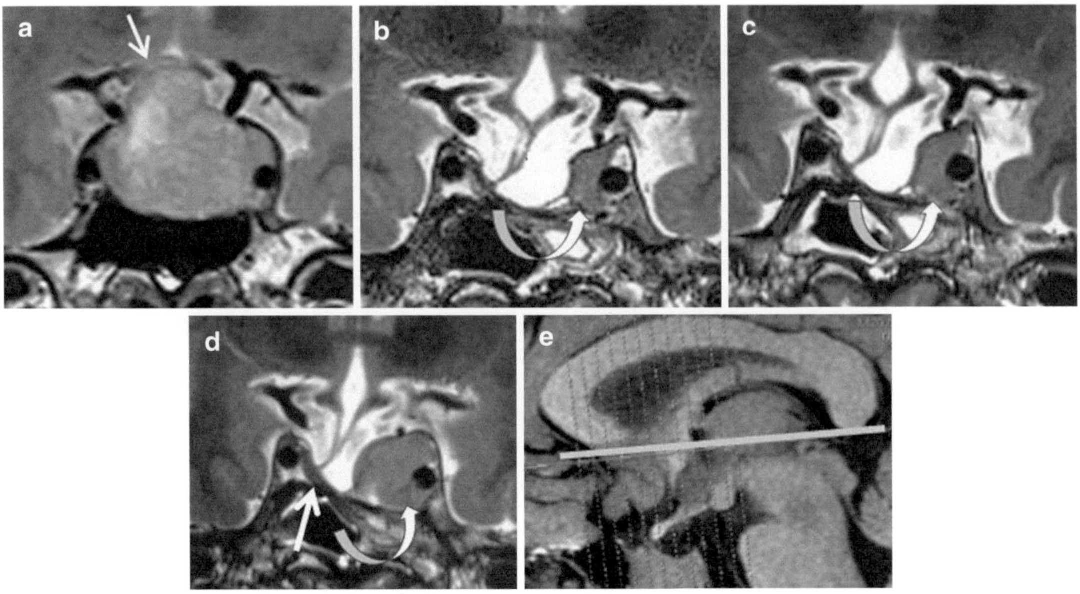

Fig. 27.1 Pituitary nonfunctioning macroadenoma remnant in a 25-year-old man. (**a–d**) Coronal T2WIs. (**a**) Pituitary adenoma with compression and T2 hypersignal of optic chiasm (*arrow*), (**b**) 3 months after surgery. Small tumoral remnant on the left (*curved arrow*). (**c**) Three months later. Discrete but indisputable rapid remnant increased volume. (**d**) Six months later. Aggressive tumoral behavior is confirmed; cavernous sinus invasion is patent. Normal residual anterior pituitary (*straight arrow*) is T2 hypointense in comparison with tumor remnant. (**e**) The use of a reference plane (here the subcallosal plane) permits an easy comparison of coronal serial MR images

affirm this stability. Volumetry obtained from 3D images can also help, but is more complicated to implement. A vasopressin storage bright spot can increase in size in both eutopic and ectopic positions with time (Fig. 27.5a, b) or even reappear after complete disappearance. Axial T1W noncontrast fat-saturated sequence is of utmost importance to detect the tiniest T1-hyperintense spot after resumption of vasopressin synthesis and storage. Descent of the optic chiasm with a V-shaped appearance is constant after surgery of intra- and suprasellar masses. Fatty degeneration of the cortical bone of the sphenoid walls occurs as soon as 6 months postoperatively and increases for years thereafter. It is observed when the neurosurgeon has removed the sphenoidal sinus mucosa to avoid mucocele formation. Such bony changes can mimic, for instance, the osteoma of a meningioma of the planum sphenoidale (Fig. 27.8).

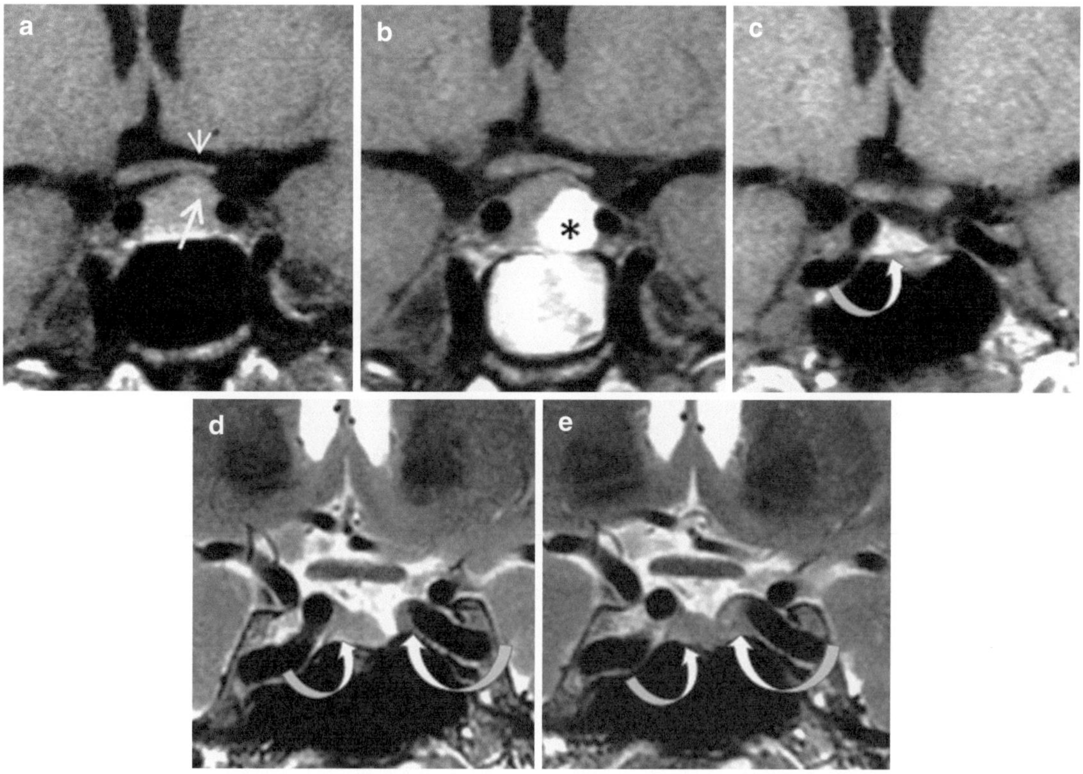

Fig. 27.2 Pituitary adenoma late recurrence. (**a**–**c**) Coronal noncontrast T1WIs. (**d**, **e**) Coronal T2WIs. (**a**) Pituitary adenoma with optic chiasm impingement (*short arrow*). (**b**) Four days postoperatively. Surgicel packing of the tumoral bed (*asterisk*). (**c**) Eighteen months after surgery. No remnant clearly visible; normal anterior pituitary is faintly T1 hyperintense (*small curved arrow*). (**d**) At 5 years. Tiny recurrent tumor suspected on the left (*long curved arrow*). (**e**) At 12 years. Recurrence is confirmed; tumoral tissue (*long curved arrow*) is slightly T2 hyperintense compared with the anterior pituitary (*short curved arrow*)

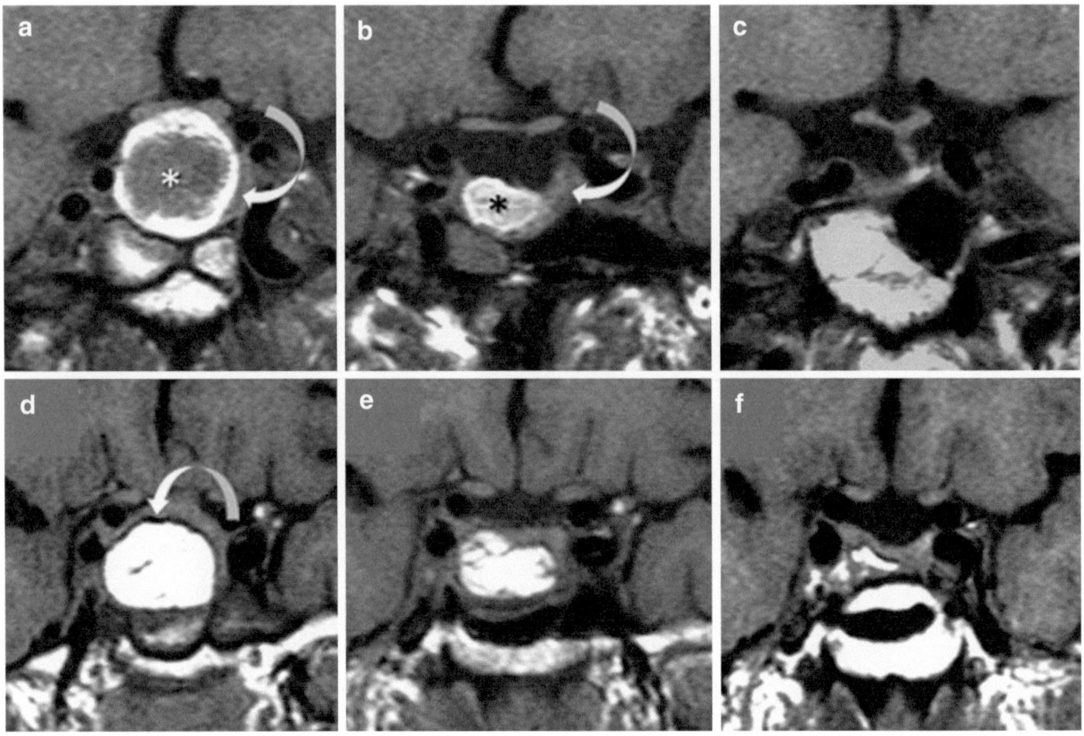

Fig. 27.3 Packing resorption. (**a–f**) Coronal T1WIs. Surgicel packing (*asterisk*) 4 days (**a**) and 3 months (**b**) after transsphenoidal surgery of a pituitary adenoma; normal anterior pituitary (*arrow*). (**c**) Follow-up at 3 years. No recurrence; the pituitary stalk is tilted toward the T1-hyperintense posterior pituitary. V-shaped deformation of optic chiasm; the sellar floor is raised. (**d**, **e**) Fat graft (*arrow*) 4 days (**d**), 6 months (**e**), and 10 years (**f**) after surgery

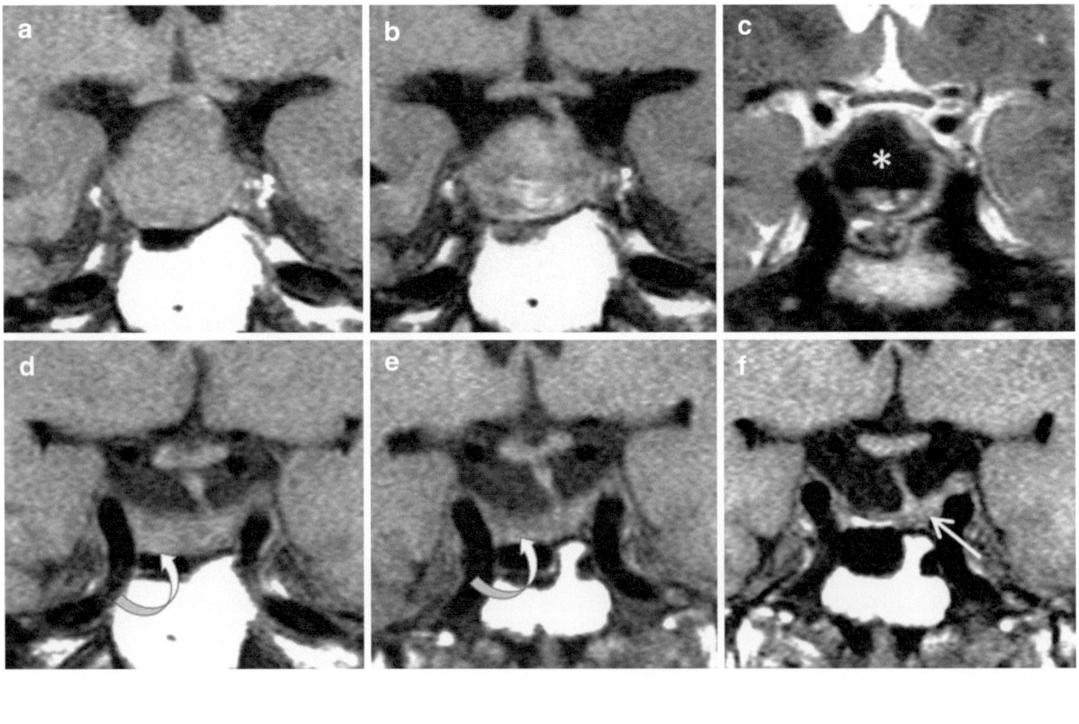

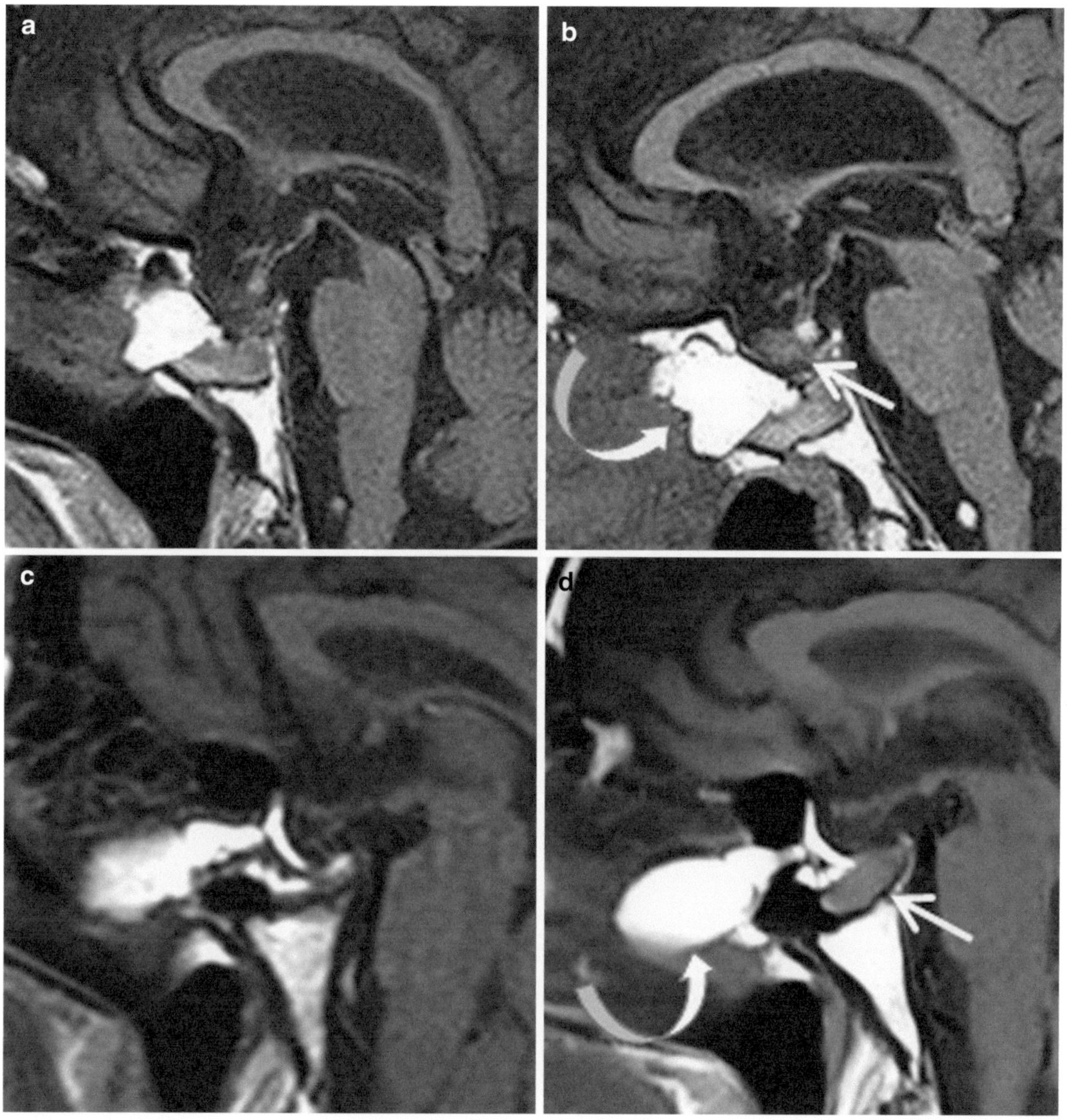

Fig. 27.5 Autologous fat graft: increased volume with time in two patients. (**a–d**) Sagittal T1WIs. (**a–c**) Persisting sphenoidal fat graft respectively 2 and 3 years after surgery of a pituitary nonfunctioning adenoma. (**b–d**) Three and 5 years later respectively. Intrasellar tumoral recurrence in both cases (*small arrow*); progressive enlargement of the ectopic posterior lobe in (**b**); increased volume of the fat graft in both cases (*curved arrow*)

Fig. 27.4 Pituitary surgery and tissue glue. (**a–f**) Coronal T1WIs. (**c**) Coronal T2WI. Pituitary macroadenoma before surgery (**a**); 4 days after surgery (**b, c**). No shrinkage of the mass; faint T1-hyperintense and marked T2-hypointense signal (*asterisk*) indicating the presence of blood. (**d–f**) Slow resorption of the sellar content (*curved arrow*) at 3, 9, and 18 months after surgery. Tilting of the pituitary stalk toward the normal pituitary gland (*straight arrow*)

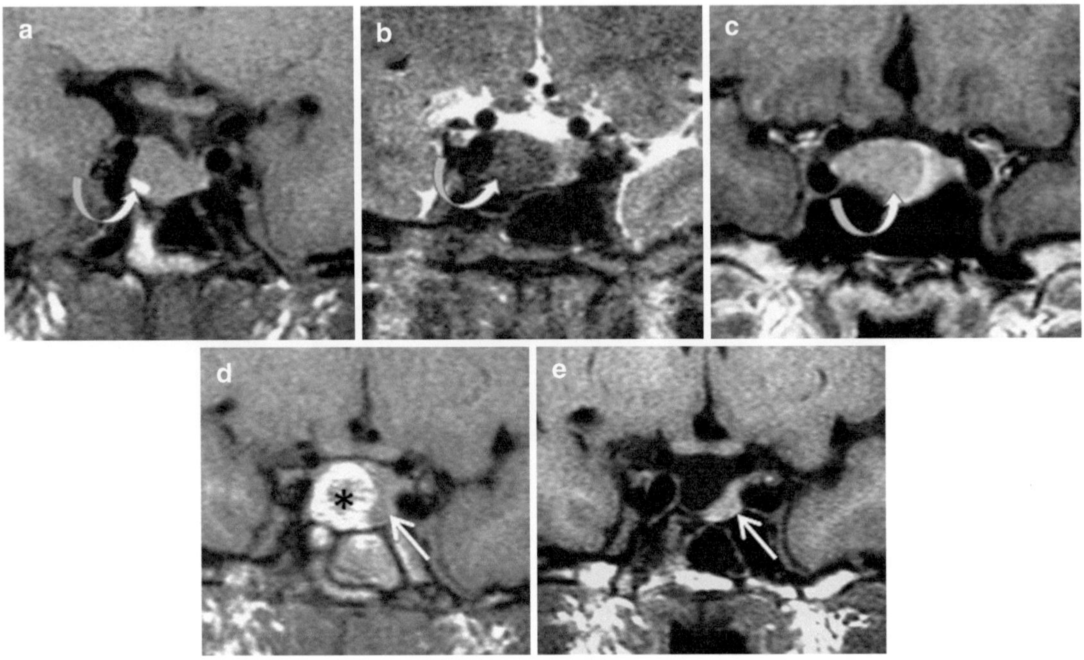

Fig. 27.6 GH-secreting intrasellar adenoma. IGF1 is 1,045 ng/ml. (**a–c**) Coronal T1, T2, and CE T1 WIs at diagnosis. Minute hemorrhage (*arrow* in **a**). T2 hypointensity of GH adenoma if compared with normal anterior pituitary (**b**) with no postgadolinium enhancement (**c**). (**d**, **e**) Coronal T1WIs 4 days (**d**) and 18 months (**e**) after surgery. Surgicel packing (*asterisk*). Remodeling of the anterior pituitary with relative T1 hyperintensity (*straight arrow*) with no tumoral remnant. IGF1 is 296 ng/ml; the patient is cured

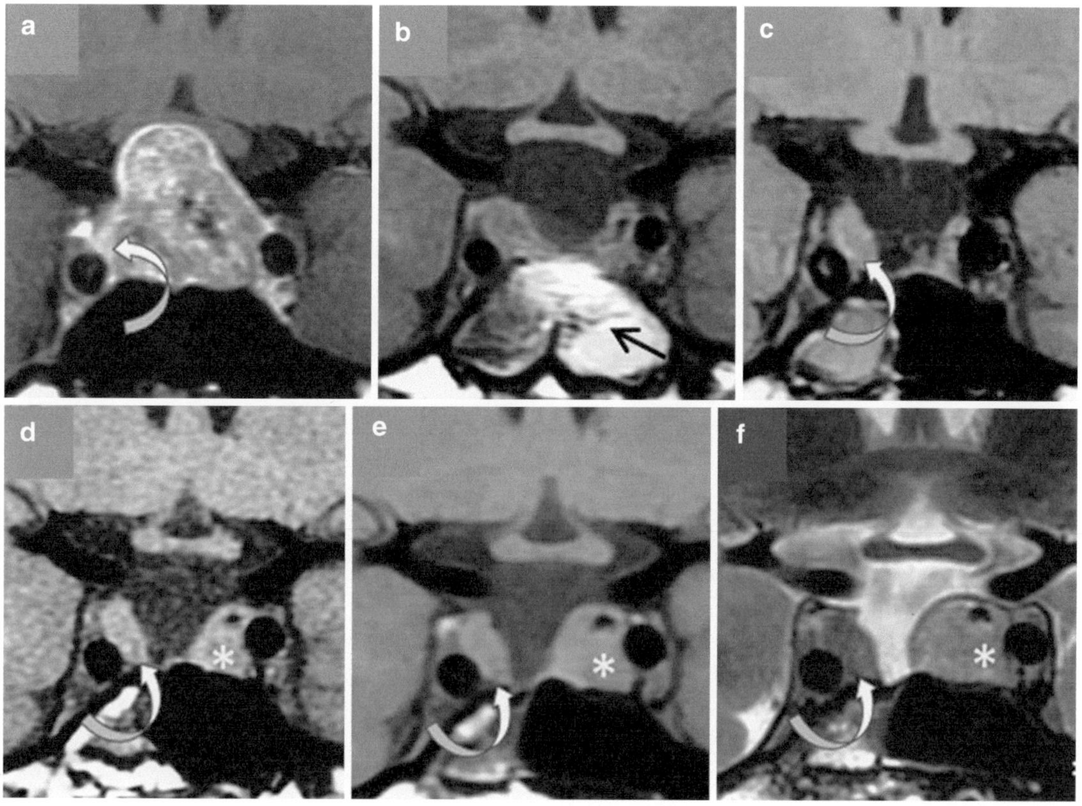

Fig. 27.7 Nonsecreting pituitary macroadenoma. (**a**) CE T1WI. The normal pituitary tissue is displaced in periphery and specially to the right side (*arrow*). (**b–e**) Coronal T1WIs at 4 days (**b**): sphenoidal Surgicel packing (*black arrow*); and at 8 months (**c**), 3 years (**d**), and 4 years (**e**). (**f**) Coronal T2WI at 5 years. Stability of the residual anterior pituitary (*curved arrow*); progressive enlargement of a tumoral remnant (*asterisk*). Difference in signal between pituitary gland and tumoral remnant is only clearly discernible on T2WI

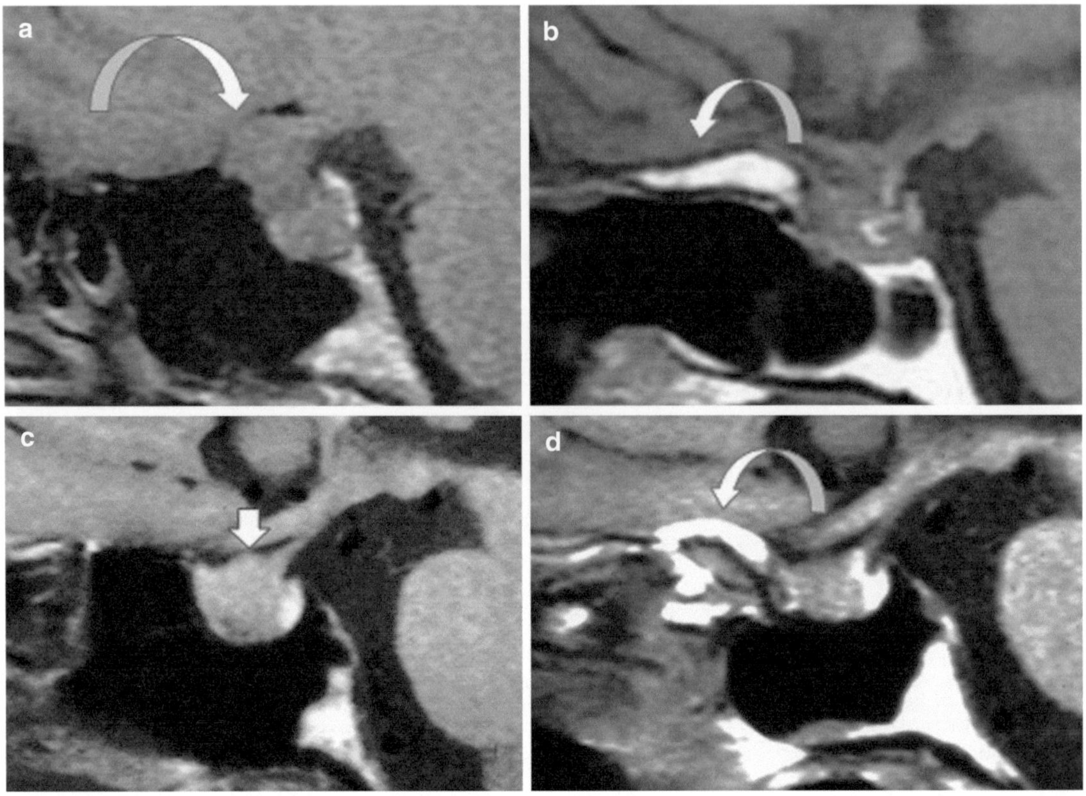

Fig. 27.8 Sphenoid bony changes after surgery in two patients; (**a**–**d**) Sagittal T1WIs. Macroadenoma (**a**) and microadenoma (**c**) at diagnosis. In both cases, the surgeon has removed the sphenoid sinus mucosa to avoid mucus retention and possible subsequent mucocele. Devascularization of periosteal bone is responsible for degenerative changes with thickening and T1 hyperintensity of the planum sphenoidale mimicking an osteoma (*curved arrows*)

Further Reading

Anis KH, Sossa DE, Castillo M et al (2013) Intrasellar fat graft gains weight with the patient. Neuroradiol J 26:301–303

Bladowska J, Bednarek-Tupikowska G, Sokolska V et al (2010) MRI image characteristics of materials implanted at sellar region after transsphenoidal resection of pituitary tumours. Pol J Radiol 75(2): 46–54

Nakasu Y, Itoh R, Nakasu S et al (1998) Postoperative sella: evaluation with fast spin echo T2-weighted high-resolution imaging. Neurosurgery 43: 440–447

28 Complications of Pituitary Surgery

Jean-François Bonneville

Complications of pituitary surgery are rare, particularly in the hands of experienced surgeons. Endoscopic transsphenoidal surgery has not significantly reduced their frequency. Cushing disease and reintervention are risk factors. Diabetes insipidus, anterior lobe dysfunction, vascular and nerve injuries, and CSF leakage can occur. Diabetes insipidus is the most frequent postoperative complication, mostly being transient. Permanent diabetes insipidus appears after manipulation or injury of the posterior lobe, pituitary stalk, or hypothalamus. Whether the preoperative presence of an ectopic posterior lobe has a protective effect against the occurrence of diabetes insipidus is a topic of debate. ADH insufficiency is correlated with loss of posterior lobe or pituitary stalk bright spot. Decreased T1 hyperintensity of the posterior lobe is best appreciated on axial T1WI and can be progressive a few days after surgery. Surgical bed hemorrhage or sellar packing can mask ADH storage and chemical shift artifact from a fatty dorsum sellae. In the latter case, axial T1W fat-saturated sequence is recommended. Late reappearance—after months—of a weak bright spot either intrasellarly or at the stalk level may announce the spontaneous cure of diabetes insipidus (Fig. 28.1). CSF fistula is usually recognized during surgery and sealed immediately, frequently with a fat graft. If unrecognized, CSF fistula can lead to rhinorrhea, intracranial hypotension, pneumocephalus (Fig. 28.2), or meningitis. Direct visualization of CSF fistula is rarely observed (see Fig. 26.4). Intracranial hypotension secondary to CSF leakage gives rise to venous congestion with bulging of the pituitary gland and enlargement of the venous compartment of the cavernous sinus, inferior coronary sinus, and retroclival venous plexus (Fig. 28.3). Visual complications are secondary to surgical bed hemorrhage or overpacking. Optic chiasm and/or intracavernous oculomotor nerve compression can occur. Slow flow of laterosellar veins attests to impaired pituitary drainage (see Fig. 26.3). Inadvertent introduction of surgical tools within the cavernous sinus may be responsible for oculomotor nerve (Fig. 28.4) or internal carotid artery injuries. Intracavernous internal carotid and, more rarely, basilar artery injuries are the most serious complications of transsphenoidal surgery. Internal carotid artery injury can manifest itself immediately during surgery or later with epistaxis. Medial position of internal carotid arteries (Fig. 28.5a–f) and extreme thinness of the carotid sulcus of the sphenoid bone are risk factors, as is acromegaly. Hard packing of cavernous sinus can lead to internal carotid artery thrombosis, which can be asymptomatic in cases of complete circle of Willis and is revealed only on serial MRI (Fig. 28.5g–i). False aneurysm of the carotid siphon is sometimes detected postoperatively; in this case, the optimal strategy remains under debate. Endovascular treatment of the false aneurysm or occlusion of the parent artery are discussed in cases of late epistaxis after surgery. Basilar artery injury, which fortunately is excep-

J.-F. Bonneville et al., *MRI of the Pituitary Gland*, DOI 10.1007/978-3-319-29043-0_28

tional, can arise with aggressive pituitary adenomas or malignant tumors involving the clivus (Fig. 28.5j–l). Aggravation of pre-existing pituitary deficiency may occur if the normal residual pituitary gland is not preserved, as in large or aggressive pituitary macroadenomas. The sella appears completely empty in these cases. Symptomatic sphenoid mucoceles are rare; risk factors include nonexcision of sphenoid sinus mucosa and obstruction of sphenoid sinus ostium (see Chap. 39).

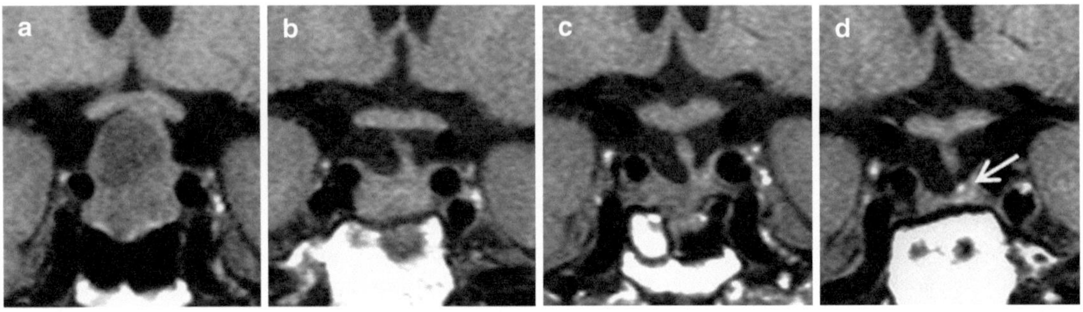

Fig. 28.1 Postoperative diabetes insipidus. (**a**–**d**) Coronal T1WIs. (**a**) Pituitary adenoma with suprasellar extension. (**b**–**d**) Serial MRIs 3, 6, and 12 months after surgery. Late reappearance of ADH storage at the pituitary stalk end (*arrow*)

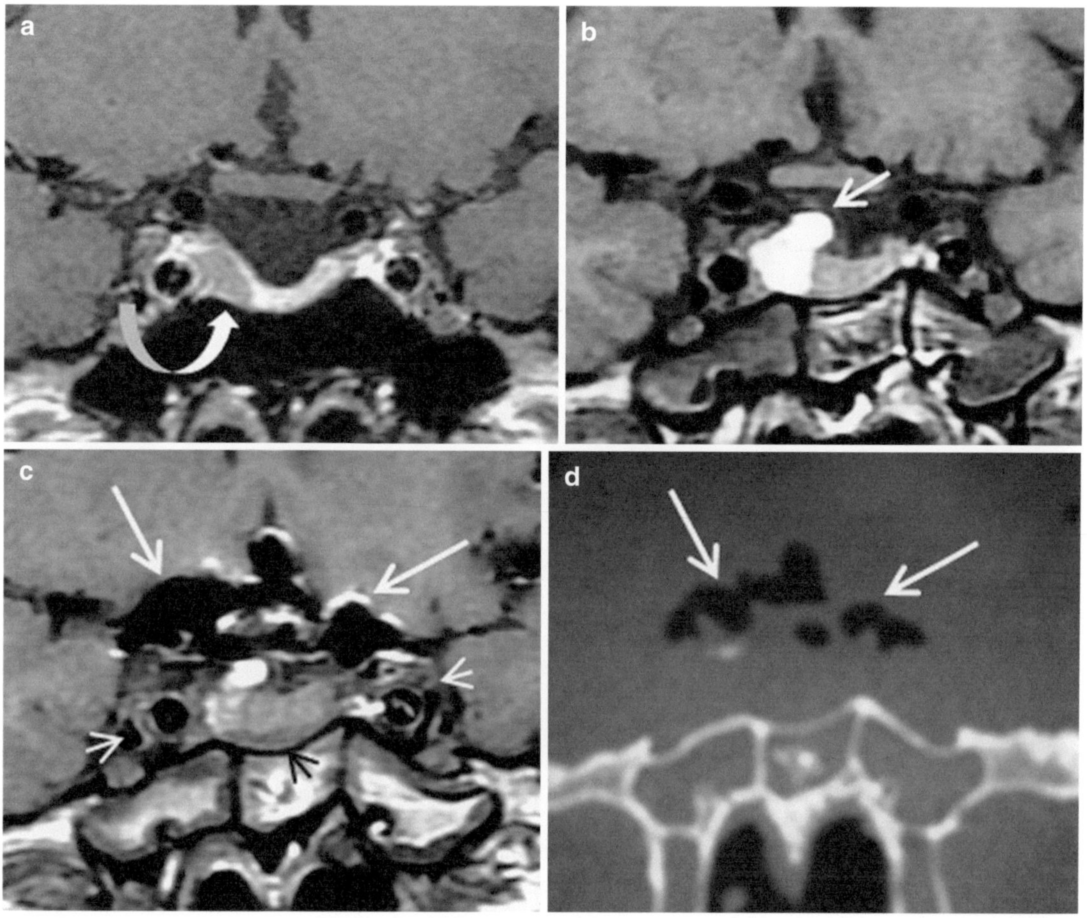

Fig. 28.2 CSF fistula and pneumocephalus. (**a**) Coronal CE TIWI. GH-secreting microadenoma in contact with the sellar diaphragm. (**b**, **c**) Coronal T1WIs. Three days after surgery (**b**), a piece of Surgicel has been put in place during surgery to plug a CSF fistula (*arrow*). Ten days later (**c**), a brutal headache occurred and pneumocephalus (*long arrows*) is detected after partial resorption of surgical packing. Note enlargement of extradural venous plexus (*small arrows*) in relation to intracranial hypotension. (**d**) CT demonstration of pneumocephalus

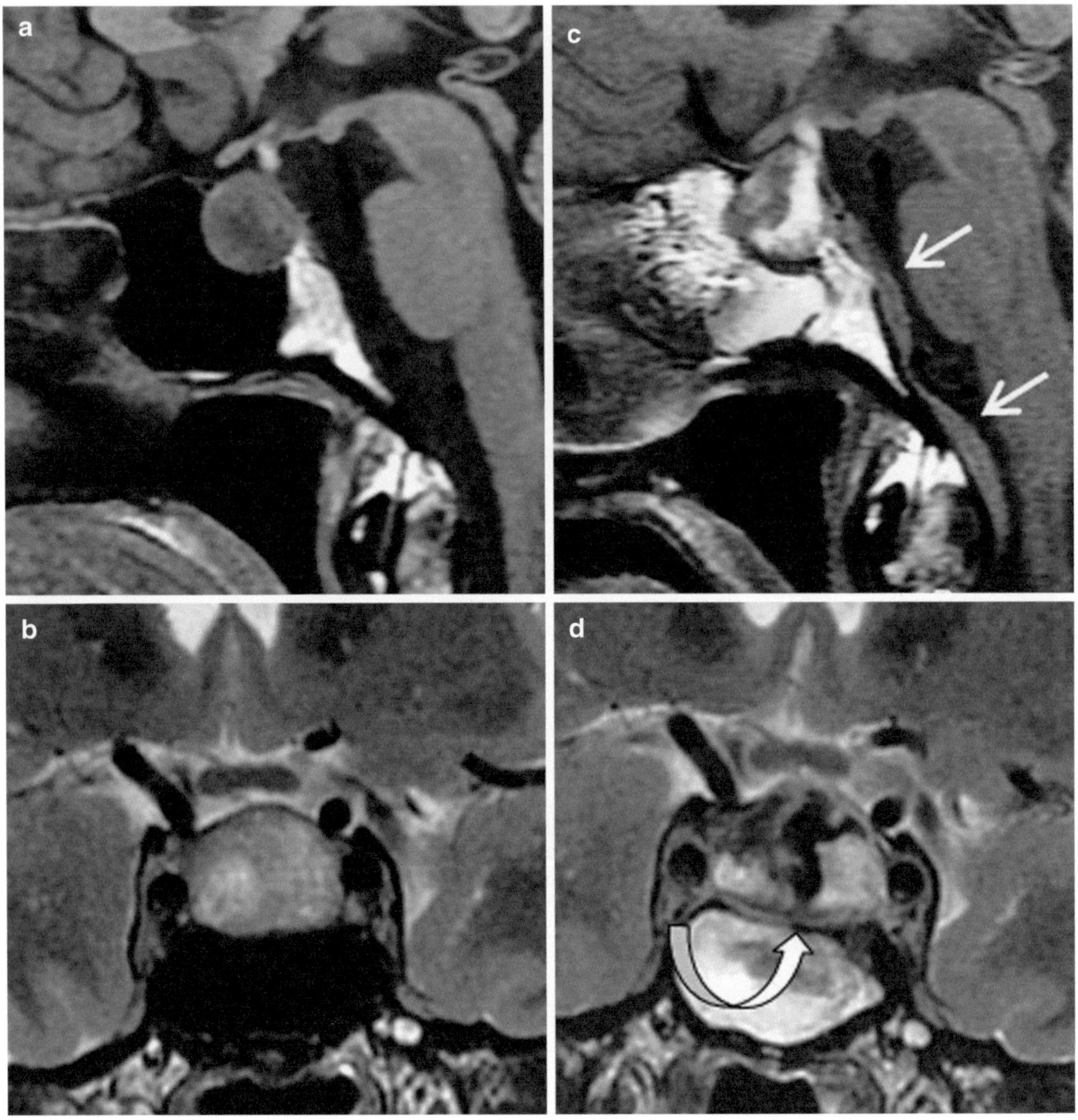

Fig. 28.3 CSF fistula and intracranial hypotension. Sagittal T1WIs (**a–c**) and coronal T2WIs (**b–d**) before (**a**, **b**) and 4 days after surgery (**c**, **d**) of a pituitary macroadenoma. Increased height of sellar content. Thickening of the retroclival venous plexus (*straight arrows*) and inferior coronary sinus (*curved arrow*). These features reveal a CSF fistula not recognized during surgery

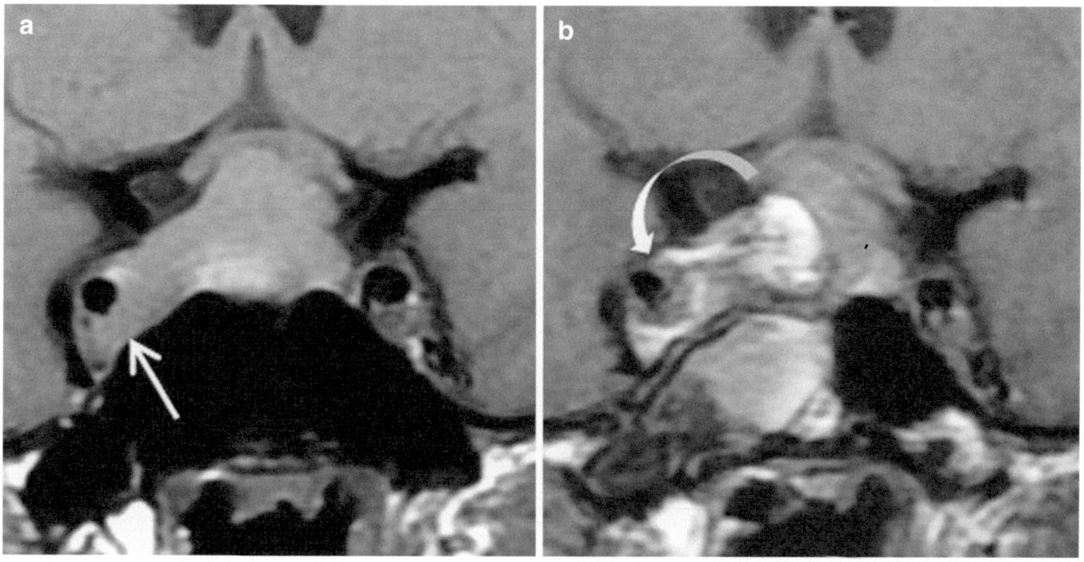

Fig. 28.4 Oculomotor nerve palsy. (**a**, **b**) Coronal T1WIs before and 4 days after surgery of a corticotropic pituitary macroadenoma invading right cavernous sinus (*straight arrow*). Inadvertent entrance of surgical tools in right cavernous sinus leads to local hemorrhage . Note a mild compression of left internal intracavernous carotid artery (*curved arrow*)

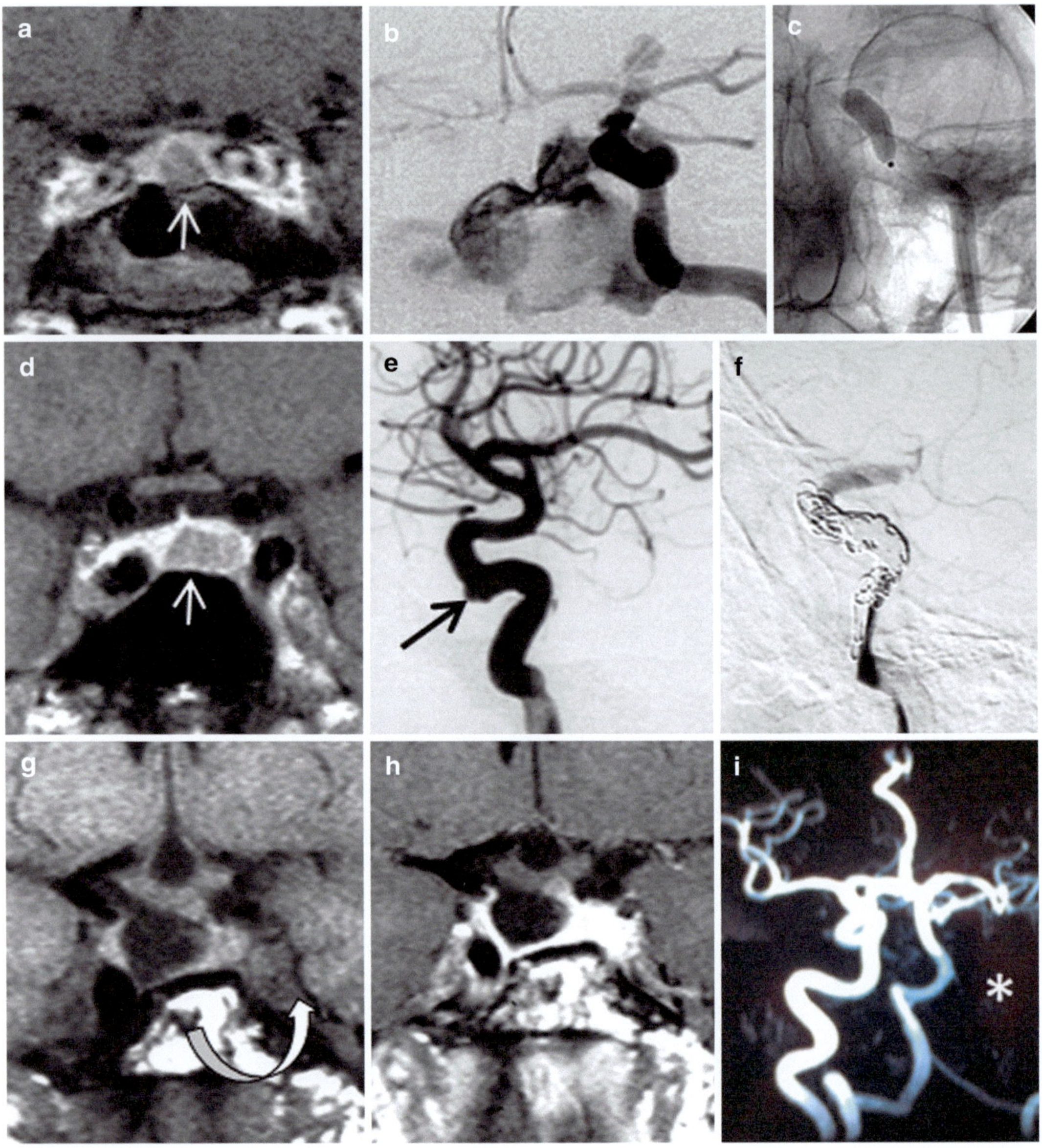

Fig. 28.5 Vascular complications of pituitary surgery in four patients. (**a**) Coronal CE T1WI. GH-secreting microadenoma (*arrow*). Narrow sella and medial position of internal carotid arteries. (**b**) Left carotid angiography. Massive bleeding from intracavernous internal carotid artery. (**c**) Balloon occlusion of left internal carotid artery. (**d**) CE T1WI. GH-secreting pituitary adenoma (*arrow*) with narrow intercarotid distance. (**e**) Carotid angiography. Small pseudoaneurysm of carotid siphon (*black arrow*) responsible for a severe epistaxis. (**f**) Coil occlusion of carotid artery. (**g–i**) Asymptomatic internal carotid artery thrombosis discovered 2 years after surgery for a GH-secreting adenoma. (**g, h**) Coronal T1 and CE T1 WIs. Left cavernous sinus looks empty (*curved arrow*); left carotid artery is absent on (**i**) MRA (*asterisk*). (**j, k**) Sagittal T1 and CE T1 WIs. Aggressive pituitary adenoma with unsuspected clival erosion (*arrow*); pseudoaneurysm of basilar artery at (**l**) control angiography

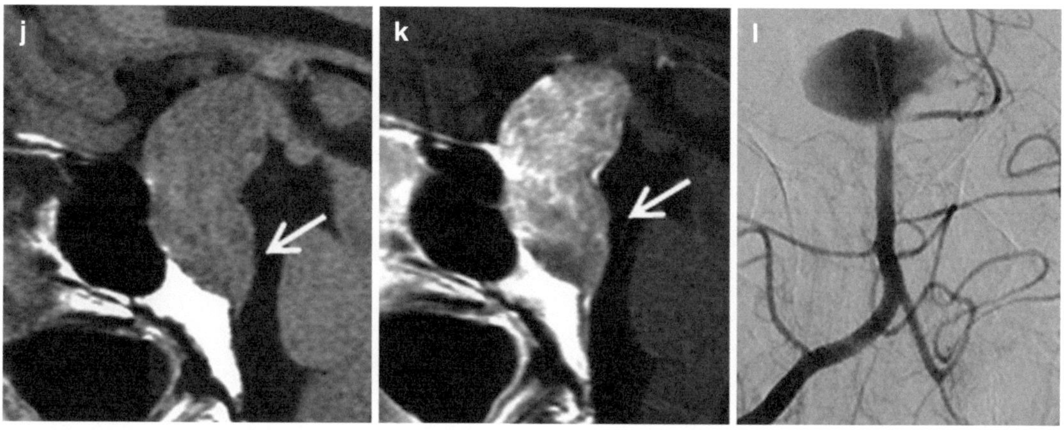

Fig. 28.5 (continued)

Further Reading

Berker M, Hazer DB, Yücel T et al (2012) Complications of endoscopic surgery of the pituitary adenomas: analysis of 570 patients and review of the literature. Pituitary 15(3):288–300

Laws ER Jr (1999) Vascular complications of transsphenoidal surgery. Pituitary 2(2):163–170

Wang F, Zhou T, Wei S et al (2015) Endoscopic endonasal transsphenoidal surgery of 1,166 pituitary adenomas. Surg Endosc 29:1270–1280

29 The Pituitary Gland After Radiation Therapy

Jean-François Bonneville

The role of radiation therapy in the management of pituitary adenomas remains controversial among endocrinologists. If radiation therapy is generally accepted in cases of obvious regrowth of a nonfunctioning pituitary adenoma remnant years after surgery if there are no further surgical options, its place is more discussed as a systematic therapeutic adjunct after partial debulking of the same adenomas. Indeed, increased volume of such a pituitary nonfunctioning adenoma remnant does not occur in all patients while pituitary radiotherapy is not without side effects, particularly hypopituitarism and its associated excess mortality. Five-year incidence of hypopituitarism is approximately 20 %, but increases to 80 % by 10–15 years. Visual complications, stroke, and secondary tumors today constitute a very low risk (Figs. 29.1 and 29.2). In general, the risk of recurrence after radiotherapy treatment is very low but not zero (Fig. 29.3). For functioning pituitary adenoma remnants observed after surgery, radiation therapy may be an option as well as medical treatment. The efficacy of radiation therapy is appreciable not only on tumoral control but mainly on hormonal normalization, which is obtained in about half of the cases. Time of remission varies from 12 to 60 months. Different modalities of radiation therapy are available. Radiosurgery delivers a high radiation dose, 12–20 Gy, in a single session. Four forms of radiosurgery are available: Gamma Knife surgery, linear accelerator, CyberKnife, and proton therapy. All four are reserved for tumoral remnants <30 mm in diameter, located at distance from the optic pathways, the ideal indication being intrasellar pituitary adenoma remnant with cavernous sinus extension. Conventional fractionated external beam radiotherapy delivers 45–50 Gy over a 5- to 6-week period and can be offered to patients with large tumors even if the tumor target is less than 5 mm remote from the optic chiasm. The role of MRI is to determine precisely the tumoral extent and tumoral volume to help the radiation oncologist decide the radiation planning; evaluation of cavernous sinus extension and visual pathway relationships are essential. After radiation therapy, MRI evaluates tumoral shrinkage, which can differ with radiation therapy modalities, dose of radiation, location of the tumor, and tumoral cell sensibility. It is accepted that an objective response rate, i.e., >25 % shrinkage, is obtained in more than 80 % of patients harboring a pituitary adenoma remnant at 4 years. There is no significant difference for nonfunctioning versus functioning pituitary adenomas. The response rate at early time points, i.e., between 6 months and 2 years after radiation therapy, is not clearly known. Nevertheless, it is important to determine as early as possible whether radiation therapy in a particular patient

J.-F. Bonneville et al., *MRI of the Pituitary Gland*, DOI 10.1007/978-3-319-29043-0_29

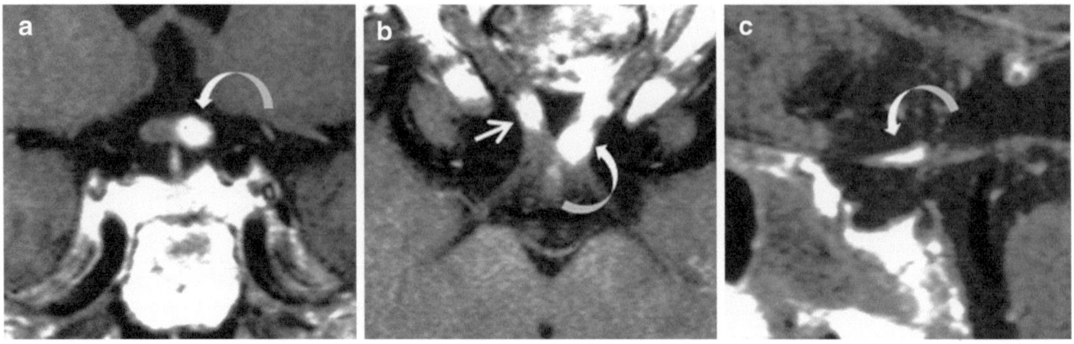

Fig. 29.1 Optic neuropathy after proton therapy in a 64-year-old diabetic patient presenting with a clival chordoma (historical). (**a–c**) Coronal, axial, and sagittal CE T1WIs. Abnormal postgadolinium enhancement of the left part of the optic chiasm (*curved arrow*) and right optic nerve (*straight arrow*). No excessive radiation dosage was applied; diabetes was held responsible for this complication

will have tumoral efficacy or not. It is our policy to track meticulously the changes in the size of pituitary tumors by using dedicated MRI techniques. Tumoral volume calculated from pituitary remnant dimensions in three orthogonal planes may not be accurate, and may lead to bias and direct volume calculation by the computer. We prefer to consider the transverse and craniocaudal dimensions only, measured on coronal T2WI, serial MRI being obtained with rigorous identical parameters and the coronal plane being strictly perpendicular to the line joining the inferior surface of the genu and the splenium of corpus callosum (Figs. 1.1 and 29.4). By this means, it seems possible to detect early tumoral shrinkage between 6 and 12 months after radiation treatment (Fig. 29.5). The use of coronal T2WI also may permit detection of tumoral signal change before any tumoral size change: in our practice, demonstration of a heterogeneous T2 hyperintensity of the pituitary adenoma remnant frequently precedes objective tumoral shrinkage and asserts that radiation therapy has begun to act (Fig. 29.6).

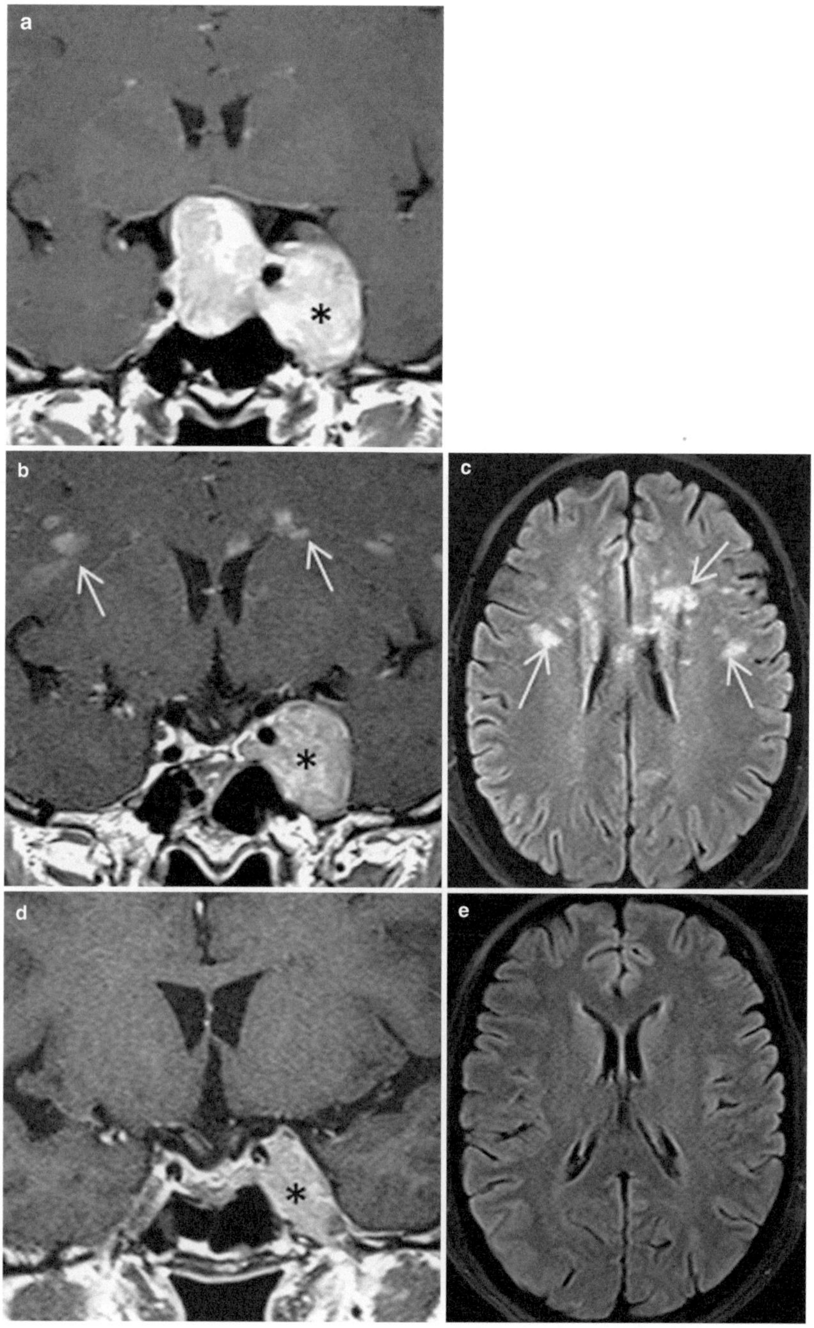

Fig. 29.2 Subacute postradiotherapy encephalitis in a 43-year-old woman with a nonfunctioning macroadenoma. (**a**) Coronal CE T1WI before radiotherapy. Postsurgical large intracavernous sinus remnant (*asterisk*) treated with conformational radiotherapy (54 Gy). Four weeks later, quadripyramidal and cerebellar syndrome, aphasia, and deep sensitivity disorders. (**b**, **c**) Coronal CE T1WI and brain axial FLAIR. Multiple enhanced hyperintense foci in the juxtaventricular and subcortical white matter (*arrows*). Favorable outcome after 6 months of corticosteroid therapy. (**d**, **e**) Same sequences as (**b**, **c**) 2 years later. Complete resolution of the brain abnormalities. Shrinkage of the cavernous sinus remnant

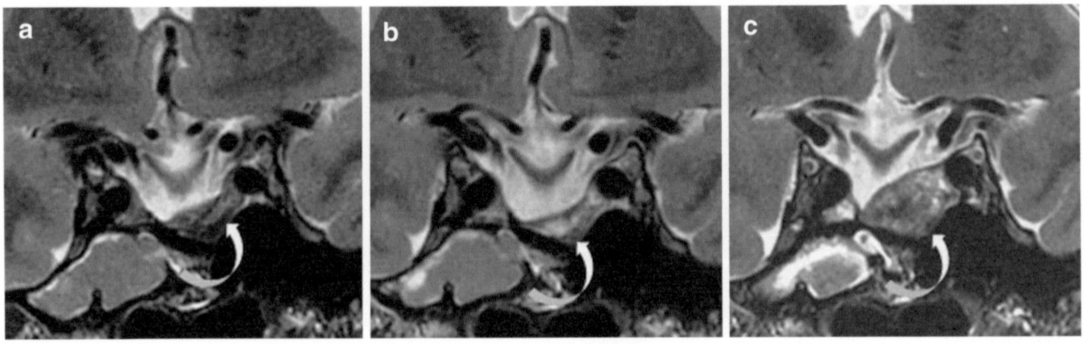

Fig. 29.3 (**a**–**c**) Coronal T2WIs. Nonfunctioning pituitary adenoma recurrence in a 36-year-old man. (**a**) Two years after surgery. (**b**) Eight months after conventional fractionated therapy. Very slight remnant shrinkage; T2 hyperintensity is more pronounced (*arrow*). (**c**) Major recurrence 8 years later

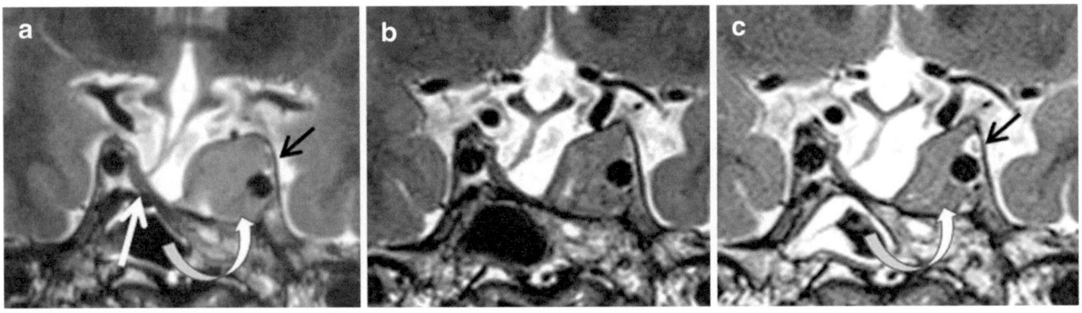

Fig. 29.4 Same patient as in Fig. 29.1. (**a**–**c**) Coronal T2WIs. (**a**) Rapid increase of a nonfunctioning pituitary adenoma remnant (*curved arrow*). The oculomotor nerve sheath is compressed (*black arrow*). Normal pituitary residual tissue (*white straight arrow*). (**b**, **c**) Four and 11 months, respectively, after CyberKnife. Shrinkage is already patent in (**b**). The third nerve sheath is no longer compressed (*black arrow*)

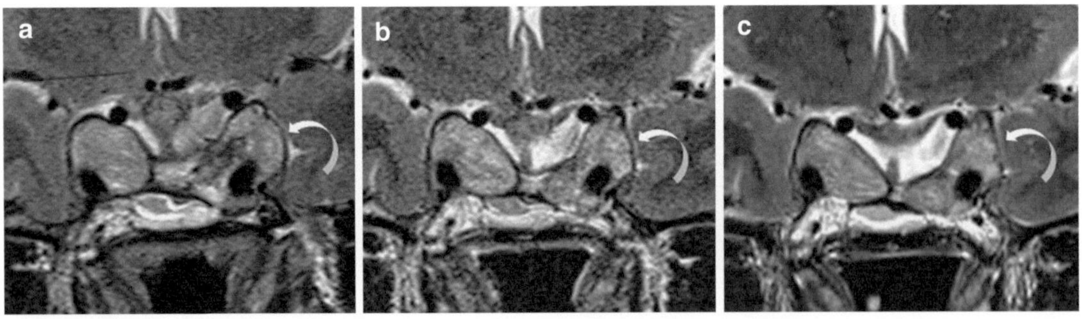

Fig. 29.5 Postsurgical remnant of a huge pituitary nonfunctioning macroadenoma invading both cavernous sinuses in a 50-year-old woman. (**a**, **c**) Coronal T2WIs respectively 2 months after surgery and 6 and 14 months after CyberKnife. Tumoral shrinkage is observed quickly after radiation therapy (**b**); additional shrinkage is very modest later (**c**)

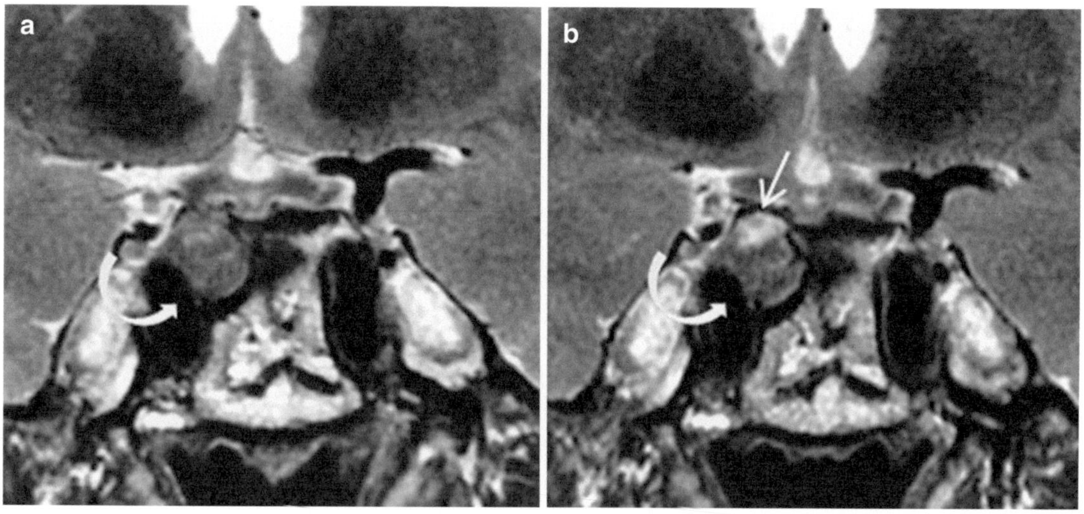

Fig. 29.6 Acromegaly in a 32-year-old man. Persistent IGF1 at high level despite surgery and somatostatin analog treatment. (**a**, **b**) Coronal T2WIs. Right cavernous sinus remnant (*curved arrow*). One year after Gamma Knife (**b**) there is no mass shrinkage, but T2 hyperintensity is noted at the upper part of the mass (*straight arrow*)

Further Reading

Castinetti F, Brue T (2010) Gamma knife radiosurgery in pituitary adenomas: why, who, and how to treat? Discov Med 10(51):107–111

Loeffler JS, Shih HA (2011) Radiation therapy in the management of pituitary adenomas. Clin Endocrinol Metab 96(7):1992–2003

Mak HK, Lai SW, Qian W, Xu S, Tong E, Vance ML et al (2015) Effective time window in reducing pituitary adenoma size by gamma knife radiosurgery. Pituitary 18(4):509–517

30 Chiasmatic and Hypothalamic Gliomas

Françoise Cattin

Chiasmatic and hypothalamic gliomas are childhood tumors, 75 % occurring in the first decade of life, and equally in boys and girls. In children, low-grade astrocytoma is the more frequent type of lesion, and 10–70 % of patients have neurofibromatosis type 1 (NF1). Visual loss with optic atrophy and growth delay are the most common signs. Intracranial hypertension syndrome with hydrocephalus in relation to obstruction of the foramina of Monro is seen in large tumors. Diencephalic syndrome characterized by emaciation, locomotor hyperactivity, euphoria, and alertness can be observed in children younger than 3 years. Optic glioma associated with NF1 is frequently asymptomatic. The precise origin of chiasmatic or hypothalamic gliomas is often impossible to determine mainly in the largest tumors. In patients with NF1, the most common site of involvement is the optic nerve, and the tumor is smaller than in non-NF1 patients. In patients without NF1, the optic chiasm and hypothalamus are the most frequent sites of involvement. The prognosis is variable: half of the tumors of NF1 patients remain stable compared with only 5 % of those of non-NF1 patients. Spontaneous regression can occur, especially in patients with NF1. Optic and hypothalamic gliomas appear as rounded or lobulated solid suprasellar masses hypointense on T1WI and hyperintense on T2WI (Figs. 30.1 and 30.2). Cystic components are much more frequent in patients without NF1. After gadolinium injection, enhancement is variable and often heterogeneous. Nonenhancement of the optic glioma is frequent in NF1 (Fig. 30.3). The enhancement pattern is often variable over time, without any clinical consequences. In the largest tumors, a posterior extension along the optic tracts to the lateral geniculate bodies is usual (Fig. 30.4). Suprasellar extension compressing the third ventricle and foramen of Monro may be responsible for hydrocephalus (Fig. 30.5). Involvement of the intraorbital optic nerve produces an enlargement and tortuosity of the nerve. Two different patterns can be observed. In some cases, the optic nerve is diffusely infiltrated and appears hypointense on T1WI and hyperintense on T2WI, with quite homogeneous enhancement after gadolinium injection. In other cases there is an infiltration of the subarachnoid spaces, sparing the optic nerve itself, with hyperintensity on T2WI and a rim of enhancement around the unaffected nerve. This pattern must be distinguished from the nontumoral enlargement of the subarachnoid spaces with no enhancement, which is frequently observed, particularly in patients with NF1. Optic-hypothalamic gliomas show a profile of choline, N-acetyl aspartate (NAA), and creatine with a choline/NAA ratio of approximately 2.5. At initial MR spectroscopy, aggressive optic or thalamic gliomas have a significantly lower myoinositol peak than the stable tumors. A decrease in myoinositol occurs before clinical and radiological deterioration. Increased permeability on perfusion imaging is suggestive of aggressive tumor. The differential diagnosis of contrast-enhancing hypothalamic

J.-F. Bonneville et al., *MRI of the Pituitary Gland*, DOI 10.1007/978-3-319-29043-0_30

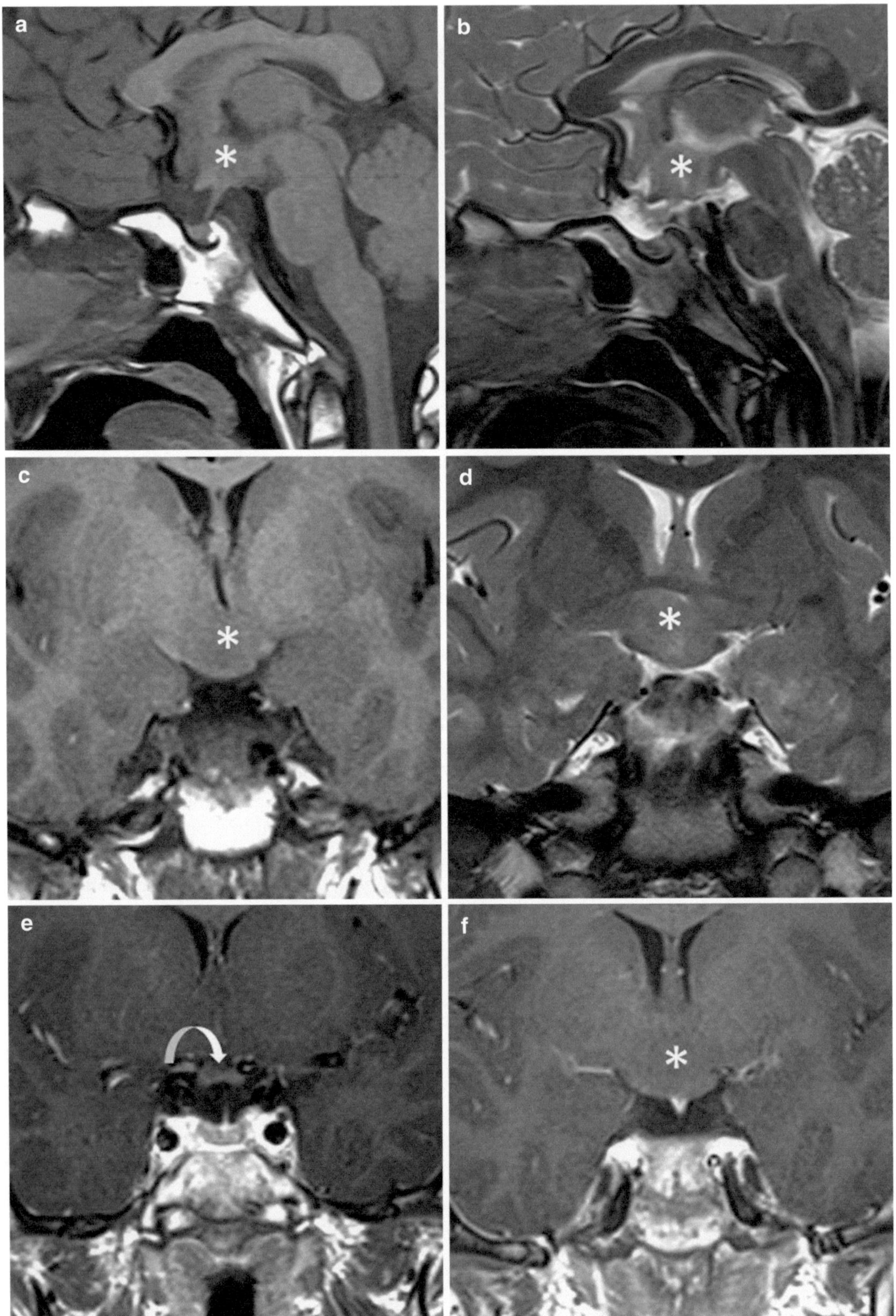
a
b
c
d
e
f

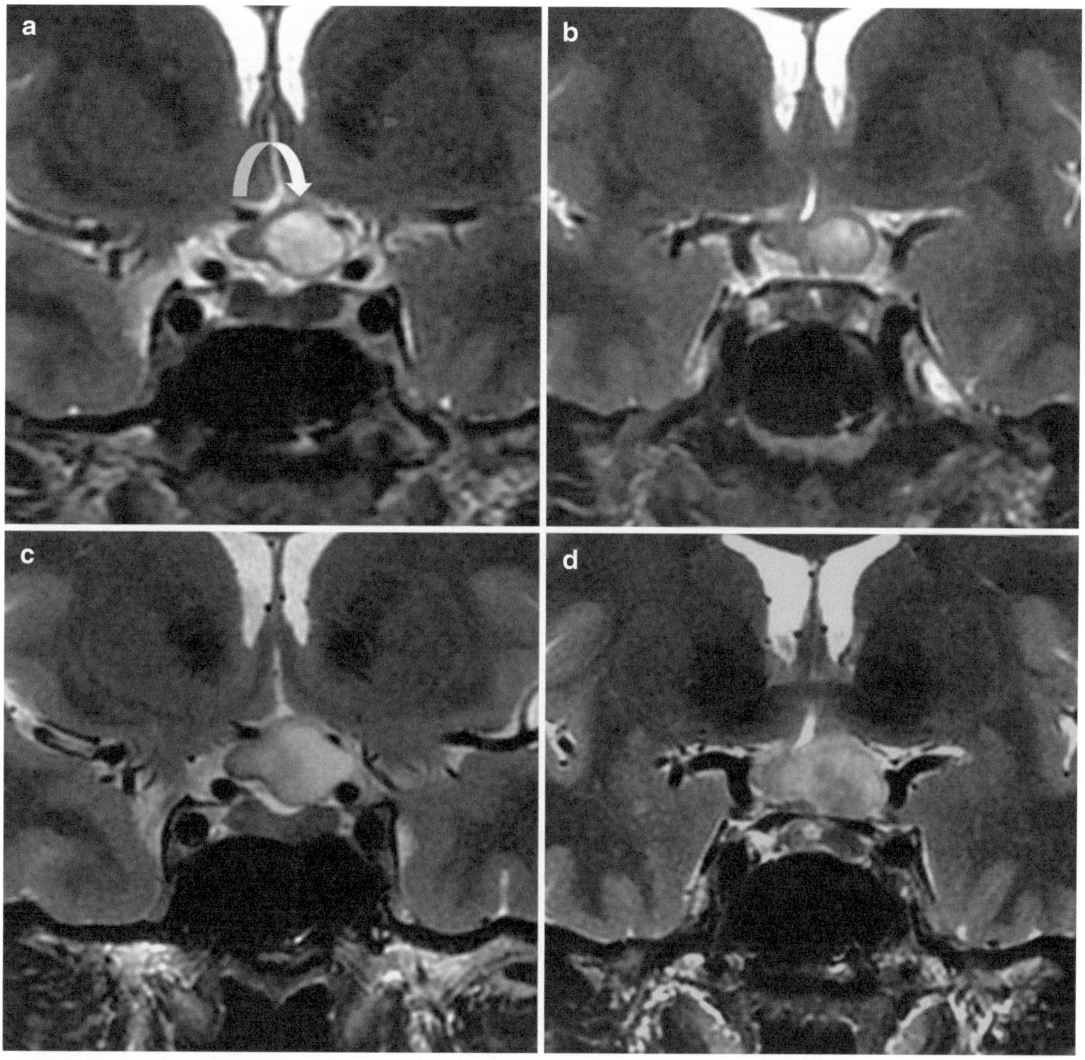

Fig. 30.2 Thirty-one-year-old woman. Left temporal hemianopia for 5 weeks. No history of NF1. (**a**, **b**) Coronal T2WIs of the sellar region separated by 4 mm. Well-circumscribed T2-hyperintense lesion (*curved arrow*) of the left part of the optic chiasm. (**c**, **d**) T2WIs at the same levels obtained 5 months later. Rapid and significant increase in size of the lesion. At biopsy, diagnosis of pilocytic astrocytoma of the optic chiasm

glioma includes, in adults, papillary craniopharyngioma, lymphoma, and metastasis; and in children, adamantinous craniopharyngioma and germinoma. In the case of nonenhancing suprasellar mass, a hamartoma of the tuber cinereum can be evoked.

Fig. 30.1 Six-year-old male with NF1. Hypothalamic glioma. (**a**, **b**) Sagittal T1 and T2 WIs. (**c**, **d**) Coronal T1 and T2 WIs. Hypothalamic poorly delineated mass, isointense to gray matter on T1WI and slightly hyperintense on T2WI (*asterisk*). (**e**, **f**) Coronal CE T1WIs. There is no enhancement of the hypothalamic mass (*asterisk*). The optic chiasm is normal (*curved arrow*)

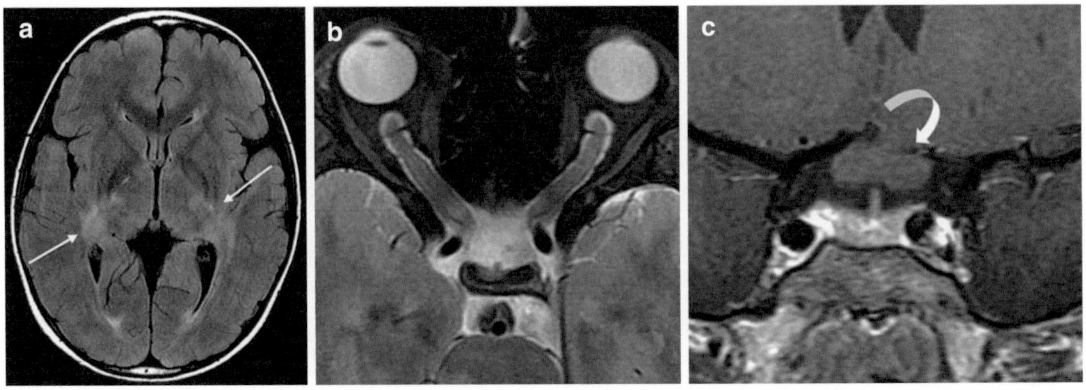

Fig. 30.3 Twelve-year-old male with NF1. (**a**) Axial FLAIR T2WI reveals multiple characteristic hyperintense lesions in the basal ganglia (*arrows*). (**b**) Axial T2WI. Bilateral enlargement of the optic nerve. (**c**) Coronal CE T1WI. The optic chiasm is thick, globulous, and does not enhance (*curved arrow*)

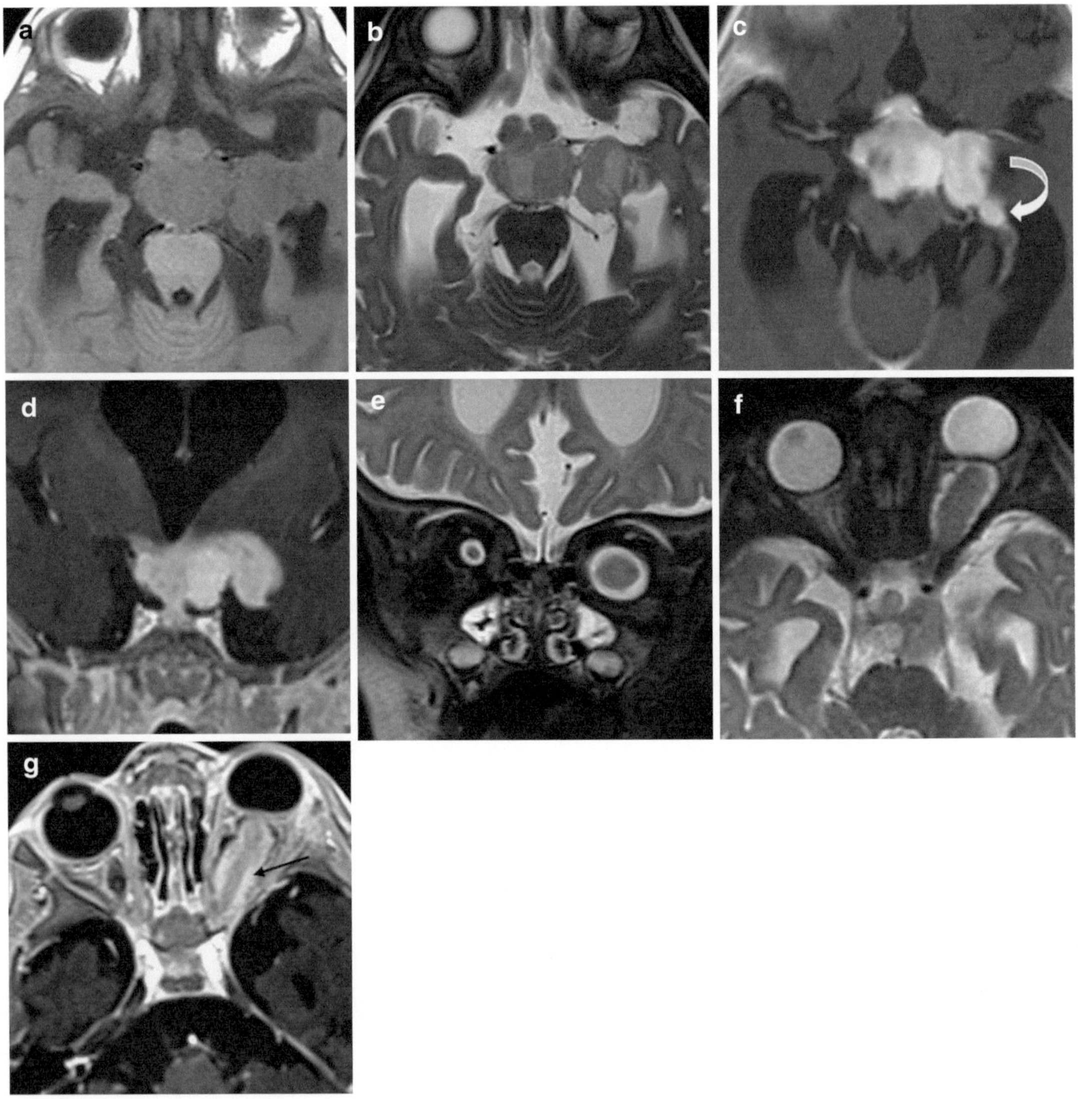

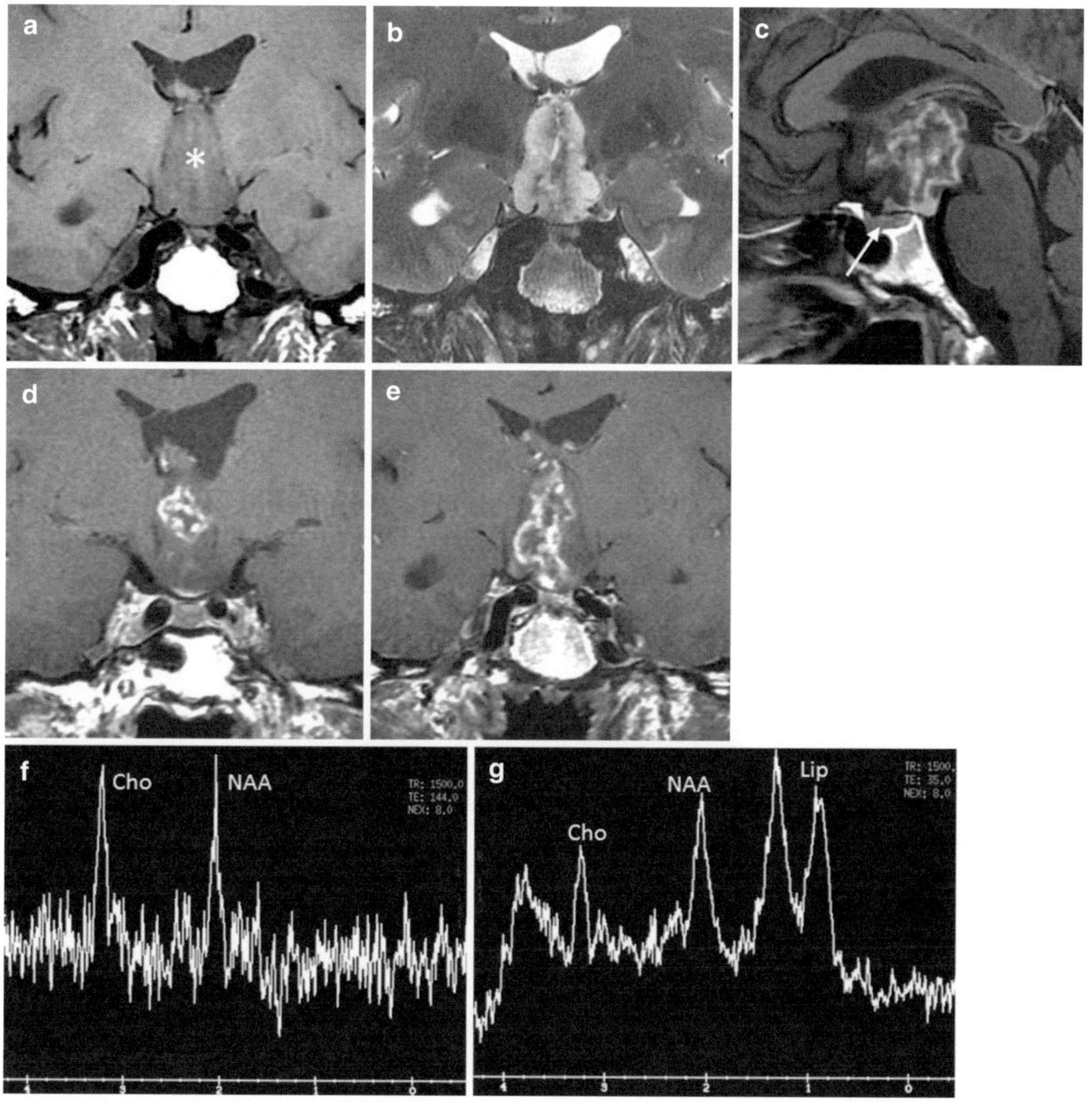

Fig. 30.5 Forty-year-old man with hypogonadism. (**a**, **b**) Coronal T1 and T2 WIs. (**c**) Sagittal CE T1WI. (**d**, **e**) Coronal CE T1WIs. Huge tumor occupying the suprasellar cistern, the hypothalamic region, and the third ventricle (*asterisk*). The anterior lobe of the pituitary gland is normal (*arrow*). The optic chiasm is not identified. The lesion appears hypointense on T1WI and hyperintense on T2WI; however, the signal is heterogeneous on both sequences. The irregular intratumoral enhancement could be related to centrotumoral necrosis. See the enlargement of the left lateral ventricle in relation to the obstruction of the foramen of Monro. (**f**) Long echo time (TE) monovoxel spectroscopy shows increase of choline and slight decrease of NAA with choline/NAA ratio of approximately 1. (**g**) Short TE spectroscopy demonstrates elevated peaks of lipids/lactate but no decrease of myoinositol. The final diagnosis is low-grade hypothalamic glioma

Fig. 30.4 Six-month-old child presenting with strabismus for 2 months and left exophthalmos with left papilledema. Suprasellar multiloculated mass associated with an enlargement of the left optic nerve. NF1 is highly suspected. (**a–c**) Axial T1, T2, and CE T1 WIs. (**d**) Coronal CE T1WI. The tumor is hypointense on T1WI, and hyperintense and heterogeneous on T2WI with strong enhancement after gadolinium injection. Posterior tumoral extension along the left optic tract (*curved arrow*). (**e**, **f**) Coronal and axial T2WIs of the orbits. Enlargement of the left optic nerve and the subarachnoid spaces. (**g**) Axial CE T1WI demonstrates a rim of marked enhancement around the optic nerve (*arrow*) indicating tumoral infiltration of the subarachnoid spaces

Further Reading

Harris LM, Davies NP, Macpherson L et al (2008) Magnetic resonance spectroscopy in the assessment of pilocytic astrocytomas. Eur J Cancer 44(17): 2640–2647

Kornreich L, Blaser S, Schwarz M et al (2001) Optic pathway glioma: correlation of imaging findings with the presence of neurofibromatosis. AJNR Am J Neuroradiol 22:1963–1969

Raelson C, Chiang G (2015) Chiasmatic-hypothalamic masses in adults: a case series and review of the literature. J Neuroimaging 25:361–364

31 Suprasellar Germinoma

Françoise Cattin

The most common germ cell tumor of the suprasellar region is the germinoma. A suprasellar germinoma can be a primitive tumoral lesion or a metastatic lesion from a pineal germinoma. Germinomas are most commonly seen in adolescents and young adults: 90 % of patients are younger than 20 years. There is no gender preference for the suprasellar location, unlike the pineal location with male predominance. Clinical symptoms include diabetes insipidus, precocious puberty, or growth failure related to hypothalamic involvement and visual loss provoked by chiasmatic compression. Large lesions can cause hydrocephalus by obstruction of the interventricular foramens. Tumoral markers such as α-fetoprotein and human chorionic gonadotropin (HCG) can be found in the serum and/or CSF. In the case of suggestive clinical and radiological patterns with presence of tumoral markers, the diagnostic biopsy can be avoided. Infundibular thickening and absence of the posterior lobe bright spot on T1WI are the more precocious radiological signs, and at this stage can simulate an inflammatory process, Langerhans cell histiocytosis, or lymphocytic infiltration (Fig. 31.1). As it grows, the lesion appears as a well-delineated round or lobulated lesion, isointense or hyperintense to gray matter on T1WI and isointense to hyperintense on T2WI (Fig. 31.2), with hyperintense necrotic foci in some cases. Calcifications, better seen on CT than on MRI, are not unusual but less frequent than in the pineal location. After gadolinium injection there is a marked and mostly speckled enhancement. The origin within the optic nerve or optic chiasm is very rare. Intraventricular extension in lateral ventricle and infiltration of the basal ganglia and the corpus callosum can occur (Fig. 31.3). Multifocal germinomas usually involve the pineal gland and the suprasellar cistern, simultaneously or not (Fig. 31.4). Leptomeningeal spread with drop metastases along the spinal cord are reported. ADC is usually decreased. MR spectroscopy shows markedly elevated choline with diminished N-acetyl aspartate. Despite the aggressive MRS pattern, a good response is observed in most cases after radiotherapy and chemotherapy. Before treatment, a complete survey of the brain and spinal canal is required because germinomas can metastasize by subarachnoid seeding. Negative MRI in children with diabetes insipidus does not exclude germinoma (Fig. 31.5). A repeat MRI examination is required in 3–6 months. Early diagnosis may reduce the risk of dissemination and the morbidity of treatment. The limited differential diagnosis includes craniopharyngioma with a more heterogeneous appearance associated with cysts, solid components and calcifications, and hypothalamic-chiasmatic glioma rarely associated with diabetes insipidus (see Chap. 30).

J.-F. Bonneville et al., *MRI of the Pituitary Gland*, DOI 10.1007/978-3-319-29043-0_31

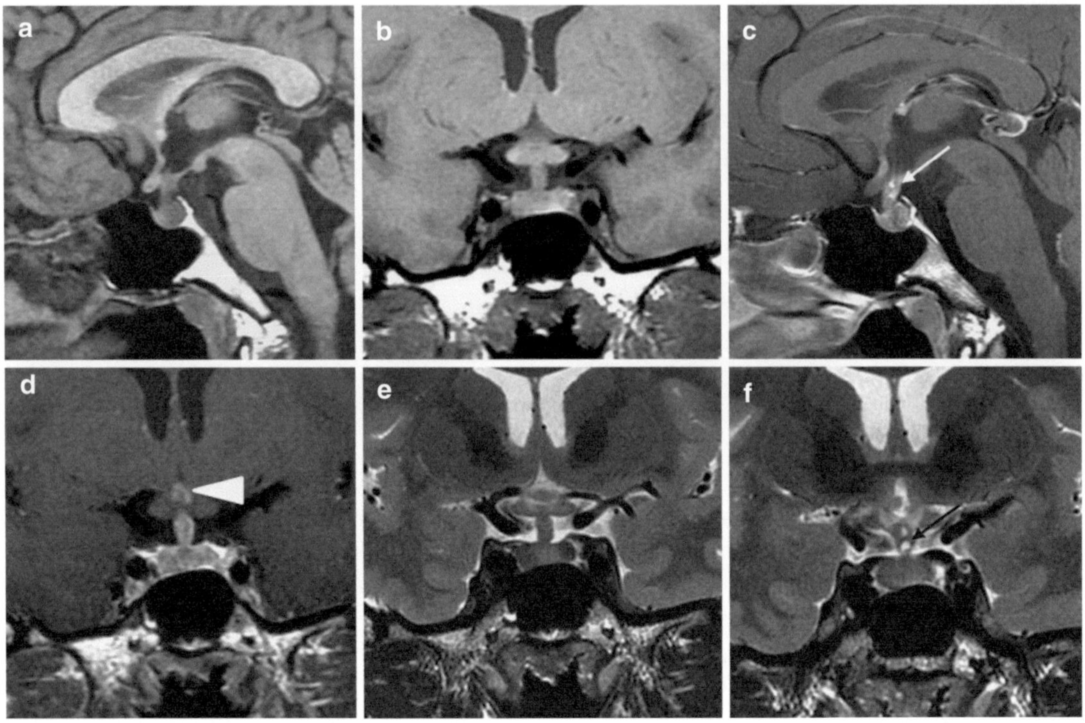

Fig. 31.1 Twenty-three-year-old man presenting with diabetes insipidus for 1 year. (**a**, **b**) Sagittal and coronal T1WIs. The hypersignal of the posterior lobe is absent and the pituitary stalk is enlarged. The anterior pituitary gland appears normal. (**c**, **d**) Sagittal and coronal CE T1WIs. Speckled enhancement of the pituitary stalk (*arrow*) and tuber cinereum (*arrowhead*). (**e**, **f**) Coronal T2WIs. Small hyperintense spots in the pituitary stalk (*black arrow*). At 3 months (not shown), there were no changes. (**g**, **h**) Sagittal and coronal CE T1WIs at 6 months. Presence of a hypointense intrasellar posterior lesion associated with significant increase in diameter of the pituitary stalk and large contrast-enhancing suprasellar sellar mass involving the optic chiasm and tuber cinereum. (**i**) Coronal T2WI. The lesion is quite homogeneous and isointense to gray matter. The diagnosis of germinoma was confirmed by the evidence of a high level of β-HCG in the CSF. (**j**) Coronal CE T1WI after corticotherapy and radiation therapy. Decrease in size of the pituitary gland. Complete shrinkage of the suprasellar tumor with marked atrophy of the pituitary stalk

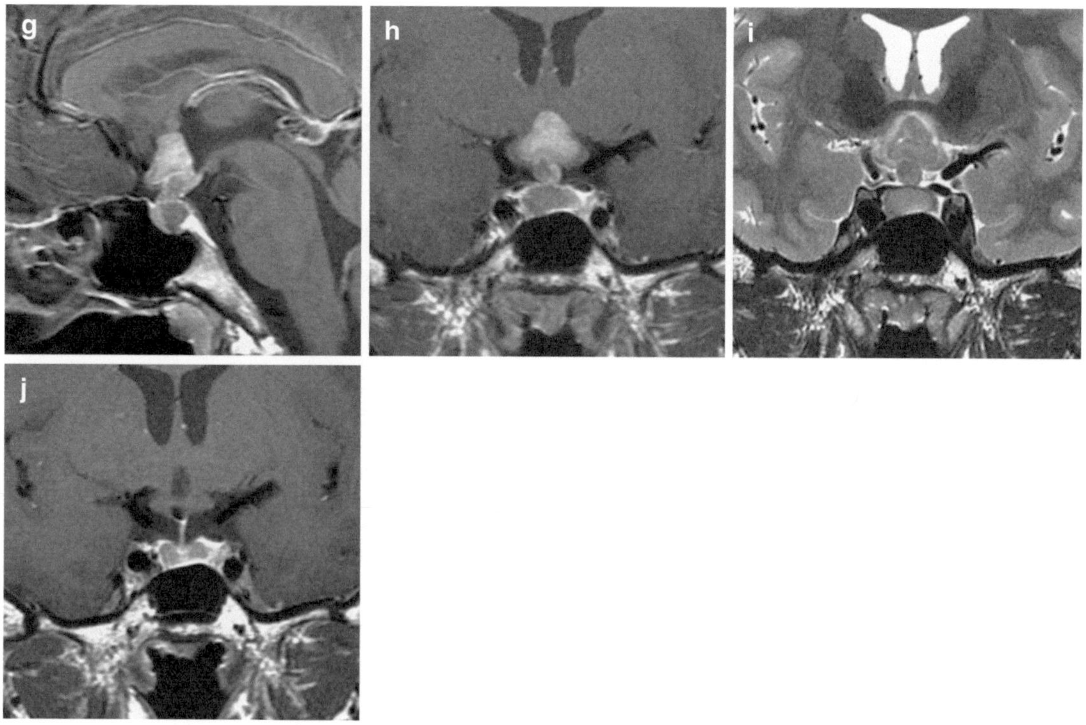

Fig. 31.1 (continued)

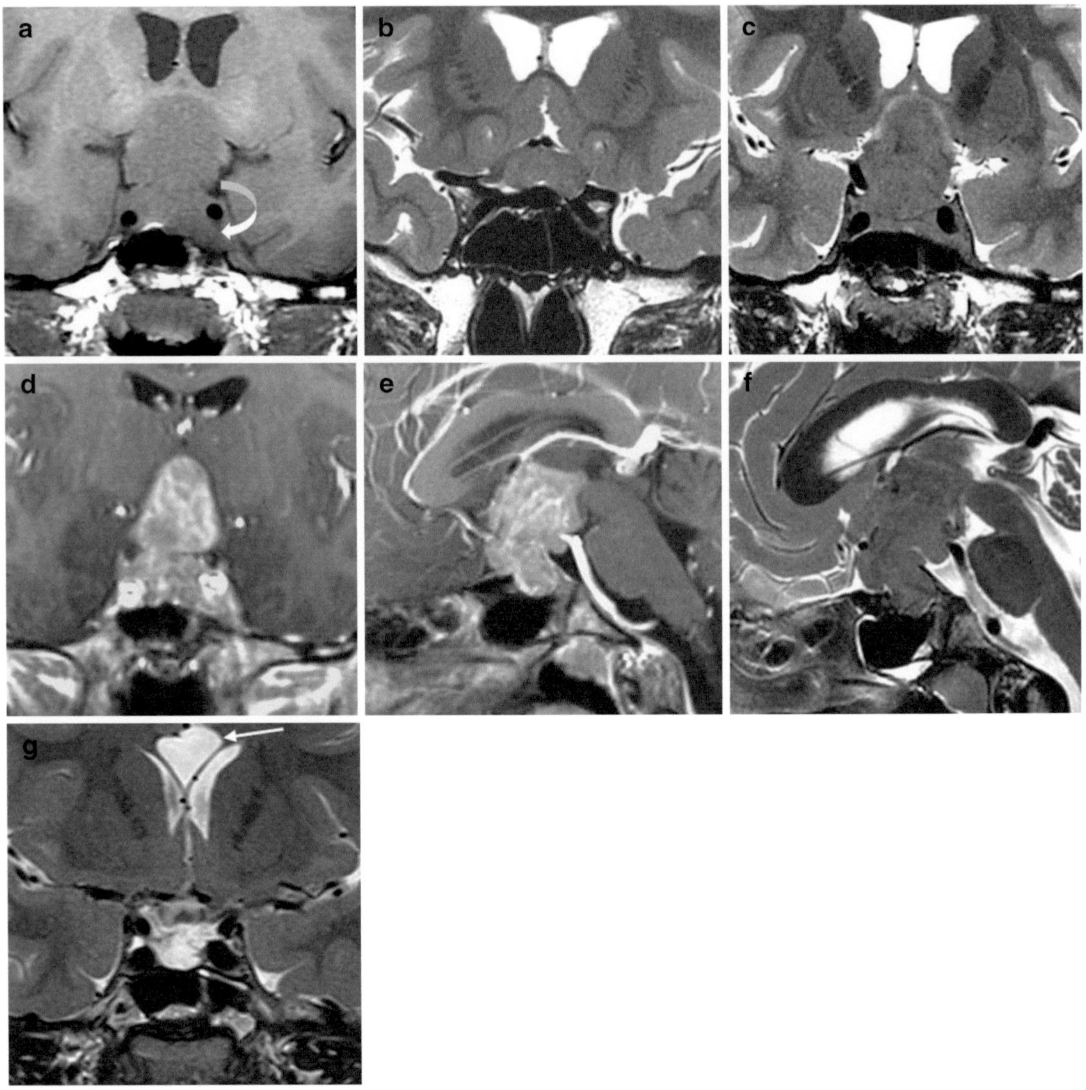

Fig. 31.2 Headaches, bitemporal hemianopia, visual loss, and diabetes insipidus in a 13-year-old girl. (**a**) Coronal T1WI. Large intra- and suprasellar tumor with invasion of the left cavernous sinus (*curved arrow*). (**b**, **c**) Coronal T2WIs. Involvement of the optic chiasm and complete obstruction of the lumen of the third ventricle. (**d**, **e**) Coronal and sagittal CE T1WIs. The enhancement is heterogeneous with multiple specks. (**f**) Sagittal T2WI. The signal is homogeneous. Note the polycyclic contours of the tumor. (**g**) Coronal T2WI. Shrinkage of the tumor after medical treatment and radiation therapy. Empty sella turcica, signal abnormalities of the optic chiasm and porencephalic cavity after transcallosal biopsy (*arrow*)

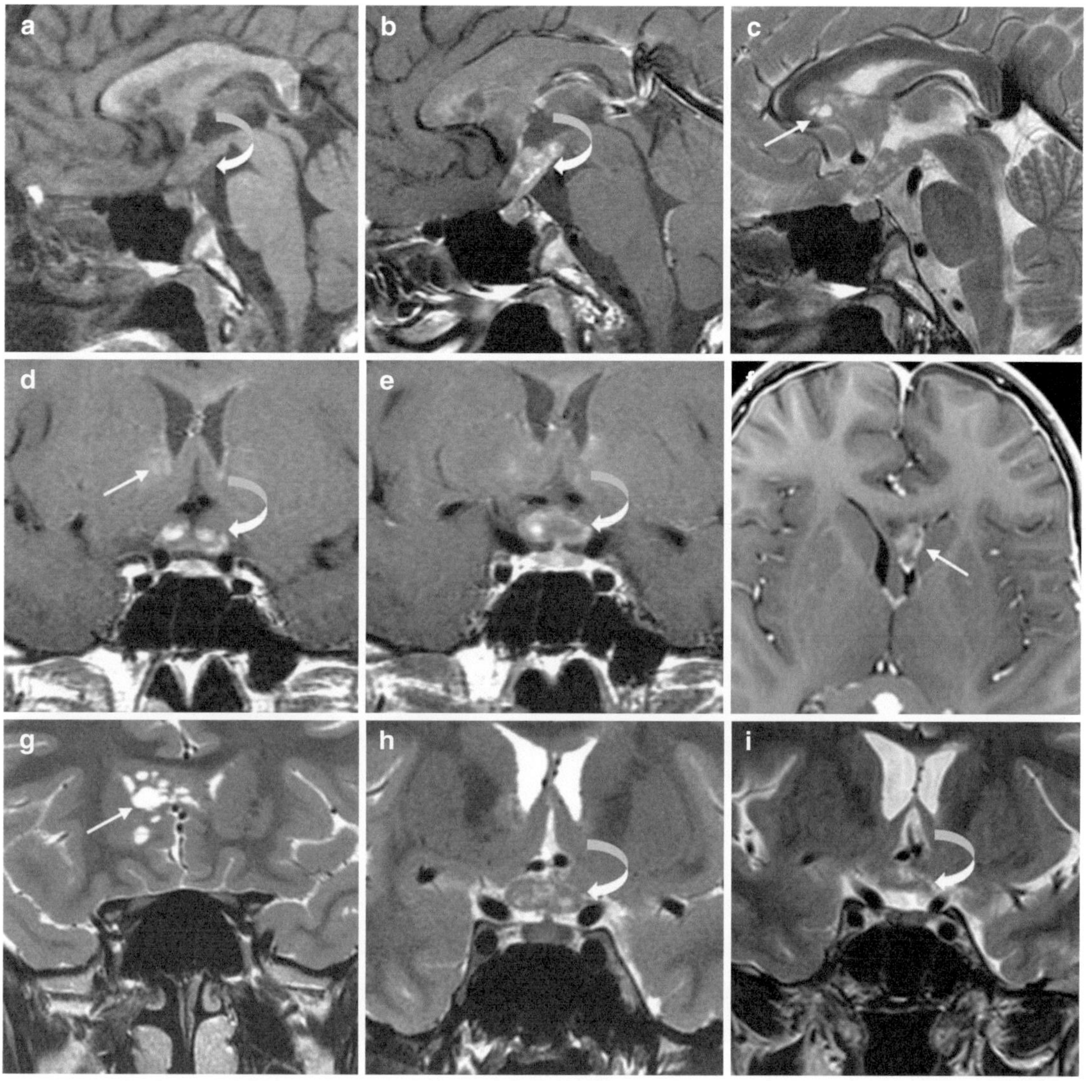

Fig. 31.3 Rapidly progressive visual loss and diabetes insipidus for 4 months in a 15-year-old boy. (**a–c**) Sagittal T1, and CE T1 and T2 WIs. The T1 hypersignal of the posterior lobe is missing. Suprasellar mass (*curved arrow*) with patchy enhancement and multiple hyperintense foci on T2WI associated with poorly delimited frontal periventricular lesions (*arrow*) presenting the same MR characteristics. (**d**, **e**) Coronal and (**f**) axial CE T1WIs. Demonstration of the contrast-enhanced intrachiasmatic lesions (*curved arrow*). The pituitary stalk is not thickened. Bifrontal periventricular tumoral infiltration (*arrow*). (**g**, **h**) Coronal T2WIs. The multicystic appearance of the optic chiasm (*curved arrow*) and periventricular lesions (*arrow*) is suggestive of germinoma. (**i**) Coronal T2WI after treatment: normalization of the optic chiasm (*curved arrow*)

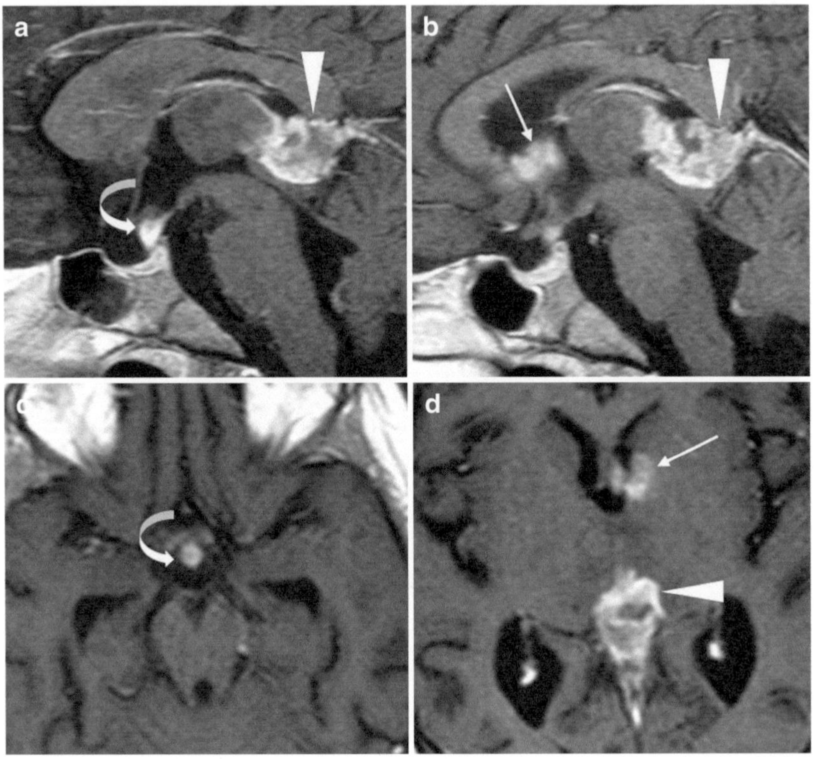

Fig. 31.4 Multifocal germinoma. (**a**, **b**) Sagittal and (**c**, **d**) axial CE T1WIs. Enlargement and marked enhancement of the superior part of the pituitary stalk (*curved arrow*), contrast-enhanced pineal mass (*arrowhead*), and involvement of the wall of the left frontal horn and surrounding parenchyma (*arrow*)

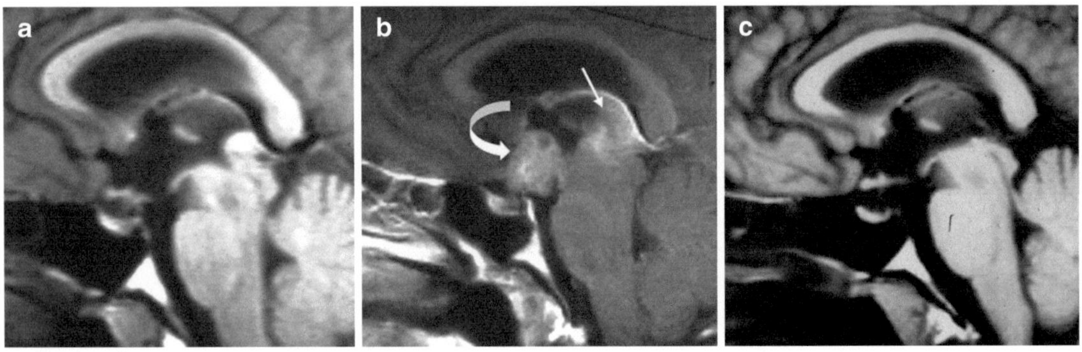

Fig. 31.5 Diabetes insipidus for 1 month. (**a**) Sagittal T1WI showing only a posterior intrasellar hyposignal instead of the physiological T1 hypersignal of the posterior lobe. (**b**) Six months later, on sagittal CE T1WI, demonstration of suprasellar (*curved arrow*) and pineal (*arrow*) lesions. (**c**) After treatment, complete radiological remission. The hypersignal of the posterior lobe is still absent

Further Reading

Kanagaki M, Miki Y, Takahashi JA et al (2004) MRI and CT findings of neurohypophyseal germinoma. Eur J Radiol 49:204–211

Phi JH, Kim SK, Lee J et al (2013) The enigma of bifocal germ cell tumors in the suprasellar and pineal regions: synchronous lesions or metastasis? J Neurosurg Pediatr 11:107–114

Sethi RV, Marino R, Niemierko A, Tarbell NJ, Yock TI, Mac Donald SM (2013) Delayed diagnosis in children with intracranial germ cell tumors. J Pediatr 163:1448–1453

32 Melanoma

Jean-François Bonneville

Although melanoma ranks fourth in the incidence of brain metastases, behind lung, breast, and unknown primary cancers, metastatic melanomas of the pituitary gland are exceedingly rare. Still rarer are primitive pituitary melanomas. Presentation is tumoral syndrome and/or pituitary insufficiency, sometimes with a history of diabetes insipidus. Apoplexy can also be revealing.

Stable free radicals of melanin are responsible for a paramagnetic effect producing hyperintensity on T1WI and hypointensity on T2WI (Figs. 32.1 and 32.2). These characteristics can mimic subacute hemorrhage, such as what is encountered in pituitary adenomas, or lipid or mucinous material present in dermoid or Rathke cleft cysts. Diagnosis of melanoma is sometimes made even more difficult before histological examination of a specimen if a tumoral hemorrhage or an apoplexia has occurred. Diagnosis is also made more challenging if the primitive melanoma is unknown. T1-hyperintense characteristics of the presence of melanin pigments can be misleading. Final diagnosis is through immunopositivity for S100 protein and HMB-45. Management of sellar melanomas consists of surgical removal followed by radiotherapy. Chemotherapy, particularly temozolomide, seems able to lead to significant survival prolongation.

J.-F. Bonneville et al., *MRI of the Pituitary Gland*, DOI 10.1007/978-3-319-29043-0_32

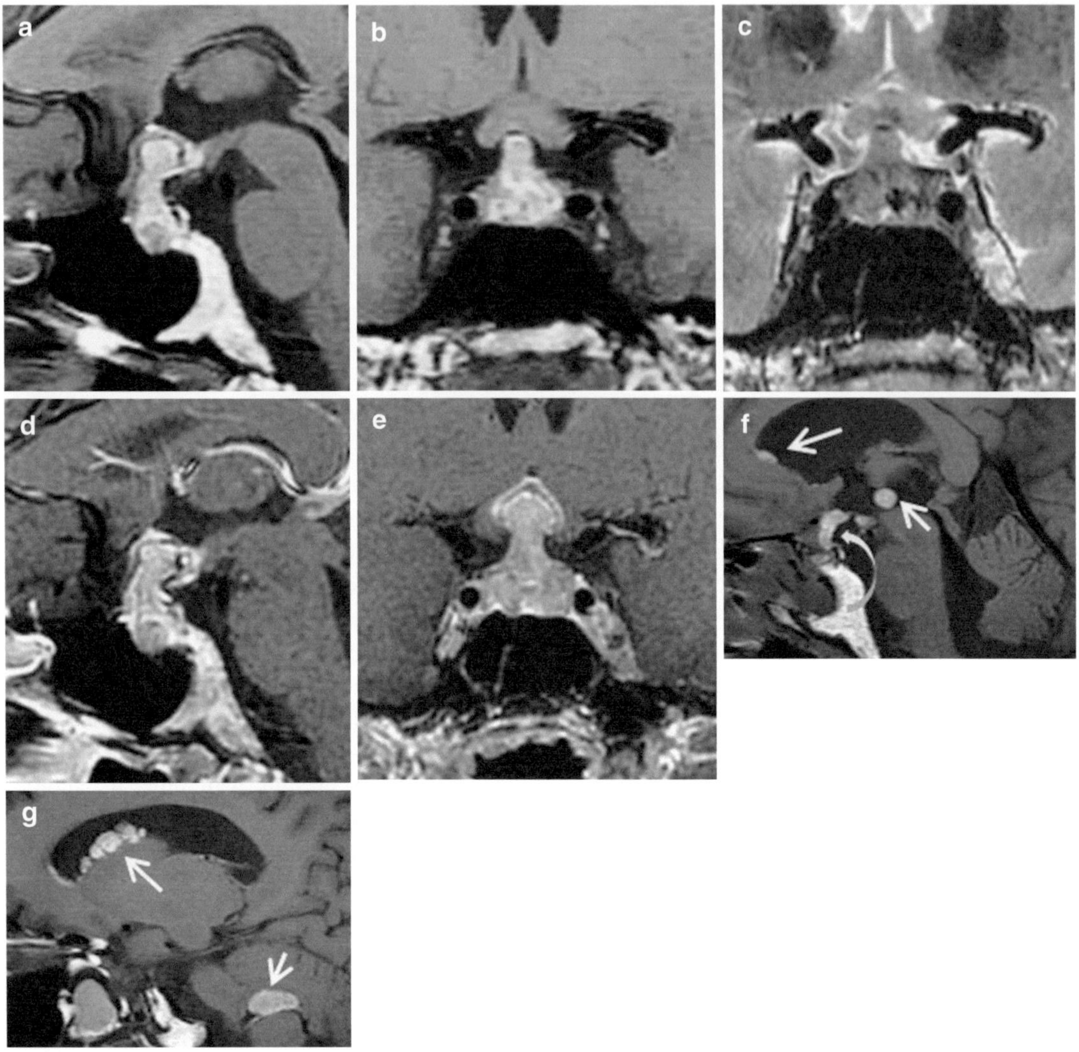

Fig. 32.1 Hemorrhagic pituitary melanoma in a 36-year-old woman. Diabetes insipidus of a few weeks' duration and brutal onset of severe headache. Hormonal status is normal except a mild hyperprolactinemia. (**a**–**c**) Sagittal and coronal noncontrast T1 and coronal T2 WIs. Spontaneous T1 hyperintense intra- and suprasellar mass involving the pituitary stalk and compressing the floor of the third ventricle. Several T2-hypointense areas within the mass. Thickening and T2 hyperintensity of the optic chiasm. (**d**, **e**) Sagittal and coronal CE T1WIs. The spontaneous T1 hyperintensity masks the postgadolinium enhancement. At surgery, a blackish tumor with a hemorrhagic component is removed and melanic pigments are found at immunochemistry. Ki-67 is 40 %. Despite radiotherapy and chemotherapy, the patient's health deteriorates and a meningeal carcinomatosis is diagnosed. (**f**, **g**) Sagittal and coronal noncontrast T1WIs 1 year after diagnosis: tumoral suprasellar remnant (*curved arrow*) and multiple subependymal nodular T1-hyperintense lesions corresponding to tumoral grafts (*arrows*). No melanoma was found elsewhere (Courtesy of B. Baltzinger MD and J.-L. Dietemann MD, PhD)

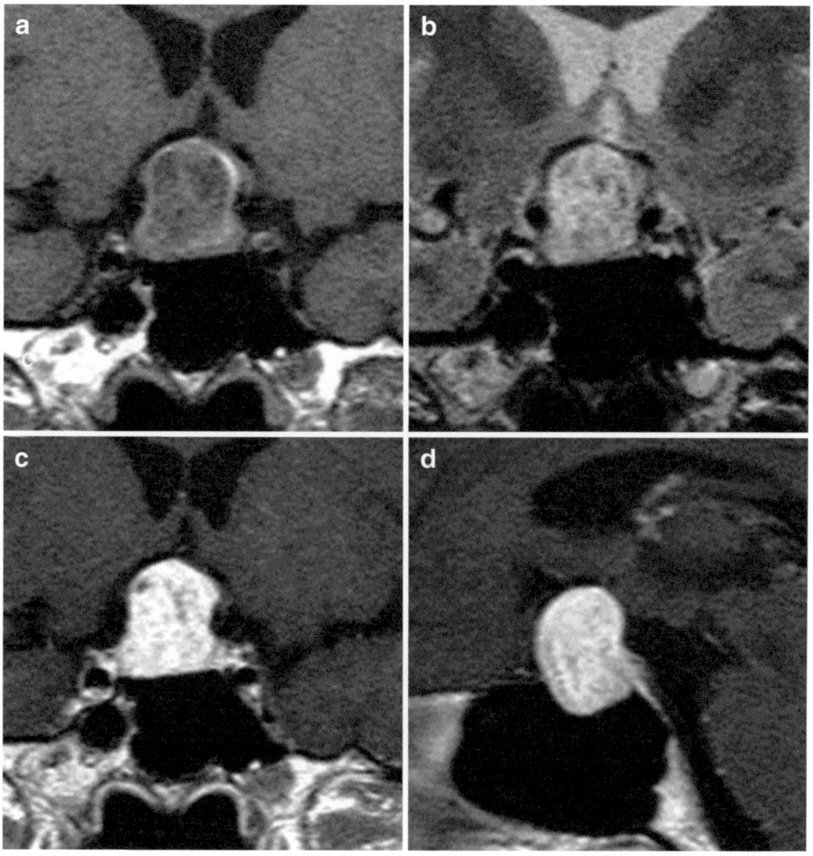

Fig. 32.2 Forty-two-year-old woman with hypopituitarism caused by primary sellar melanocytic tumor. (**a–c**) Coronal T1, T2, and CE T1 WIs and (**d**) sagittal CE T1WI show an intra- and suprasellar lesion harboring subtle spontaneous T1 hyperintensity and heterogeneous T2 hyperintensity. The mass lesion homogeneously and strongly enhances after gadolinium injection, more than would an adenoma. Note the lack of visible residual normal pituitary and absence of neighboring dural enhancement

Further Reading

Masui K, Yonezawa T, Shinji Y et al (2013) Pituitary apoplexy caused by hemorrhage from pituitary metastatic melanoma: case report. Neurol Med Chir (Tokyo) 53(10):695–698

Sidiropoulos M, Syro LV, Rotondo F et al (2013) Melanoma of the sellar region mimicking pituitary adenoma. Neuropathology 33(2):175–178

Wang YY, Norris A, du Plessis D et al (2011) Melanoma of the sellar region. J Clin Neurosci 18(1):154–156

Pituitary Metastases 33

Jean-François Bonneville

Pituitary metastases are found frequently in autopsy series of cancer patients, particularly in breast and lung cancer patients, but much more rarely in living patients The pituitary gland can be reached by metastatic deposits via hematogenous spread, via the skull base, or by meningeal spread. The posterior lobe is the most frequently involved, probably because of its direct arterial blood supply by the inferior hypophyseal arteries (Figs. 33.1 and 33.2). Localization to the infundibulum is less frequent (Figs. 33.3 and 33.4). In fact, symptomatic pituitary metastases are so rare that some have suggested sparing the pituitary gland and infundibulum areas in the setting of whole brain therapy while treating the rest of the brain, thus avoiding late endocrinologic and vascular sequelae. Nevertheless, pituitary metastases have been more frequently reported since the advent of high-resolution MRI. Most cases are associated with multiple, particularly bone, metastases. Breast and lung cancers are responsible for one-third and one-fourth of pituitary metastases, respectively; metastases of prostate, renal cell, gastrointestinal, thyroid, and pancreatic cancers are far less common. Most pituitary metastases are asymptomatic, but can represent the initial presentation of an unknown primary tumor. Diabetes insipidus is by far the most frequent symptom. Anterior pituitary deficiency was initially considered rare but is more frequently found when sensitive immunochemistry tests are used, particularly in the setting of renal cell carcinoma. It is noteworthy that diabetes insipidus can be concealed if mineralocorticoid function is reduced. Oculomotor nerves palsies can represent the initial symptom if the cavernous sinus is involved. Loss of vision is rare. In the absence of diabetes insipidus and if a primary tumor is unknown, the clinical setting of a pituitary metastasis can mimic a pituitary macroadenoma discovered by chance. Precise analysis of imaging studies can help. Diagnosis of pituitary metastasis is made easier if the tumor is still confined to the posterior part of the sella. Loss of hyperintensity in the posterior pituitary is constant, and more faithfully shown on axial T1W fat-saturated images than on sagittal T1WI. Demonstration of erosion or destruction of the dorsum sellae, better appreciated on CT, favors the diagnosis of metastasis. The MR signal of metastasis is variable, mostly hyperintense on T2WI. Hemorrhage is unusual, but cases of apoplexy have been described in the setting of concomitant pituitary adenoma. In a few cases of metastatic melanomas, a spontaneous T1 high signal has been described. Postgadolinium enhancement can be intense or not. Isolated thickening of the infundibulum can be encountered in different pathologies and is much less specific than the involvement of the posterior pituitary. Rapid growth of the lesion on sequential MRI suggests a malignant disease. In large tumors, this rapid growth has been reported as responsible for an intra- and supra-dumbbell-shaped tumor caused by indentation of the mass by the sellar diaphragm; in fact, this pattern is frequently observed with pituitary macroadenomas

J.-F. Bonneville et al., *MRI of the Pituitary Gland*, DOI 10.1007/978-3-319-29043-0_33

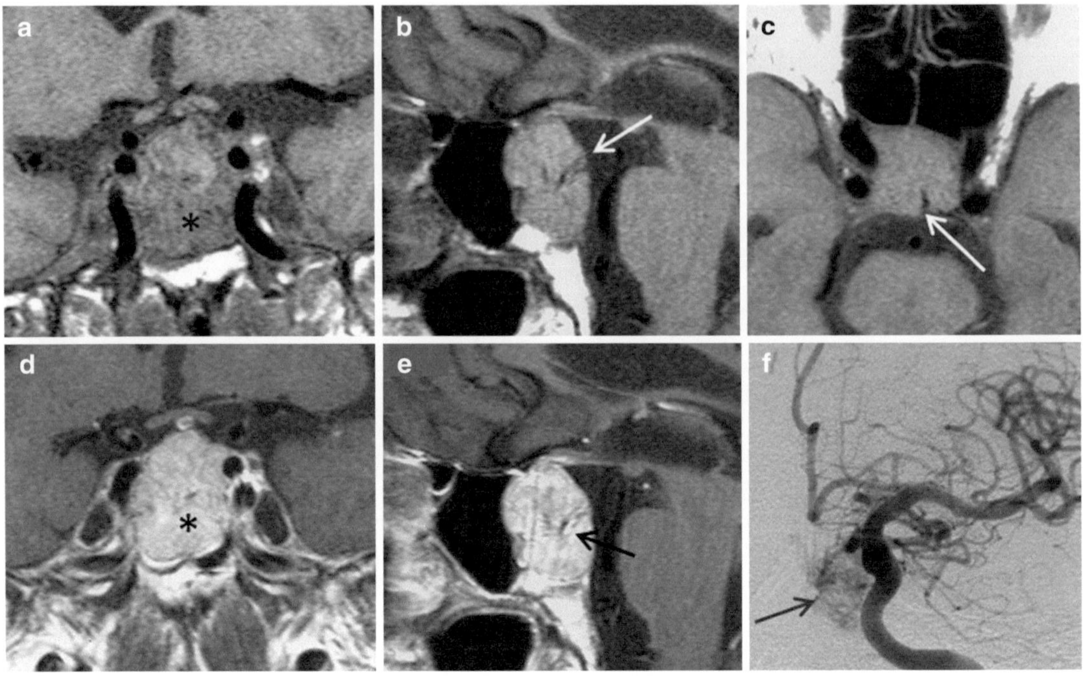

Fig. 33.1 Pituitary metastasis in a 68-year-old man with renal cell cancer. Diabetes insipidus. (**a**–**c**) Coronal, sagittal, and axial T1WIs. (**d**, **e**) Coronal and sagittal CE T1WIs. (**f**) Left internal carotid angiography. Highly vascular sellar mass invading sphenoid sinus (*asterisk*). The sellar floor is destroyed. Tumoral arteries are demonstrated on MRI as rapid flow vessels, and on angiography (*arrows*)

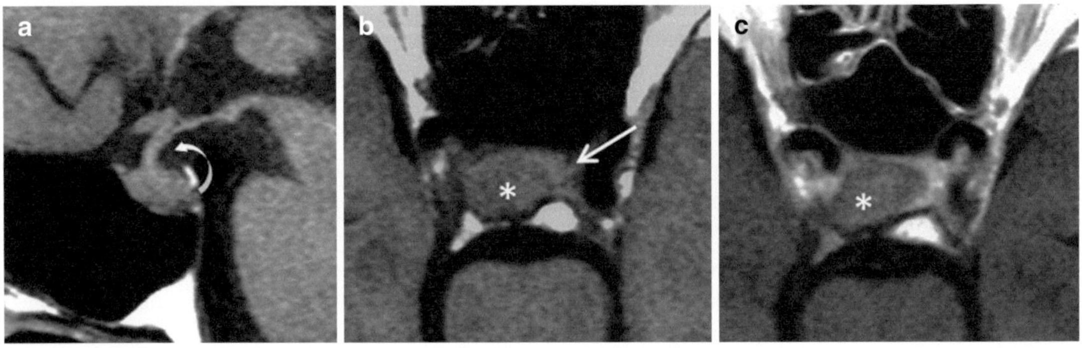

Fig. 33.2 Pituitary metastasis in a 65-year-old man with lung epithelioma and isolated diabetes insipidus. (**a**–**c**) Sagittal T1, axial T1, and CE T1WIs. The pituitary stalk is pushed forward (*curved arrow*) by a T1-hypointense centimetric lesion (*asterisk*) which is less enhanced if compared with the normal anterior pituitary (*straight arrow*). The normal posterior pituitary bright spot is not demonstrated

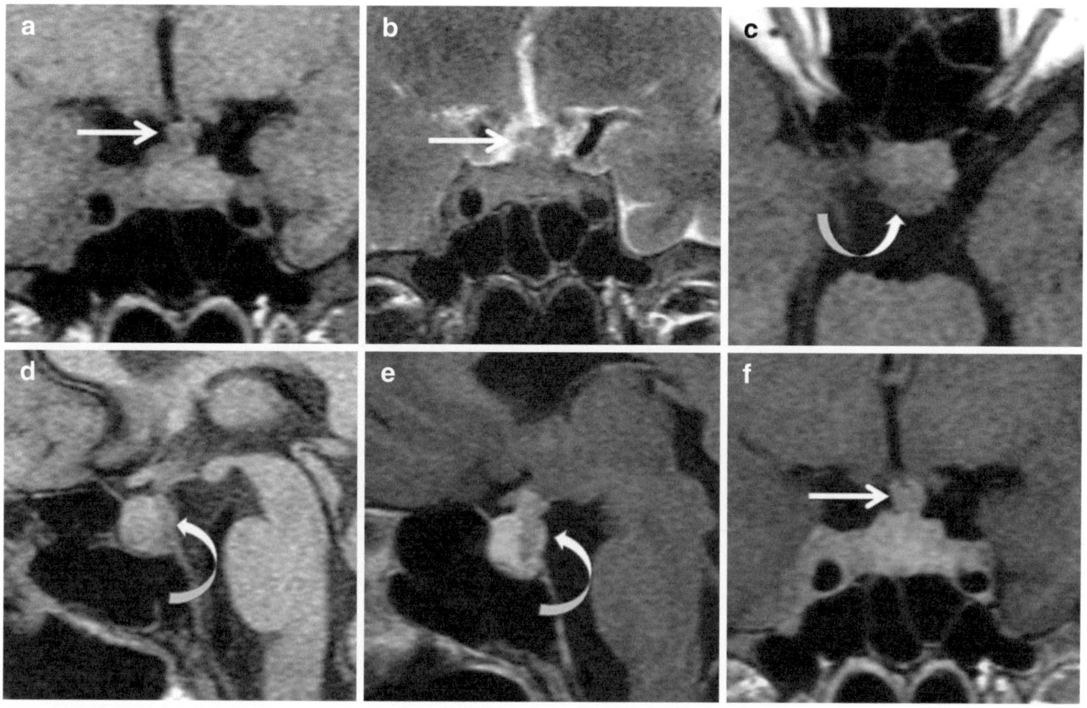

Fig. 33.3 Pituitary metastasis in a 42-year-old woman with breast cancer. Diabetes insipidus and right sixth nerve palsy for a month. (**a**, **b**) Coronal T1 and T2 WIs. (**c**) Axial T1WI. (**d**, **e**) Sagittal T1 and CE T1 WIs. (**f**) Coronal CE TIWI. Demonstration of a mass involving mainly the posterior lobe (*curved arrows*) and the infundibulum (*straight arrow*); the lesion is T1 hypointense if referred to the anterior lobe and is less enhanced

and is then not specific. Invasion of cavernous sinus (Fig. 33.5) can be uni- or bilateral, the latter being somewhat rare with pituitary adenomas. Visual pathway edema, never observed in pituitary adenomas but not infrequent in craniopharyngiomas, is a good indicator of malignancy (Fig. 33.6). Metastatic seeding to pituitary adenoma exists, mainly to nonfunctioning adenoma and prolactinoma, and can complicate the diagnosis, but tumor-to-tumor metastasis remains exceptional. Allowing exceptions (Fig. 33.7), evolution of pituitary metastasis is rapidly pejorative. In cases of a sellar mass discovered incidentally, it must be borne in mind that the best criterion for differentiation of pituitary metastasis from pituitary adenoma is diabetes insipidus.

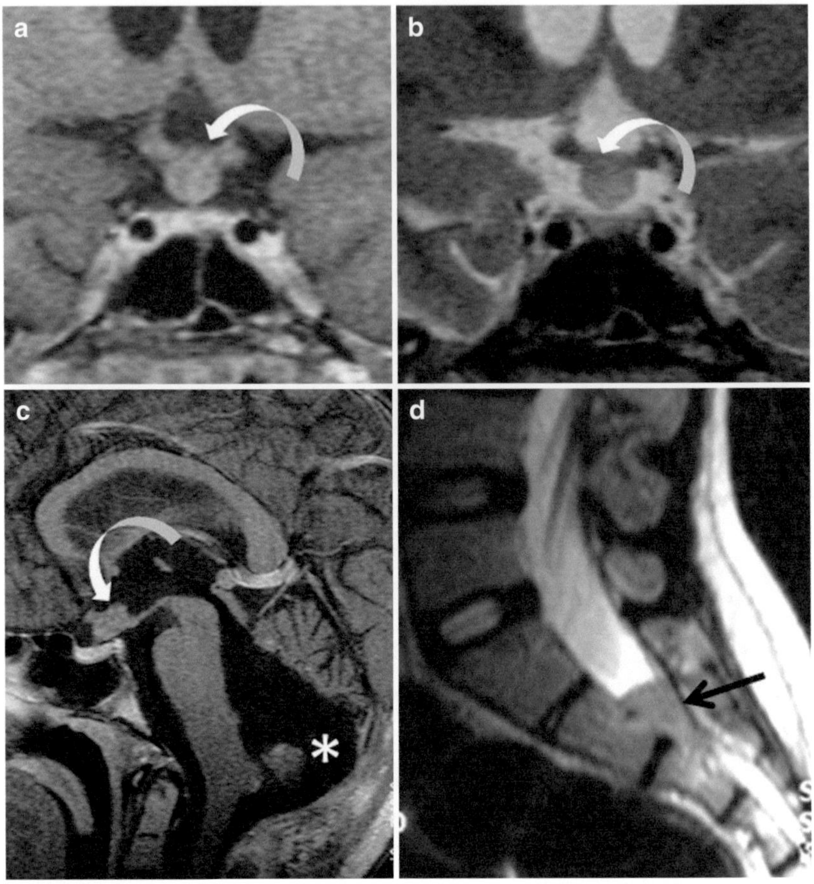

Fig. 33.4 Infundibulum metastasis in a 16-year-old boy with diabetes insipidus 2 years after surgery of a fourth ventricle ependymoma. (**a**, **b**) Coronal CE T1 and T2 WIs. Nodular enlargement of the pituitary stalk without postcontrast enhancement (*arrows*). (**c**) Sagittal CE T1WI. Postsurgical sequelae after resection of a fourth ventricle ependymoma (*asterisk*). (**d**) Lumbar spine sagittal T2WI. Intracanalar metastasis (*black arrow*)

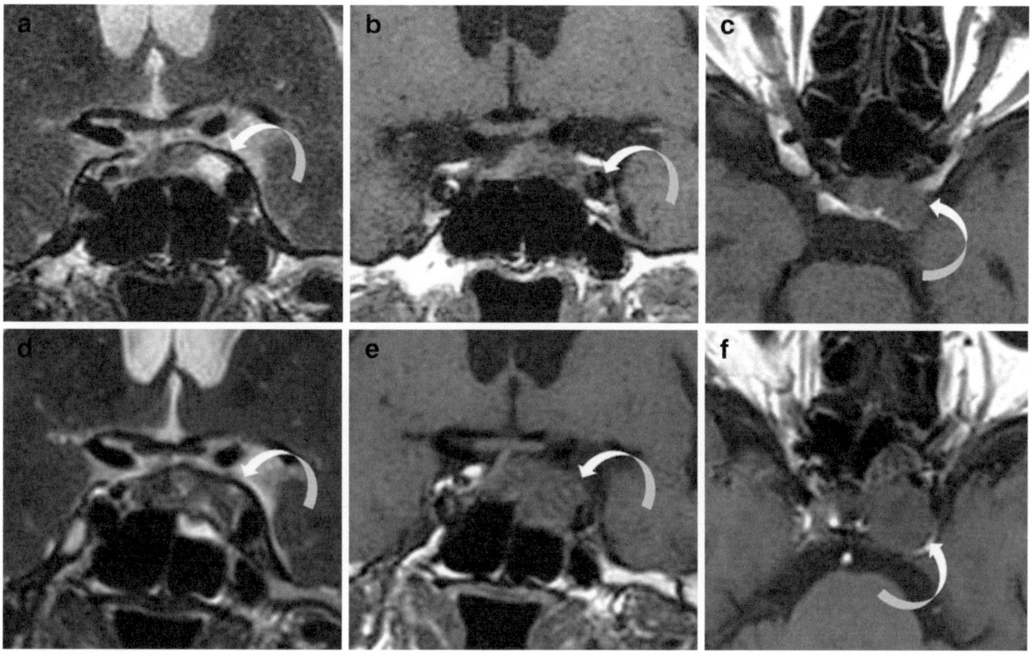

Fig. 33.5 Cavernous sinus metastasis in a 62-year-old man with a previously undiagnosed lung carcinoid. Brutal onset left of third oculomotor nerve palsy. (**a–c**) coronal T2, T1, and axial T1 WIs. Nonspecific T1-hypointense and T2-hyperintense mass invading left cavernous sinus (*arrows*). (**d–f**) Same MR sequences 2 months later. Very rapid evolution (*arrow*) signing the malignant nature of the tumor

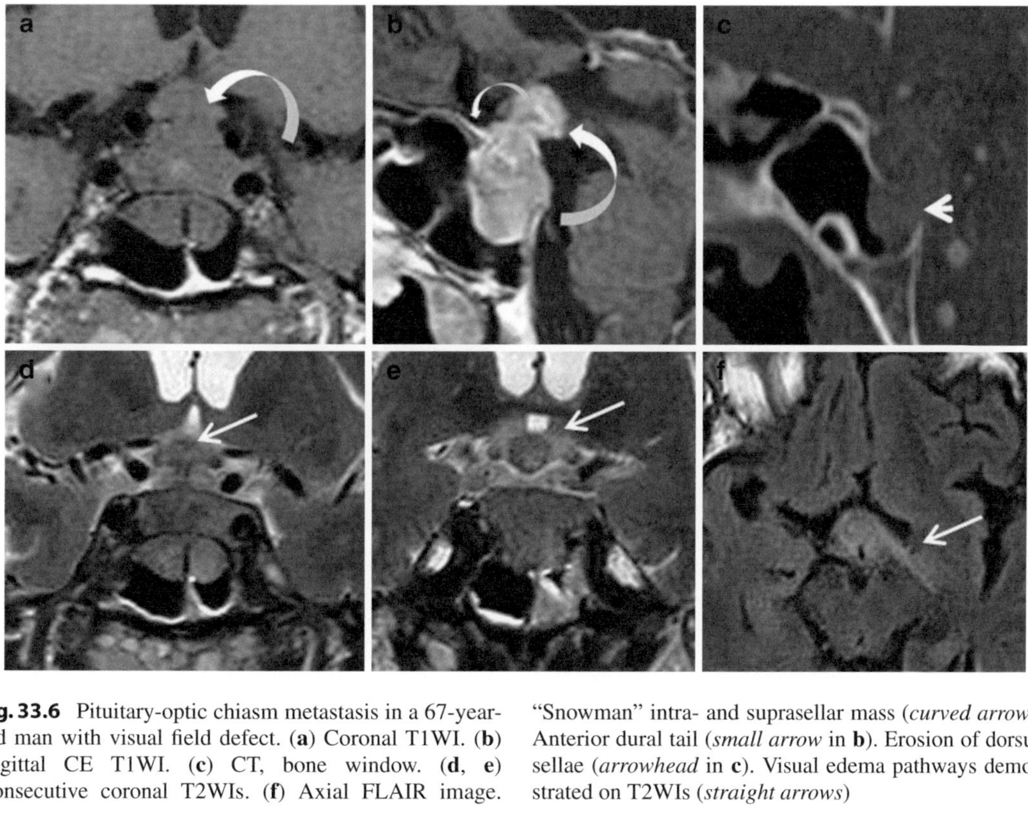

Fig. 33.6 Pituitary-optic chiasm metastasis in a 67-year-old man with visual field defect. (**a**) Coronal T1WI. (**b**) Sagittal CE T1WI. (**c**) CT, bone window. (**d, e**) Consecutive coronal T2WIs. (**f**) Axial FLAIR image. "Snowman" intra- and suprasellar mass (*curved arrows*). Anterior dural tail (*small arrow* in **b**). Erosion of dorsum sellae (*arrowhead* in **c**). Visual edema pathways demonstrated on T2WIs (*straight arrows*)

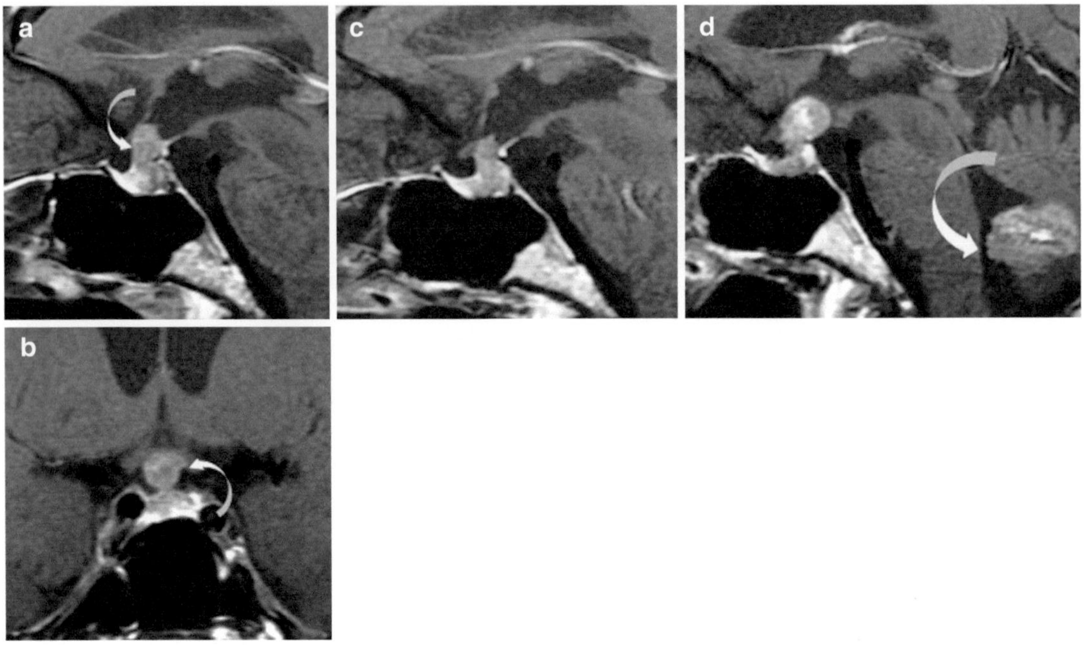

Fig. 33.7 Infundibulum metastasis in a 59-year-old woman with breast cancer considered cured 20 years previously. Isolated diabetes insipidus. (**a**, **b**) Sagittal and coronal CE T1WIs. Thickened pituitary stalk (*small arrow*). Sarcoidosis is suspected and corticotherapy is given. (**c**, **d**) Sagittal CE T1WIs. Four months later (**c**), infundibulum size is decreased and the diagnosis seems confirmed. Two years later (**d**), marked increased thickening of the stalk; a previously not demonstrated cerebellar metastasis is revealed (*large arrow*)

Further Reading

He W, Chen F, Dalm B et al (2015) Metastatic involvement of the pituitary gland: a systematic review with pooled individual patient data analysis. Pituitary 18(1):159–168

Komninos J, Vlassopoulou V, Protopapa D et al (2004) Tumors metastatic to the pituitary gland: case report and literature review. J Clin Endocrinol Metab 89(2): 574–580

Marsh JC, Garg S, Wendt JA et al (2010) Intracranial metastatic disease rarely involves the pituitary: retrospective analysis of 935 metastases in 155 patients and review of the literature. Pituitary 13(3): 260–265

34 Sellar and Suprasellar Lymphoma

Sonia Nagi and Maha Mahmoud

Primary central nervous system lymphoma (PCNSL) is rarely limited to the sellar region. Sellar and suprasellar locations represent a diagnostic challenge.

The mean age of patients is 55 years. Sixty percent of patients are males. The most common presentation is hypopituitarism, followed by headache, diplopia, diabetes insipidus, and hyperprolactinemia. Lymphoma is the most common neoplasm causing fever of unknown origin. Prognosis is generally poor and the disease rapidly progresses. Histologically similar to PCNSL, most lymphomas of the sellar and suprasellar region are B-cell non-Hodgkin lymphomas. PCNSL can arise from the suprasellar and hypothalamic regions (Fig. 34.1). Septal (Fig. 34.2) or ependymal extension may be noticed. Possible spread to the infundibular region, the cavernous sinus, or the clivus (Figs. 34.3 and 34.4) has been reported. Lymphoma of the sella and the pituitary gland can mimic a pituitary adenoma (Fig. 34.5). Unenhanced CT typically reveals hyper- or iso-attenuated lesions with homogeneous marked contrast enhancement in most cases. On MRI, there are no significant distinctive radiological characteristics. The common MRI finding is a mass lesion that is iso- to hypointense on T1 and T2 WIs. On T1 and T2 WIs, this tumor appears hypointense to gray matter (Fig. 34.2). This low intensity results from the dense cellularity and high nucleus-to-cytoplasm ratio of lymphoma, and it may help in the differentiation of primary CNS lymphoma from other brain tumors. In immunocompetent patients, contrast enhancement is typically intense and homogeneous (Fig. 34.1), but is more likely to be inhomogeneous or ring-like in immunocompromised patients. Associated vasogenic edema and mass effect are usually present. Mild or moderate T2-hyperintense peritumoral edema is a common feature of PCNSL, generally less pronounced than in metastases or high-grade gliomas. Non-acquired immune deficiency syndrome (AIDS) PCNSL typically presents as a solitary homogeneously enhancing parenchymal mass. Multiple lesions are reported in 20–40 % of non-AIDS PCNSLs.

However, PCNSL may be also present with necrotic (Fig. 34.2) and even hemorrhagic lesions primarily in immunocompromised, usually human immunodeficiency virus patients. Contrast enhancement can also vary and in very rare cases may even be completely absent, more frequently after steroid treatment. Vasogenic edema and mass effect can sometimes also be minimal.

A pituitary tumor with a propensity for perineural spread and an infiltrative growth pattern, with rapid growth on two successive examinations, is suggestive of lymphoma (Figs. 34.1 and 34.5), particularly in immunocompromised patients or in the elderly. CNS lymphomas usually have characteristic imaging findings on CT and conventional MRI; nevertheless, they cannot be unequivocally differentiated from other brain lesions. In the large majority of reported cases,

J.-F. Bonneville et al., *MRI of the Pituitary Gland*, DOI 10.1007/978-3-319-29043-0_34

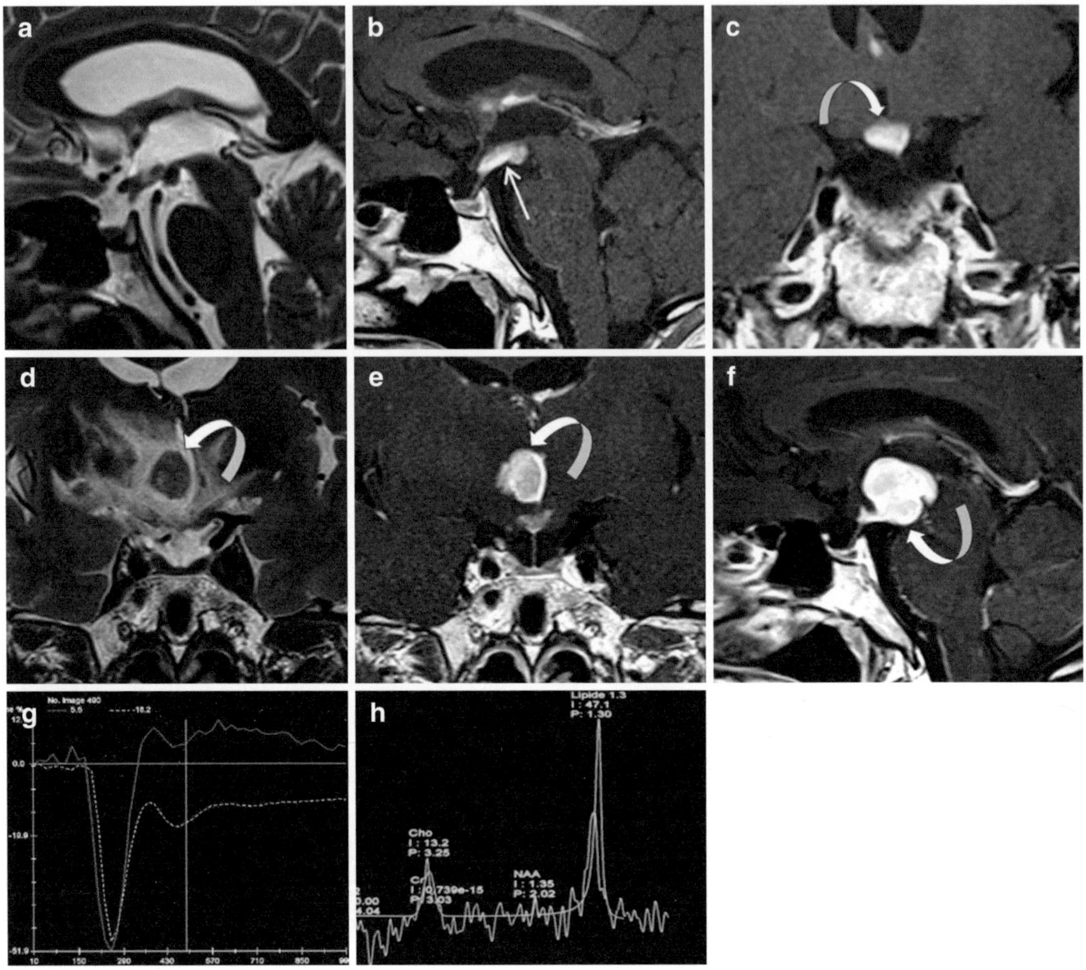

Fig. 34.1 Suprasellar lymphoma in a 46-year-old man with central diabetes insipidus, nausea, and vomiting. (**a–c**) Sagittal T2, coronal, and sagittal CE T1 WIs: thickening of the infundibulum, the tuber cinereum, the mammillary bodies and the optic chiasm (*curved arrow*). Marked enhancement of the infundibulum and tuber cinereum (*straight arrow*), thin pituitary stalk. (**d**) Coronal T2WI and (**e**, **f**) Coronal and sagittal CE T1WIs 1 month later. No improvement despite corticotherapy and antituberculosis treatment. T2 iso-hypointense hypothalamic mass with important peritumoral edema and marked homogeneous contrast enhancement (*curved arrow*). (**g**) Perfusion MRI. Low maximum rCBV. The first-pass perfusion curve remains below the baseline at 3 T. (**h**) Proton MR spectroscopy. Elevated lipid peaks

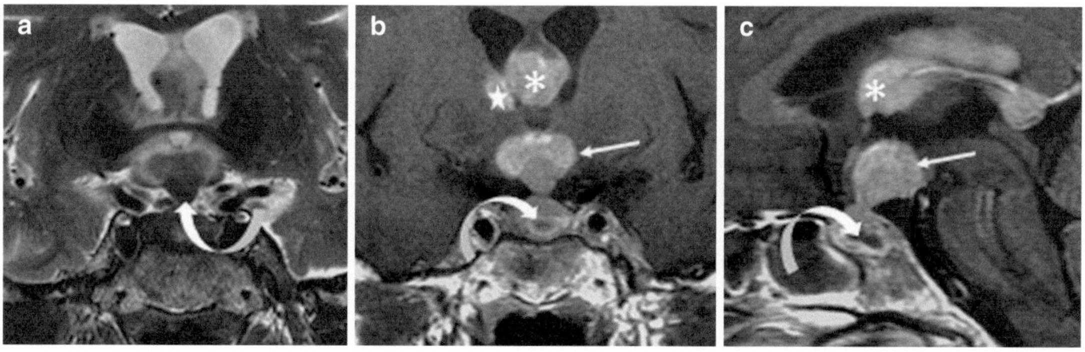

Fig. 34.2 Sellar and suprasellar lymphoma with trigonoseptal and thalamic extension in a 62-year-old woman. (**a**) Coronal T2WI. Well-circumscribed dumbbell-shaped sellar and suprasellar mass extending through the diaphragma sellae with hypointense signal (*curved arrow*). (**b**, **c**) Coronal and sagittal CE T1WIs: enhancing sellar mass with central necrosis (*curved arrow*), tissular suprasellar lesion with homogeneous enhancement (*straight arrow*), trigonoseptal (*asterisk*) and right thalamic (*star*) spread

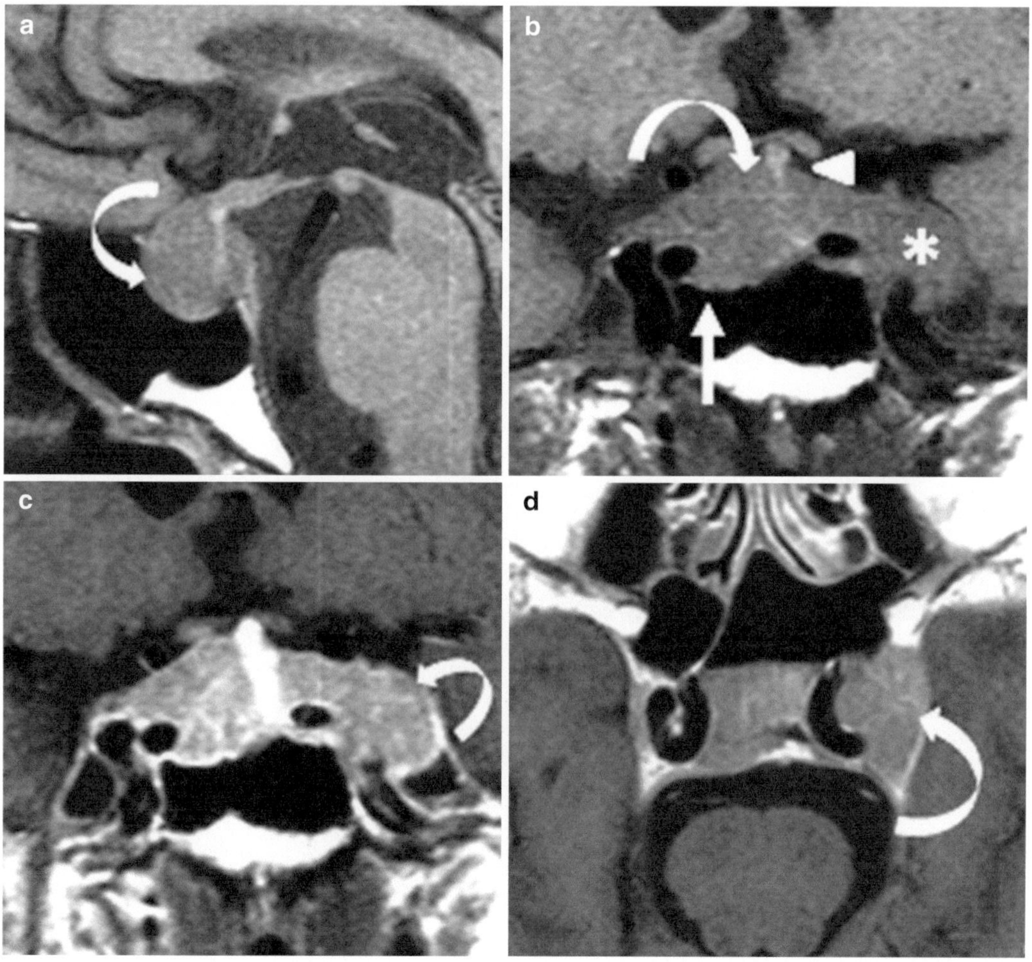

Fig. 34.3 Sellar lymphoma in an 81-year-old man. (**a**, **b**) Sagittal and coronal T1WIs. Isointense pituitary mass (*curved arrow*), bulging of the sellar floor (*straight arrow*), pituitary stalk deviation (*arrowhead*), extension into the left cavernous sinus surrounding the left internal carotid artery (*asterisk*), absence of the bright signal normally seen in the posterior lobe. (**c**, **d**) Coronal and axial CE T1WIs. Inconspicuous and homogeneous enhancement of the mass pushing outward the lateral wall of left cavernous sinus (*curved arrow*)

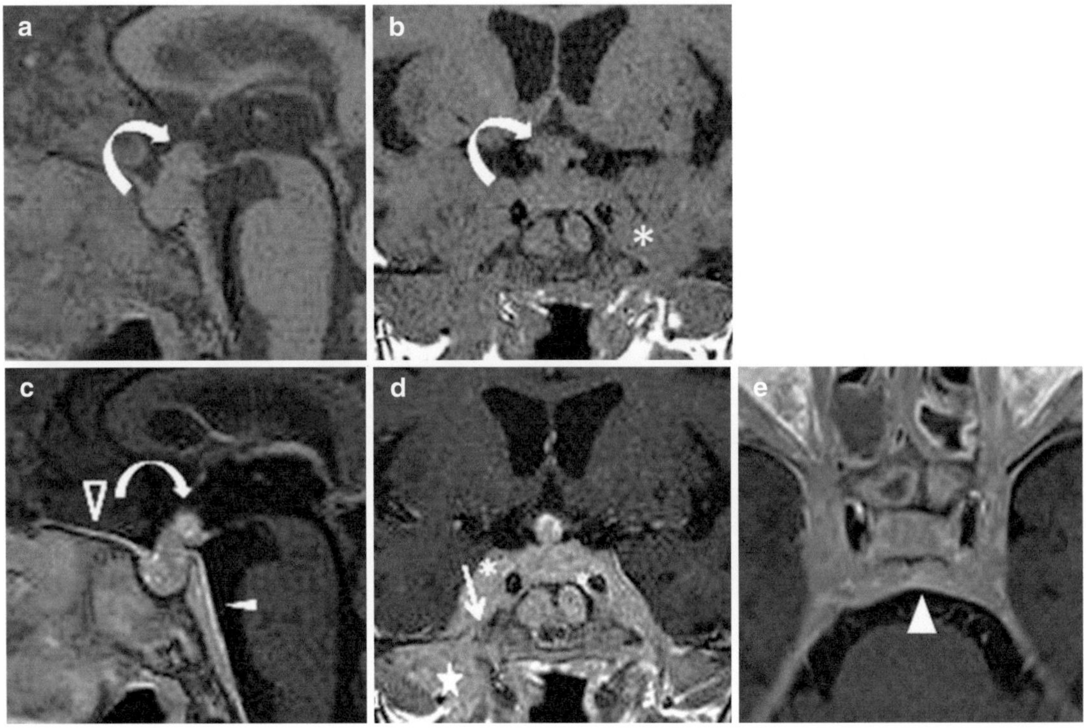

Fig. 34.4 Pituitary gland and infundibular lymphoma. (**a**, **b**) Sagittal and coronal T1WIs. Isointense pituitary stalk mass (*curved arrow*), bilateral parasellar tissular infiltration (*asterisk*), absence of the normal T1 hyperintensity of the posterior lobe. (**c–e**) Sagittal, coronal, and axial CE T1WIs. Gadolinium uptake of the pituitary stalk mass and the pituitary gland (*curved arrow*), bilateral cavernous sinus involvement (*asterisk*) with extension through the foramen ovale (*straight arrow*) and right lateral pterygoid muscle infiltration (*star*), dural thickening and abnormal enhancement along the clival dura (*arrowhead*), presellar dural tail (*empty arrowhead*)

presumptive diagnosis was pituitary adenoma (Fig. 34.5). Confirmation of diagnosis was most frequently obtained after surgery. DWI, perfusion MRI, and MR spectroscopy may help to differentiate CNS lymphomas from other brain lesions.

Because CNS lymphomas are highly cellular tumors, water diffusion is often restricted, making them appear hyperintense on DWI with characteristic dark appearance on ADC maps. PCNSL lesions often have more restricted diffusion and lower ADC values than high-grade gliomas and metastases. Perfusion MRI does not show neovascularization on a cerebral blood volume map. Regional rCBV is close to 1, and the first-pass perfusion curve exceeds the baseline after gadolinium bolus, related to a massive leakage of contrast medium into the interstitial space. This first-pass perfusion curve may remain below the baseline at 3 T (Fig. 34.1).

In PCNSL, proton MR spectroscopy demonstrates elevated lipid peaks combined with high choline/creatinine ratios.

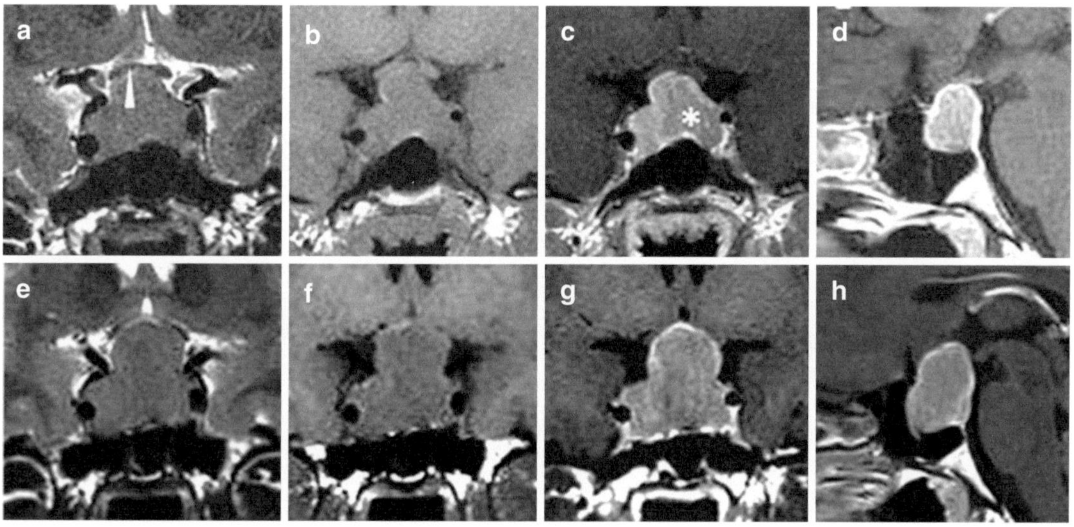

Fig. 34.5 Pituitary gland lymphoma in a 31-year-old man with chronic fever. Prolactin is 150 ng/ml. (**a**, **b**) Coronal T2 and T1 WIs. Pituitary mass with suprasellar extension compressing the optic chiasm (*arrowhead*) and eroding the sellar floor. (**c**, **d**) Coronal and sagittal CE T1WIs. Heterogeneous enhancement with lesser enhancement on the left (*asterisk*). A macroprolactinoma is suspected and a treatment with cabergoline instituted. Five months later, prolactin is normal and an MRI follow-up is systematically performed. (**e–h**) Coronal T2, T1, coronal and sagittal CE T1 WIs. Unexpected increase of the mass with major compression of the optic chiasm. The diagnosis of B lymphoma was obtained at surgery

Further Reading

Fadoukhair Z, Amzerin M, Ismaili N et al (2010) Symptomatic hypopituitarism revealing primary suprasellar lymphoma. BMC Endocr Disord 10:19

Haldorsen IS, Espeland A, Larsson EM (2011) Central nervous system lymphoma: characteristic findings on traditional and advanced imaging. Am J Neuroradiol 32:984–982

Kaufmann T, Lopes MB, Laws ER et al (2002) Primary sellar lymphoma: radiologic and pathologic findings in two patients. Am J Neuroradiol 23: 364–367

35 Cavernous Sinus Lesions

Fabrice Bonneville and Françoise Cattin

Cavernous sinuses are a pair of extradural spaces located laterally on both sides of the sella turcica. These interperiostodural spaces are very similar to the orbits and the anterior spinal epidural space, all of them being limited by meninges and periostea, and containing fat, vessels, and nerves. More precisely, cavernous sinuses contain on each side a large venous network draining the orbit and the cerebral temporal fossa, cranial nerves III, IV, V1, V2, and VI, the intracavernous internal carotid artery, and some fat. Cavernous sinuses communicate with each other via coronary sinuses. Lesions of cavernous sinus are numerous and are listed in Table 35.1. They may originate directly from the cavernous sinus itself or its walls, or invade secondarily the cavernous sinus from the neighboring structures. Of note, invasion by a pituitary adenoma is by far the most frequent lesion encountered in the cavernous sinus and has been extensively described in Chap. 11. Similarly, most cavernous sinus lesions are described in dedicated chapters throughout this book, and only those not presented elsewhere or that need further details are illustrated here.

Table 35.1 Gamut of cavernous sinus lesions

(A) Tumoral lesions
1. Intracavernous tumors
Meningioma
Schwannoma/neurofibroma
Malignant peripheral nerve sheath tumor
Lymphoma
Metastasis
Other rare tumors (sarcoma, neuroblastoma, angioleiomyoma)
2. Neighboring lesions invading the sinus
Adenoma
Chordoma/Chondrosarcoma
ENT carcinoma
Paraganglioma
Juvenile nasopharyngeal angiofibroma
3. Cystic lesions
Epidermoid cyst
Dermoid cyst
Arachnoid cyst
(B) Vascular lesions
Aneurysm
Cavernous hemangioma
Carotid cavernous fistula
Thrombosis
(C) Inflammatory lesions
Tolosa-Hunt syndrome and pseudotumor
Sarcoidosis
Wegener granulomatosis
Infection/tuberculoma

35.1 Aneurysm

Aneurysms have been detailed in Chap. 60. In the cavernous sinus, aneurysms almost never bleed. They are usually discovered incidentally on CT or MRI when small. They produce mass effect and compression of the adjacent structures when large or giant, resulting in unspecific symptoms of cavernous sinus syndrome, such as facial

J.-F. Bonneville et al., *MRI of the Pituitary Gland*, DOI 10.1007/978-3-319-29043-0_35

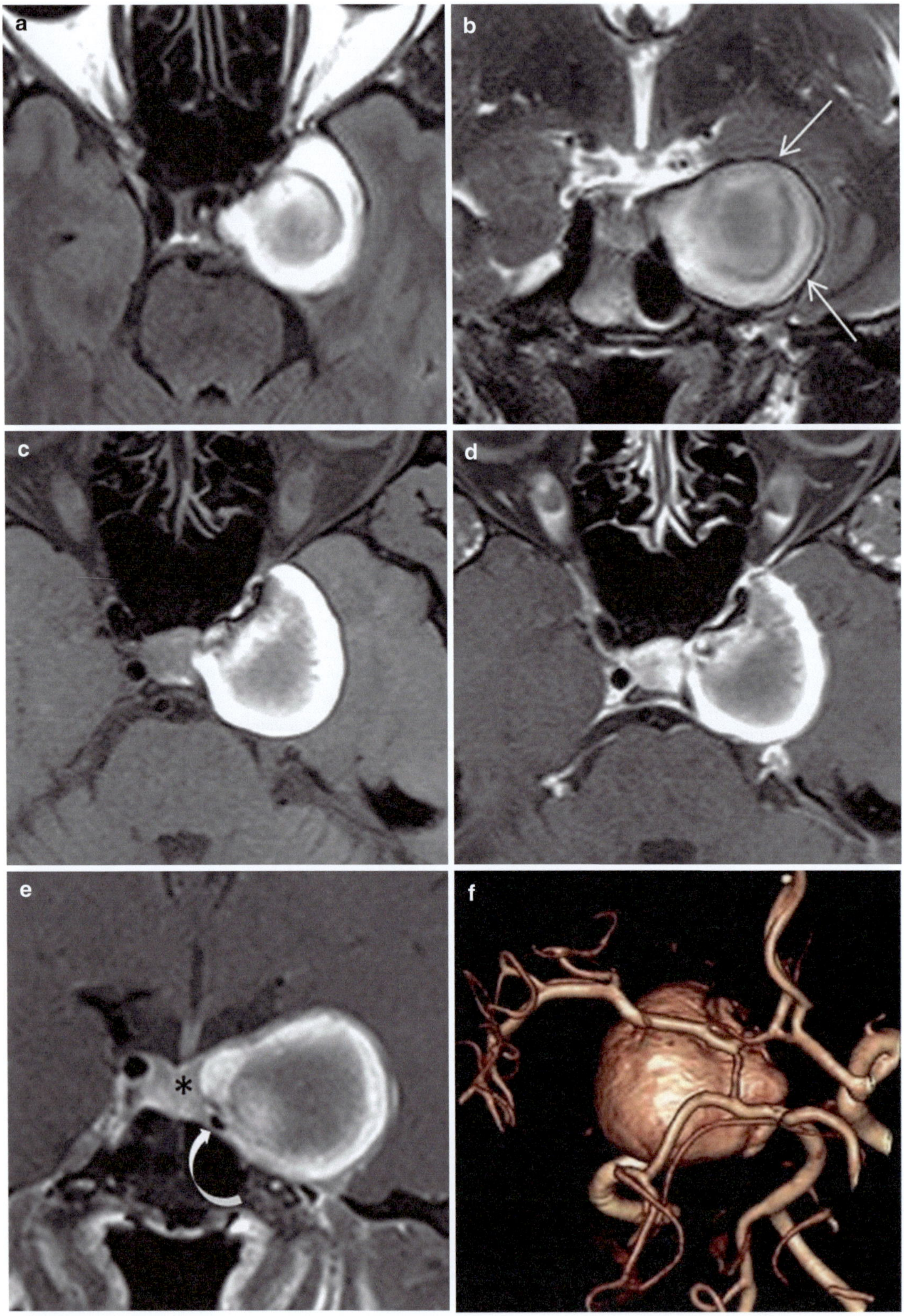
a
b
c
d
e
*
f

neuralgia and diplopia. An aneurysm should always be evoked facing a round T2-hypointense lesion. However, a large aneurysm may be partially thrombosed and contain clot with various signal intensities that may mimic another lesion. Circumferential layers of thrombus of different ages and lack of enhancement after gadolinium injection are clues to the diagnosis of such thrombosed aneurysms on MRI (Fig. 35.1). A patent portion of the lumen of the aneurysm sac should be carefully sought to confirm the diagnosis. This should appear as a signal void on spin-echo sequences and with high signal on axial source images of MRA and other gradient echo techniques.

35.2 Cavernous Hemangioma

Cavernous sinus cavernous hemangioma is a rare, extra-axial vascular lesion formed by sinusoidal spaces that contain slow-flowing or stagnant blood. This tumor is important to recognize preoperatively because of its propensity to bleed during eventual surgery. It is often mistaken for a cavernous sinus meningioma, but a close look at MR images allows one to reliably distinguish these two completely different entities. A rapid description of cavernous hemangioma will relate whether they present as well-demarcated hypo- to isointense lesions on T1WI, are markedly hyperintense on T2WI, and enhance intensely and homogeneously after gadolinium administration (Fig. 35.2). Such may also be true for meningiomas. However, looking at details, hemangiomas demonstrate remarkable ultra-high homogeneous signal intensity on T2WI, similar to CSF or the eyeball. They may also contain intratumoral septa that appear as dark lines on T2WI (Fig. 35.3). Because they are extradural within the cavernous sinus, cavernous hemangiomas are outlined by the lateral wall of the cavernous sinus, which also appears as a T2-hypointense line. Those lesions are soft and barely erode the adjacent skull base, and never go through it to invade the sphenoid sinus, as meningiomas can do. Neither do they narrow the diameter of the internal carotid artery. They may invade medially the sella and displace the pituitary, thus mimicking a macroadenoma, and may also demonstrate foci of T1 hyperintensity corresponding to areas of limited focal thrombosis. On CE T1WIs, cavernous hemangiomas demonstrate a singular centripetal enhancement. If dynamic acquisition is performed, one can see a progressive enhancing process from heterogeneous to uniform, from the edges of the lesion to the center, from mild to intense. Of note, no dural tail enhancement accompanies this lesion.

35.3 Cavernous Sinus Thrombosis

Cavernous sinus thrombosis may be secondary to infection of the face, paranasal sinuses, orbits, and temporal bone. Clinically the diagnosis can be evoked in the presence of chemosis, eyelid edema, exophthalmos, or cranial nerve deficit. MR signs of cavernous sinus thrombosis include changes in signal intensities and enlargement of the occluded cavernous sinus. Acute thrombus is isointense on T1 and T2 WIs, while subacute thrombus exhibits high signal intensity on all sequences and is easily recognized. After gadolinium injection, visualization of a filling defect in the cavernous sinus associated with enhancement of the peripheral margins of the enlarged cavernous suggests

Fig. 35.1 Patient with intracavernous internal carotid artery thrombosed aneurysm and acute left facial neuralgia and diplopia. (**a**) Axial FLAIR and (**b**) Coronal T2WI demonstrate a large, well-defined, round intracavernous lesion with unusual circumferential layers of variable signal intensities. Note the thin outlying hypointense line surrounding the lesion that corresponds to the distended lateral wall of the cavernous sinus (*arrows*). Axial fat-saturated T1WIs (**c**) before and (**d**) after gadolinium injection reveal a thick rim of spontaneous hyperintensity corresponding to older peripheral thrombosis, while the hypointense center represents acute clot. (**e**) Coronal fat-saturated CE T1WI illustrates the relationship between the cavernous mass lesion, the pituitary (*asterisk*), and the tiny residual compressed patent intracavernous carotid artery (*curved arrow*). Of note, no enhancement is depicted in this completely thrombosed aneurysm, as confirmed on (**f**) 3D rendering reformatted MR angiogram

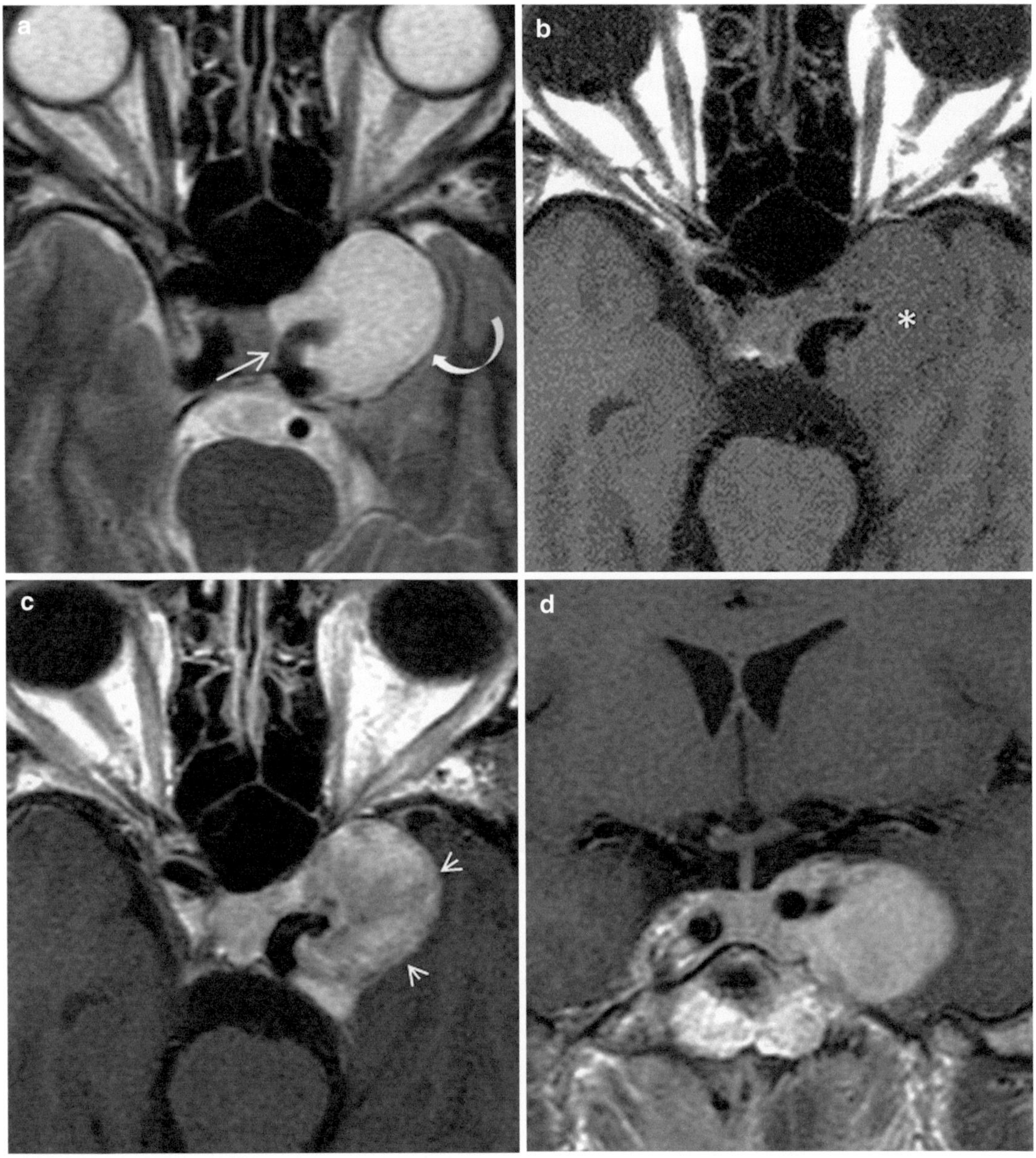

Fig. 35.2 Patient with typical cavernous hemangioma of the left cavernous sinus and diplopia. (**a**) Axial T2WI reveals a homogeneous well-defined cavernous sinus mass lesion with ultra-high signal intensity, similar to that of the ocular globe. Additional features are normal diameter of the wrapped internal carotid artery (*arrow*) and distension of the hypointense lateral wall of the cavernous sinus (*curved arrow*). (**b**) Axial T1WI demonstrates a homogeneous isointense lesion (*) that on (**c**) axial CE T1WI progressively enhances from periphery to center (*shorts arrows*), to finally show uniform and intense enhancement on (**d**) coronal CE T1WI, without any adjacent dural tail enhancement

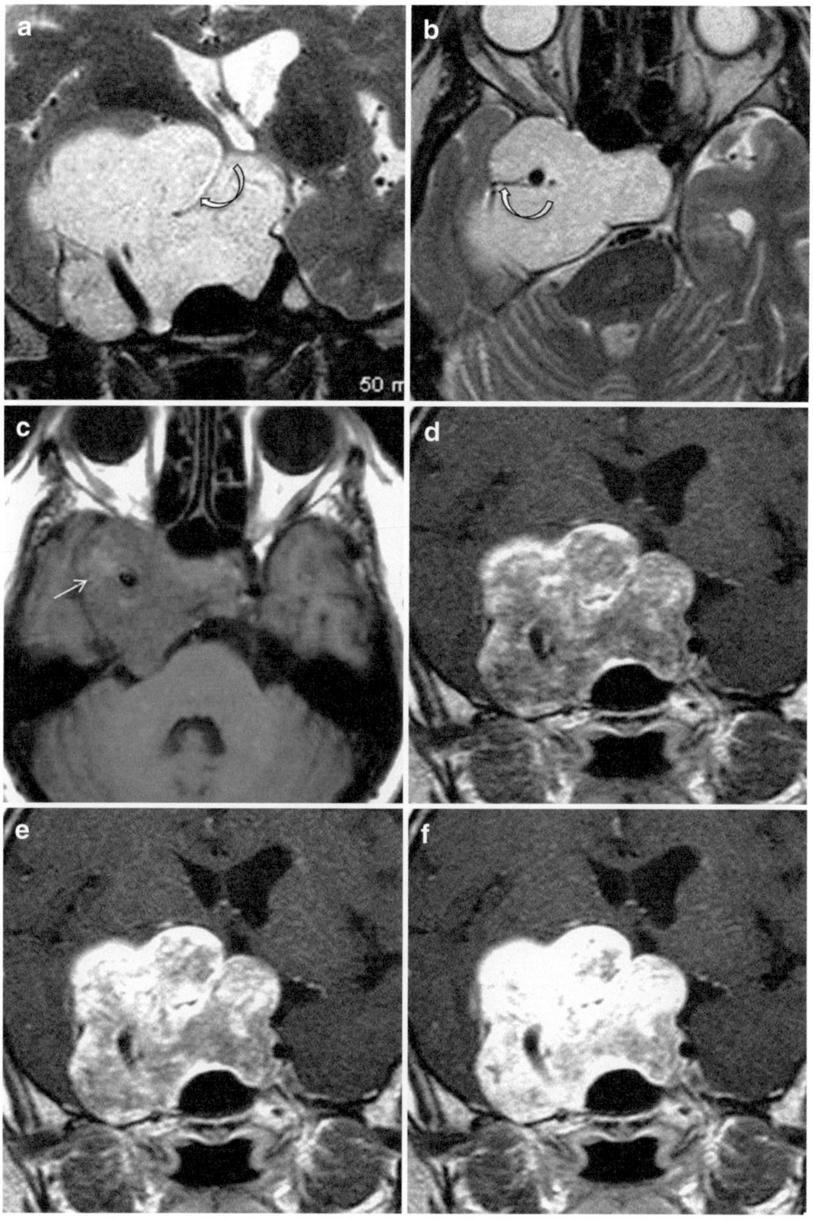

Fig. 35.3 Patient with huge cavernous hemangioma, headaches, and hypopituitarism. (**a**) Coronal and (**b**) axial T2WIs show a giant intra-, latero-, and suprasellar homogeneous hyperintense lesion with intratumoral septation (*curved arrows*). Note the lack of infrasellar extension in the sphenoid sinus. (**c**) Axial T1WI demonstrates subtle foci of hyperintensities interpreted as area of focal thrombosis (*arrow*). (**d–f**) Coronal dynamic CE T1WIs illustrate the progressive centripetal enhancement of this hemangioma from the periphery to the center

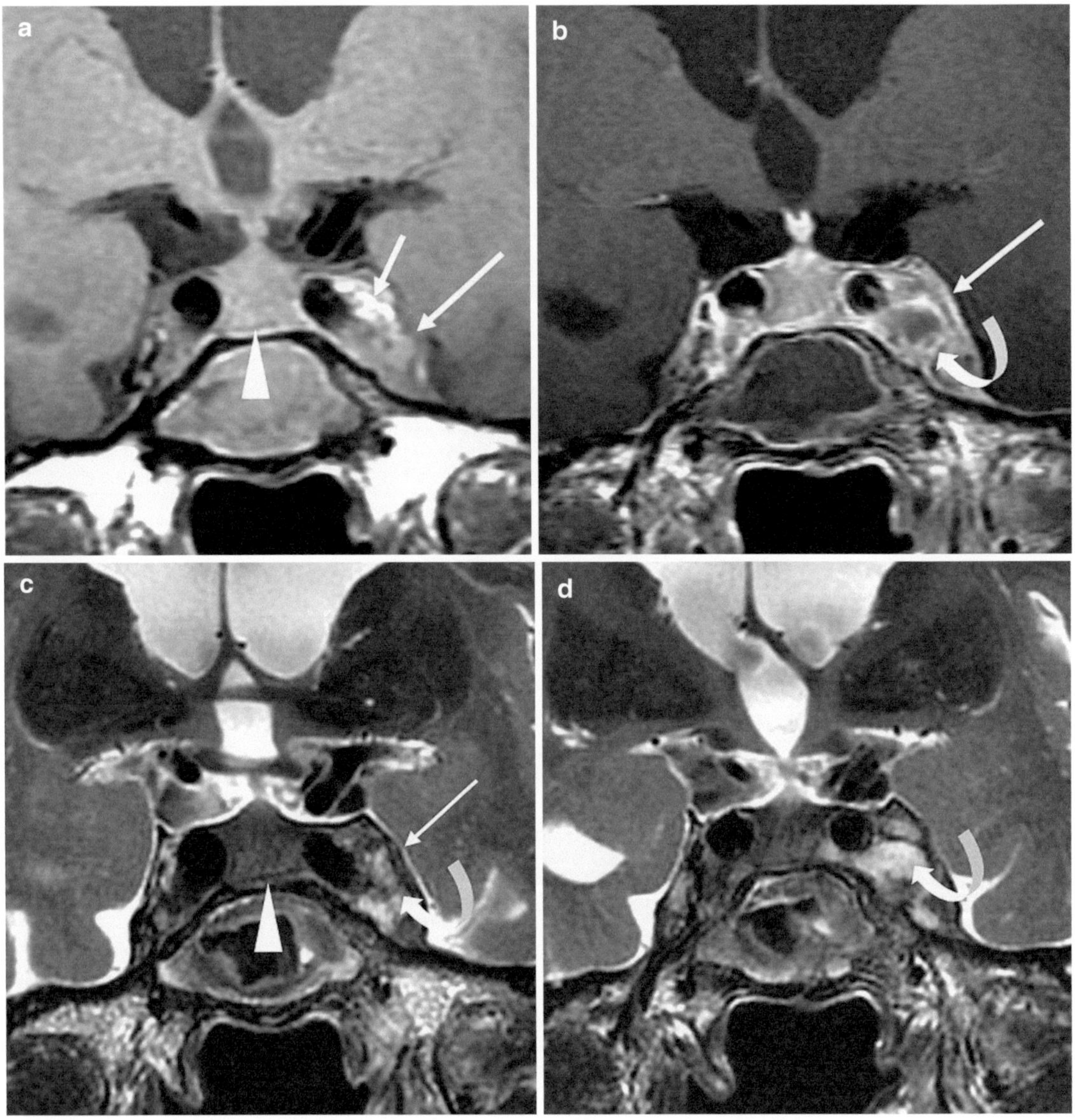

Fig. 35.4 An 80-year-old woman with headaches, vomiting, and left oculomotor and abducens nerves palsy. Cavernous sinus thrombosis. (**a–d**) Coronal T1, CE T1, and T2 WIs. Enlargement of the left cavernous sinus (*long arrow*) and demonstration of the inferior intercavernous sinus (*arrowhead*). Bulging of the upper surface of the pituitary gland. The signal of the left cavernous sinus is heterogeneous on all sequences, but hyperintensity predominates on T2WI. On T1WI, some veins appear spontaneously hyperintense (*small arrow*). The intracavernous thrombus (*curved arrow*) is well delineated after contrast injection and on T2WI. (**e**) Diffusion imaging showing restricted diffusion evoking the presence of pus in the sphenoid sinus (*arrow*). (**f**) Sagittal T1WI. Complete filling of the sphenoid sinus (*asterisk*). (**g**) Axial T2WI. Dilation of the left superior ophthalmic vein (*arrow*) and left exophthalmos. (**h**) Axial CE 3D gradient echo T1WI. Filling defect in the left cavernous sinus (*curved arrow*) and marked enhancement of the left free edge of the tentorium (*arrowhead*)

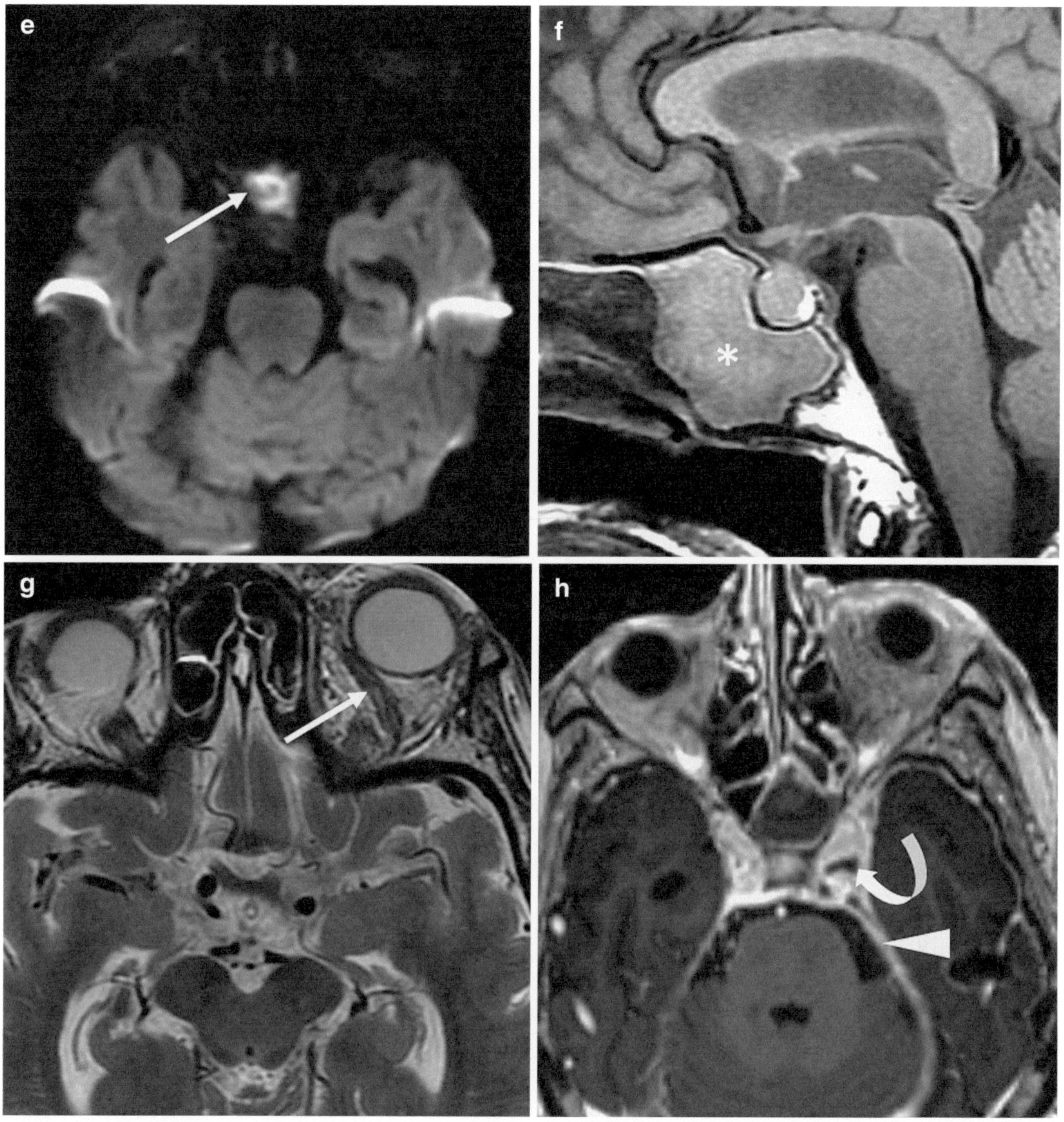

Fig. 35.4 (continued)

thrombosis (Fig. 35.4). Indirect signs such as dilation of the superior ophthalmic veins, orbital cellulitis, exophthalmos, and increased dural enhancement along the lateral border of cavernous sinus are crucial for the diagnosis. The origin of the infection responsible for cavernous sinus thrombosis is often indicated by DWI. This sequence also indicates subacute sinus thrombosis by showing focal abnormal hyperintensity and restricted diffusion.

Diffusion imaging is also crucial to detect cerebral infarcts downstream of focal narrowing of the intracavernous internal carotid artery trapped in the septic thrombosis (Fig. 35.5). In this setting, MRA should be performed for artery assessment.

35.4 Tolosa-Hunt Syndrome

Tolosa-Hunt syndrome is due to granulomatous inflammation involving the cavernous sinus, the superior orbital fissure, or the orbital apex. The etiology of Tolosa-Hunt syndrome remains unknown.

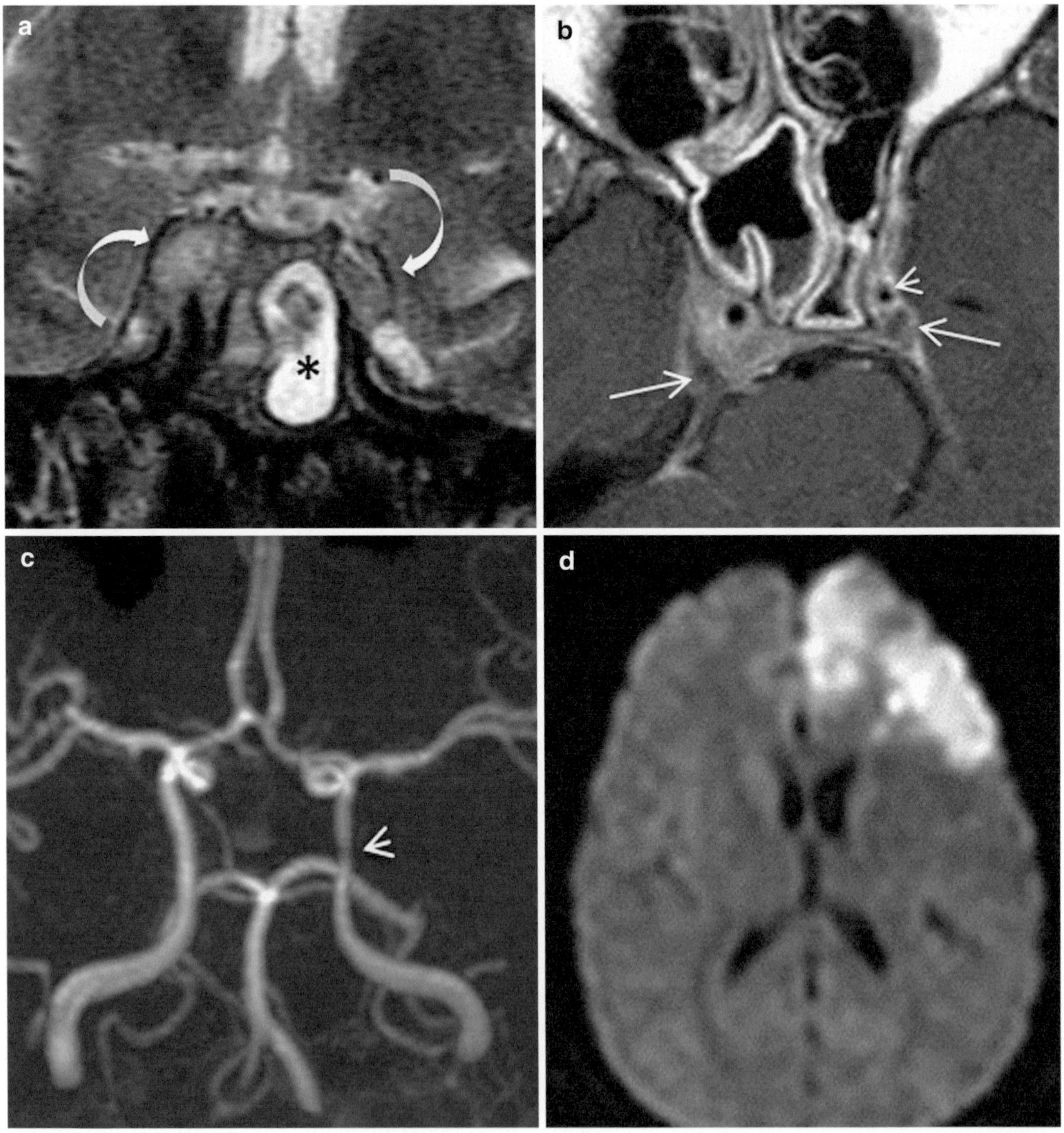

Fig. 35.5 A 16-year-old patient with cavernous sinus thrombosis and sphenoid sinusitis, fever, and headaches followed by right hemiparesis. (**a**) Coronal T2WI shows enlargement of the posterior aspect of both cavernous sinuses (*curved arrows*) together with partial filling of the sphenoid sinus by secretion (*asterisk*). (**b**) Axial CE T1WI depicts corresponding filling defects, thus confirming areas of cavernous sinus thrombosis (*straight arrows*). Note the focal reduction of the diameter of the intracavernous ICA (*shorts arrow*), a finding demonstrated by (**c**) 3D time-of-flight (TOF) MRA. This stenosis consequently led to a large left frontal stroke, as illustrated by (**d**) DWI

The clinical diagnosis is evoked in the presence of relapsing-remitting unilateral painful ophthalmoplegia with rapid favorable response to systemic corticosteroids. Tolosa-Hunt syndrome is usually unilateral, although bilateral alternate involvement is possible. MRI demonstrates enlarged cavernous sinus with abnormal soft tissue extending to the superior orbital fissure, isointense to temporal white matter on T1WI and isointense to mildly hypointense on T2WI, which markedly enhances after gadolinium injection. The granulomatous tissue encircling the intracavernous internal carotid artery can be at the origin of a narrowing of the arterial lumen (Fig. 35.6).

35.5 Trigeminal Schwannoma

Trigeminal schwannomas are encapsulated tumors arising from Schwann cells of the nerve sheath which displace, but not invade, the nerve fascicles. They can occur at any age with a peak during the third and fourth decades. The most frequent symptom is trigeminal nerve dysfunction, including pain, numbness, and paresthesias. Tumor arises from the cisternal segment of the trigeminal nerve in 20 % of the cases, in the Meckel cave in 50 %, and both segments in 25 %; in this last case, the tumor has a typical dumbbell shape. The remaining 5 % arise from distal branches and extend extracranially.

Bone changes due to the slow growth of the tumor can be better appreciated on CT scanning with bone window than on MRI: erosion of the petrous apex, erosion of the middle fossa floor, enlargement of the foramen ovale, foramen rotundum, and superior orbital fissure (Fig. 35.7). On MRI, schwannomas are isointense to hypointense masses on T1WI, and markedly enhance after gadolinium injection with sharp demarcation between the margin of the tumor and adjacent structures because of the peripheral capsule. The small lesions have slight to moderate low signal on T2WI in relation with their high cellularity. The large tumors are mostly hyperintense on T2WI and tend to be heterogeneous owing to intratumoral necrosis, cystic components or, less frequently, hemorrhagic components (Fig. 35.8).

Though extremely rare, nerve sheath tumors could be malignant. Ill-defined infiltrative margins, rapid growth, and extensive lysis of the skull base may suggest an underlying malignant nature, confirmed by histology.

35.6 ENT Lesions

Nasopharyngeal carcinoma, juvenile angiofibroma, or even paragangliomas can be large and aggressive enough to invade intracranially the cavernous sinus. This is of major importance for surgical planning and outcome, as an intracavernous component usually precludes complete and successful treatment.

Nasopharyngeal carcinoma invades the intracranial space in 5–15 %, with a predilection for the cavernous sinus. This extension may occur directly via skull-base erosion or by perineural spread along branches of the trigeminal nerve. The tumor is usually large at this stage and is present in the nasopharynx. ENT carcinomas are rather hypointense on T1 and T2 WIs and show moderate to intense contrast enhancement (Fig. 35.9).

Juvenile nasopharyngeal angiofibroma is a highly vascular tumor responsible for epistaxis and nasal obstruction in male adolescents. Such tumors originate in the posterolateral wall of the nasopharynx and are centered by the sphenopalatine foramen, but can present with significant skull-base involvement and intracranial extension, and even invade the cavernous sinus by erosion of the pterygoid bone (Fig. 35.10). On MRI, juvenile nasopharyngeal angiofibroma appears as a large heterogeneous mass with T2 hyperintensities and signal voids consistent with the highly vascular nature of this tumor. Therefore, it enhances intensely after gadolinium administration.

Jugulotympanic or vagal paragangliomas can similarly extend intracranially and invade the cavernous sinus (Fig. 35.11). Although tumoral signal intensities of this highly vascularized lesion are rather identical to those of juvenile angiofibroma, including intratumoral flow voids and marked enhancement, the epicenter of the

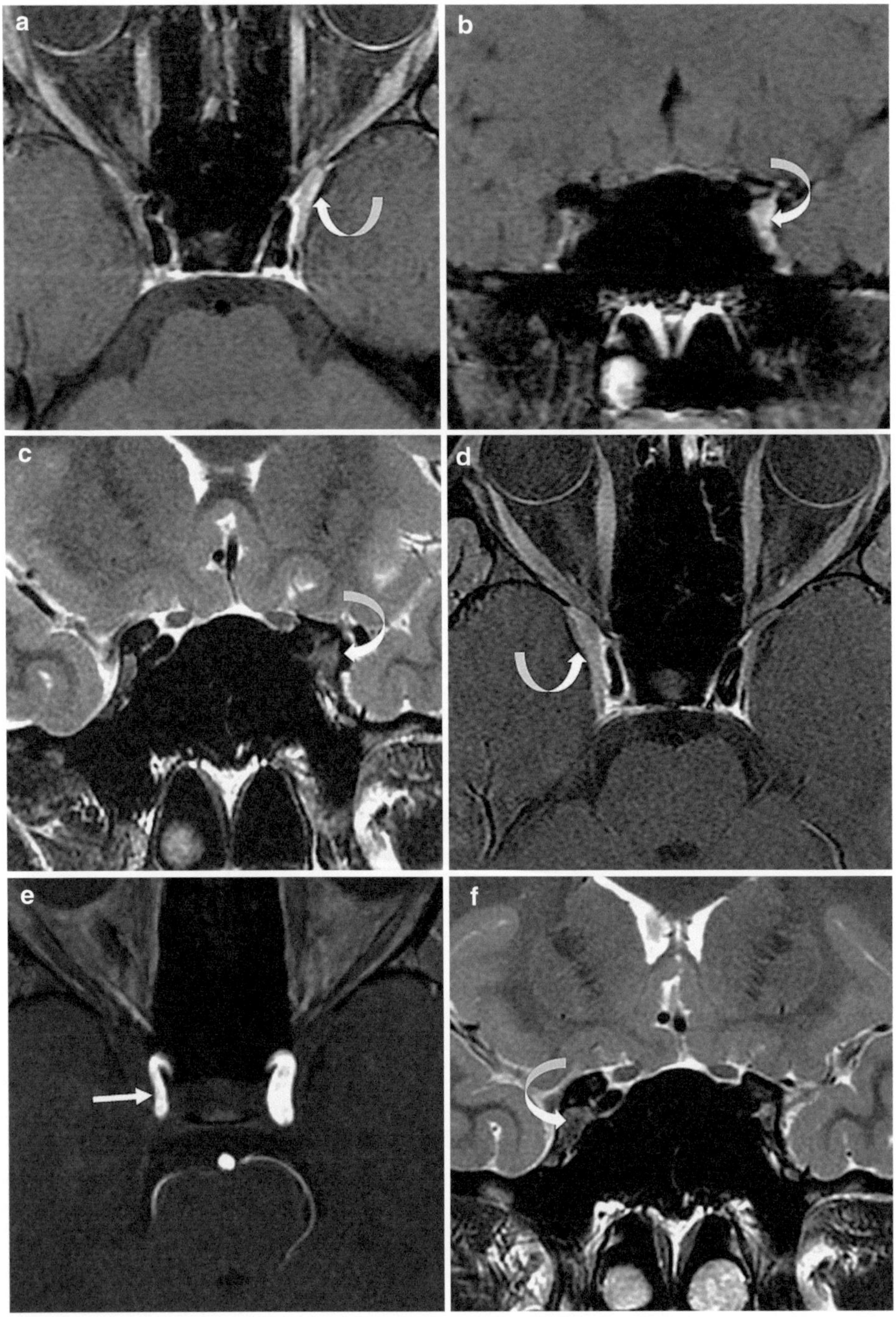

Fig. 35.6 Tolosa-Hunt syndrome. A 14-year-old girl presenting with progressive continuous orbital-periorbital pain and frontotemporal headaches for 10 days. Sudden onset of left oculomotor nerve palsy. (**a**, **b**) Axial and coronal fat-saturated CE T1WIs. Discrete enlargement and mild enhancement of the anterior part of the left cavernous sinus (*curved arrow*). (**c**) Coronal T2WI. The signal of the infiltrative tissue is similar to that of the temporal white matter (*curved arrow*). Corticosteroid therapy resolved both the clinical and radiological findings of Tolosa-Hunt syndrome after 2 months (not shown). One year later, new attack of headaches and periorbital pain with paresis of the right abducens nerve. (**d**) Axial CE T1WI. Enlargement and marked enhancement of the right cavernous sinus (*curved arrow*). (**e**) 3D TOF MRA showing a narrowing of the right intracavernous internal carotid artery (*arrow*). (**f**) Coronal T2WI. Abnormal slightly hypointense tissue in the anterior part of the cavernous sinus (*curved arrow*). Prompt response to corticosteroid treatment

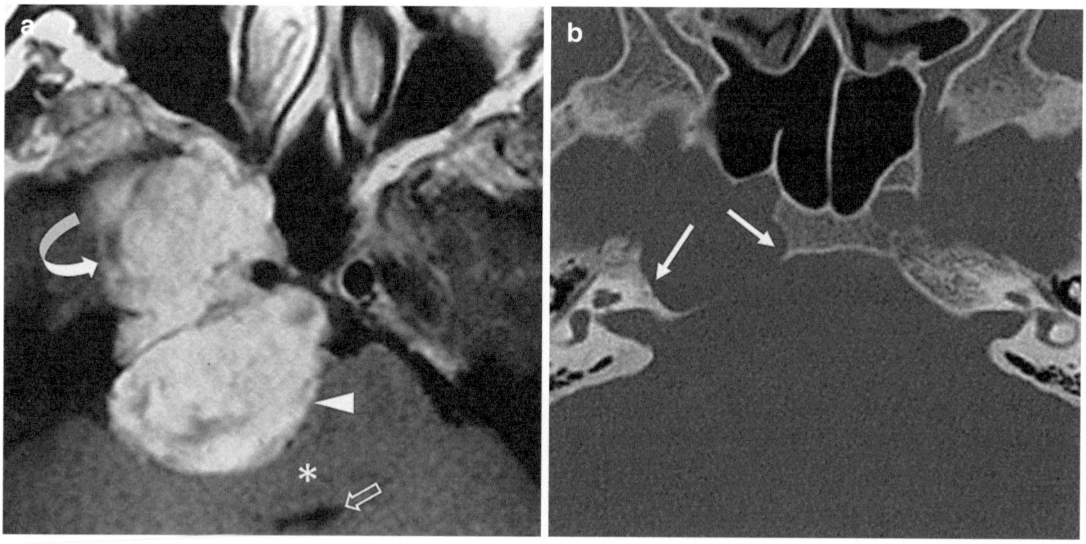

Fig. 35.7 A 49-year-old man with incidentally found erosion of the petrous bone on CT scan of the skull base. Trigeminal schwannoma extending to the posterior fossa with dumbbell shape. (**a**, **b**) Axial CE T1WI and CT scan (bone window). Large tumor occupying the right cavernous sinus (*curved arrow*) with a prominent posterior extension along the cisternal segment of the trigeminal nerve (*arrowhead*). Marked and heterogeneous enhancement. Mass effect on the pons (*asterisk*) and fourth ventricle (*opened arrow*). The smooth margins of the petrous bone erosion are characteristic of slow-growing tumor (*arrows*)

mass lesion is different and located at the jugular foramen.

35.7 Metastases

Metastases to the cavernous sinus result from hematogenous dissemination of a remote cancer (breast, lung, lymphoma, kidney, thyroid) or from retrograde perineural extension along the branches of the trigeminal nerve of a local cancer (adenoid cystic or squamous cell carcinoma, melanoma). MRI demonstrates cavernous sinus enlargement and outward bowing of its lateral wall, with additional filling of the Meckel cave and potential enlargement and enhancement of the cisternal segment of the trigeminal nerve. Searching for other metastases in the brain, meninges, or skull helps in evoking the diagnosis (Fig. 35.12).

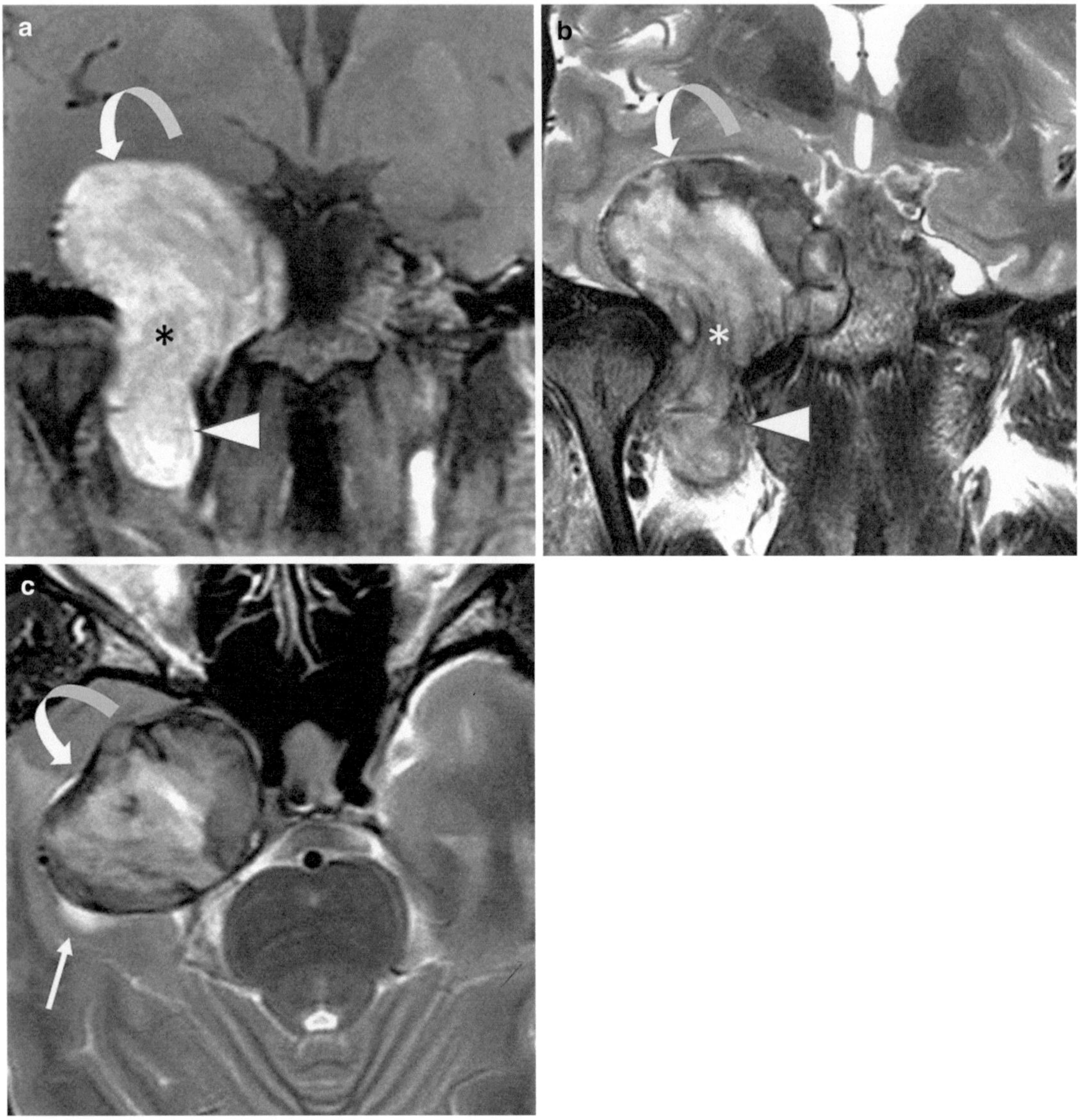

Fig. 35.8 A 55-year-old woman with sensory disturbance in the right V1 and V2 territories. Trigeminal schwannoma with inferior extension. (**a–c**) Coronal CE T1WI, coronal and axial T2WIs. Huge tumor of the right cavernous sinus extending laterally to the temporal fossa (*curved arrow*) and inferiorly to the pterygoid fossa along the mandibular division of the trigeminal nerve (*arrowhead*), through a widened foramen ovale (*asterisk*). There is no extension to the prepontine cistern. The signal of the tumor is very heterogeneous, mainly on T2WI. Note a discrete peritumoral edema in the temporal white matter (*arrow*)

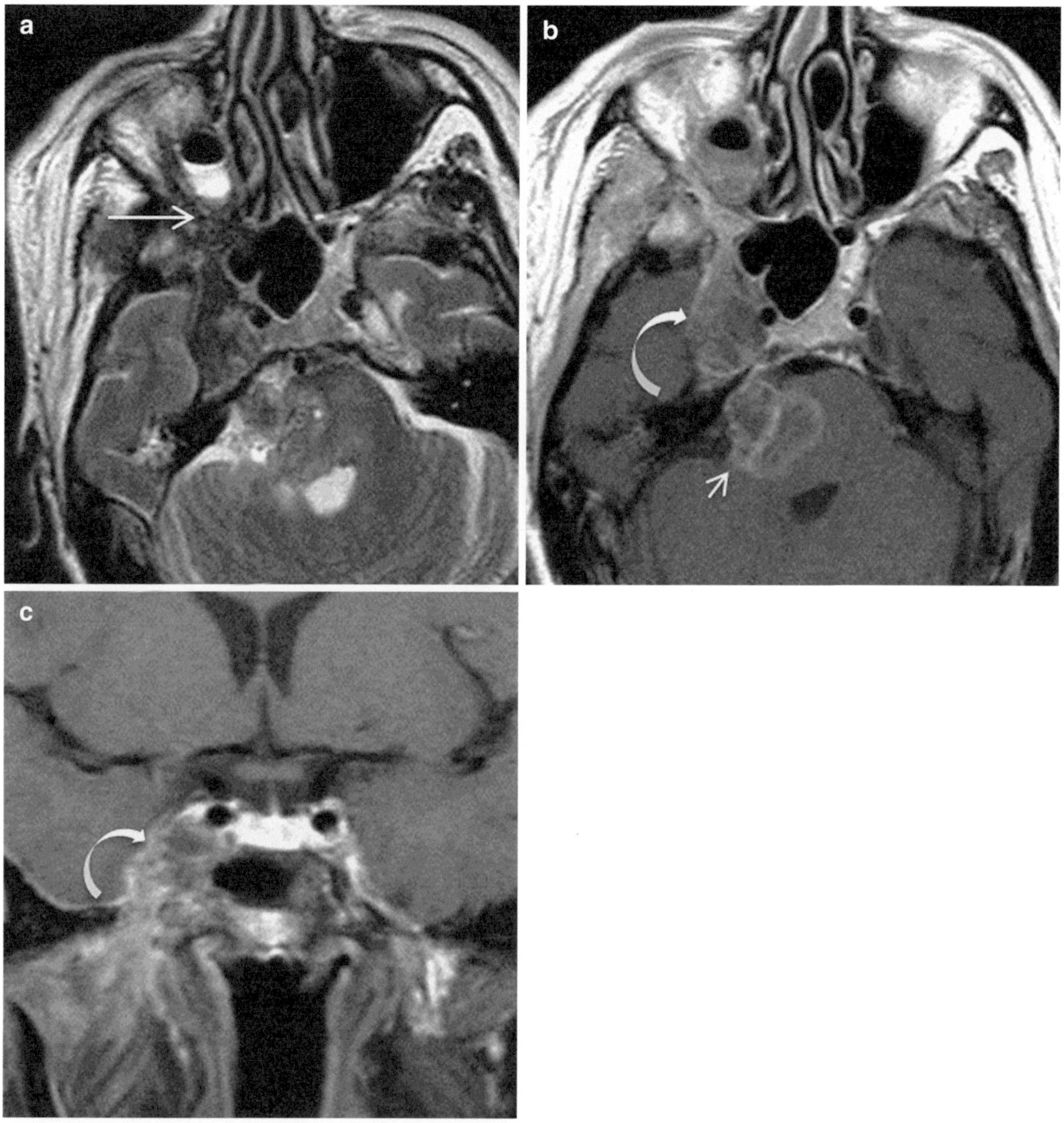

Fig. 35.9 Patient with maxillary sinus carcinoma, retrograde perineural spread, and intracranial extension. (**a**) Axial T2WI, (**b**) axial and (**c**) coronal CE T1WIs show a T2-hypointense lesion that moderately enhances after gadolinium injection, thickens the posterior aspect of the right maxillary sinus, fills the pterygopalatine fossa (*arrow*), spreads backward along the maxillary nerve, enlarges the Meckel cave and the cavernous sinus (*curved arrow*), and extends further along the trigeminal nerve and even infiltrates the brainstem (*short arrow*)

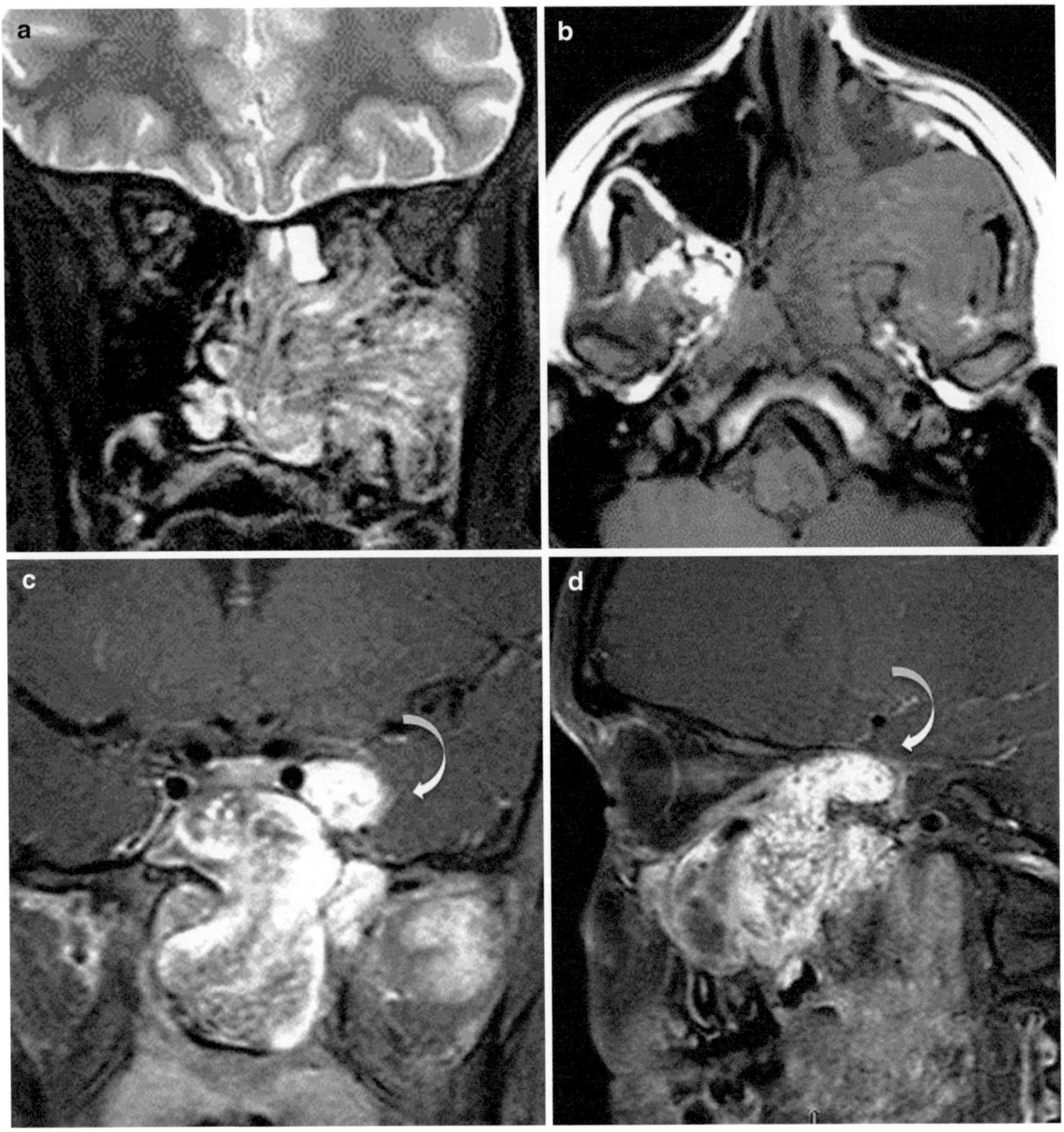

Fig. 35.10 An 18-year-old male patient with giant juvenile nasopharyngeal angiofibroma and unilateral recurrent epistaxis. (**a**) Coronal T2, (**b**) axial T1WI, (**c**) coronal and (**d**) sagittal CE T1WIs. Large heterogeneous mass lesion with flow voids filling the left nasal fossa, the maxillary sinus, the nasopharynx, and the sphenoid sinus. The lesion also extends intracranially in the left cavernous sinus (*curved arrows*)

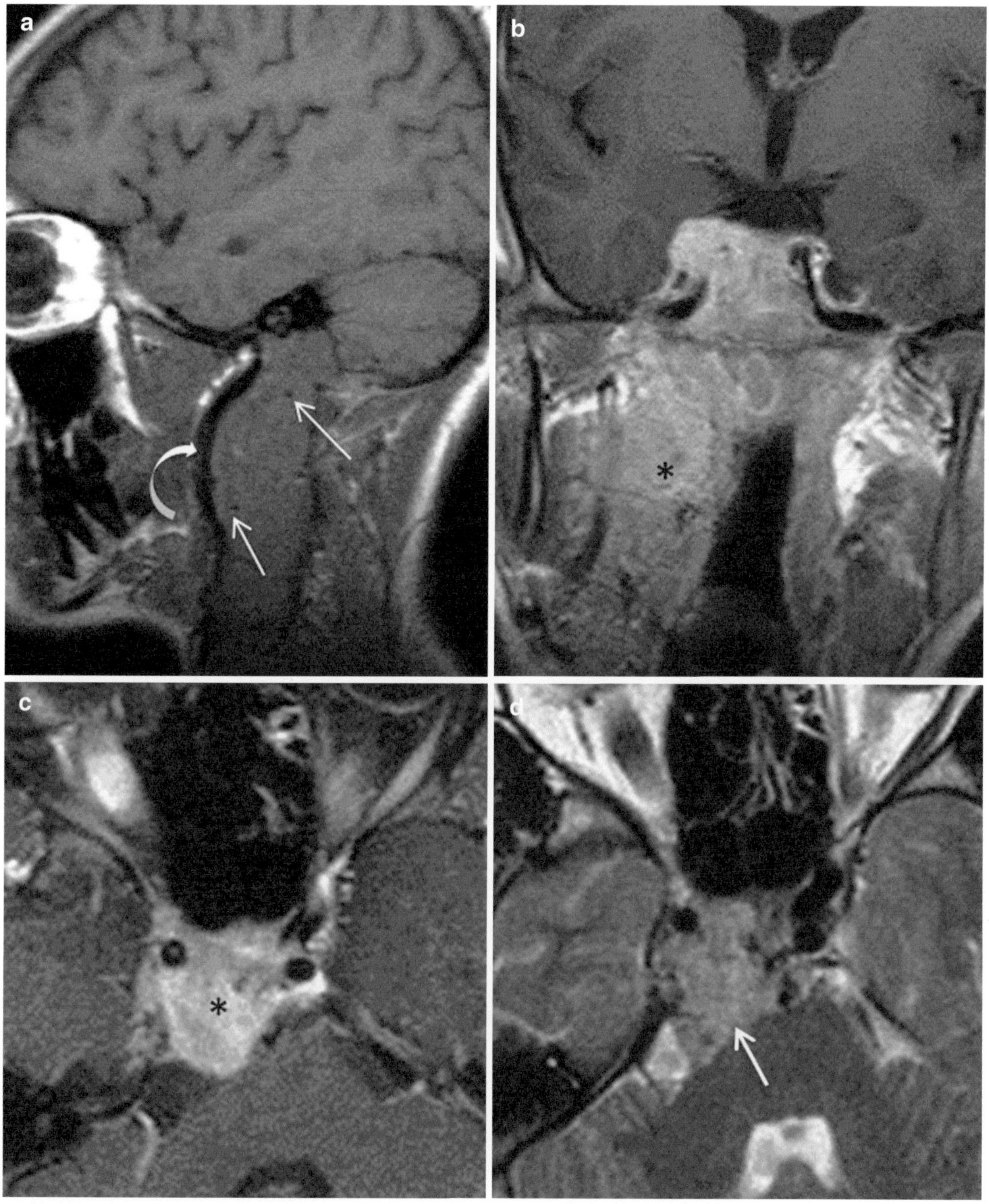

Fig. 35.11 Patient with giant paraganglioma, neck pain, and diplopia. (**a**) Sagittal T1WI reveals an enormous laterocervical mass extending from the neck up to the jugular foramen, displacing anteriorly the cervical internal carotid artery (*curved arrow*), with dots of flow voids (*arrows*), a feature very suggestive of paraganglioma. (**b**, **c**) Coronal and axial CE T1WIs demonstrate marked enhancement of this highly vascular tumor (*asterisks*). (**d**) Axial T2WI depicts the cranial extent of this aggressive lesion that invades the clivus and the right cavernous sinus (*thick arrow*)

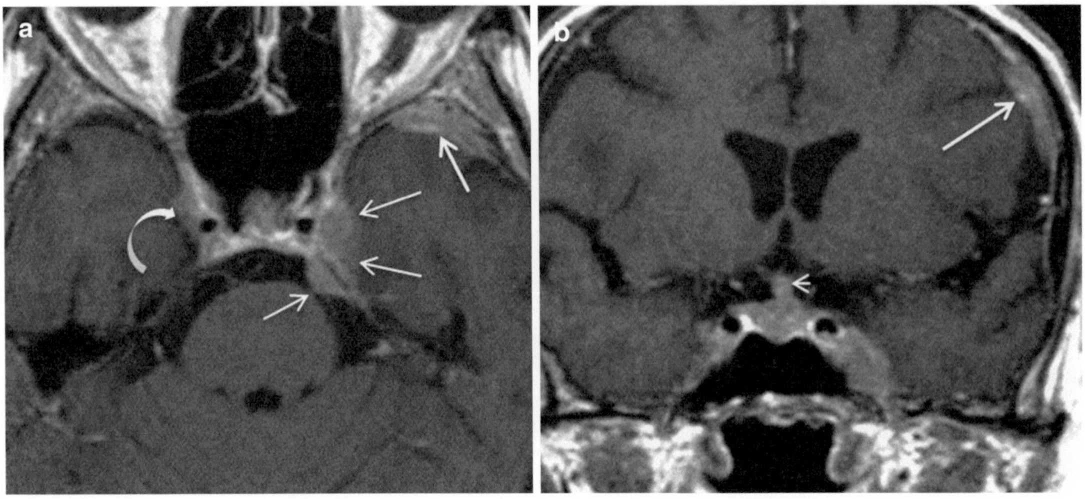

Fig. 35.12 Patient with bilateral cavernous sinus metastases from breast cancer. (**a**, **b**) Axial and coronal CE T1WIs demonstrate on the left side an obvious unspecific enhancing lesion enlarging the fifth cranial nerve, the Meckel cave, and the cavernous sinus (three *arrows*). Diagnosis of metastasis becomes easy when additional similar lesions are depicted in multiple other sites such as the dura at the left temporal pole and the left convexity (*thick arrows*), the lateral wall of the opposite cavernous sinus (*curved arrow*), and the stalk (*short arrow*), which is abnormally broadened

Further Reading

Agarwal A (2015) Intracranial trigeminal schwannoma. Neuroradiol J 28:36–41

Hanak BW, Zada G, Nayar VV et al (2012) Cerebral aneurysms with intrasellar extension: a systematic review of clinical, anatomical, and treatment characteristics. A review. J Neurosurg 116:164–178

Hao R, He Y, Zhang H et al (2015) The evaluation of ICHD-3 beta diagnostic criteria for Tolosa-Hunt syndrome: a study of 22 cases of Tolosa-Hunt syndrome. Neurol Sci 36:899–905

He K, Chen L, Zhu W et al (2014) Magnetic resonance standard for cavernous sinus hemangiomas: proposal for a diagnostic test. Eur Neurol 72:116–124

Press CA, Lindsay A, Stence NV et al (2015) Cavernous sinus thrombosis in children: imaging characteristics and clinical outcomes. Stroke 46:2657–2660

Primary Neurohypophyseal Glial Tumors

36

Sonia Nagi and Cyrine Drissi

The pituitary stalk and the posterior pituitary gland are composed of specialized glial cells called pituicytes. Hence, it is understandable that the neurohypophysis can be a host to all of the neoplastic processes that originate from the glial cell series. These primary neurohypophyseal glial tumors are rare. We distinguish astrocytoma, tanycytoma, and granular cell tumor (GCT). Tanycytoma and astrocytomas, which include pituicytoma and pilocytic astrocytoma, are specific to the neurohypophysis, whereas GCT is less specific as it has been described elsewhere in the CNS. In addition, very few cases of neurohypophyseal ependymoma, pleomorphic xanthoastrocytoma, and primitive neuroectodermal tumors have been reported. Pituicytoma, formerly called infundibuloma, is considered grade I glial neoplasm by the 2007 WHO classification. Because it arises from pituicytes, it is highly specific to neurohypophysis. When arising from the infundibulum it is suprasellar, whereas when arising from the posterior lobe or both it is intrasellar. Suprasellar extension may induce optic chiasm and hypothalamus compression. Pituicytoma is seen in adults with a mean age of 50 years, without gender predilection. Only a few cases have been described in children. The main clinical signs are visual impairment, headache, hypopituitarism, and fatigue. Paradoxically, diabetes insipidus is an uncommon symptom in pituicytoma. It can also be incidentally discovered in asymptomatic patients. On MRI , the normal bright spot on T1WI of the posterior pituitary is typically absent. The pituicytoma appears as a solid, well-circumscribed mass with an average size of 16 mm, ranging between 5 and 30 mm. It can be suprasellar, intra- and suprasellar, or, rarely, purely intrasellar in location, with occasional cavernous invasion. This tumor is hyperintense on T2WI, and iso- or hypointense to gray matter on T1WI (Figs. 36.1 and 36.2). The presence of a cystic component is uncommon. After gadolinium administration, the tumor will typically show an intense and homogeneous enhancement (Fig. 36.2). Uncommonly, it will show moderate and heterogeneous enhancement (Fig. 36.1). A nonspecific pre- and postsellar dural enhancement can be seen (Fig. 36.2). When seen, the anterior displacement of the adenohypophysis by the tumor is an affirmative sign suggesting the neurohypophyseal origin (Fig. 36.1). Sellar enlargement, though uncommon, can help to differentiate pituicytoma from pituitary adenoma. Diagnosis may be improved by better morphological characterization but most importantly by clinical correlation (visual impairment and headache without diabetes insipidus). However, the final diagnosis is made by immunohistochemistry and electron microscopy. A total surgical resection is curative, with no recurrence or need for adjuvant therapy. Pituitary pilocytic astrocytoma is indistinguishable from pituicytoma on imaging. The differential diagnosis is made on pathology. Tanycytoma is a hypothalamic–suprasellar tumor that can also involve the pituitary stalk. It is clinically aggressive with a high recurrence rate, and is characterized by its large size. Tumor encasement of the arteries of the circle

J.-F. Bonneville et al., *MRI of the Pituitary Gland*, DOI 10.1007/978-3-319-29043-0_36

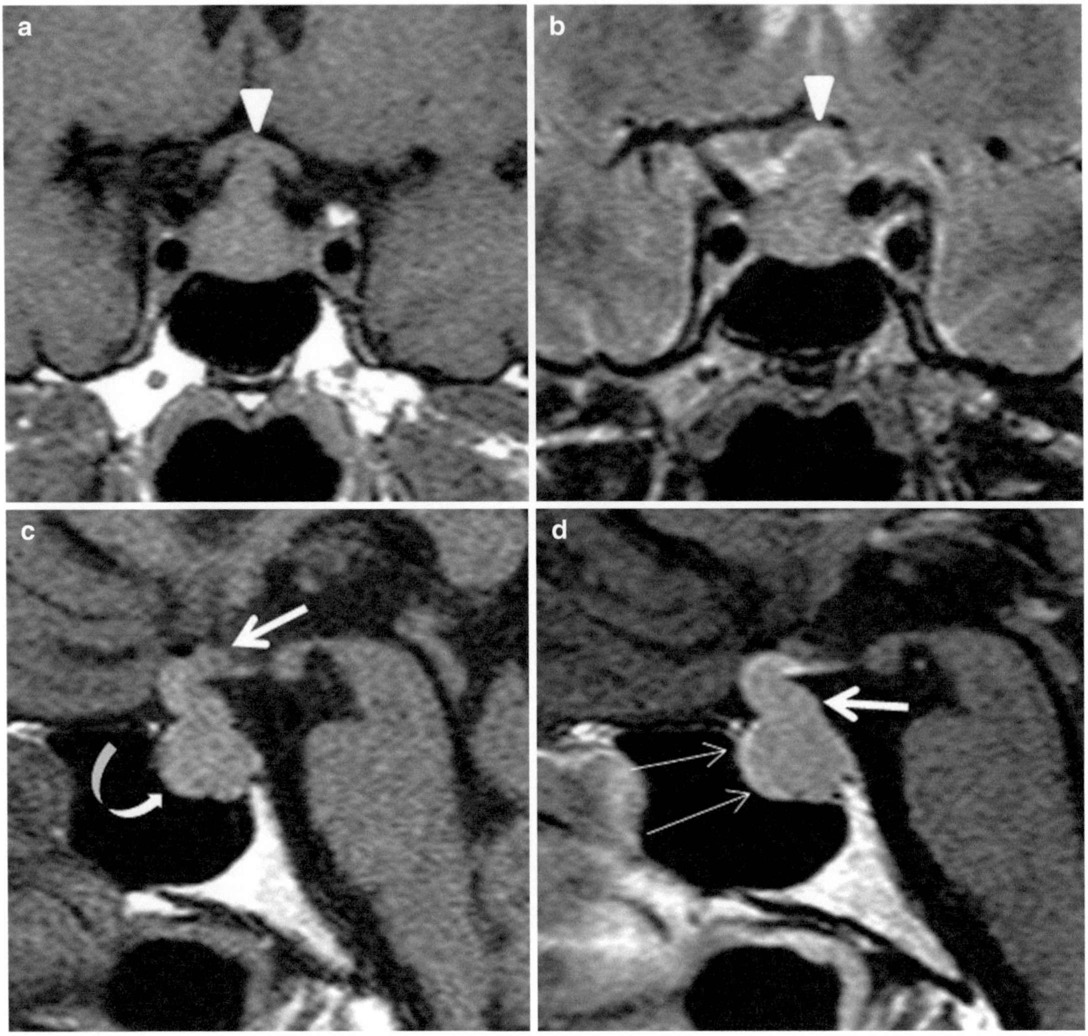

Fig. 36.1 A 55-year-old man with central diabetes insipidus and hypopituitarism. (**a**, **b**) Coronal T1 and T2 WIs. The mass is slightly hyperintense on T2WI and the suprasellar extension distorts the optic chiasm (*arrowhead*). (**c**) Sagittal T1WI. Intrasellar tumor (*curved arrow*) isointense to gray matter with pituitary and infundibular stalk involvement (*thick arrows*). No posterior lobe bright spot. (**d**) Sagittal CE T1WI. Slight homogeneous enhancement of the tumor. Anterior displacement and compression of the normally enhancing anterior pituitary (*thin arrows*). Histopathological findings: pituicytoma

of Willis with possible infarction, extension beneath the frontal lobes, and third ventricle obstruction are common features in children. Tanycytoma appears hyperintense on T2WI and hypointense on T1WI with cystic and solid components. Intense enhancement of the solid portion is seen after contrast administration. The prognosis in children is worse than in adults. GCT is a rare and benign tumor of the neurohypophysis, considered a WHO grade I glial neoplasm. Previously called granular cell myoblastoma or choristoma, it arises from granular cell type pituicytes, although structurally identical tumors have been described elsewhere in the CNS. This tumor is usually diagnosed in the fifth decade and twice as often in females than in males. In most cases, GCT consists of small nests of tumor cells that do not have any space-occupying effects, and patients are asymptomatic. When symptomatic, symptoms are related to very large size and mass effect. These signs consist of

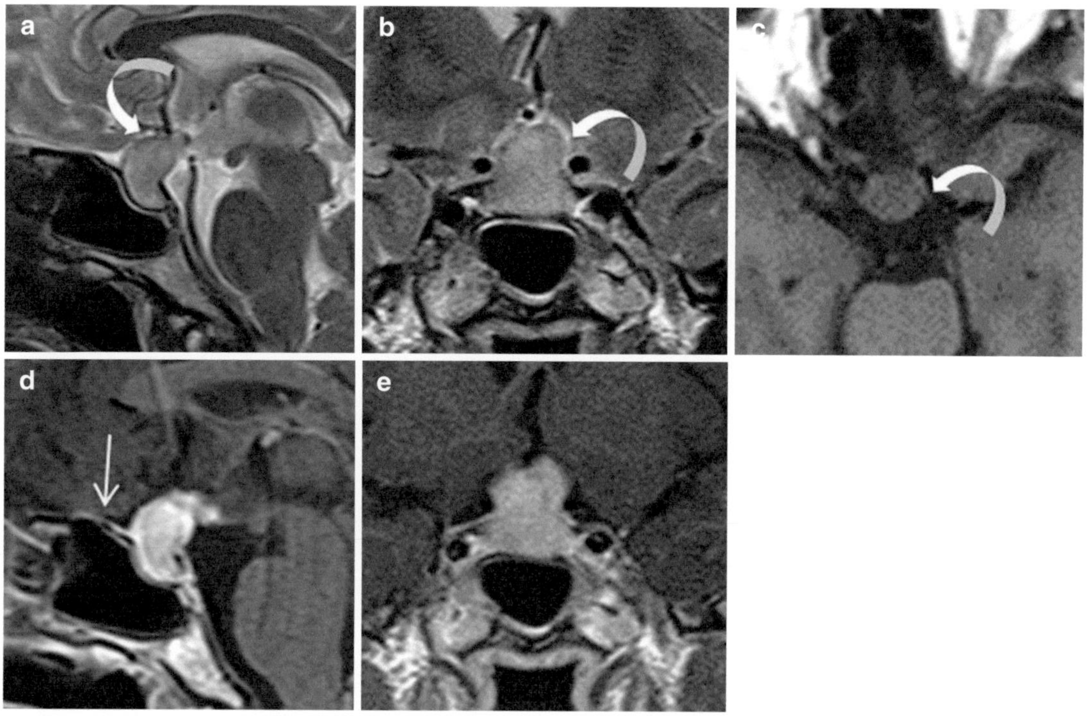

Fig. 36.2 A 58-year-old woman with central diabetes insipidus and hypopituitarism. (**a**, **b**) Sagittal and coronal T2WIs. Hyperintense intrasellar mass with suprasellar expansion (*curved arrow*). Pituitary stalk and infundibulum are indistinguishable. (**c**) Axial T1WI. The tumor is isointense to gray matter (*curved arrow*). No posterior lobe bright spot. (**d**, **e**) Sagittal and coronal CE T1WIs. Strong homogeneous enhancement of the tumor. Note presellar dural tail (*thin arrow*). Histopathological findings: pituicytoma

visual disturbances, hypopituitarism, hyperprolactinemia, and headache. The appearance of GCT on MRI is nonspecific, with an enhancing suprasellar or supra- and intrasellar mass which is isointense to gray matter on both T2 and T1 WIs. Homogeneous or heterogeneous but intense enhancement is possible and reflects its high vascularity. Calcifications may be seen. Absence of the normal pituitary bright spot may be a clue that the tumor is of neurohypophyseal origin, but this finding is not specific. Treatment for symptomatic GCT is surgical; postoperative irradiation is controversial. Germ cell tumors are described in Chap. 31.

Further Reading

Huang BY, Castillo M (2005) Non adenomatous tumors of the pituitary and sellar turcica. Top Magn Reson Imaging 16:289–299

Liebermann KA, Wasenko JJ, Schelper R et al (2003) Tanycytomas: a newly characterized hypothalamic suprasellar and ventricular tumors. Am J Neuroradiol 24:1999–2004

Zygourakis CC, Rolson JD, Lee HS et al (2015) Pituicytomas and spindle cell oncocytomas: modern case series from the university of California, San Francisco. Pituitary 18:150–158

37 Chordoma and Chondroma/Chondrosarcoma

Sonia Nagi and Cyrine Drissi

Both CT scanning and MRI are usually necessary for the complete evaluation of these tumors because of the involvement of both soft tissue and bony structures at the skull base. Chordomas are rare tumors that derive from embryonic remnants of the notochord. Cranial chordomas arise mainly from the clivus and are locally destructive. Clival chordomas represent less than 0.2 % of all intracranial tumors. They can be encountered in all age groups, with a peak in the fourth decade of life. Gender ratio is 2:1 (male/female) and there is no racial predilection. Cranial chordomas most often originate from the spheno-occipital synchondrosis, and thus typically have a midline location. Occasionally chordomas may arise unilaterally in the skull base from the petrous apex. They may spread to sellar and parasellar area, posterior fossa, and nasopharynx. Clinical symptoms depend on the direction of tumor growth. Sellar chordomas usually present with hypopituitarism and chiasmal compression. Parasellar chordomas present with hypopituitarism, oculomotor nerve palsy, and optic tract compression. Purely clival chordomas are characterized by headache, cranial nerve palsy, and brainstem compression. The abducens nerve is the most commonly affected. They usually are locally aggressive and frequently recur, but metastases are very rare. Sarcomatous degeneration and dedifferentiation have been reported. There are three histological subtypes of chordomas: classic, chondroid, and dedifferentiated. Chordomas are characterized by foamy, vacuolated, physaliferous cells within a myxoid stroma, and usually cause extensive bone destruction of the skull base, best analyzed on CT. CT will also show frequent intratumoral sequestered bone fragments. MRI typically shows a destructive invasive soft tissue mass arising from the clivus. At an early stage, bone expansion indicates that the tumor originates from bone and not adjacent structures. The extension of chordomas is primarily posterior, with involvement of the pontine cistern and, occasionally, the premedullary cistern. On MRI, posterior extension may show as a thumb indenting the pons and/or of the medulla (Fig. 37.1). Extension can be upward to the sella turcica, displacing the pituitary gland, downward to the nasopharynx, or laterally to the middle cranial fossa. Most chordomas demonstrate T1 hypointensity and T2 hyperintensity, with suggestive hypointense intratumoral septations (Fig. 37.2). Foci of T1 hyperintensity may be depicted within the tumor or at its periphery, which represent residual bony fragments, calcifications, mucoid material, or hemorrhage (Fig. 37.3). Following gadolinium administration, chordomas usually show lobulated areas with a honeycomb appearance. Enhancement is variable: it can be mild, intense, or absent. Overall, the signal in chordomas is heterogeneous on all sequences on T1 and T2 WIs and after gadolinium administration (Fig. 37.4). Low ADC values have been found in the dedifferentiated histological variant ecchordosis physaliphora, also derived from notochord remnants. Knowledge of this entity is merited because it is considered as a benign congenital malformation and thus differs from chordoma,

J.-F. Bonneville et al., *MRI of the Pituitary Gland*, DOI 10.1007/978-3-319-29043-0_37

which is a true tumor. It is usually asymptomatic. Pontine hemorrhage or CSF fistula associated with ecchordosis physaliphora have been reported. Ecchordosis physaliphora is a midline intradural retro-/intraclival lesion inducing a bony clival defect without aggressive features. Its signal is similar to CSF on T2 and T1 WIs with no enhancement after gadolinium infusion (Fig. 37.5). When detected, the bony stalk attachment to the clivus is considered a characteristic sign. It can be seen on

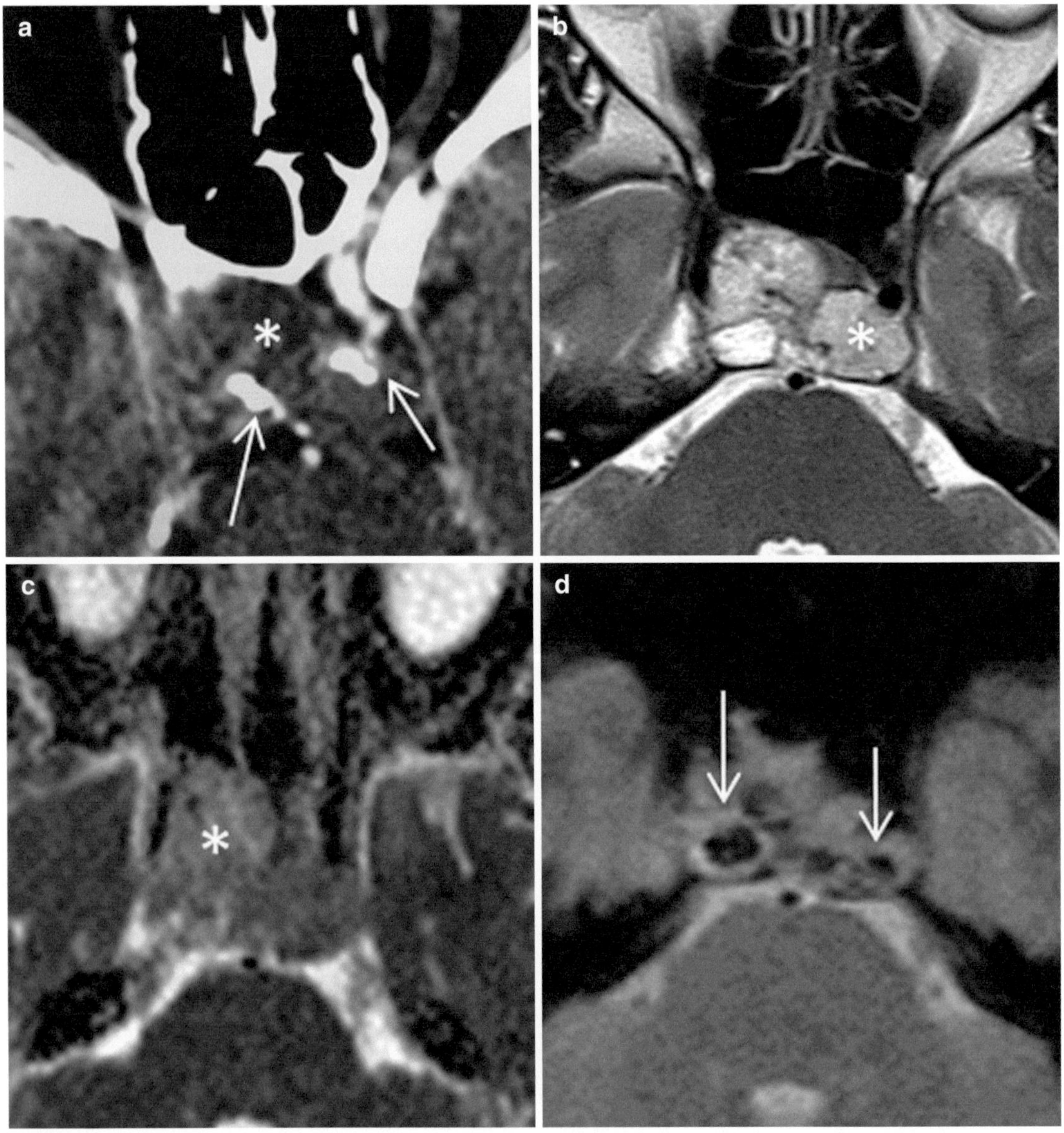

Fig. 37.1 A 37-year-old man with headaches, insidious right visual disturbance, and abducens nerve. Clival chordoma. (**a**) Axial CT after contrast administration. Iso- to hypodense midline mass (*asterisk*) arising from the clivus. Entrapped bone fragments (*arrows*). (**b–e**) Axial T2, ADC map, and T2* and CE T1 WIs. Heterogeneous bright signal on T2 without diffusion restriction. Heterogeneous enhancement, more intense in periphery and in septa with "honeycomb" pattern (*asterisk*). Intralesional marked hypointensities due to bone fragments (*arrows*). (**f, g**) Sagittal T2 and CE T1 WIs. The basilar artery is displaced posteriorly (*thick arrow*). The mass indents the anterior pons as a thumb (*curved arrow*). The pituitary gland is displaced anteriorly (*short arrow*)

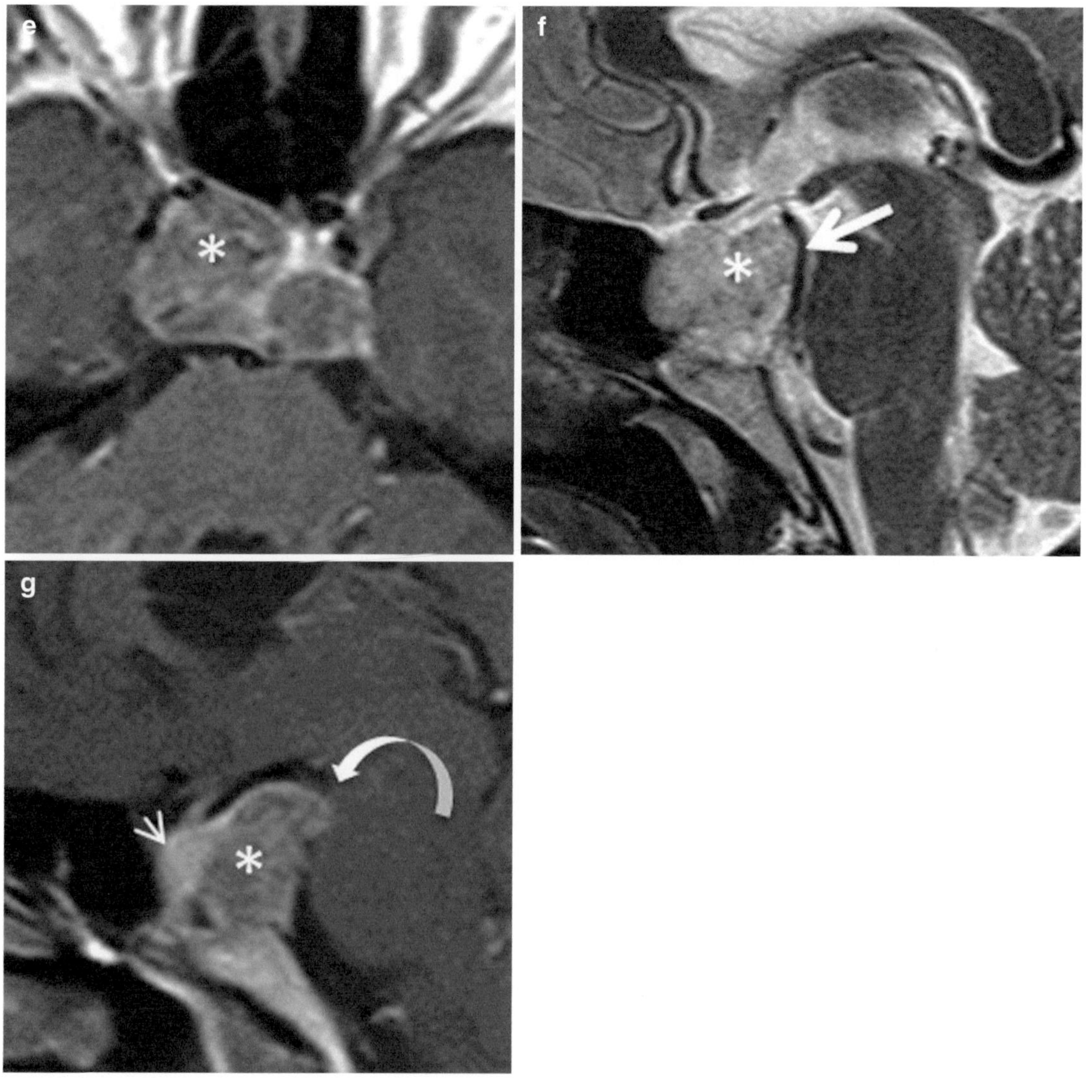

Fig. 37.1 (continued)

CT or on thin high-resolution MR sequences. Chondromas and chondrosarcomas of the skull base are uncommon cartilaginous tumors that develop from embryonic cartilaginous remnants enclosed in the cranial base synchondroses. They most often arise from the petro-occipital synchondrosis and have a lateral location in the parasellar area, at the foramen lacerum level. They may also arise from the spheno-occipital synchondrosis with a midline location. Chondromas of the sella turcica have been reported, for which there is no gender predilection; they are often diagnosed between the third and fourth decade. Chondromas and chondrosarcomas occur at higher frequency in Ollier disease and Maffucci syndrome. The most common presentation symptoms are deficits of the cranial nerves, including the abducens, optic, acoustic-facial, and lower cranial nerves, and headaches. The onset of symptoms is usually gradual. Endocrine dysfunction has been reported in sellar chondromas. On histologic examination, chondromas consist of mature, well-differentiated hyaline cartilage. Total excision is curative, with no recurrence. Chondrosarcomas are malignant tumors composed of atypical chondrocytes, whose nuclei are hyperchromatic and enlarged. There are

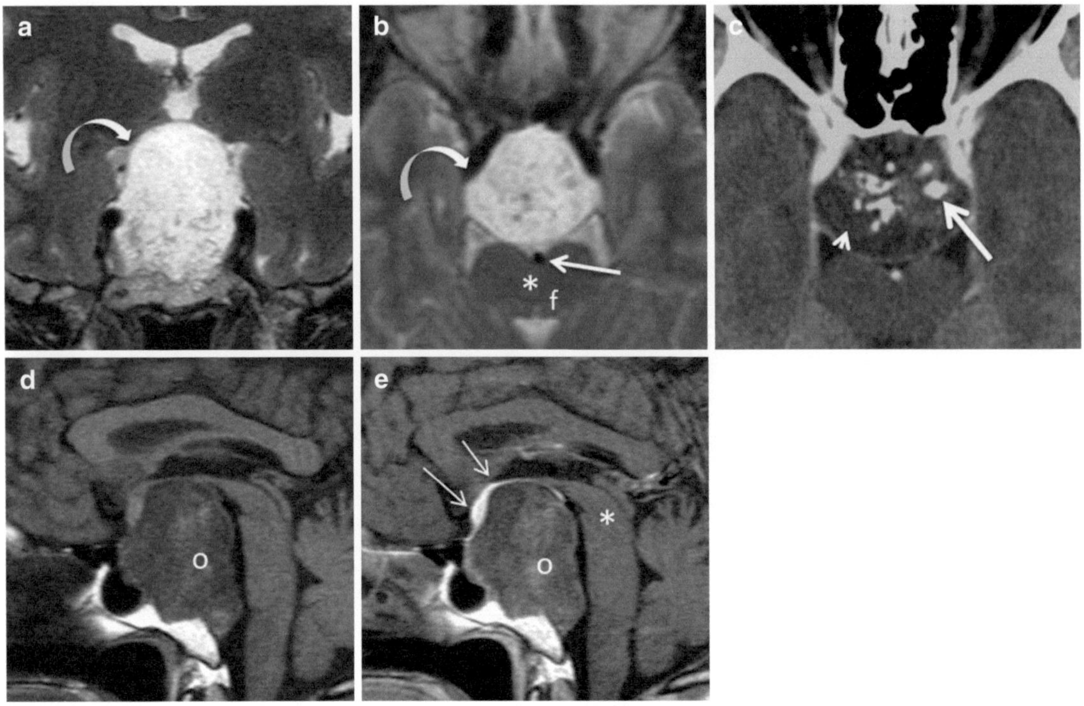

Fig. 37.2 A 49-year-old woman with intracranial hypertension, bilateral decrease of visual acuity, right ophthalmoplegia, and galactorrhea. Clival chordoma. (**a**, **b**) Coronal and axial T2WIs. destructive midline expanding tumor arising from the clivus with bright signal (*curved arrow*). Superior and posterior extension displacing the midbrain (*asterisk*) and the basilar artery (*long arrow*). (**c**) Axial CT after contrast administration. Intratumoral bone sequestra (*thick arrow*). Hypodense myxoid areas (*short arrow*). (**d**, **e**) Sagittal T1 and CE T1 WIs: low signal with spontaneous slightly hyperintense areas, and subtle and partial tumoral enhancement (*circle*). The pituitary gland is elevated (*double arrows*); pons and midbrain are displaced (*asterisk*)

three histological subtypes of chondrosarcomas, ranging from grade I (well differentiated) to grade III (poorly differentiated). They display chondroid calcifications in more than half of the cases. CT is required to evaluate intratumoral calcification and bone erosion (Fig. 37.6). On MRI, these tumors appear hypointense or isointense on T1WI and heterogeneously brightly hyperintense on T2WI (Fig. 37.7). They enhance poorly in a heterogeneous fashion, with linear and nodular areas (Fig. 37.8). The typical chondroid calcifications are curvilinear and usually appear hypointense on MR spin-echo sequences. However, they may appear hyperintense T1WIs depending on the degree of mineralization. On ADC maps these tumors are usually bright, reflecting high diffusion.

Distinguishing chordomas from chondromas/chondrosarcomas using imaging criteria can be difficult. Chordomas are typically located more centrally. Chondroid calcifications are characteristic of chondromas and chondrosarcomas. Histology with immunohistochemistry allows reliable differentiation. Other differential diagnoses for chordoma include ecchordosis physaliphora, invasive adenoma, metastasis, and plasmacytoma. Metastasis and plasmacytoma do not usually appear hyperintense on T2WIs. The main differential diagnoses for lateral chondroma and chondrosarcoma are schwannoma, aneurysm, and nasopharyngeal carcinoma.

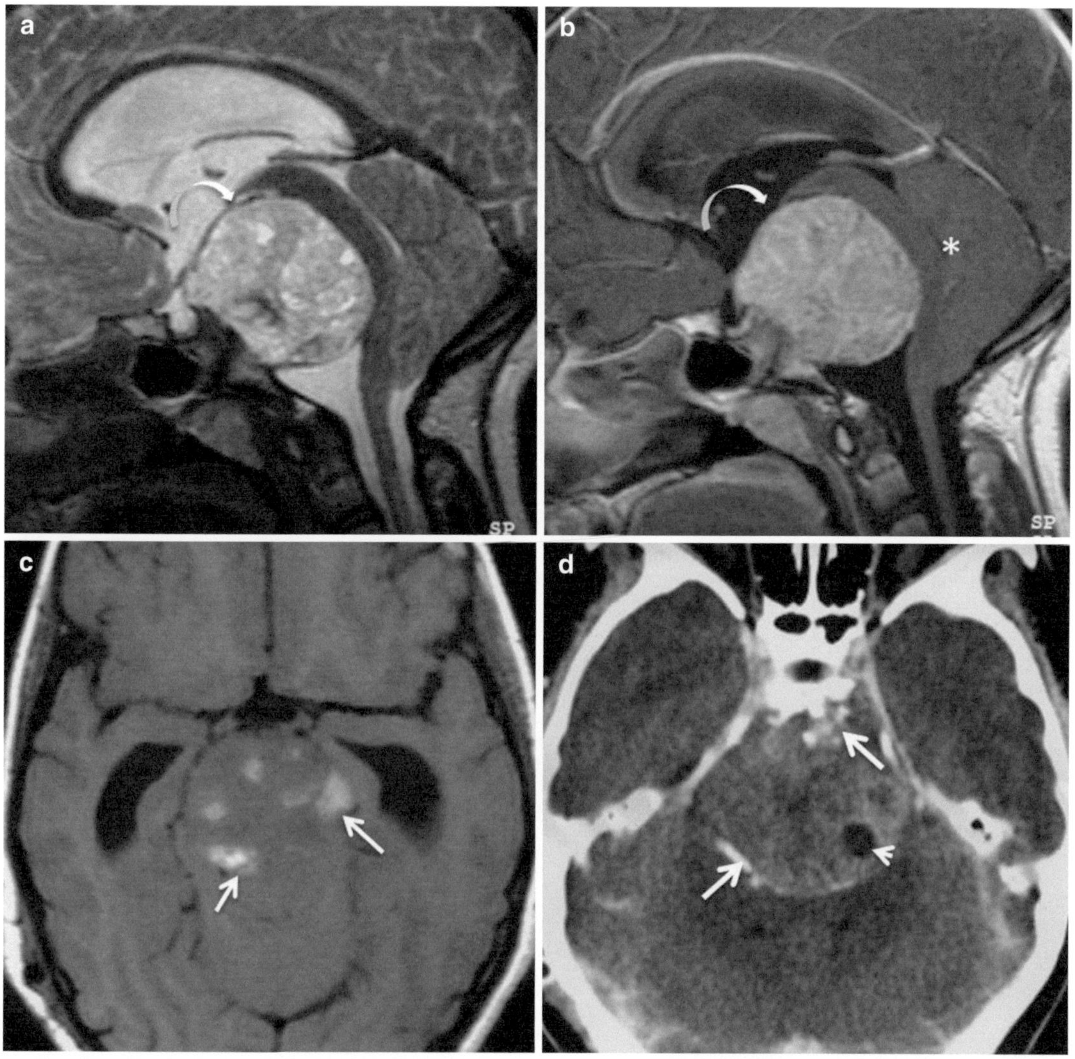

Fig. 37.3 An 11-year-old girl with intracranial hypertension for 1 month, bilateral papillary edema, and paresis of abducens nerves. Clival chordoma. (**a**, **b**) Sagittal T2 and CE T1 WIs. Midline heterogeneous hyperintense round mass centered on the upper part of the clivus with heterogeneous enhancement (*curved arrow*). The lesion compresses brainstem, fourth ventricle, and cerebellum (*asterisk*) inducing hydrocephalus. (**c**) Axial T1WI. Hyperintense foci due to myxoid areas (*arrows*). (**d**) Axial CT after contrast administration. Nonenhanced cyst-like areas (*short arrow*). Bone fragments at the periphery and the base of implantation of the chordoma (*thick arrows*)

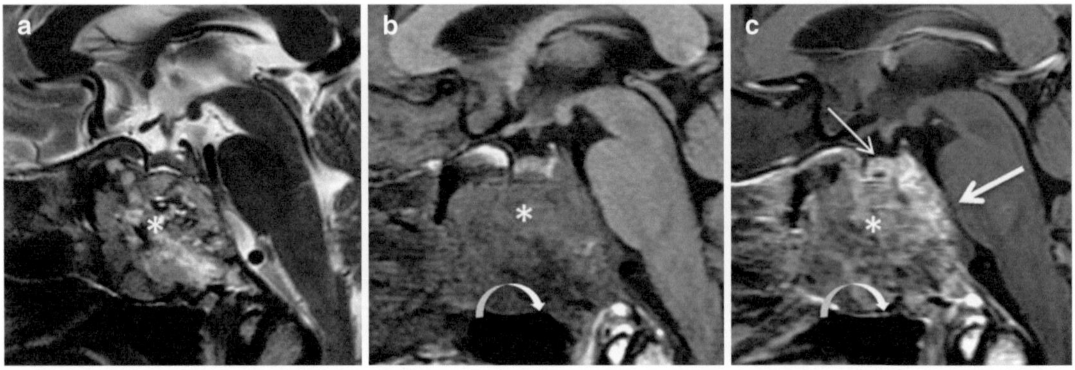

Fig. 37.4 A 55-year-old man with headaches, nasal obstruction, and dysphagia. Clival chordoma. (**a–c**) Sagittal T2, T1, and CE T1 WIs. Destructive clival mass with predominantly intrasphenoidal extension. Heterogeneous hyperintense signal before and after gadolinium administration (*asterisk*). The tumor invades the nasopharynx with a downward bowing of the hard palate (*curved arrow*). Thickening of the clivus (*thick arrow*). Pituitary gland (*arrow*)

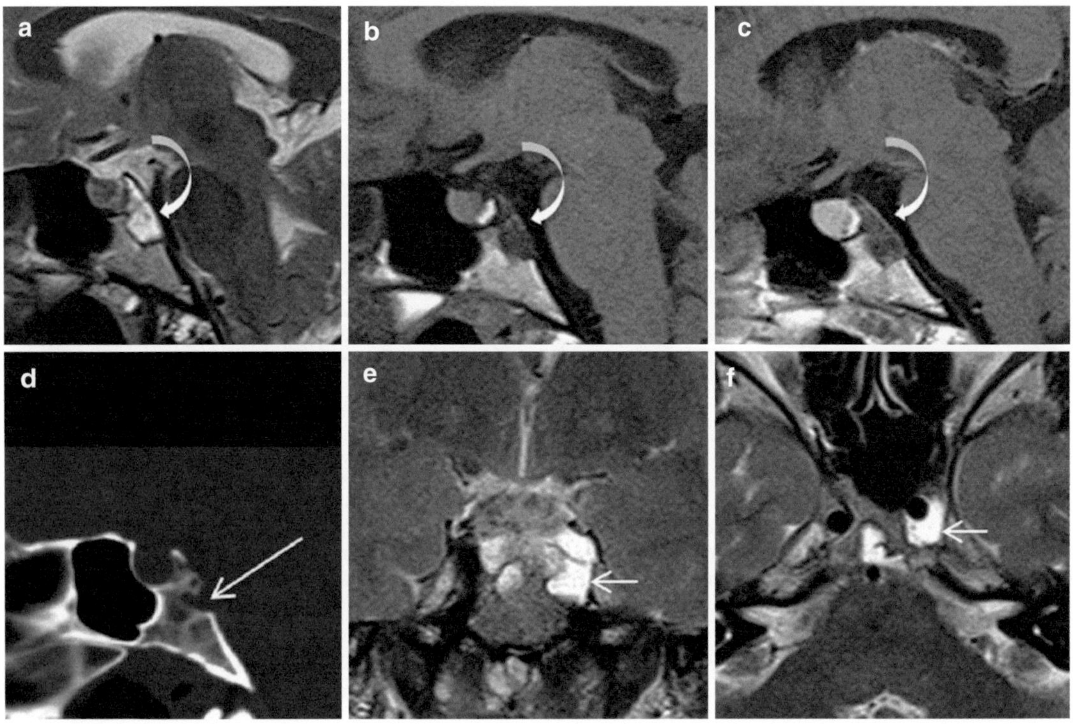

Fig. 37.5 A 36-year-old woman. Clival ecchordosis physaliphora. Unchanged MRI and CT pattern for 10 years. (**a–c**) Sagittal T2, T1, and CE T1 WIs. (**e**, **f**) Coronal and axial T2WIs. (**g**) Axial CE T1WI. Dorsal clival lobulated cyst-like lesion (*curved arrows*) extended to left cavernous sinus (*short arrows*). The signal is more hyperintense on T2 and less hypointense on T1 if compared with CSF. No postgadolinium enhancement. (**d**, **h**) Sagittal reformatted and axial CT. Bony clival defect with mild osteosclerosis (*long arrow*)

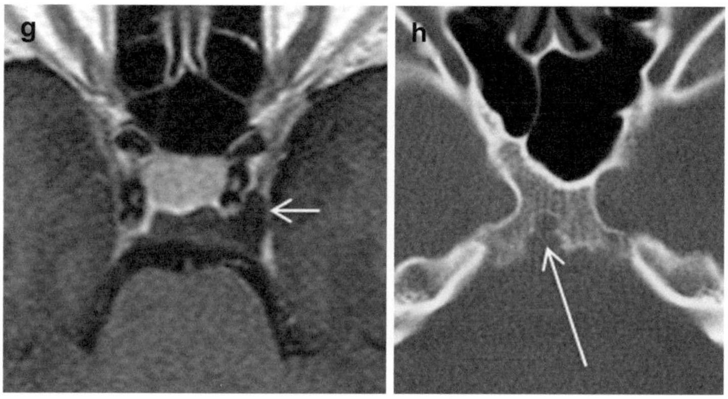

Fig. 37.5 (continued)

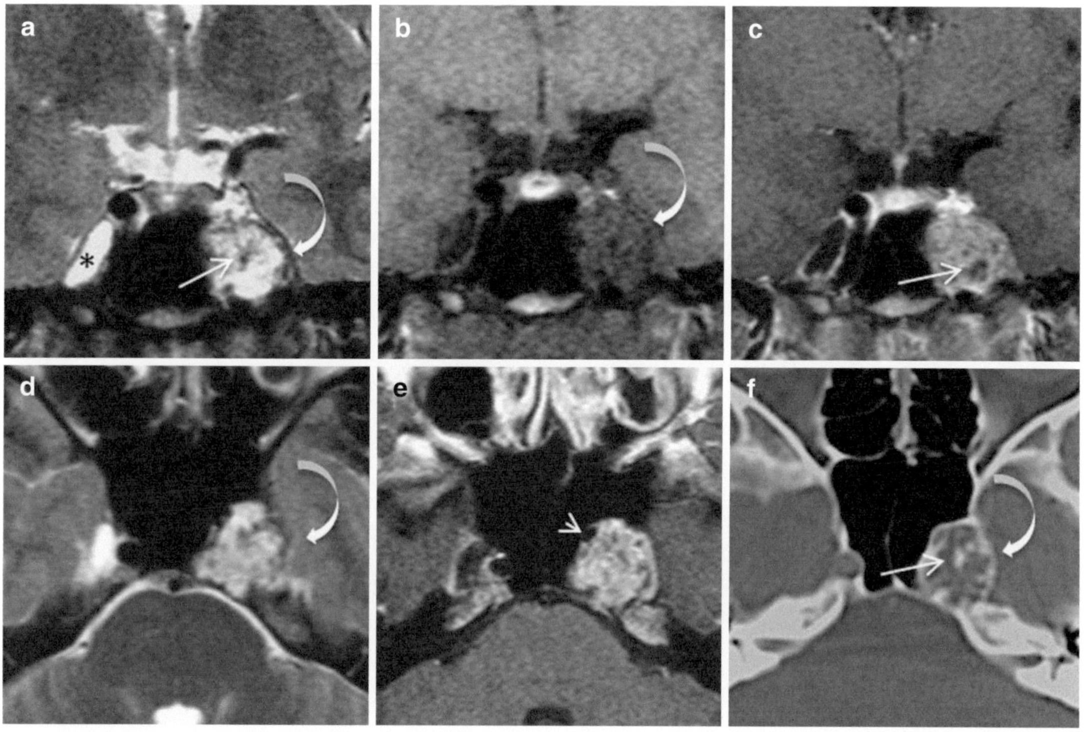

Fig. 37.6 A 22-year-old man with convergent strabismus of the left eye gradually evolving for 4 years, left abducens nerve palsy, and hypoesthesia in the territory of the left trigeminal nerve. Chondroma. (**a–c**) Coronal T2, T1, and CE T1 WIs. Heterogeneous hyperintense T2 and isointense T1 lobulated mass centered by the left Meckel cave (*curved arrow*) with hypointense linear and nodular areas (*thin arrow*). Heterogeneous enhancement spearing these linear and nodular areas. Note normal right Meckel cave filled with CSF (*asterisk*). (**d**, **e**) Axial T2 and T1 CE WIs. The lobulated aspect is well seen (*curved arrow*). The left internal carotid artery is displaced forward (*short arrow*). (**f**) Axial CT with bone window. Calcified wall with septated calcifications within the mass (*thin arrow*). Lateral sphenoid sinus wall is eroded

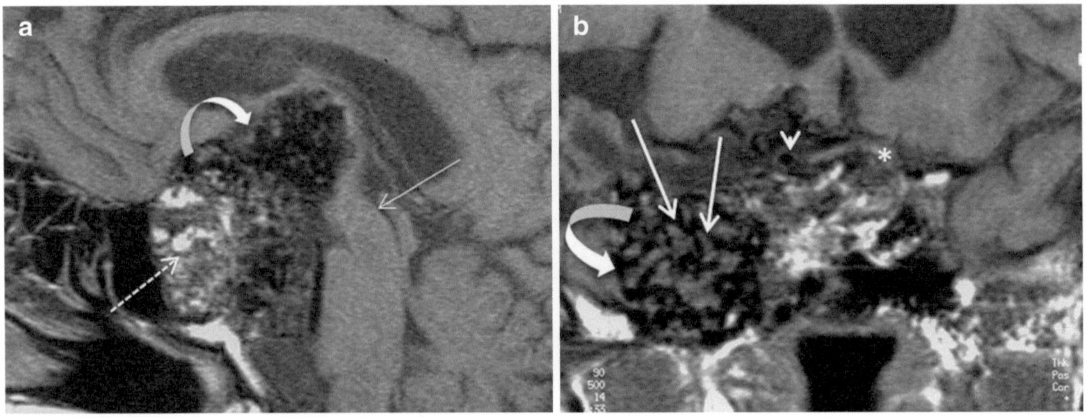

Fig. 37.7 A 52-year-old man with headaches. Chondroma. (**a**, **b**) Sagittal and coronal T1WIs. Heterogeneous huge mass centered on the right petroclival fissure with lobulated margins (*curved arrow*). Nodular bright areas (*dotted line*) with markedly low signal foci corresponding to chondroid calcifications (*thick arrows*). Optic chiasm (*asterisk*) and brainstem (*thin arrow*) are displaced. The internal carotid artery is displaced upward (*short arrow*)

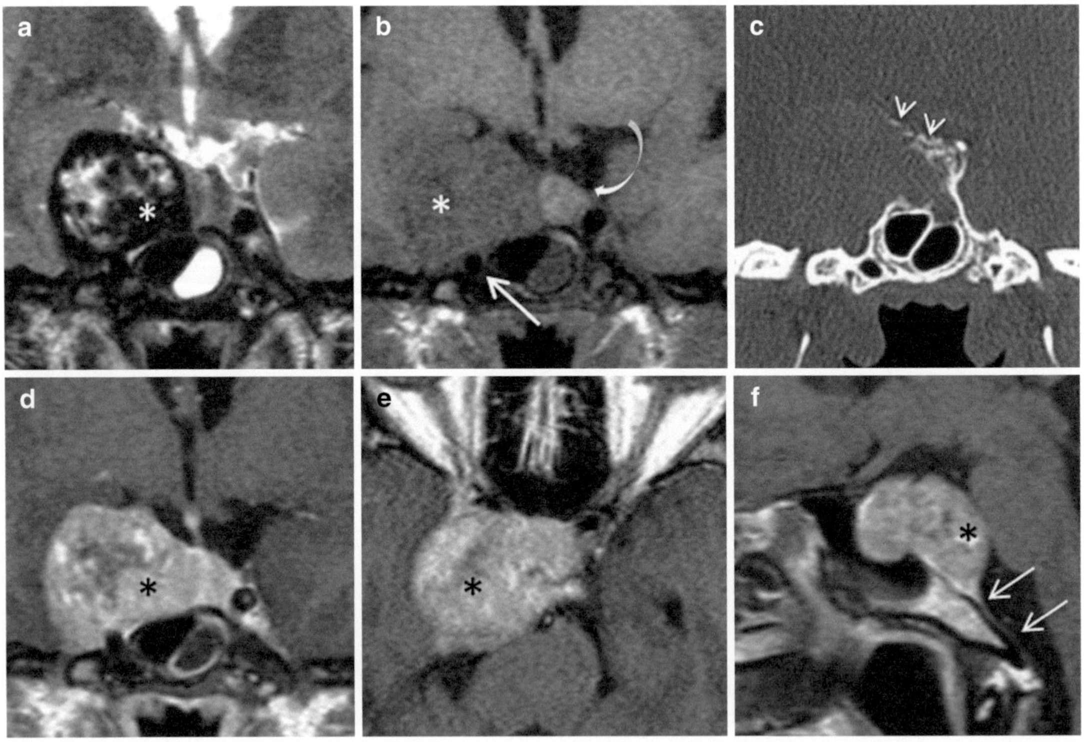

Fig. 37.8 A 20-year-old woman with headaches and right abducens nerve palsy. Chondrosarcoma. (**a**, **b**) Coronal T2 and T1 WIs. Round mass lateral to the pituitary fossa with heterogeneous appearance on T2, composed of a bright signal with markedly hypointense wall and central components (*asterisk*). Intermediate signal on T1 with central nodular hypointensities (*asterisk*). The internal carotid artery is displaced downward (*arrow*). Pituitary gland is displaced to the left (*curved arrow*). (**c**) Coronal reformatted CT in bone algorithm and bone window. Superior and internal peripheral calcifications (*short arrows*). Absence of central chondroid calcifications suggests that the marked hypointense foci seen within the mass on T2WI correspond to fibrocartilaginous components. (**d**–**f**) Coronal, axial, and sagittal CE T1WIs. Heterogeneous enhancement (*asterisk*). Clival dural tail (*double arrow*)

Further Reading

Chiara C, Korogi Y, Kakeda S et al (2013) Ecchordosis physaliphora and its variants: proposed new classification based on high-resolution fast MR imaging employing steady-state acquisition. Clin Neuroradiol 23:2854–2860

Geng S, Zhang J, Zhang LW et al (2014) Diagnosis and microsurgical treatment of chondromas and chondrosarcomas of the cranial base. Oncol Lett 8:301–304

Pamir MN, Özduman K (2006) Analysis of radiological features relative to histopathology in 42 skull-base chordomas and chondrosarcomas. Eur J Radiol 58:461–470

Hamartoma of the Tuber Cinereum 38

Françoise Cattin

Hamartomas of the tuber cinereum are not true tumoral lesions but rather congenital malformations formed by accumulation of normal neurons and glia from the tuber cinereum in an unusual location. The tuber cinereum, part of hypothalamus, is a hollow eminence of gray matter located between the optic chiasm and the mammillary bodies. Hamartomas of the tuber are usually revealed by a very early precocious puberty and gelastic seizures; less frequently, the only clinical manifestation is a developmental delay in relation with isolated GH deficit or a panhypopituitarism. Cognitive impairment and behavioral disorders including aggressiveness are infrequent and less known. The relationships of the hamartoma to the third ventricle, infundibulum, and mammillary bodies are appreciated on multiplanar MR studies. Association of hamartoma to the mammillary bodies is a particularly important radiological finding, as the anterior thalamic nuclei included in mammillary bodies are involved in the generation of seizures. There is no correlation between the clinical symptoms and the size of the hamartoma. Arita classified the hypothalamic hamartomas into two categories: the parahypothalamic type when the hamartoma is attached to the floor of the third ventricle at the origin of precocious puberty without seizures, and the intrahypothalamic type when the hamartoma is enveloped by the hypothalamus causing medically intractable seizures, behavioral disturbances, mental retardation, and precocious puberty. On MR studies, the hypothalamic hamartoma appears as a round suprasellar mass, sessile or pedunculated. The size is variable, from a few millimeters to 5 cm in diameter. The signal is similar to that of gray matter on all sequences (Figs. 38.1 and 38.2). However, T2-hyperintense foci are occasionally seen (Fig. 38.3); in these cases, the differential diagnosis with hypothalamic glioma can be difficult. There is no enhancement after gadolinium injection. Cysts and calcifications are exceptional. Diagnosis of intrahypothalamic hamartoma is a challenge: coronal high-resolution T2WI focused on the hypothalamic region is mandatory in young patients presenting with intractable seizures and/or isolated severe behavioral troubles even in the absence of precocious puberty (Fig. 38.4). MR spectroscopy can be normal or shows a slight decrease in N-acetylaspartate, and an increase in choline and myoinositol (Fig. 38.5). Non-enhancing hypothalamic-chiasmatic glioma is the only differential diagnosis of hamartoma.

J.-F. Bonneville et al., *MRI of the Pituitary Gland*, DOI 10.1007/978-3-319-29043-0_38

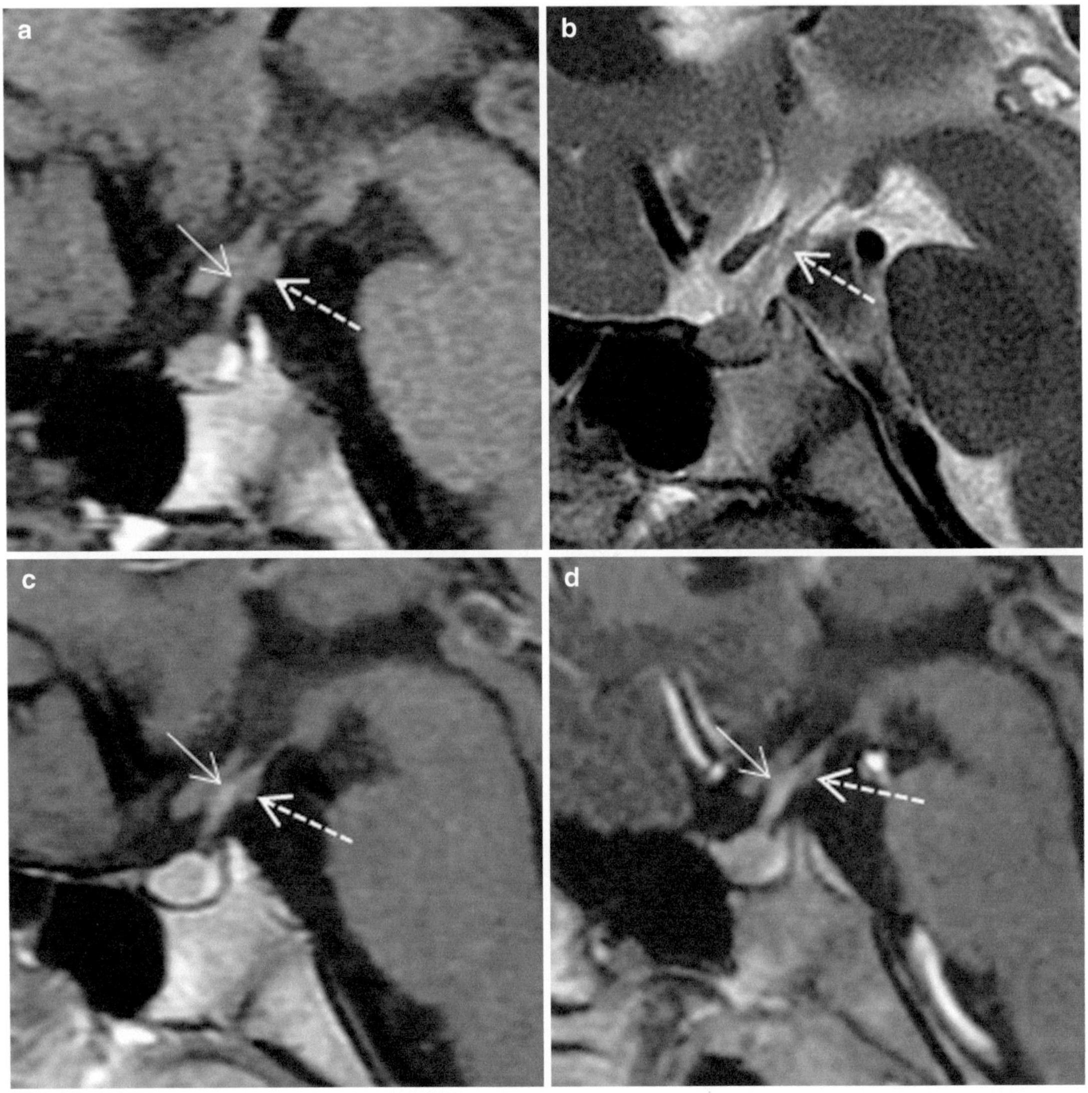

Fig. 38.1 Precocious puberty in an 8-year-old girl. (**a–d**) Sagittal T1, T2, CE T1 WIs, and CE GE T1WI. Mild swelling of the tuber cinereum (*arrow*). The inframillimetric hamartoma (*dotted line*) is nonenhanced on thin reformatted image in (**d**)

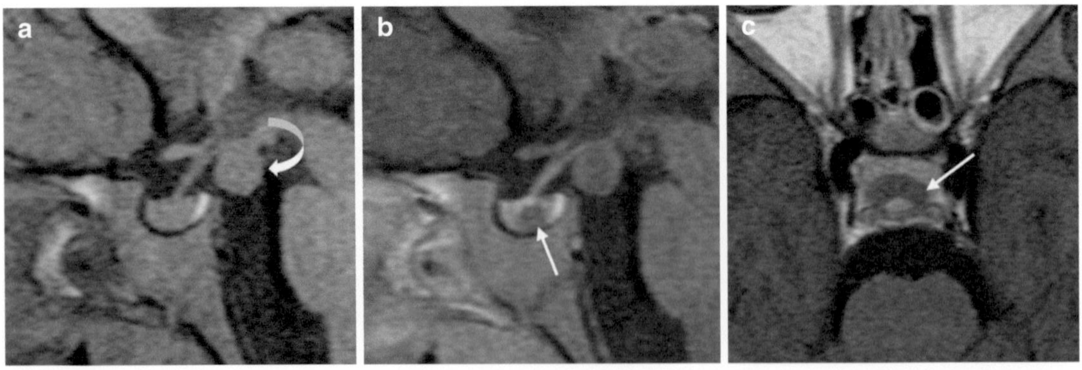

Fig. 38.2 Precocious puberty in a 3-year-old male. (**a**) Sagittal T1WI. Large pediculated hamartoma in the interpeduncular cistern (*curved arrow*). (**b**, **c**) Sagittal and axial CE T1WIs. The hamartoma is associated with an intrasellar Rathke cleft cyst (*arrow*)

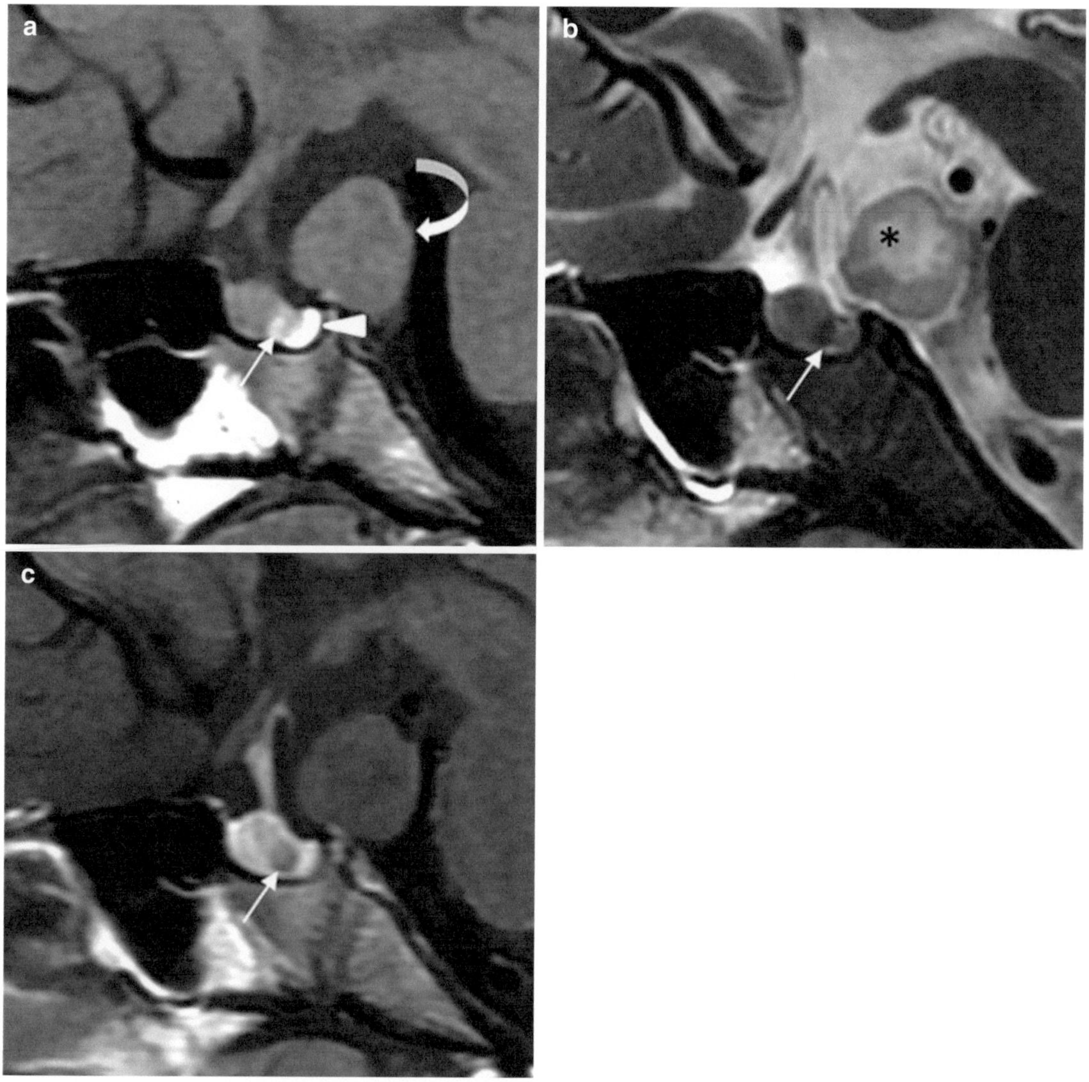

Fig. 38.3 Five-year-old girl presenting with precocious puberty. (**a**) Sagittal T1WI. Large supra-retrosellar mass isointense relative to the gray matter (*curved arrow*). The pituitary stalk is pushed anteriorly. Note the presence of a small mucous Rathke cleft cyst (*arrow*) between the posterior lobe (*arrowhead*) and the normal anterior lobe of the pituitary gland. (**b**) Sagittal T2WI. The lesion is heterogeneous with intralesional hyperintense foci (*asterisk*). The Rathke cleft cyst appears hypointense (*arrow*) (**c**) Sagittal CE T1WI. The mass does not enhance. Normal enhancement of the pituitary stalk and pituitary gland. The hypointense intrasellar nodule corresponds to the incidental Rathke cleft cyst (*arrow*). No change for 10 years: the diagnosis of hamartoma is very likely

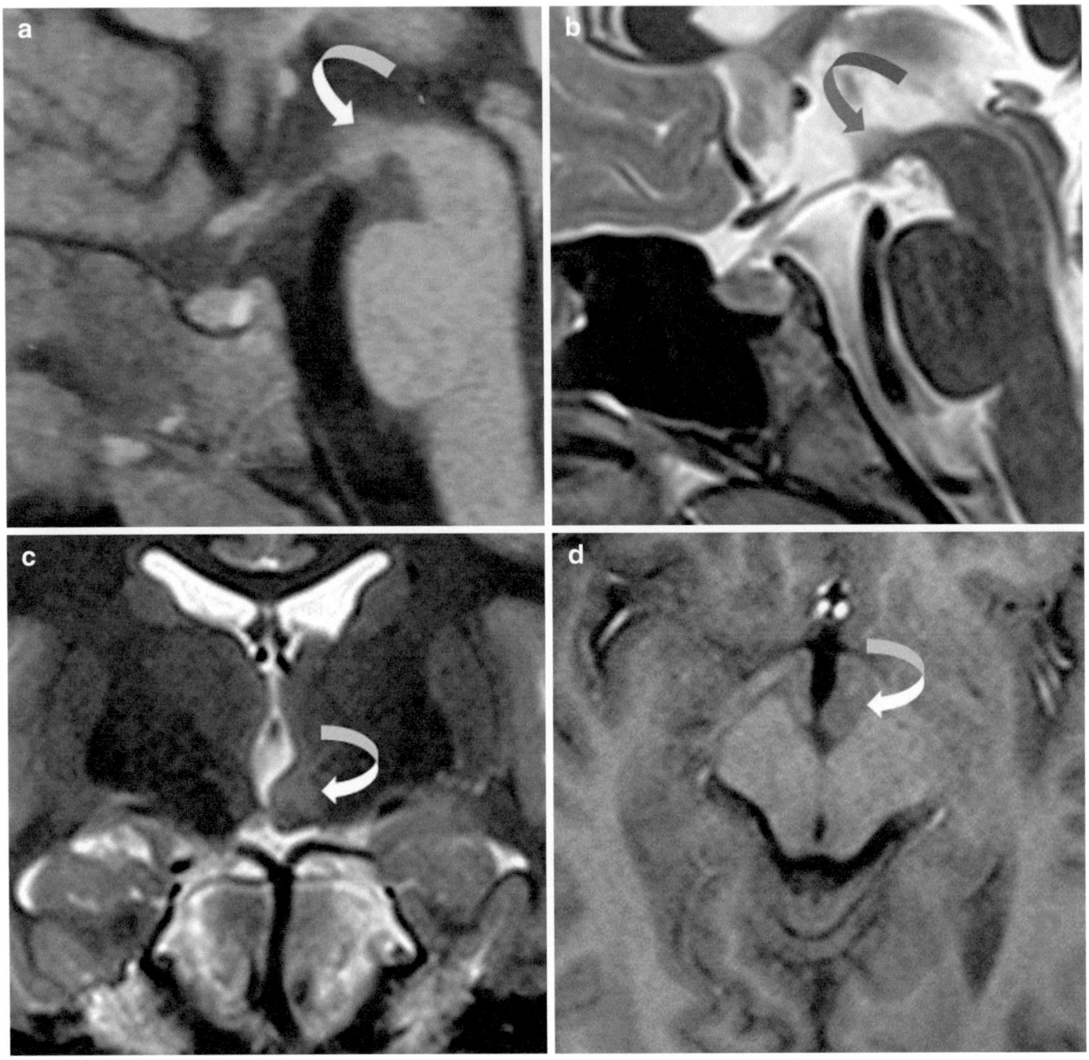

Fig. 38.4 Nine-year-old male presenting with severe behavior disorders, without precocious puberty or epilepsy. (**a**, **b**) Sagittal T1 and T2 WIs. In these medial sagittal planes, the identification of the hamartoma in the wall of the third ventricle is very difficult (*curved arrow*). (**c**) Coronal T2WI. The hamartoma (*curved arrow*), slightly hyperintense, is developed into the wall of the third ventricle and is protruding into the ventricular cavity. (**d**) Axial T1WI. The lesion is visualized on the left of the interpeduncular cistern (*curved arrow*)

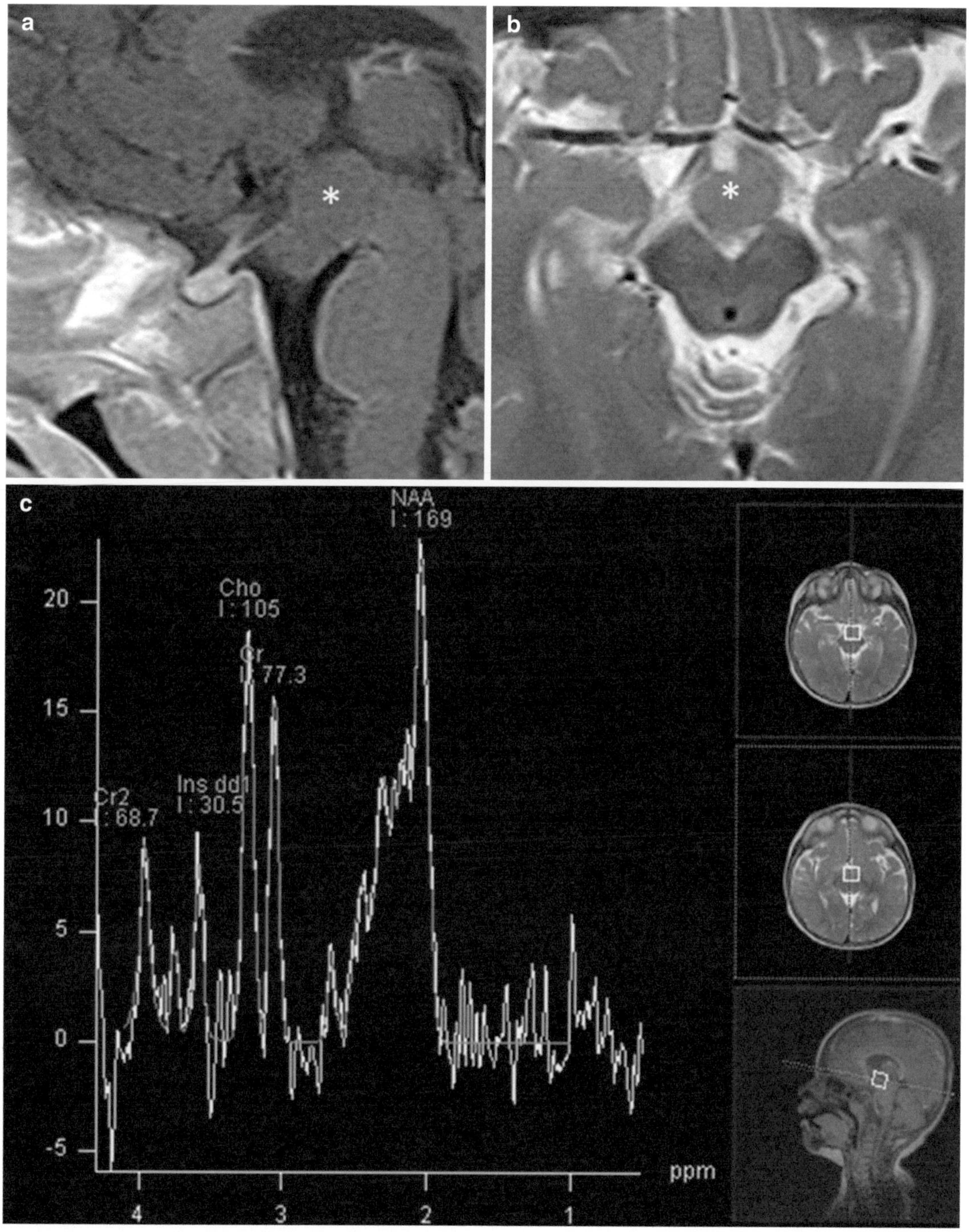

Fig. 38.5 Large pediculated hamartoma of the tuber cinereum (*asterisk*). (**a**) Sagittal CE T1WI and (**b**) Axial T2WI. (**c**) Single-voxel MR spectroscopy with short echo time (35 ms). The MR spectrum of the hamartoma is quite similar to that of the normal brain

Further Reading

Arita K, Ikawa F, Kurisu K et al (1999) The relationships between magnetic resonance findings and clinical manifestations of hypothalamic hamartoma. J Neurosurg 91:212–220

Boyko OB, Curnes JT, Oakes WJ, Burger PC (1991) Hamartomas of the tuber cinereum: CT, MR and pathologic findings. AJNR Am J Neuroradiol 12:309–314

Martin DD, Seeger U, Ranke MB, Grodd W (2003) MR imaging and spectroscopy of a tuber cinereum hamartoma in a patient with growth hormone deficiency and hypogonadotropic hypogonadism. AJNR Am J Neuroradiol 24:1177–1180

39 Sphenoid Mucocele

Jean-François Bonneville

Sphenoid mucocele is defined as the accumulation and retention of mucoid secretion within the sphenoid sinus, leading to thinning, distension, and erosion of its bony walls. Sphenoid sinus mucoceles must be differentiated from simple retentional cysts frequently observed after transsphenoidal surgery (Fig. 39.1) Several mechanisms have been proposed for the formation of mucocele: primary mucoceles can develop as retention cysts of the mucous glands of the sinus epithelium; secondary mucoceles are caused by obstruction of the sinus ostium, possibly from tumors extending inside the sphenoid sinus such as nasopharyngeal carcinoma, after trauma, radiotherapy, or transsphenoidal surgery. If impaired permeability of the antigravitational sphenoid sinus ostium seems always necessary for mucocele formation, it is probably not sufficient: an associated chronic inflammatory process, as attested by the presence of cytokines in the mucocele, constitutes a better explanation for the bone resorption and erosion phenomenon resulting in sphenoid sinus wall expansion and pseudotumoral development. Clinical features are related to mass effect, mainly headache and optic nerve compression, the latter being favored by anterior clinoid process pneumatization. Third and sixth cranial nerve palsies can also occur (Fig. 39.2) as well as chiasm compression and invasion of the pituitary fossa (Fig. 39.3). Intracranial extension caused by mucocele rupture in the subarachnoid spaces is rare (Figs. 39.4 and 39.5). On MRI, mucocele appears as a T1-hyperintense mass with regular contours occupying the whole or the main part of the sphenoid sinus. T1 intensity depends on the proteinic concentration and mucus viscosity. T2 signal is more variable, from hyperintense to hypointense in cases of high proteinic concentration. Concomitant aspergillosis can result in signal heterogeneity. After gadolinium injection, enhancement of the mucocele wall, but not of the mucocele itself, can be observed. Bulging or ballooning of sphenoid sinus walls is constantly observed. Diagnosis is usually easy except when the sphenoid mucocele is secondary to a sphenoid tumor. In cases of transsphenoidal surgery history, a T1WI fat-saturated sequence can be useful to differentiate fatty surgical packing from mucocele. Prevention of postsurgical sphenoid mucocele is based on excision of the sphenoid sinus mucosa and on a large sphenoidotomy to avoid mucus accumulation. Surgical treatment consists of endoscopic transnasal marsupialization.

J.-F. Bonneville et al., *MRI of the Pituitary Gland*, DOI 10.1007/978-3-319-29043-0_39

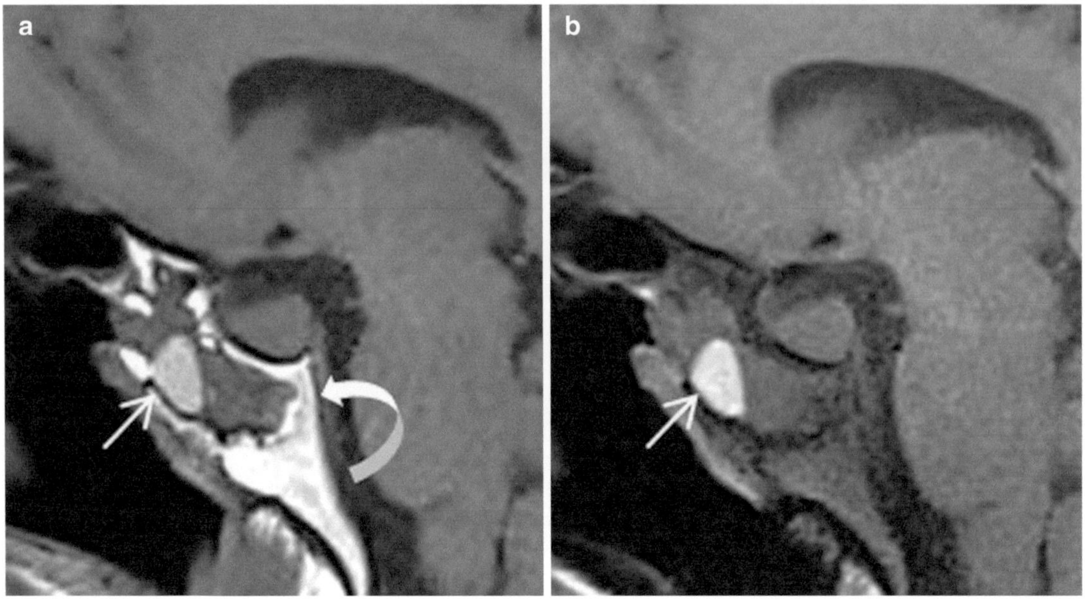

Fig. 39.1 Retentional mucoid cyst seen 1 year after surgery (*arrow*). (**a**) Sagittal T1WI. Hyperintensity of the sphenoid sinus walls (*curved arrow*) corresponding to fatty bone degeneration, as seen usually after surgical excision of the sinus mucosa. The proteinic nature of the cyst is confirmed with a T1W fat-saturated image (**b**)

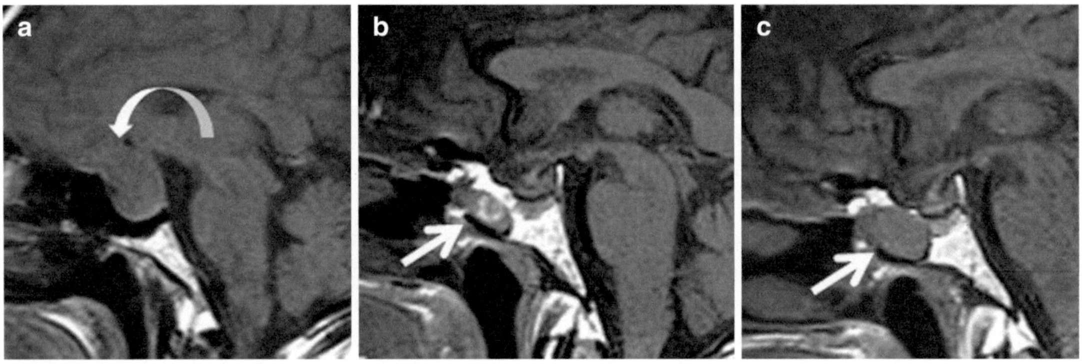

Fig. 39.2 From retentional cyst to sphenoid mucocele. (**a–c**) Sagittal T1WI. (**a**) Pituitary adenoma with extrasellar extension (*arrow*) before surgery. The sphenoid sinus is clear. (**b**) Five years after transsphenoidal surgery, postoperative changes with fatty degeneration of the sphenoid bone; limited retentional cyst (*thick arrow*). (**c**) Two years later, increased size of the retentional cyst or sphenoid mucocele? A follow-up is recommended

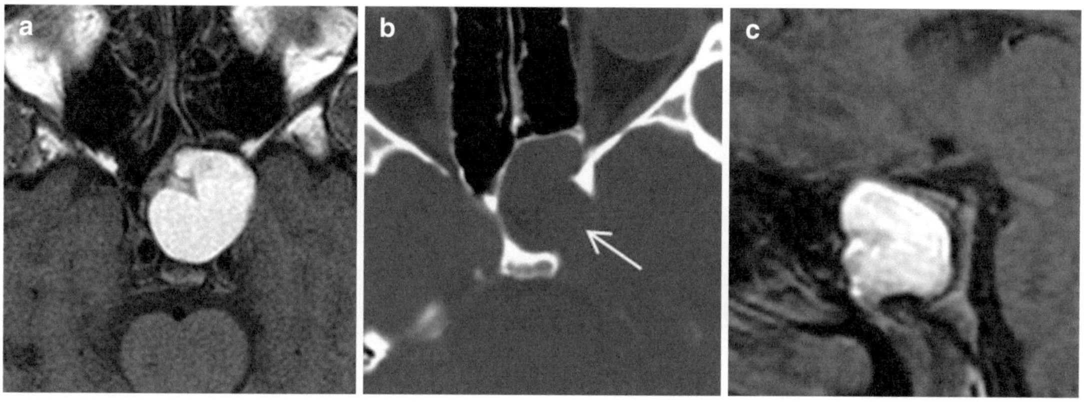

Fig. 39.3 Sphenoid mucocele revealed by headache and left oculomotor nerve palsy in a 68-year-old man. (**a**, **c**) Axial and sagittal T1WIs. The whole sphenoid sinus is occupied by a T1-hyperintense well-demarcated mass. (**b**) Axial CT demonstrates bone erosion (*arrow*)

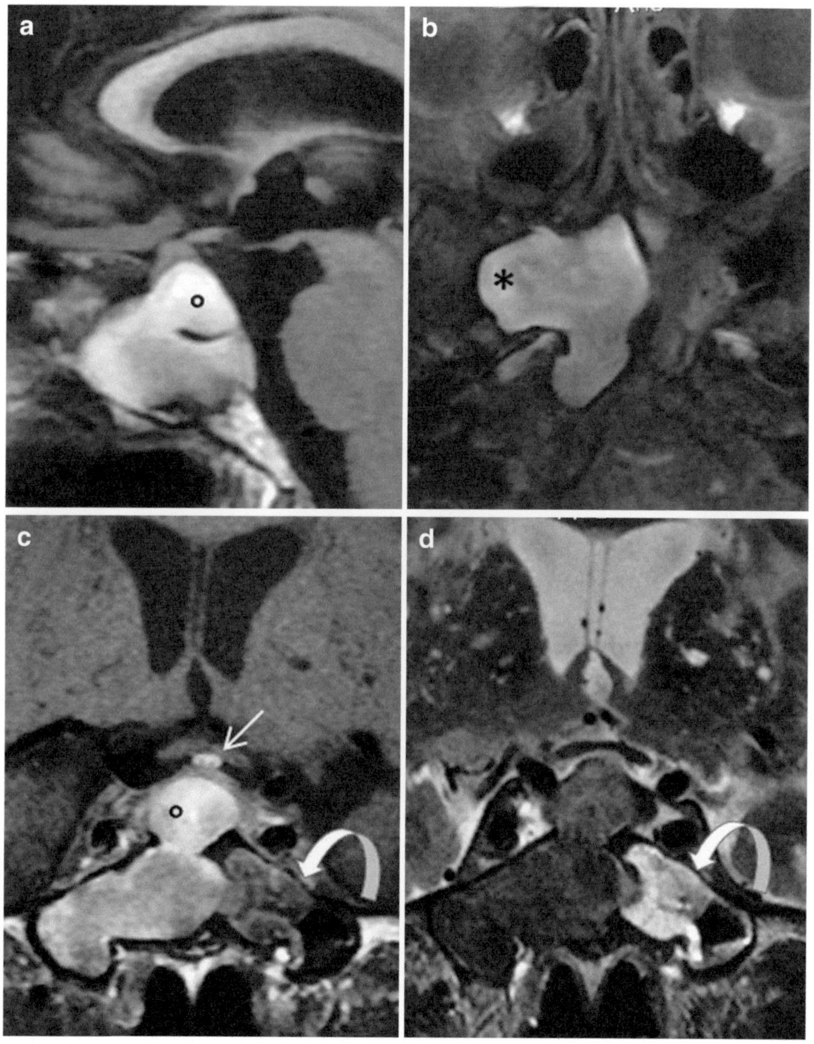

Fig. 39.4 A 78-year-old woman. Headache and right sixth nerve palsy. (**a**, **c**) Sagittal and coronal T1WIs. (**b**) Axial T1W fat-saturated image. (**d**) Coronal T2WI. Huge sphenoid mucocele compressing right cavernous sinus (*asterisk*) and invading pituitary fossa (*circle*). Note an ectopic posterior lobe (*small arrow*). The mucocele is hyperintense on T1WI and hypointense on T2WI except for a left sphenoid sinus cell (*curved arrow*) where T1 and T2 signals indicate a lower protein concentration

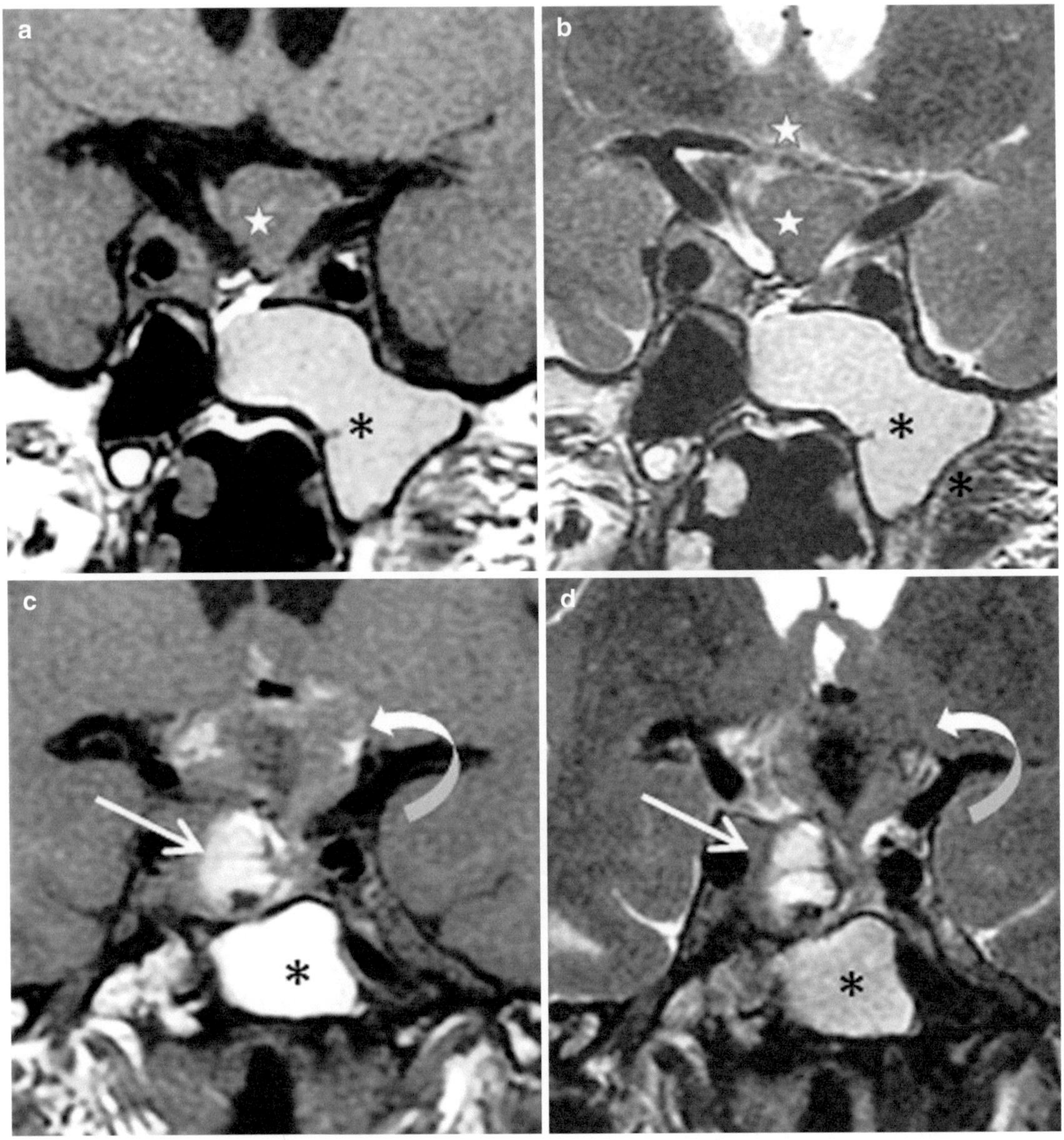

Fig. 39.5 A 67-year-old man. Mucocele rupture and apoplexy of a pituitary adenoma remnant. History of transsphenoidal surgery of a nonfunctioning pituitary macroadenoma. (**a**, **b**) Coronal T1 and T2 WIs. Intra- and suprasellar remnant (*star*) and uncomplicated sphenoid sinus mucocele (*asterisk*) stable for years. The patient is admitted to the emergency room for sudden severe headache, nausea, and partial loss of vision. (**c**, **d**) Coronal T1 and T2 WIs. Increased volume of intra-/suprasellar remnant in parallel with decreased size of sphenoid mucocele. Mixed signal intensity of the intrasellar (*straight arrow*) and suprasellar mass (*curved mass*) related to concomitant hemorrhage and mucus expulsion from the sphenoid sinus.

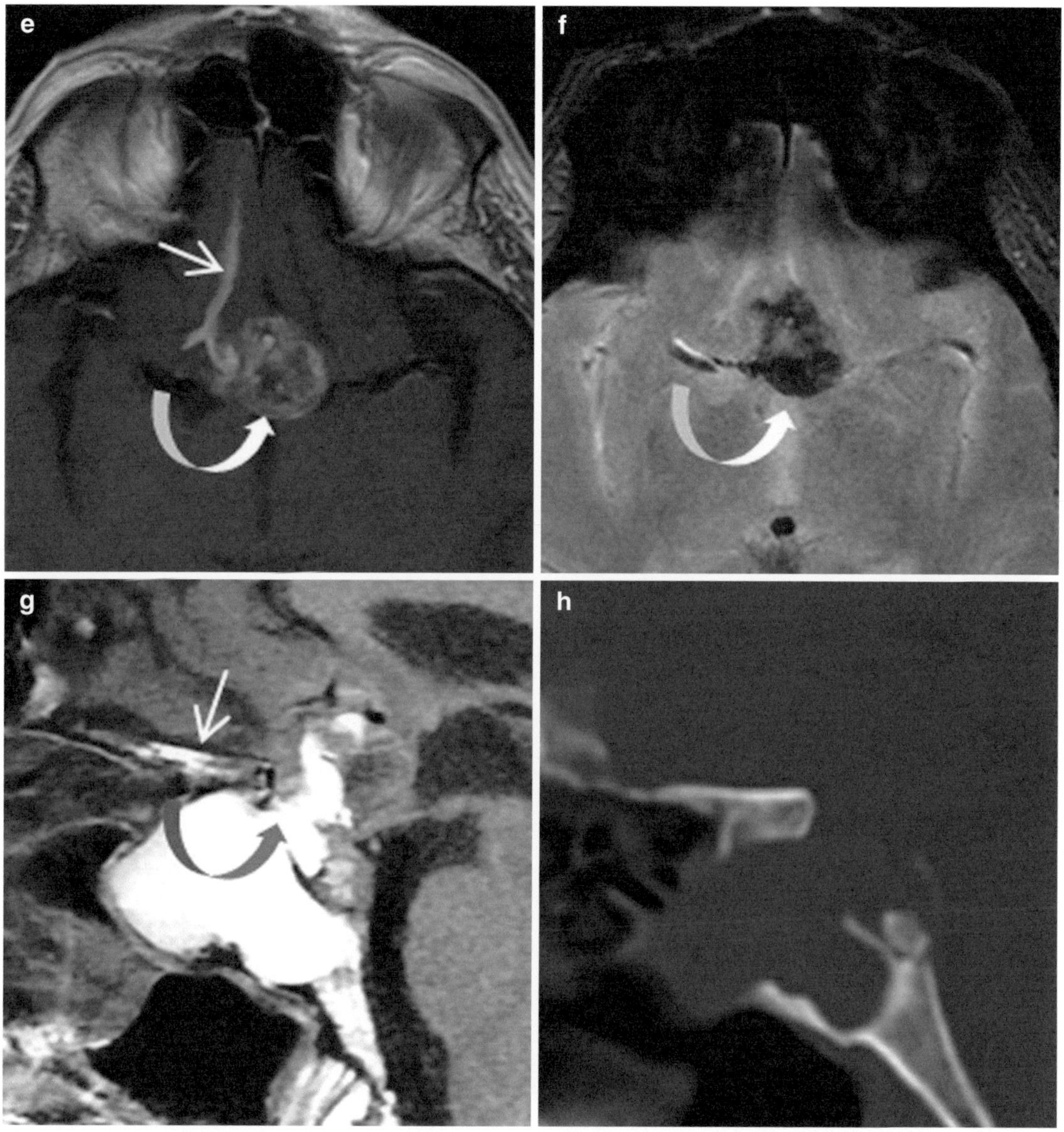

Fig. 39.5 (continued) (**e**) Axial T1WI. Hyperintensity of the suprasellar mass (*curved arrow*) and the right olfactory groove (*short arrow*). (**f**) Axial T2W GE image. Low signal of the hemorrhagic suprasellar mass, but not of the olfactory groove, thus confirming the presence of a proteinic-mucoid substance in the olfactory groove responsible for a chemical meningitis. (**g**) Sagittal T1WI. Expulsion of mucoid material from sphenoid sinus toward the pituitary fossa (*gray arrow*) and anterior cranial fossa is clearly shown (*short arrow*). (**h**) Bone destruction of sphenoid sinus and sella turcica walls demonstrated on sagittal CT reformatted image (Courtesy L. Rivail, MD)

Further Reading

Barrat JL, Marchat JC, Bracard S et al (1990) Mucoceles of the sphenoidal sinus. J Neuroradiol 17:135–151
Herman P, Lot G, Guichard JP, Marianowski R et al (1998) Mucocele of the sphenoid sinus: a late complication of transphenoidal pituitary surgery. Ann Otol Rhinol Laryngol 107:76–78
Kösling S, Hintner M, Brandt S et al (2004) Mucoceles of the sphenoid sinus. Eur J Radiol 51(1):1–5

Primary Hypophysitis

40

Sonia Nagi

Hypophysitis, a chronic inflammation of the pituitary gland, is a rare condition which can be classified as secondary or primary. Secondary hypophysitis includes the cases where an etiological agent is identified, whereas primary hypophysitis refers to those that do not currently have identifiable causes. Primary hypophysitis is the most common form of hypophysitis and comprises five histologic forms: lymphocytic, granulomatous, xanthomatous, necrotizing, and immunoglobulin G4 (IgG4) plasmacytic. The two main types are lymphocytic and granulomatous hypophysitis. IgG4-related hypophysitis is a recently reported new variant. Although lymphocytic hypophysitis is the most common form of primary hypophysitis, it is rare, representing less than 1 % of pituitary masses and estimated to be the cause of hypopituitarism in 0.5 % of cases. Lymphocytic hypophysitis predominantly affects women, particularly during late pregnancy or in the early postpartum period. However, cases in men, menopausal women, and children have been described. Available data strongly suggest an autoimmune pathogenesis: association with autoimmune conditions affecting other organs in 50 % of cases (thyroid, parathyroid, and adrenal glands), histopathological findings comprising fibrosis and lymphocytic infiltration, with antipituitary antibodies described in a few cases. Granulomatous hypophysitis represents less than 1 % of all operated cases of hypophysitis. It is usually diagnosed in middle- to old-age patients without gender predominance. Primary granulomatous hypophysitis is rare and its pathogenesis is still not understood. The secondary form of granulomatous hypophysitis is more common, associated with tuberculosis, sarcoidosis, syphilis, Langerhans cell histiocytosis, or Rathke cleft cyst (RCC) rupture. Pathology demonstrates the formation of granulomas, aggregates of lymphocytes, and epithelioid histiocytes with multinucleated giant cells. It usually involves the anterior lobe but may extend to involve the posterior lobe, the stalk, and even the hypothalamus. Xanthomatous hypophysitis predominantly affects young females. Its cause remains unknown, although autoimmune, infectious, and localized endothelial dysfunction have been suggested. It is pathologically characterized by mixed inflammatory infiltrate of foamy histiocytes called xanthoma cells and mature lymphocytes with cyst-like areas typically confined to the anterior pituitary. The basic structure of anterior pituitary is usually preserved without alteration of the pituitary stalk. Necrotizing hypophysitis is pathologically characterized by a marked mononuclear infiltrate showing significant necrosis. It involves the adenohypophysis, pituitary stalk, infundibuloneurohypophysitis, and hypothalamus. The pathogenesis of this rare hypophysitis variant remains unknown. IgG4-related hypophysitis is part of a multifocal systemic disease of unknown etiology called “IgG4-related autoimmune disease.” This disease, which mainly affects middle-aged to

J.-F. Bonneville et al., *MRI of the Pituitary Gland*, DOI 10.1007/978-3-319-29043-0_40

elderly males, is characterized by elevated serum IgG4 concentration and tissue infiltration by IgG4+ plasma cells with fibrosis and sclerosis . Diagnostic criteria include involvement of various organs such as the CNS, salivary glands, lacrimal glands, thyroid gland, lungs, pancreas, bile ducts, kidneys, prostate, lymph nodes, retroperitoneum, mesentery, gastrointestinal tract, skin, breast, and arteries. Adenohypophysitis, infundibuloneurohypophysitis, or panhypophysitis may be distinguished according to the anatomic involvement of the gland. Classical manifestations of adenohypophysitis may be tumoral or endocrine symptoms. Tumoral syndrome consists of headaches and visual impairment. The sudden onset of these signs is related to the rapid pituitary volume increase. Oculomotor disorders caused by cavernous sinus involvement are seldom seen. Endocrine symptoms consist of partial or total anterior hypopituitarism. ACTH secretion is most frequently impaired, followed by TSH and LH/FSH secretion. Hyperprolactinemia caused by pituitary stalk compression can be seen. Hypogonadism is typically encountered in xanthomatous hypophysitis. A few cases of aseptic meningitis with meningeal syndrome have been reported. Infundibuloneurohypophysitis occurs in older patients without gender predilection, and typically presents with diabetes insipidus. Young age at onset (<30 years), vasopressin-cell antibodies, and association with other autoimmune diseases support the autoimmune hypothesis for pathogenesis. Diabetes insipidus is seldom encountered in xanthomatous hypophysitis. The role of MRI in primary hypophysitis is to eliminate a pituitary adenoma. Diffuse and symmetric enlargement of the pituitary gland is seen in adenohypophysitis, with frequent upward tongue-like extension. Optic chiasm compression is inconstant. This tumoral syndrome contrasts with a normal-sized pituitary fossa. Signal intensity is usually hypointense on T1WI and more or less hyperintense on T2WI. Postgadolinium enhancement is usually homogeneous and intense but can be moderate and heterogeneous (Fig. 40.1). The pseudocapsule formed by compressed normal pituitary gland is sometimes not seen after gadolinium administration. A nonspecific perisellar dural enhancement is frequent (Fig. 40.2). This feature, classically described in hypophysitis and meningiomas, can also be encountered in pituitary macroadenomas. A noticeable delay in pituitary enhancement compared with the normal gland (<60 s) has been described on dynamic CE studies. In contrast, we have observed during dynamic MRI an intense and early enhancement of some foci presenting a pronounced hyperintensity on T2WI and probably corresponding to a localized inflammatory process (Fig. 40.3). Enhancement of the diaphragm has been reported in a few cases. A peripheral enhancement pattern seems more common in xanthomatous hypophysitis than in other types of hypophysitis. Restitutio ad integrum is rare (Fig. 40.4). Recurrence can be observed after treatment withdrawal (Fig. 40.5). Anterior pituitary atrophy is frequently the final outcome of adenohypophysitis. Another more specific but later sign has been described by Nakata in lymphocytic hypophysitis, appearing 2–20 months after the initial MR examination. It consists of a dark fibrotic rim encircling the pituitary gland on T2WI (Fig. 41.4). Infundibuloneurohypophysitis is characterized by a thickened pituitary stalk and a loss of the posterior pituitary bright spot as seen on axial noncontrast T1WI. Pituitary stalk thickening usually resolves with time, sometimes very quickly. In the end, atrophy takes place with a threadlike pituitary stalk and a decrease in size of the anterior lobe (Fig. 40.6). However, recurrence of the stalk thickening can be seen. Loss of the posterior lobe bright spot is usually permanent. In cases of panhypophysitis, signs of both entities will be seen. The main differential diagnosis is pituitary adenoma. Other nonadenomatous pituitary masses and secondary hypophysitis can be difficult to distinguish from primary hypophysitis. Approximately 40 % of patients are misdiagnosed as having pituitary macroadenoma and undergo unnecessary surgery. Hence, distinguishing primary hypophysitis from pituitary adenoma is very important. On MR scans,

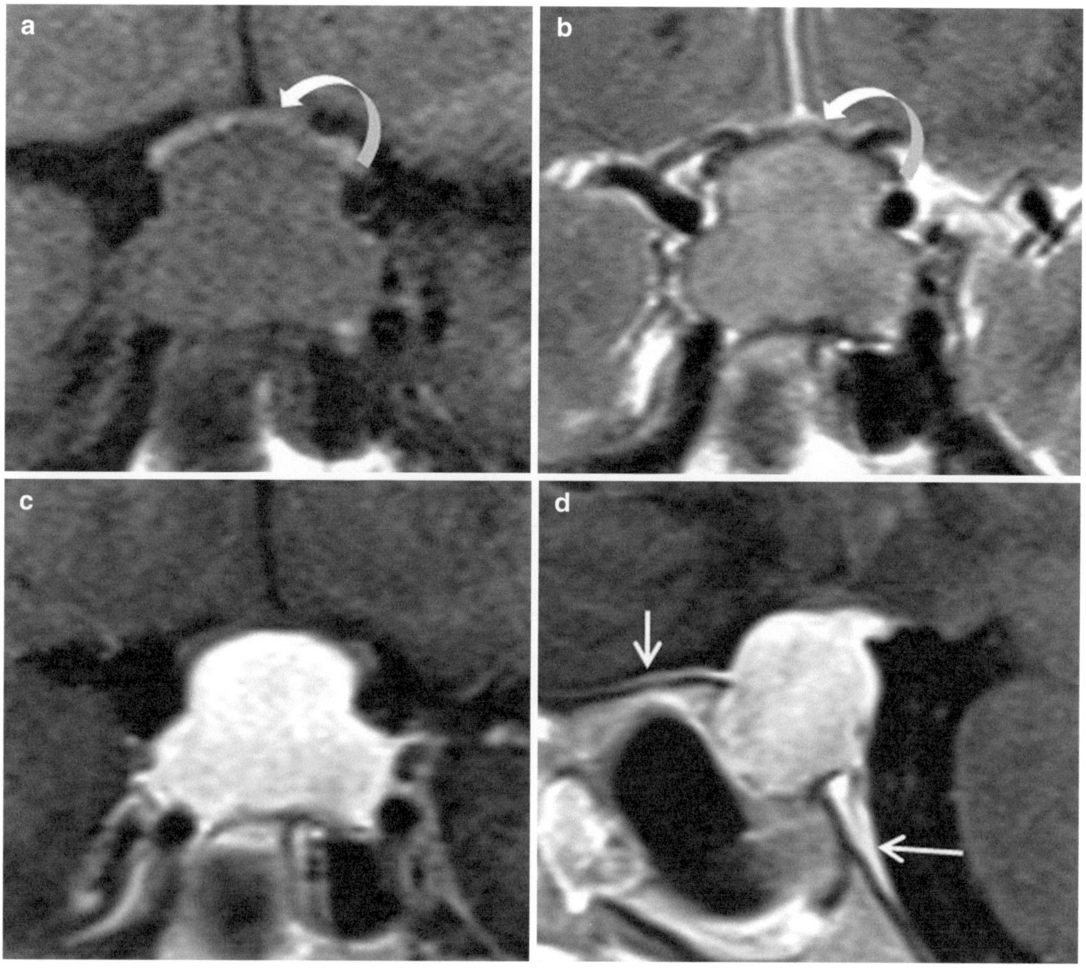

Fig. 40.1 A 43-year-old woman with headache, corticotropic insufficiency, and hyperprolactinemia. (**a**, **b**) Coronal T1 and T2 WIs. Symmetric intra- and suprasellar mass, hypointense on T1, hyperintense on T2, with compression of the optic chiasm (*curved arrow*). (**c**, **d**) Coronal and sagittal CE T1WIs. Intense, diffuse, and homogeneous enhancement of the mass. Presellar and retrosellar dural enhancement along the clivus (*straight arrows*). A pituitary adenoma was initially suspected and the patient underwent surgery. Histopathological examination revealed a lymphocytic hypophysitis

pituitary adenoma can easily be distinguished from normal pituitary parenchyma. The normal pituitary gland is most often located at the upper part of the sella, anteriorly or lateral to the adenoma. It is best seen as a pseudocapsule on coronal T1WI after contrast administration. Another distinctive feature is the absence of thickening of the pituitary stalk. Diabetes insipidus is seldom encountered in adenomas and the posterior bright spot is present, although often ectopic. The other nonadenomatous pituitary masses are germinoma, choristoma, and pituitary metastases. Another differential diagnosis to consider is pituitary hyperplasia secondary to hypothyroidism. In this case, the posterior bright spot is present, the pituitary stalk is normal, and there is no delayed enhancement on dynamic postcontrast scans. Distinguishing primary hypophysitis from secondary hypophysitis is a diagnosis of exclusion (Fig. 40.7). Investigations are required to rule out numerous etiologies; administration of immunomodulatory drugs such as CTLA-4

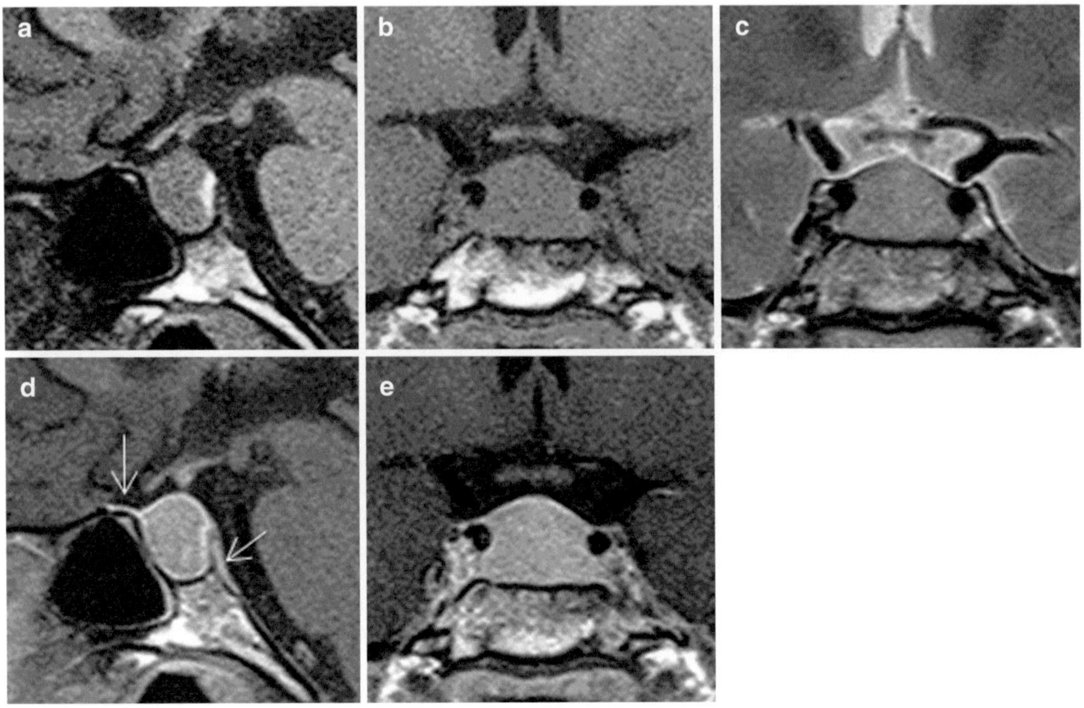

Fig. 40.2 A 46-year-old-woman with headache, corticotropic insufficiency, central hypothyroidism, and moderate hyperprolactinemia. Diagnosis of Hashimoto's thyroiditis was made by detection of high levels of anti-thyroid peroxidase antibodies. (**a**) Sagittal T1WI. Enlarged pituitary gland in a normal-sized pituitary fossa. (**b**, **c**) Coronal T1 and T2 WIs. Symmetric enlarged pituitary gland with suprasellar extension. The mass is slightly hyperintense on T2 and relatively hypointense to temporal white matter on T1WI. (**d**, **e**) Sagittal and coronal CE T1WIs. Homogeneous enhancement. Presellar and retrosellar dural enhancement (*arrows*)

blocking antibody (ipilimumab) or interferon-α, Wegener granulomatosis, tuberculosis, sarcoidosis, syphilis, tuberculosis, and Langerhans and non-Langerhans cell histiocytosis (see Chap. 41). Other etiologies may induce a secondary hypophysitis such as ruptured RCC, pituitary abscess, and Takayasu disease. The T2 dark fibrotic rim around the pituitary gland and along the dura mater, seen in the chronic stage of lymphocytic and IgG4-related hypophysitis (Figs. 40.8 and 40.9) is not a distinctive sign for secondary hypophysitis and can be observed in granulomatosis, sarcoidosis, or tuberculosis. Primary hypophysitis management remains controversial. Surgery may be indicated when the tumoral syndrome is important. Otherwise, when the diagnosis of primary hypophysitis is the most likely, medical treatment is initiated. Medical treatment consists of corticosteroid therapy and hormonal replacement therapy. This treatment should be carried out under clinical, biological, and neuroradiological supervision. Different outcomes have been reported. The disease may be self-limited, show a relapsing and remitting course, or progress to permanent hypopituitarism. In cases where the tumoral syndrome persists, surgery is indicated to avoid complications.

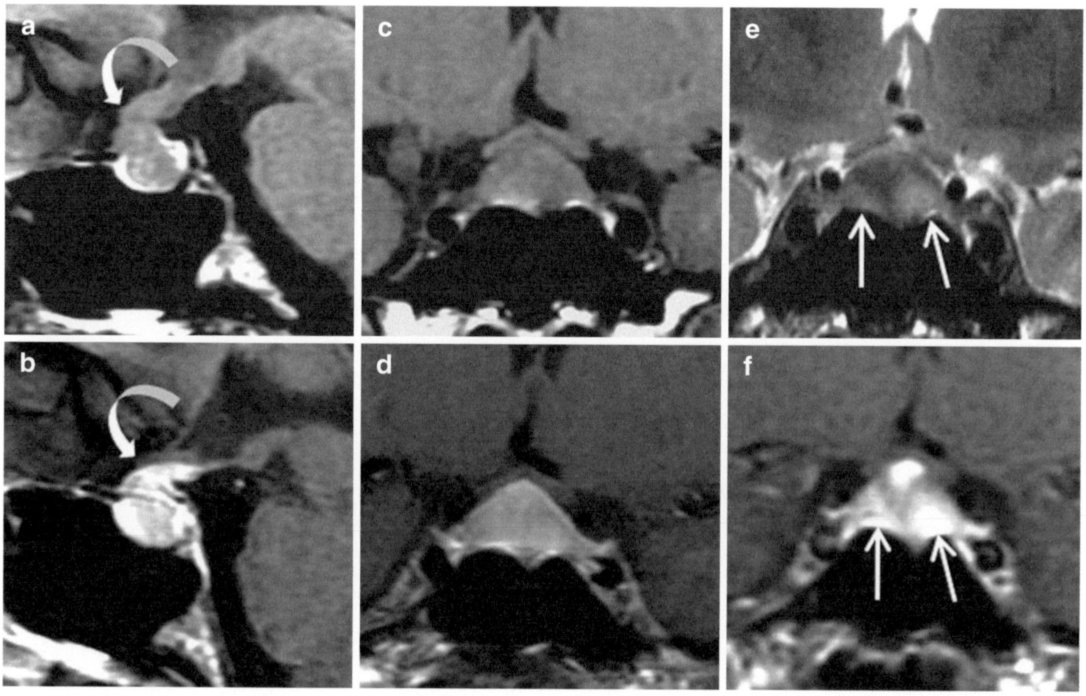

Fig. 40.3 Presumed lymphocytic hypophysitis in a 27-year-old woman presenting with severe unusual retro-orbital headache at the fifth month of a first pregnancy. No pituitary deficit. No visual field defect. (**a**, **b**) Sagittal T1 and CE T1 WIs. Pituitary mass with suprasellar tongue-like extension (*curved arrows*) and strong enhancement after gadolinium perfusion. (**c**, **d**) Coronal T1 and CE T1 WIs. Symmetrical enlargement of the lesion and compression of the optic chiasm. (**e**) Coronal T2WI detects two areas of hyperintensity (*straight arrows*) exactly corresponding to foci of marked enhancement during dynamic MRI (*straight arrows* in **f**)

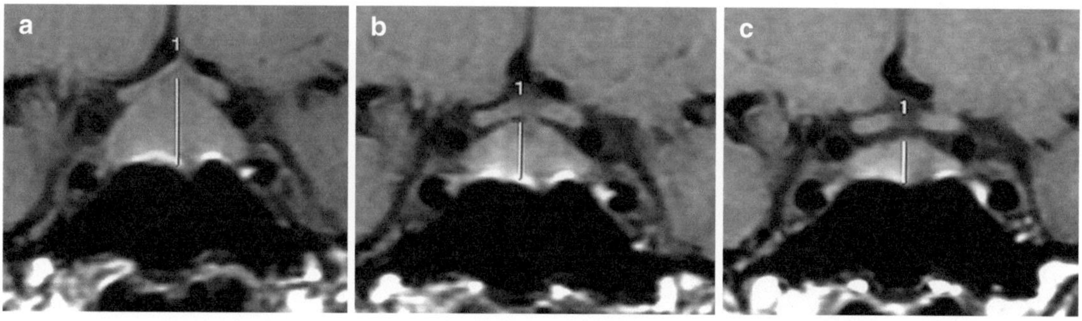

Fig. 40.4 Same patient as in Fig. 40.3. (**a–c**) Coronal T1WI at diagnosis, 2 and 6 months later with conservative management. Normalization of the sellar content. The patient is asymptomatic after a normal delivery

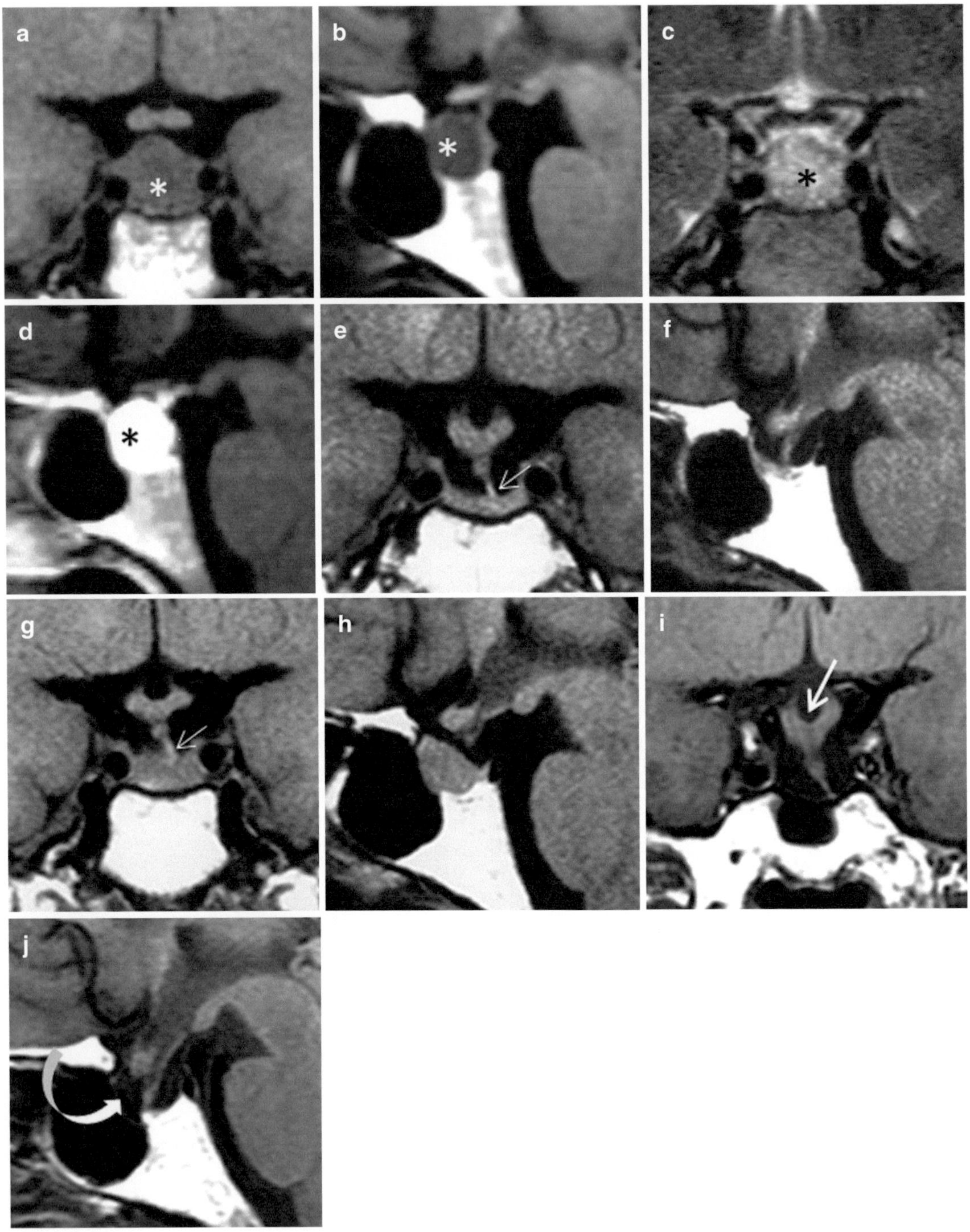

Fig. 40.5 Relapsing panhypophysitis in a 48-year-old woman with anterior pituitary deficit and diabetes insipidus. (**a**, **b**) Coronal and sagittal T1WIs. Enlarged and hypointense pituitary gland (asterisk). (**c**) Coronal T2WI. Heterogeneous hyperintensity of the mass. (**d**) Sagittal CE T1WI. Intense enhancement after contrast administration. (**e**, **f**) Coronal and sagittal T1WIs 1 month after initiation of medical therapy (a new MRI was performed for immediate preoperative evaluation of what was diagnosed as a pituitary macroadenoma). Rapid shrinkage of the pituitary content; atrophy of the pituitary stalk; ectopic ADH storage (*small arrow*). (**g**, **h**) Coronal and sagittal T1WIs at 3 months. Clinical relapse with recurrence of pituitary gland enlargement. (**i**, **j**) Coronal and sagittal T1WIs. MR follow-up 6 years later showing an empty sella (*curved arrow*) and ptosis of the optic chiasm (*thick arrow*)

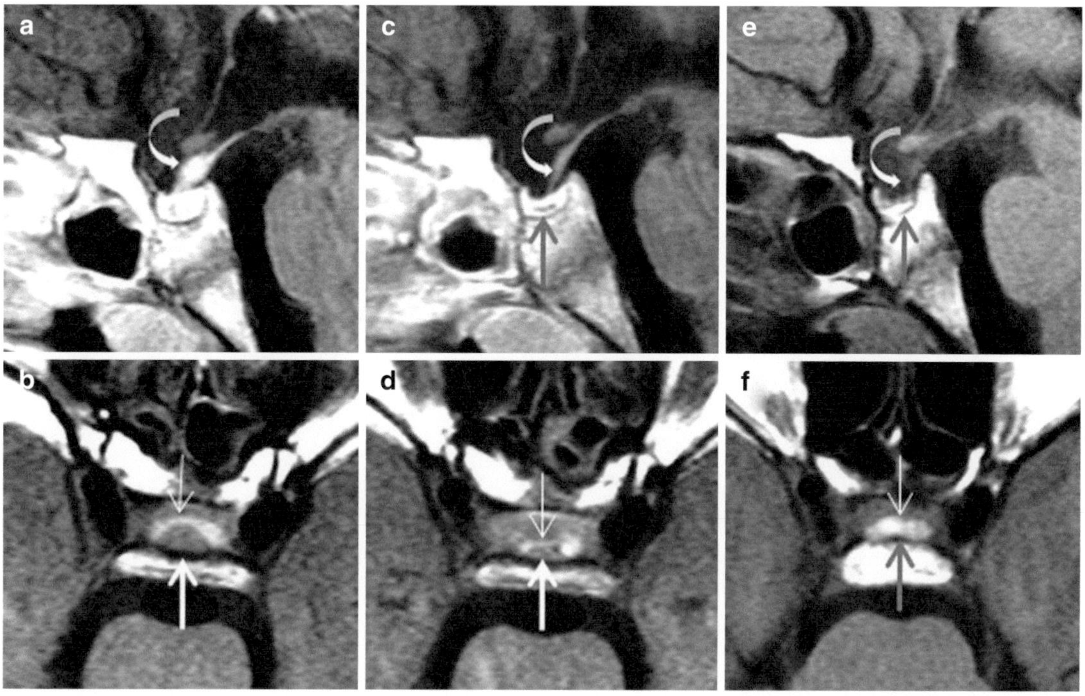

Fig. 40.6 Infundibuloneurohypophysitis in a 3-year-old boy presenting with diabetes insipidus. Incidental intrasellar RCC. (**a**, **b**) Sagittal CE T1WI and axial noncontrast T1WI at diagnosis. Enlarged pituitary stalk (*curved arrow*). The posterior lobe (*thick arrow*) is not T1 hyperintense but clearly enlarged and outlined by a compressed arch-like RCC (*thin arrow*). (**c**, **d**) Same sequences 1 month later. Shrinkage of the pituitary stalk and posterior lobe (*thick arrow*). The small RCC is represented by a thin linear nonenhanced area (*straight arrow* in **c**). (**e**, **f**) Sagittal and axial noncontrast T1WIs 3 years later. Further atrophy of the pituitary stalk (*curved arrow*) and posterior lobe (*thick arrow*). Enlarged T1-hyperintense RCC (*thin arrow*)

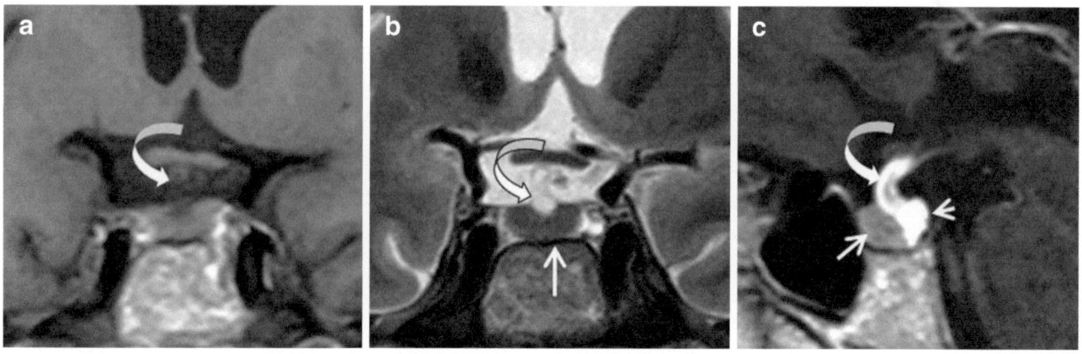

Fig. 40.7 Secondary hypophysitis. Presumed autoimmune hypophysitis after treatment with ipilimumab in a patient with metastatic melanoma. (**a**, **b**) Coronal T1 and T2 WIs. (**c**) Sagittal CE T1WI. Thickened pituitary stalk, T1 hypointense, T2 hyperintense: the stalk is quite transparent, but strongly enhanced after gadolinium administration (*curved arrows*), as is the posterior pituitary (*short arrow*). Size and signal of the anterior pituitary are normal (*straight arrows*) (Courtesy of G. Raverot, MD, PhD)

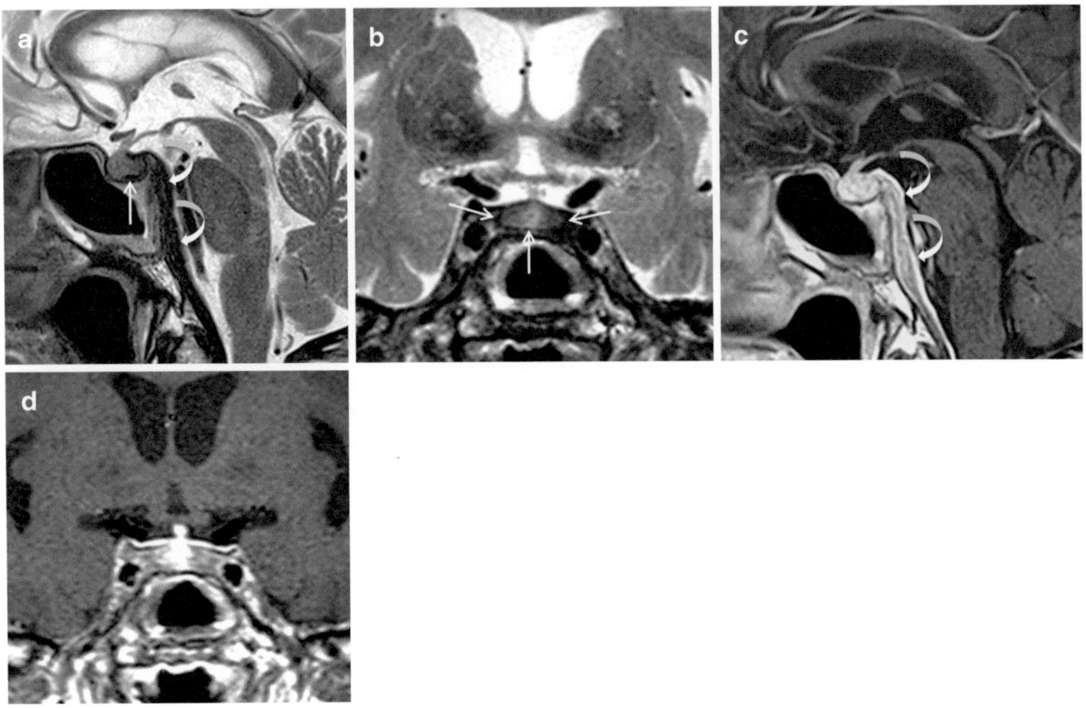

Fig. 40.8 An 80-year-old man with hypopituitarism due to IgG4 hypophysitis. Past history of infiltrative lesions in the lungs and kidneys whose biopsy led to the diagnosis of IgG4 disease. (**a**) Sagittal and (**b**) coronal T2WIs demonstrate a perisellar hypointense infiltrate gliding along the clivus (*curved arrow*) and encircling the pituitary gland itself (*arrows*). This inflammatory lesions enhance markedly after gadolinium administration, as seen on (**c**) sagittal and (**d**) coronal CE T1WIs

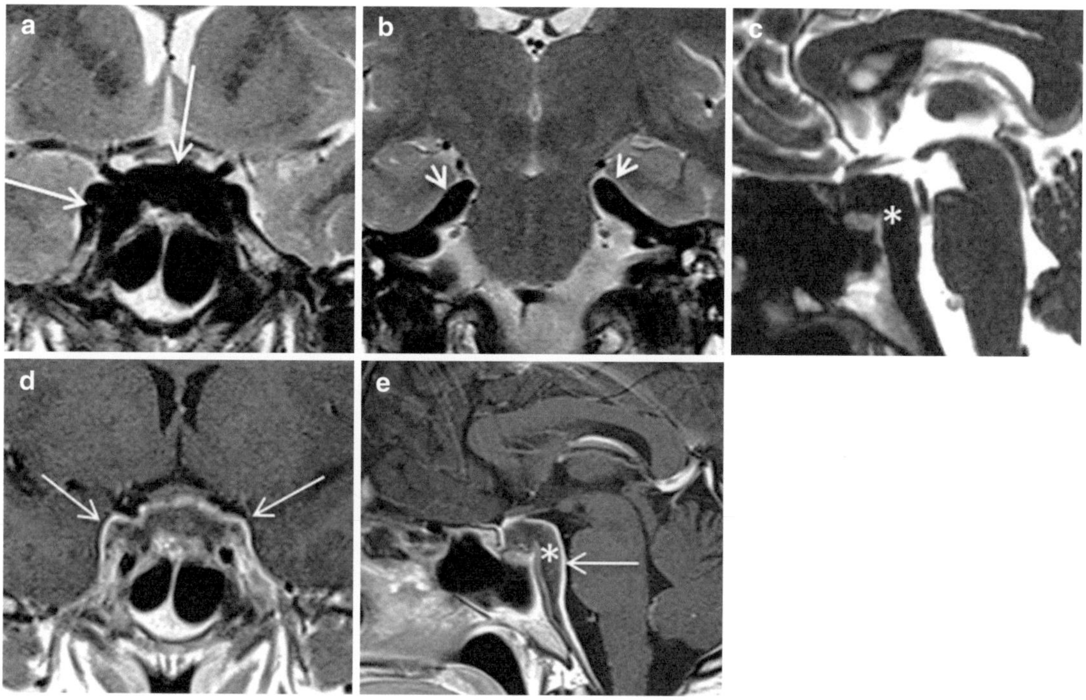

Fig. 40.9 A 30-year-old man with history of pulmonary and renal lesions related to IgG4-related disease. Four years later, occurrence of an anterior pituitary deficit and diabetes insipidus. (**a**, **b**) Coronal T2WI. (**c**) Sagittal heavily T2WI. (**d**, **e**) Coronal and sagittal CE T1WIs. Marked peripheral T2 hypointensity encircling the pituitary gland and the cavernous sinuses (*long arrows*), extending to the clivus (*asterisk*) and the tentorium cerebelli (*short arrows*) due to fibrous pachymeningitis (*asterisk*). Peripheral enhancement (*thin arrows*) sparing the center (*asterisk*)

Further Reading

Khare S, Jaktab VS, Budyal SR et al (2015) Primary (autoimmune) hypophysitis: a single centre experience. Pituitary 18:16–22

Nagi S, Megdiche H, Nouira K et al (2002) Hypophysite granulomateuse idiopathique: aspects cliniques et radiologiques. J Neuroradiol 29:43–48

Nakata Y, Sato N, Masumoto T et al (2010) Parasellar T2 dark sign on MR imaging in patients with lymphocytic hypophysitis. Am J Neuroradiol 31:1944–1950

41 Pituitary in Systemic Diseases

Fabrice Bonneville

Systemic diseases represent a group of diseases of unknown origin that affect the body as a whole. Therefore, they are known to develop in multiple organs and may sometimes involve the sellar region. There, they can be located within the anterior pituitary lobe, resulting in hypophysitis and hypopituitarism; in the stalk or the infundibulum, being a source of diabetes insipidus and sometimes mimicking a suprasellar tumor; a combination thereof; or in the parasellar meninges, cavernous sinus, skull base, or neighboring brain. Two opposite situations may lead to the diagnosis of a systemic disease lesion in the sellar region: first, the diagnosis is straightforward when the underlying systemic disease is already known and MRI depicts a lesion there; second, which is more delicate, when a lesion is depicted in the sellar region and the radiologist has to evoke the diagnosis of a specific systemic disease. Clues hopefully exist, and together with the knowledge of particular patterns suggestive of each disease, make the diagnosis feasible or, at least, help the radiologist to suggest it. In general, in patients with a sellar/suprasellar mass and unusual clinical presentation such as diabetes insipidus or associated neurological deterioration, granulomatous lesions should be carefully considered in differential diagnosis. Systemic diseases are numerous and encompass various autoimmune diseases, connective tissue diseases, granulomatosis, and vasculitis. Autoimmune hypophysitis have been detailed in Chap. 40. Here, granulomatous hypophysitis and other lesions located in the sellar region in the setting of nonautoimmune systemic diseases, such as sarcoidosis, histiocytosis, or Wegener granulomatosis, are illustrated.

41.1 Sarcoidosis

Sarcoidosis is a multisystemic granulomatosis, characterized by the presence of epithelioid granulomas, without caseous necrosis. Intracranial sarcoidosis lesions develop on the meninges, the brain, and the cranial nerves, with a predilection for the optic chiasm and hypothalamus-pituitary regions. There, lesions can be asymptomatic and only depicted by MRI in front of diffuse neurosarcoidosis, or can be responsible for endocrine disorders. Diabetes insipidus is the most frequent clinical symptom and is found in 25–50 % of neurosarcoidosis, followed by signs attributable to hyperprolactinemia and hypogonadism.

On MRI, lesions of neurosarcoidosis are often multiple and diffused, affecting the meninges, the brain, and the cranial nerves at variable degrees. In detail, lesions of sarcoidosis in the sellar region may be encountered in the hypothalamus, the infundibulum, the stalk, the adenohypophysis, the cavernous sinus, and the optic chiasm. Classic features are stalk thickening, stalk nodule, or enlargement of the adenohypophysis, and evoke the diagnosis of neurosarcoidosis when associated to other intracranial lesions. The leptomen-

J.-F. Bonneville et al., *MRI of the Pituitary Gland*, DOI 10.1007/978-3-319-29043-0_41

ingeal lesions are suggestive of the diagnosis and appear as micronodular or linear gadolinium uptake along the surface of the brain, with a predilection for the suprasellar area and the base of the brain. Thus, infiltration of the hypothalamic-pituitary axis is common in neurosarcoidosis (Fig. 41.1). Leptomeningeal lesions subsequently penetrate the brain through the perivascular Virchow-Robin spaces where they form remote micronodular enhancing lesions, or T2 hyperintensities in the basal ganglia or the cerebral white matter. Intracerebral lesions are also frequently observed on the walls of the ventricles, along the ependyma. Hydrocephalus may exist, owing to this meningeal sheathing. Intra-axial lesions of sarcoidosis are usually surrounded by edema. Therefore, the combination of micronodular or linear enhancing lesions along the surface of the brain and within the brain is very suggestive of neurosarcoidosis, especially if located at the base of the brain, i.e., the hypothalamus-hypophysis axis, the basal ganglia, and the ventricles (Fig. 41.2). Differential diagnoses include tuberculous meningitis and carcinomatous meningitis. However, in granulomatosis, lesions often appear with evocative T2-low or -isosignal intensity. This may be of precious help when the systemic disease is unknown, or when only a single lesion is depicted on MRI. Although most lesions of neurosarcoidosis are small and appear as dots of enhancement, they may sometimes act as large macronodules giving a pseudotumor appearance. In our experience, a single macronodule is found on the stalk or the infundibulum in about 25 % of neurosarcoidosis cases (Fig. 41.3). In this specific setting, differential diagnosis includes all the tumors of the stalk such as germinoma, metastasis, lymphoma, or pituicytoma. Overall, this pattern may be identical to lesions of histiocytosis, and it is impossible to distinguish these two entities according to MRI only, especially when the lesion shows T2-low signal intensity. The age of the patient may help as histiocytosis often occurs in childhood or in young adults, while sarcoidosis develops a little later in life, but large overlap of disease onset exists between sarcoidosis and histiocytosis. Neurosarcoidosis may also be located along the dura, with a diffuse spreading, or may be focal, thus mimicking a meningioma. Again, such lesions often appear with a characteristic T2-hypointense signal, a feature unusual in meningioma. Specific infiltration of the meningeal layers surrounding the pituitary gland is also observed, further detailed in the histiocytosis section in this chapter (Fig. 41.4). All of these intracranial lesions are presumed to

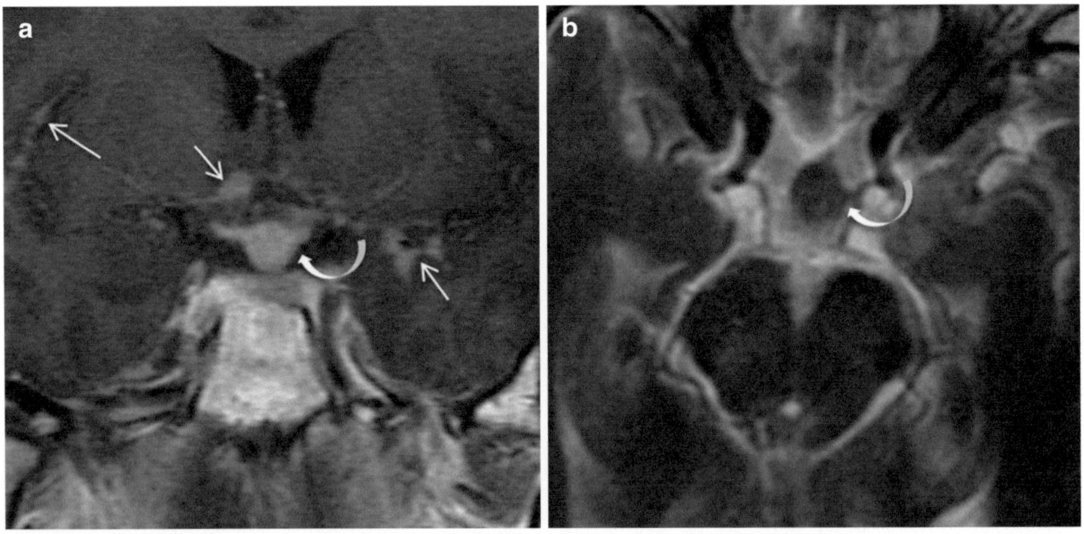

Fig. 41.1 Neurosarcoidosis in a patient with diabetes insipidus. (**a**) Coronal CE T1WI demonstrates an enhancing lesion on the pituitary stalk (*curved arrow*) associated with multiple micronodular and linear leptomeningeal enhancing lesions (*straight arrows*) spread at the surface of the base of the brain. (**b**) On axial T2WI the nodular lesion of the infundibulum appears isointense (*curved arrow*)

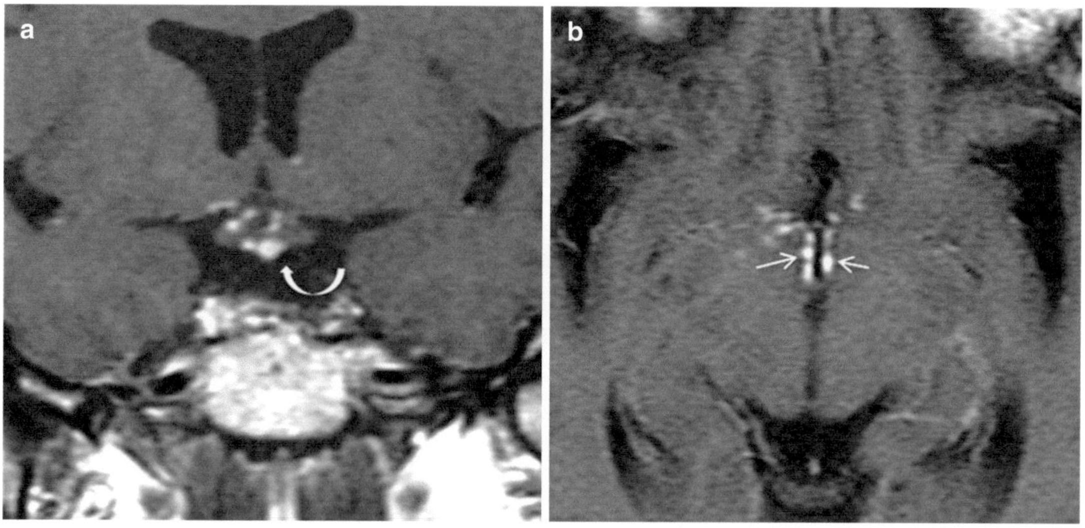

Fig. 41.2 Typical neurosarcoidosis illustrated on (**a**, **b**) Coronal and axial CE T1WIs. As may happen, these classic leptomeningeal micronodular enhancing lesions are located only along the hypothalamus-pituitary axis, at the infundibulum (*curved arrow*), and laterally on the walls of the third ventricle (*arrows*)

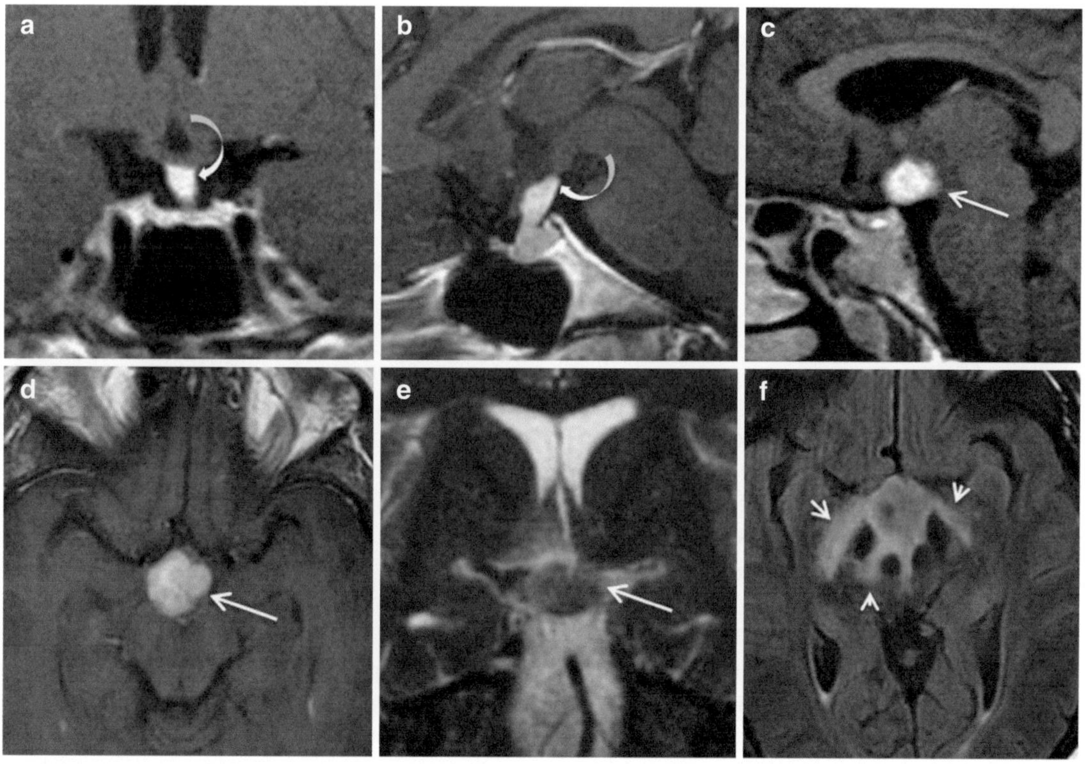

Fig. 41.3 Two examples of neurosarcoidosis with single lesion limited to the suprasellar area. These lesions are rather nonspecific and may be misdiagnosed as histiocytosis or suprasellar tumor such as germinoma, lymphoma, or metastasis. (**a**, **b**) Coronal and sagittal CE T1WIs show a unique lesion thickening the stalk (*curved arrow*). (**c**, **d**) Sagittal and axial CE T1WIs demonstrate in another patient a large, suprasellar, well-defined macronodule limited to the infundibulum (*arrow*). (**e**) Coronal T2 reveals isointensity of the mass lesion, which is surrounded by extensive edema along the optic tracts and the adjacent mesencephalon (*short arrows*), as observed on (**f**) FLAIR image

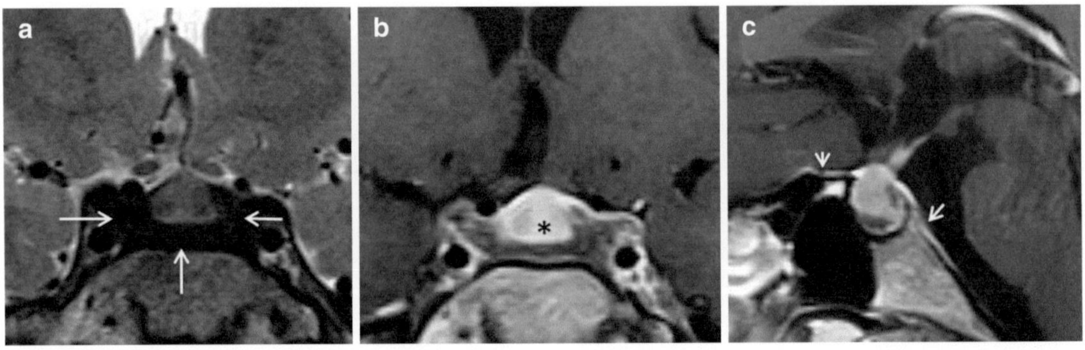

Fig. 41.4 Neurosarcoidosis with intrasellar extrahypophyseal lesion as the sole intracranial manifestation. (**a**) Coronal T2WI depicts abnormal T2 hypointensity along the lateral and inferior edges of the pituitary (*arrows*). This may be interpreted either as a fibrous thickening of the pituitary capsule, as described after hypophysitis, or more likely as a direct infiltration by sarcoidosis of the dural layers of the cavernous sinuses walls adjacent to the adenohypophysis, as suggested by the marked T2 hypointensity. Note that on (**b**) coronal and (**c**) sagittal CE T1WIs, the adenohypophysis (*asterisk*) is convex but normal in size, signal intensity, and gadolinium uptake, only upward shifted and raised by the underlying abnormal nonenhancing thickening. On the sagittal CE T1WI, enhancement of the pre- and postsella dura mater (*short arrows*) confirms actual inflammation, while the patient suffers from headaches but no endocrine symptoms such as hypopituitarism

regress partially or fully under treatment with corticosteroids or other immunosuppressive therapy.

41.2 Histiocytosis

Different types of histiocytosis are associated with tissue accumulation of histiocytes: Langerhans cell histiocytosis (LCH) and non-Langerhans histiocytosis. Lesions of LCH and Erdheim-Chester disease, a rare non-Langerhans histiocytosis, are observed in the sellar area. LCH mainly develops in children aged 1–5 years but a second peak occurs in adulthood. LCH is a multiorgan disease that mostly affects the cranial region, liver, spleen, lymph nodes, and bone. LCH also touches the endocrine system, principally the hypothalamic-pituitary axis, with a predilection for the pituitary stalk, where it can cause deficiencies of both anterior and posterior pituitary functions. Diabetes insipidus is the most frequent endocrine disorder associated with LCH. The stalk involvement in histiocytosis may also be responsible of hyperprolactinemia in 33–50 %, hypopituitarism, and hypogonadotropic hypogonadism.

On MRI, absence of the posterior pituitary bright spot is noticed with or without an associated suprasellar abnormality. The latter may be an infundibular thickening, a stalk enlargement, a small nodule, or even a large hypothalamic mass (Figs. 41.5 and 41.6). Such lesions demonstrate T1 isointensity and enhance markedly after gadolinium administration. Similarly to what is described in sarcoidosis, these granulomatous lesions show T2-low signal intensity, a feature suggestive of the diagnosis, and perilesional edema. Specific additional lesions observed on brain MRI may help to evoke the diagnosis. Although supratentorial intra-axial masses and cerebellar hemisphere T2 hyperintensities can occur in all of these types of histiocytosis, in LCH infiltrative lesion in the pons and lytic lesions of the vault should be sought, while in Erdheim-Chester disease intra-orbital enhancing mass lesions (Fig. 41.7), pachymeningeal thickening, and osteosclerosis of the walls of the sinus are indicative of the diagnosis (Fig. 41.8). Furthermore, in the sella turcica, a peripheral dark rim surrounding the adenohypophysis may also be observed during histiocytosis on T2WI (Fig. 41.8). This sign, described in lymphocytic hypophysitis as a sequel of the

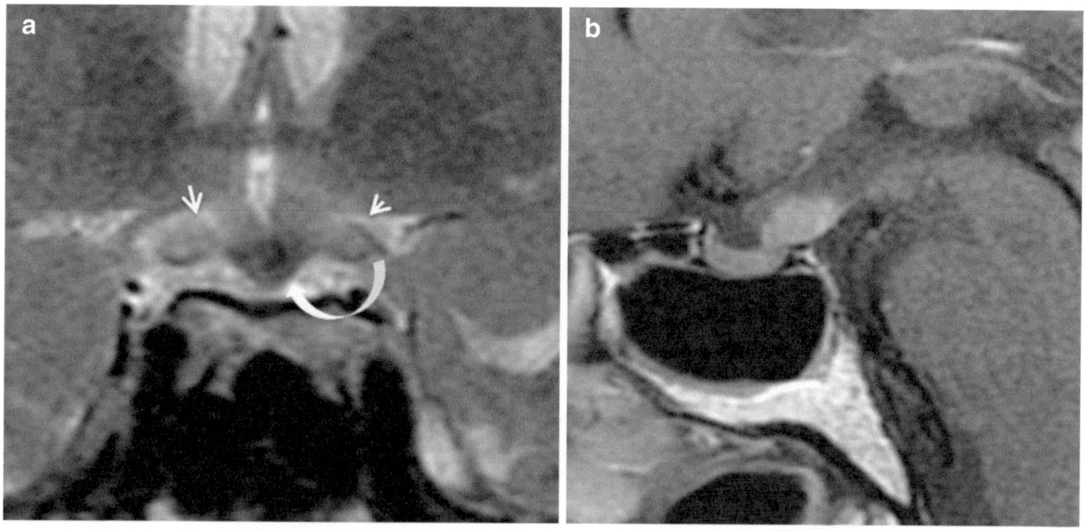

Fig. 41.5 Histiocytosis in a patient with diabetes insipidus. (**a**) Coronal T2WI depicts a hypointense mass lesion of the infundibulum (*arrow*), together with edema in the optic tracts (*short arrows*). The lesion enhances homogeneously after gadolinium administration, as seen on (**b**) sagittal CE T1WI. Note the marked T2 hypointensity of the lesion, a feature suggestive of granulomatosis. The lesion of histiocytosis resembles those of sarcoidosis illustrated in Fig. 41.3

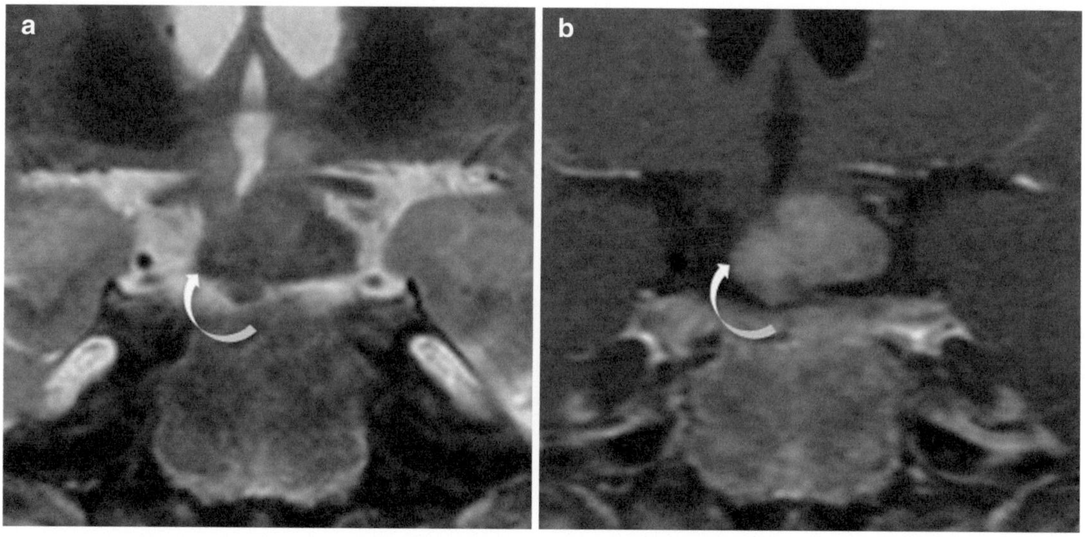

Fig. 41.6 Diabetes insipidus in a patient with already known Erdheim-Chester disease. (**a**) Coronal T2WI depicts a large hypointense mass lesion of the infundibulum (*arrow*) that enhances homogeneously after gadolinium administration, as seen on (**b**) coronal CE T1WI. Similarly to what is observed in other granulomatoses, the lesion also appears with evocative T2 hypointensity in non-Langerhans cell histiocytosis

inflammatory tissue changes, may be consistent with fibrosis. In the setting of granulomatosis that may involve the pachymeninges, such as sarcoidosis and histiocytosis, one may also surmise that these abnormalities could correspond to direct involvement of the disease in the dural layers wrapping the pituitary anterior lobe. Radiation therapy, chemotherapy, or a combination of both are usually proposed to patients with histiocytosis.

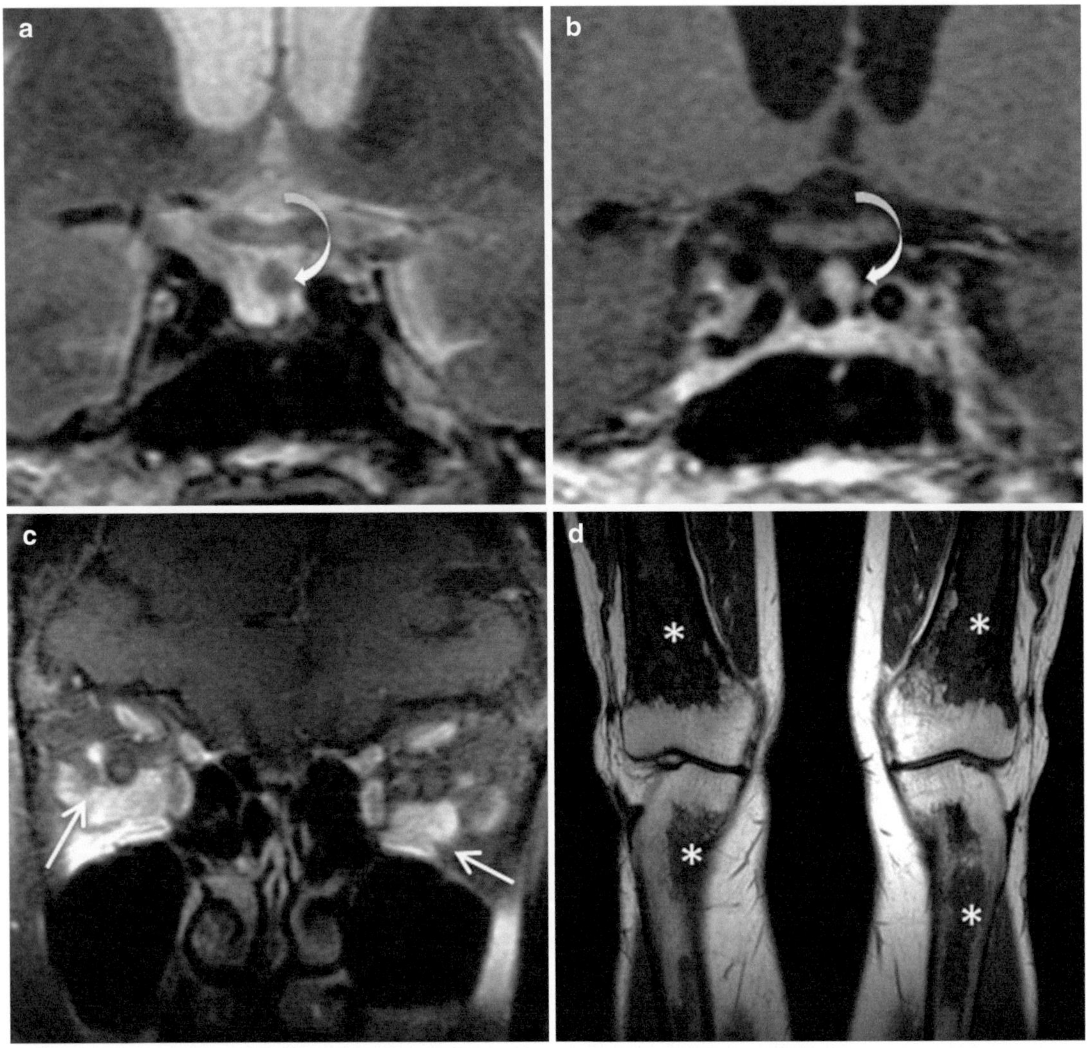

Fig. 41.7 Patient with typical multisystemic lesions in Erdheim-Chester disease. (**a**) Coronal T2WI shows a small hypointense nodule of the stalk (*curved arrow*), that enhances homogeneously after gadolinium administration, as seen on (**b**) coronal CE T1WI. This lesion is not particular and may correspond to sarcoidosis or histiocytosis. Additional specific lesions such as bilateral intraorbital retro-ocular enhancing masses (*arrows*), as seen on (**c**) coronal fat-saturated T1WI, and osteosclerosis of the long bones (*stars*) depicted on (**d**) coronal T1WI, allow establishment of the appropriate diagnosis

41.3 Wegener Granulomatosis

Granulomatosis with polyangiitis (GPA), also known as Wegener granulomatosis, is a granulomatosis associating necrotizing small-vessel vasculitis and giant-cell necrotizing extravascular granulomas. It is known to involve the respiratory tracts, the kidneys, and the ear/nose/throat (ENT) area. Pituitary involvement is usually a late manifestation of GPA, and is associated with ENT lesions. Direct pituitary involvement is extremely rare in GPA, reported in about 1 %, mostly leading to diabetes insipidus and gonadotropin deficiency. The sellar region is more often affected by contiguous extension of an ENT lesion necrotizing the skull base

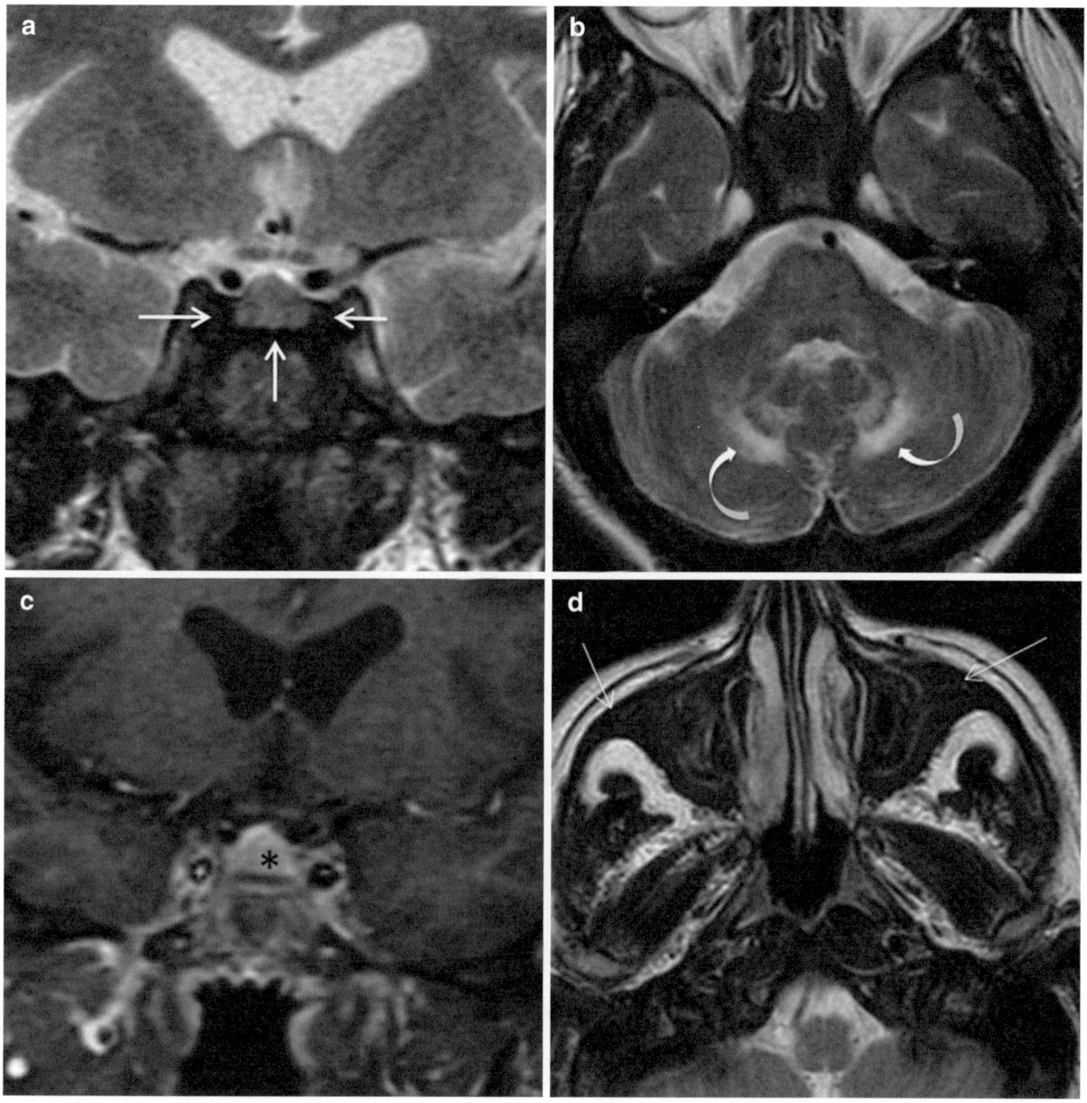

Fig. 41.8 Brain MRI of a patient with Erdheim-Chester disease, ataxia, and headaches, but without pituitary disorders. (**a**, **b**) Coronal T2 and CE T1 WIs demonstrate findings similar to those of sarcoidosis as illustrated in Fig. 41.4, namely an abnormal T2 hypointensity along the lateral and inferior edges of the pituitary (*arrows*), which barely enhances after gadolinium injection, while the adenohypophysis (*asterisk*) is convex but normal in size, signal intensity, and enhancement. On (**c**, **d**) axial T2WIs, other cardinal features of Erdheim-Chester disease are visible and allow one to confirm the diagnosis, such as symmetrical T2 hyperintensities in the peridentate regions (*curved arrows*) and osteosclerosis and dark thickening of the maxillary sinus walls (*thin arrows*)

(Fig. 41.9). When affected by this mechanism, the sella turcica content itself becomes abnormal and demonstrates a pseudoadenoma pattern (Fig. 41.10).

On MRI, similarly to any other granulomatosis, GPA lesions appear with a suggestive T2-low signal intensity and enhance after gadolinium administration. However, lesions of GPA located to the pituitary gland are rather nonspecific and may be similar to lymphocytic hypophysitis or neuroinfundibulohypophysitis (Fig. 41.11). Pituitary enlargement and stalk thickening are the most frequent features, together with and loss of posterior pituitary bright spot on T1WI.

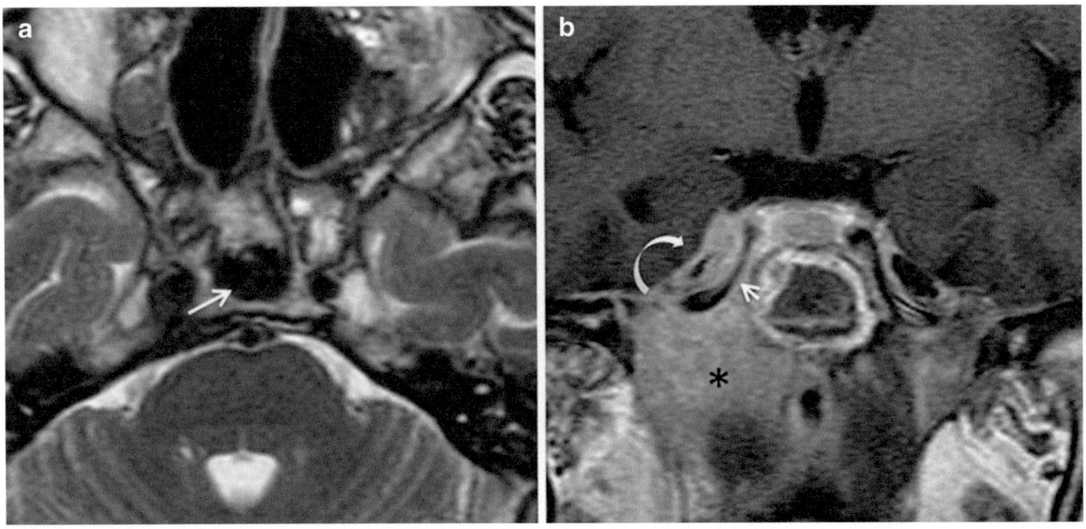

Fig. 41.9 Patient with known Wegener granulomatosis and right facial neuralgia. (**a**) Axial T2WI demonstrates sphenoidal sinus invasion by an ill-defined T2-hypointense lesion (*arrow*). (**b**) Coronal CE T1WI reveals the aggressiveness of the lesion with intracranial extension by contiguity from the parapharyngeal soft tissues (*asterisk*). The right laterosellar region is invaded with partial filling of the Meckel cave (*curved arrow*) and narrowing of the internal carotid artery (*short arrow*), while the adenohypophysis appears normal

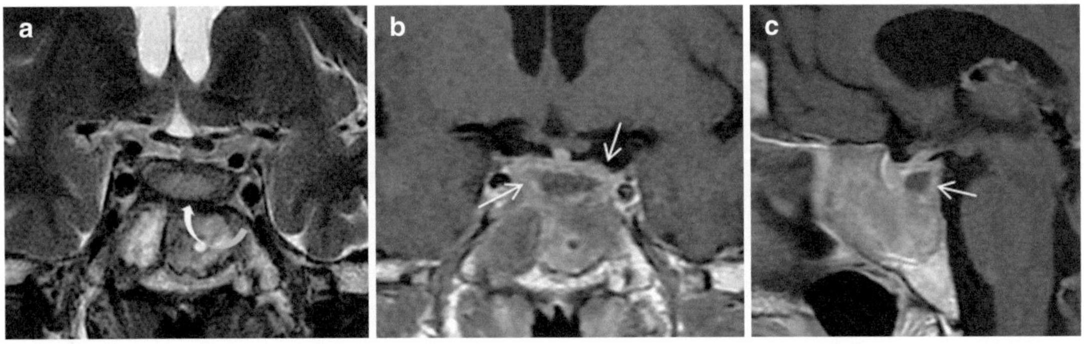

Fig. 41.10 Patient with known Wegener granulomatosis and hypopituitarism. (**a**) Coronal T2WI demonstrates abnormal filling of sphenoidal sinus and a contiguous central hyperintense lesion within the adenohypophysis (*curved arrow*). (**b**, **c**) Coronal and sagittal CE T1WIs demonstrate a rim of peripheral enhancement giving a pseudoadenoma pattern (*arrows*), which in fact may correspond to pituitary necrosis rather than granulomatous infiltration of the gland

41.4 Crohn Disease

Pituitary lesions of Crohn disease are exceptional. They have no specific pattern and appear in our experience as a granulomatous and heterogeneous hypophysitis (Fig. 41.12). We believe that no clue exists to evoke this entity if the underlying disease is unknown.

41.5 IgG4-Associated Multifocal Systemic Fibrosis

Details of this entity are presented in Chap. 40.

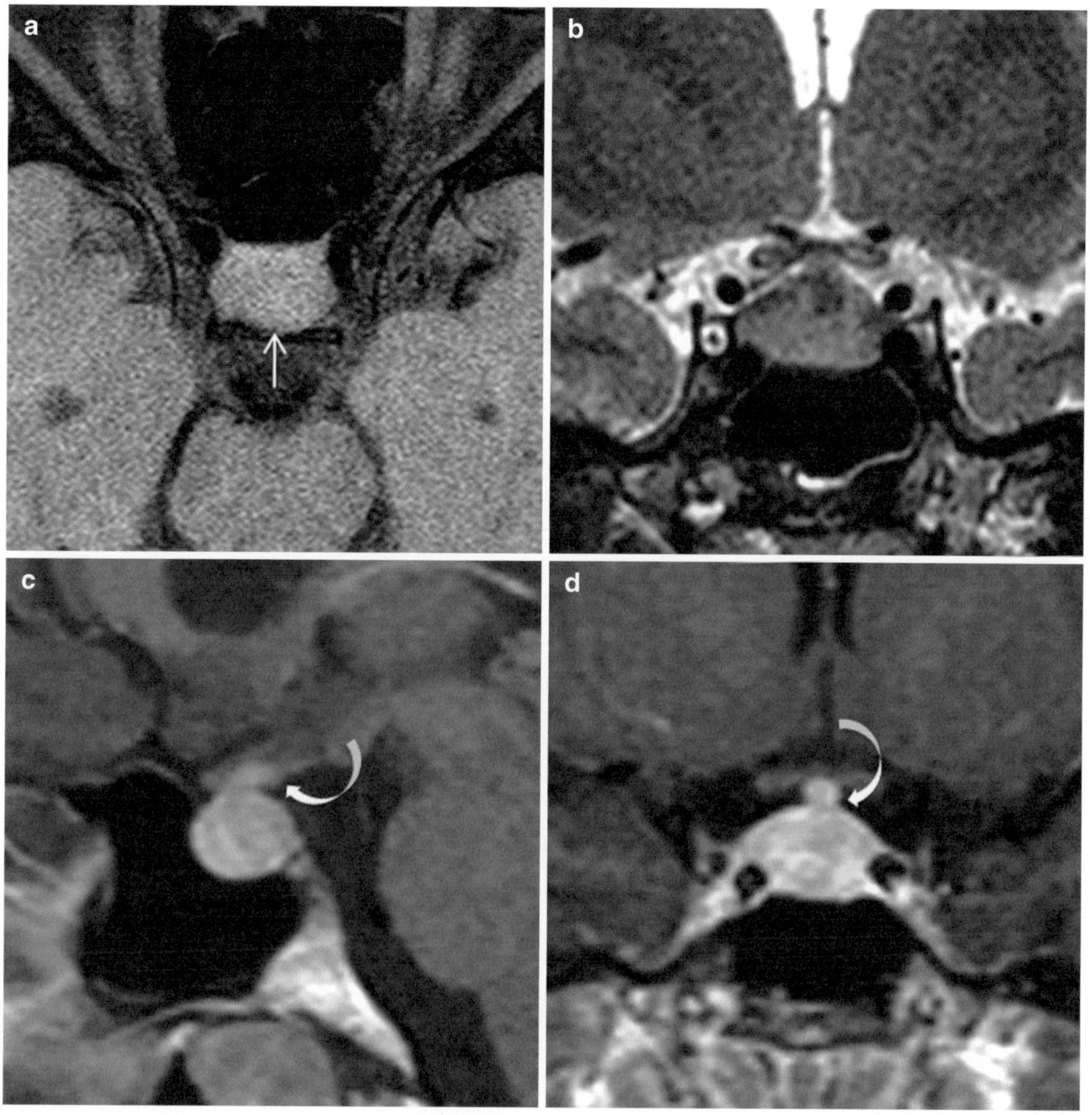

Fig. 41.11 Patient with known Wegener granulomatosis and diabetes insipidus. (**a**) Axial fat-saturated T1WI confirms the central origin of the diabetes insipidus with loss of posterior pituitary bright spot in front of the dorsum sellae (*arrow*). (**b**) Coronal T2WI demonstrates a swelling of the pituitary gland that is abnormally convex. (**c**, **d**) Sagittal and coronal CE T1WIs show an enlargement of both anterior and posterior pituitary lobes together with a thickening of the stalk (*curved arrows*)

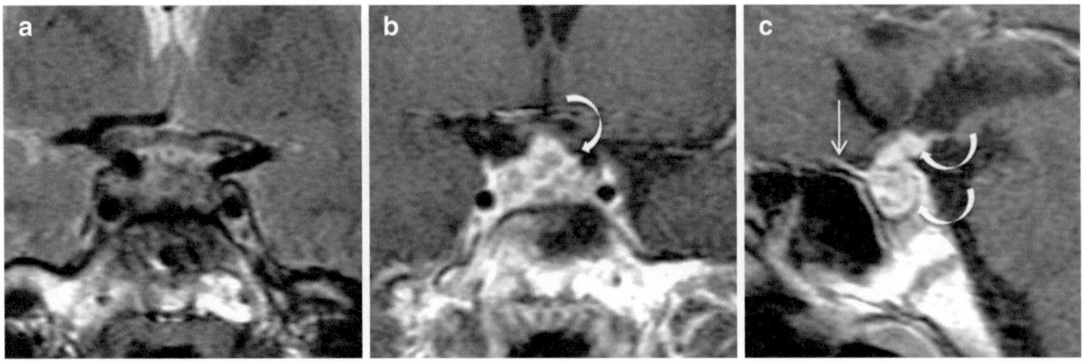

Fig. 41.12 Patient with proven Crohn disease and rapid onset of headaches and hypopituitarism. (**a**) Coronal T2WI shows a heterogeneous infiltration of the adenohypophysis. (**b**, **c**) Coronal and sagittal CE T1WIs demonstrate a granulomatous infiltrative lesion enlarging both the anterior pituitary lobe and the neurohypophysis (*curved arrows*), with heterogeneous enhancement. Note also the abnormal presellar dural enhancement (*arrow*), a feature described in hypophysitis

Further Reading

De Parisot A, Pue'chal X, Langrand C et al (2015) Pituitary involvement in granulomatosis with polyangiitis. Report of 9 patients and review of the literature. Medicine 94:e748

Kurtulmus N, Mert M, Tanakol R, Yarman S (2014) The pituitary gland in patients with Langerhans cell histiocytosis: a clinical and radiological evaluation. Endocrine 48:949–956

Langrand C, Bihan H, Raverot G et al (2012) Hypothalamo-pituitary sarcoidosis: a multicenter study of 24 patients. Q J Med 105:981–995

Pituitary Abscess

42

Fabrice Bonneville

Intracranial infectious pathologies mainly include meningitis, encephalitis, brain abscesses, and ventriculitis. Infectious processes located in the sellar region are rare, and even rarer when abscesses limited to the pituitary gland itself are considered. Pituitary abscesses represent less than 1 % of all pituitary lesions. Pathophysiology of pituitary abscesses consists in a contiguous spreading of a local infection arising from the sphenoid sinus, the surrounding meninges of the basal cisterns or a thrombophlebitis of the cavernous sinus. Direct hematogenous seeding to the gland itself also exists. Patients with pituitary abscess usually present with either sudden or long-lasting headaches or anterior pituitary deficiency. Fever is rarely present, and symptoms of bacteremia are usually absent. Other symptoms related to the mass effect of large abscesses may be observed, such as visual disturbances and diabetes insipidus. Pituitary abscesses are primary lesions of the pituitary gland, but about one-third develop on a pre-existing lesion such as pituitary adenoma, Rathke cleft cyst (RCC), or craniopharyngioma. Necrosis and hemorrhage in pituitary adenoma may facilitate their secondary infection (Fig. 42.1). Abscesses may also complicate transsphenoidal surgery.

While streptococci and staphylococci are the most common infectious agents leading to pituitary abscesses, a wide variety of Gram-positive and Gram-negative bacteria, anaerobic bacteria, and fungi might also be the source of pituitary abscess. Mycobacterial tuberculosis and fungal pituitary abscess have also been observed in patients receiving chemotherapy or in immunosuppressed patients (Fig. 42.2). However, cultures of abscess material have been negative in approximately 50 % of cases reported in the literature. Broad-spectrum antibiotic therapy effective against Gram-negative, Gram-positive, and anaerobic bacteria should thus be started as soon as the diagnosis of pituitary abscess is suspected or confirmed by surgery.

While the diagnosis of pituitary abscess is usually made subsequent to surgery, the typical MRI findings may be important for the preoperative diagnosis of this potentially life-threatening disorder. Suggestive features of a pituitary abscess are a sellar/suprasellar cystic mass that appears hypointense or isointense on T1WI and hyperintense or isointense T2WI, and always show peripheral ring enhancement after gadolinium administration. The peripheral capsule may demonstrate spontaneous T1 hyperintense signal (Fig. 42.3). Of note, no internal enhancement is depicted in pituitary abscess. The ring enhancement is regular in pituitary abscess, while noncomplicated cystic adenoma and craniopharyngioma usually show thick and nodular wall enhancement. RCCs lack peripheral enhancement when not complicated. In satellites to the sellar abscess, abnormal signals are also observed in the suprasellar or parasellar regions, representing local edema, brain abscesses, or thickening of the adjacent meninges. DWI may also be useful to differentiate pituitary abscesses from other cystic or necrotic

J.-F. Bonneville et al., *MRI of the Pituitary Gland*, DOI 10.1007/978-3-319-29043-0_42

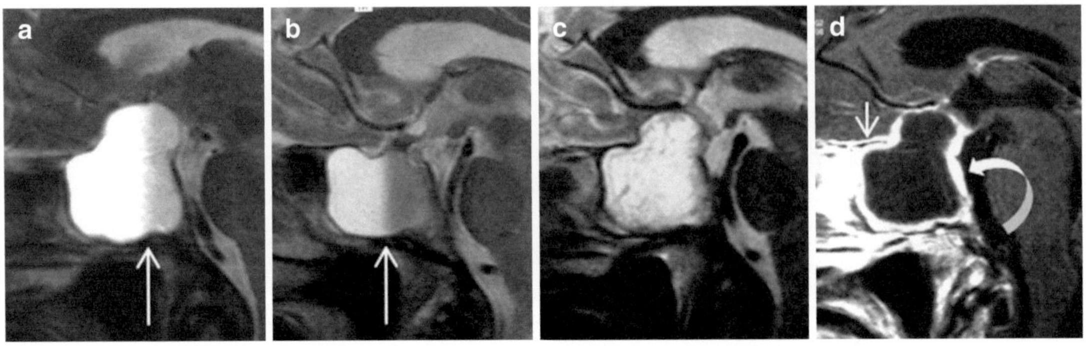

Fig. 42.1 Pneumococcus pituitary abscess. (**a–c**) Sagittal T2WIs. (**a**) Hemorrhagic macroprolactinoma invading sphenoid sinus in a 62-year-old-woman. Prolactin level is 200 ng/ml. Fluid-fluid level (*long arrow*). (**b**) Rapid adenoma shrinkage after cabergoline 1 mg/week. Prolactin is 30 ng/ml. (**c**) Six months later, meningitis with pneumococcus found in CSF. Re-expansion of the sellar content with caseous pattern T2 signal. (**d**) Sagittal CE T1WI. Marked enhancement of a thick peripheral rim (*curved arrow*) and dural enhancement (*short arrow*)

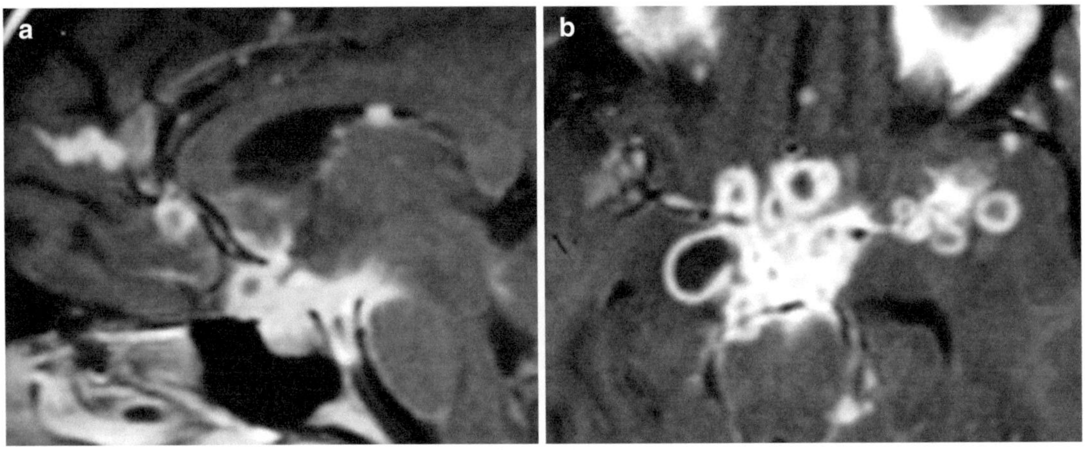

Fig. 42.2 Mycobacteria tuberculosis meningoencephalitis with suprasellar location. (**a**, **b**) Sagittal and axial CE T1WIs show typical features suggestive of tuberculosis, with grape-like confluence of multiple tuberculomas gathered in the basal cisterns and the suprasellar region, but also spread, with hematogenous distribution in the brain cortex

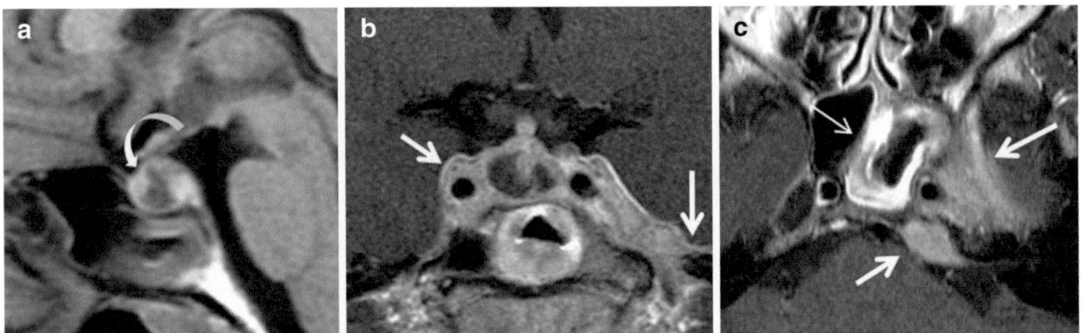

Fig. 42.3 *Klebsiella* pituitary abscess in an immunocompromised patient. (**a**) Sagittal T1WI shows a heterogeneous isointense sellar lesion with hyperintense edges (*curved arrow*). (**b**) Coronal CE T1WI demonstrates peripheral enhancement of the lesion. Note abnormal thickening of the lateral walls of both cavernous sinuses spreading along the dura beneath the left temporal lobe (*thick arrows*). (**c**) Axial CE T1WI confirms the left extension of the process with focal thickening at the petrous apex and filling of the adjacent Meckel cave. Note also the abnormal thickening of the mucosa of the sphenoid sinus (*thin arrows*)

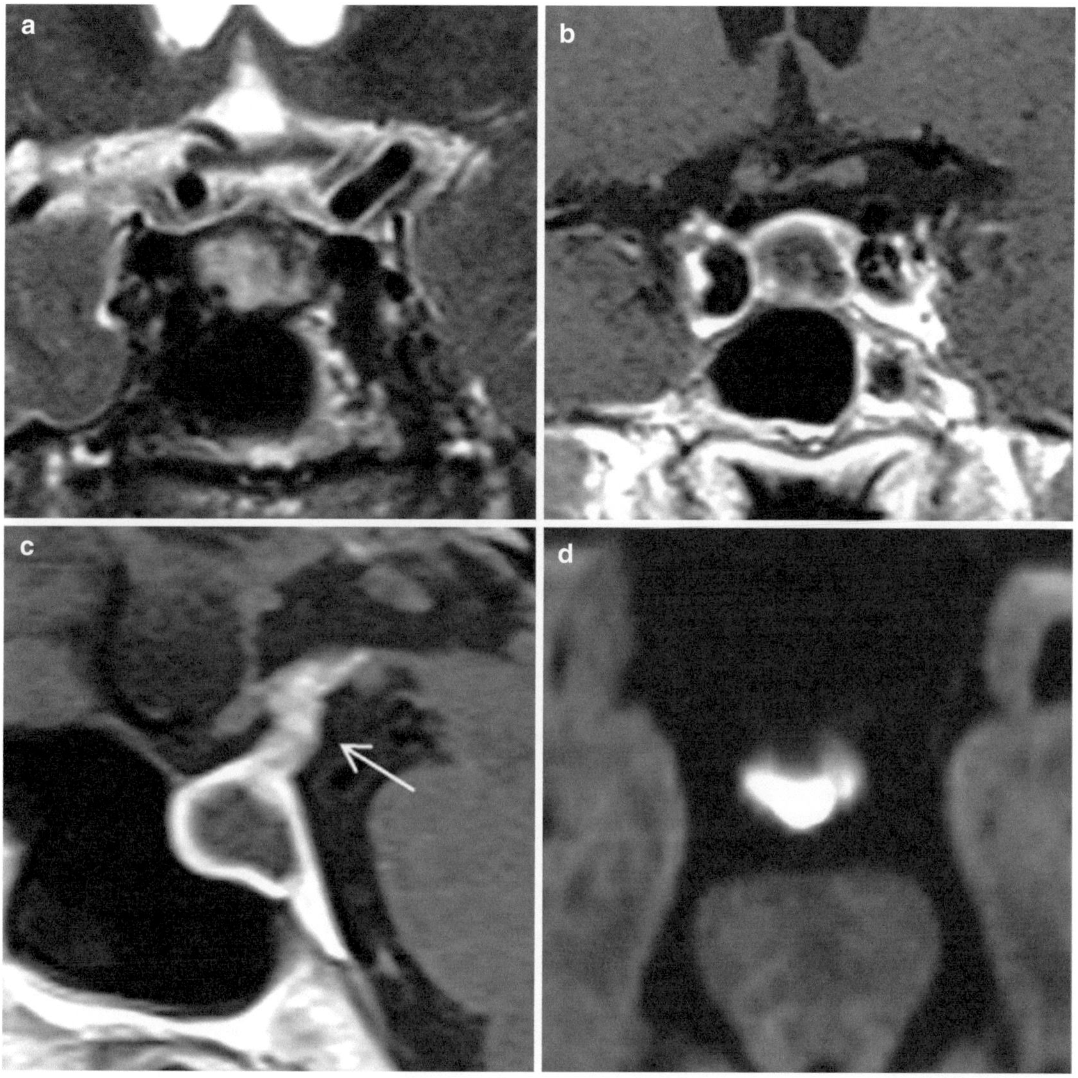

Fig. 42.4 *Staphylococcus* pituitary abscess. (**a**) Coronal T2WI shows heterogeneous nonspecific hyperintense sellar lesion. (**b**, **c**) Coronal and sagittal CE T1WIs reveal peripheral enhancement of this intrasellar lesion with unusual thickening of the stalk (*arrow*). Note the lack of other abnormalities such as mucosal thickening in the sphenoid sinus or enhancement of the adjacent meninges. (**d**) DWI returns a hyperintense signal of the purulent content of the abscess, a finding usually not observed in cystic adenoma, RCC, or craniopharyngioma (Courtesy of Ch. Magni, MD)

sellar lesions (Fig. 42.4). While pituitary abscesses demonstrate a very suggestive content with hyperintense signal and reduction of apparent diffusion coefficient, necrotic tumors show a low diffusion-weighted signal intensity and corresponding elevated ADC values.

Therefore, physicians should consider the existence of pituitary abscess in patients with a recent history of paranasal sinusitis, meningitis, or inflammatory syndrome, who develop manifestations of anterior pituitary insufficiency or diabetes insipidus, and in whom MRI demonstrates a ring-enhancing cystic pituitary lesion with locoregional abnormalities such as mucosal thickening in the sphenoid sinus, brain edema, or gadolinium enhancement of the adjacent meninges.

Finally, in endemic regions, one should consider neurocysticercosis when facing multiple nonenhancing CSF-like cysts of the subarachnoid spaces on MRI (Fig. 42.5). Such a racemous form of the disease may involve the basal cisterns and the sellar region.

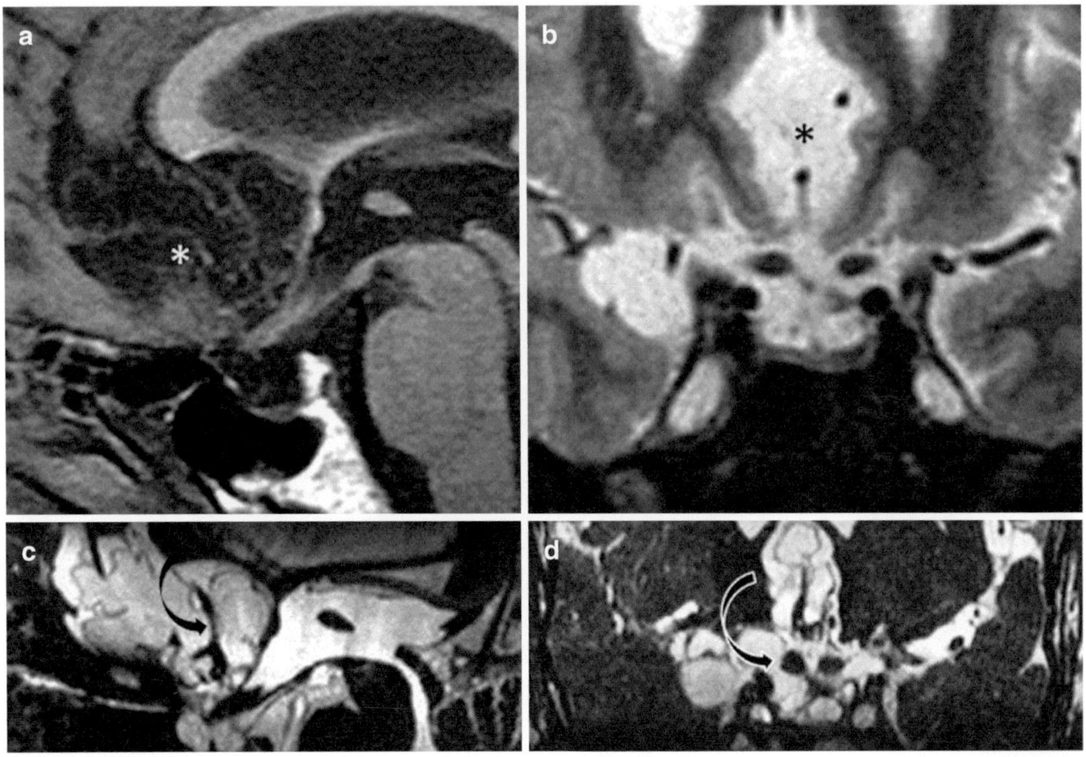

Fig. 42.5 Racemous form of neurocysticercosis. (**a**) Sagittal T1WI shows suprasellar hypointense lesions impinging the suprasellar cistern and the basofrontal region (*asterisk*). (**b**) Coronal T2 WI demonstrates the extra-axial location of these multiple cysts invading the optochiasmatic cistern and interhemispheric fissure (*asterisk*). Signal intensity is similar to that of CSF, as shown in arachnoid cyst. (**c**, **d**) Sagittal and coronal reformatted heavily T2WIs nicely depict the membranes delineating those cysts. Anterior cerebral arteries (*black arrow*) and optic chiasm and optic nerves (*black and white arrow*) are encased by the cysts, a feature not seen in arachnoid cyst, which gently push away neurovascular structures (Courtesy of H. Siqueira Lima, MD)

Further Reading

Fuyi L, Giulin L, Yong Y et al (2011) Diagnosis and management of pituitary abscess: experiences from 33 cases. Clin Endocrinol 74:79–88

Wan L, Yao Y, Feng F et al (2014) Pituitary abscess following transsphenoidal surgery: the experience of 12 cases from a single institution. Clin Neurol Neurosurg 124:66–71

Zhang X, Sun J, Shen M et al (2012) Diagnosis and minimally invasive surgery for the pituitary abscess: a review of twenty nine cases. Clin Neurol Neurosurg 114:957–961

43 Empty Sella

Jean-François Bonneville

The term empty sella refers to the extension of the subarachnoid space within the sella turcica; therefore, the sella is not really empty but filled with CSF: the term "intrasellar arachnoidocele" is sometimes preferred, but "empty sella" remains the customary term. Differential diagnosis includes intrasellar cysts and necrotic pituitary adenomas. The clue is demonstration of a CSF-filled sella with an elongated pituitary stalk attached to a flattened pituitary gland at the level of the sellar floor. The pituitary stalk is frequently pressed against the dorsum (Fig. 43.1) and better seen on coronal T1WI. It can be blurred by flow artifacts on T2WI (Fig. 43.2). These flow artifacts from CSF pulsations are not seen in cysts or intrasellar tumors. An incomplete sellar diaphragm can sometimes be visualized. Demonstration of an empty sella during an imaging checkup is frequent and raises questions. Is it a primary or secondary empty sella? Can it be responsible for headache, visual symptoms, or endocrinologic disorders? Is a "partial empty sella" a true abnormality or should it be ignored in the radiological report? It is worth remembering here that a flattened pituitary gland and, therefore, a partial empty sella, is common in the elderly without any hormonal deficit. Diagnosis of secondary empty sella is easy in cases of a history of pituitary tumor shrinkage, occurring spontaneously or more frequently after medical treatment, apoplexy, surgery, or radiotherapy. In these cases, the sella is usually enlarged. Diagnosis of secondary empty sella is less simple if there is no known definite pathological process involving the pituitary gland; it can be after undiagnosed postpartum pituitary necrosis, hypophysitis, or complicated Rathke cleft cyst (RCC). In these cases, the sella can be of normal size. In most cases of secondary empty sella, a small normal pituitary gland remnant can be found at the bottom of the sella, and hormonal deficit may or may not be present. The posterior lobe is either ectopic or pressed against the dorsum sellae, and only visible on axial T1WI. Diabetes insipidus is rare. Mild hyperprolactinemia (<50 ng/ml) resulting from stalk effect may be noted. In large empty sella, ptosis of optic nerves or even of the inferior part of third ventricle may be rarely responsible for unclear visual symptoms (Fig. 43.3). Headache, if present, is usually unrelated to the presence of empty sella except in the context of benign chronic intracranial hypertension (Fig. 43.4). Bone erosion can exceptionally lead to a CSF fistula and rhinorrhea (Fig. 43.5).

Primary empty sella is unrelated to any pathology of the sellar region. In most patients, primary empty sella is an incidental finding while in 20 % of patients, mainly men, some degree of anterior pituitary deficiency, particularly growth hormone deficiency, may be noted. For this reason, an endocrine evaluation can be recommended in adult

J.-F. Bonneville et al., *MRI of the Pituitary Gland*, DOI 10.1007/978-3-319-29043-0_43

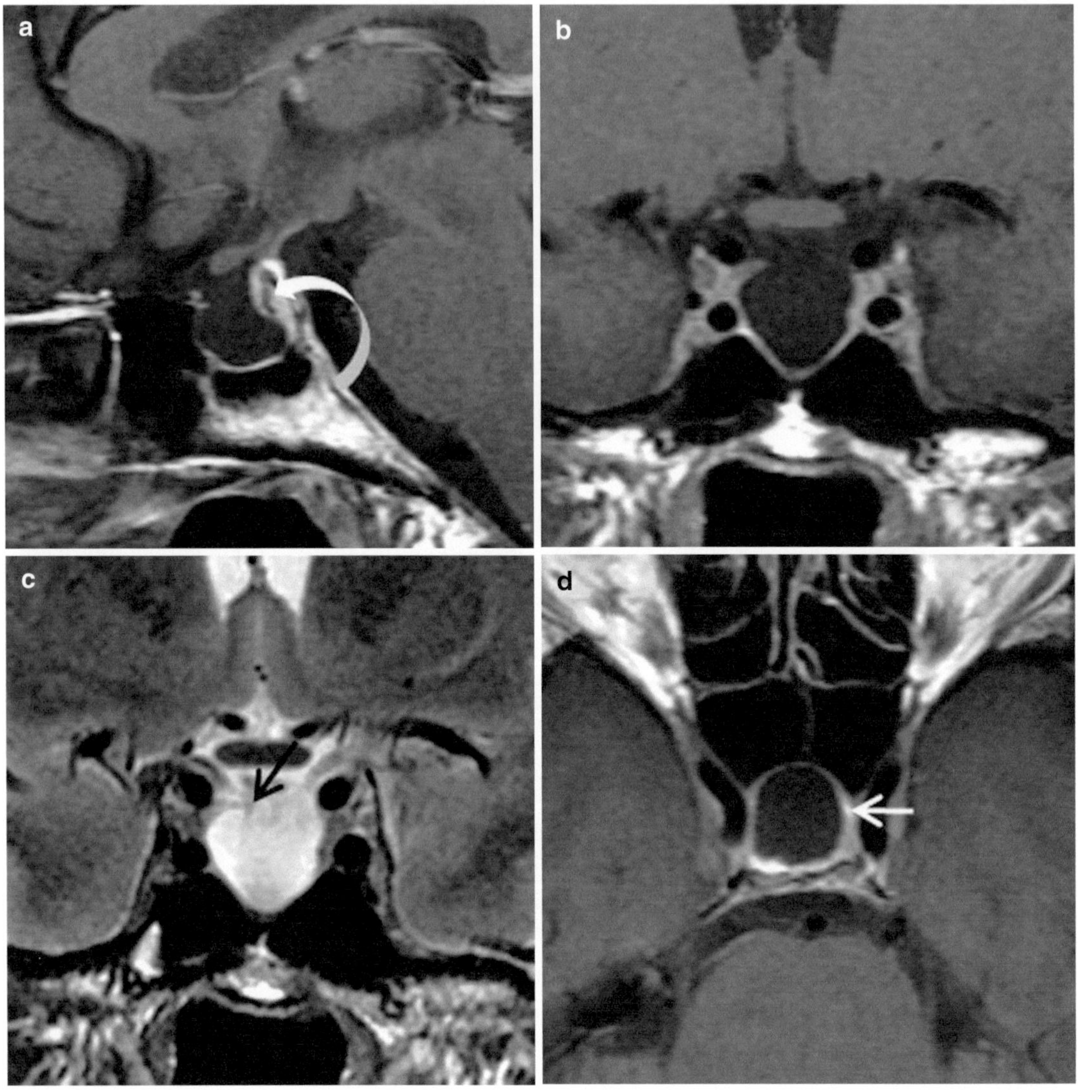

Fig. 43.1 Primary empty sella. (**a**–**d**) Sagittal T1, coronal CE T1, coronal T2, and axial CE T1 WIs. Incompetent sellar diaphragm (*black arrow*). Thin residual anterior pituitary tissue (*white arrow*). Pituitary stalk pressed against the dorsum sellae (*curved arrow*)

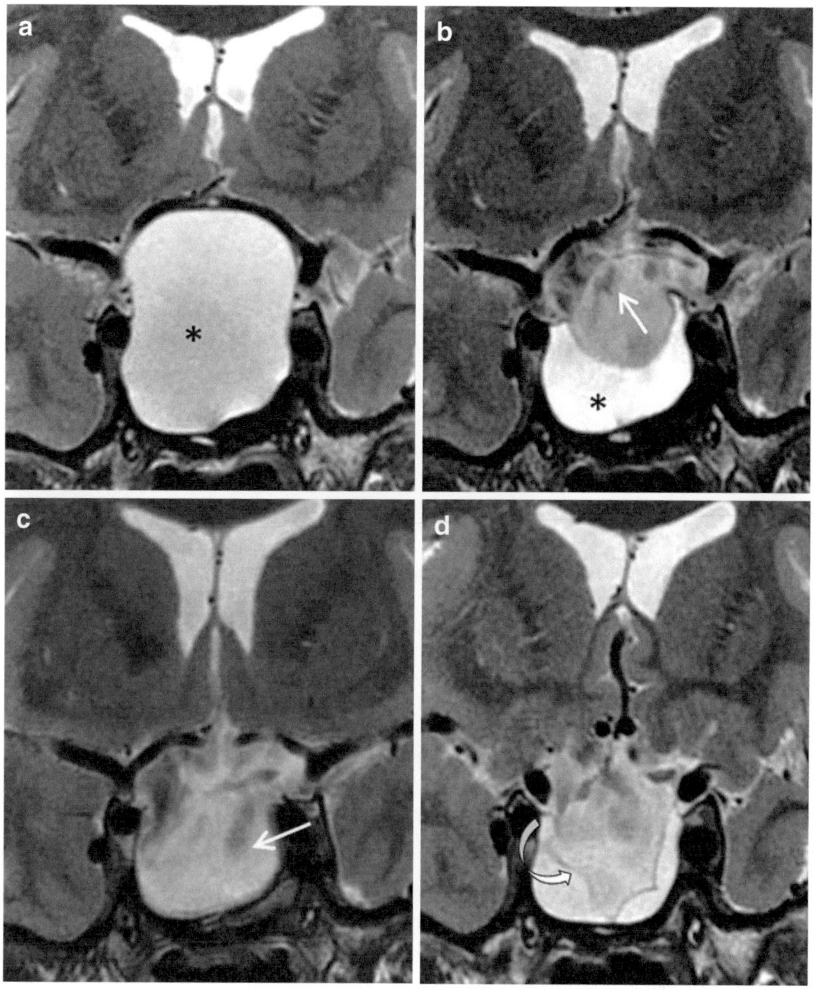

Fig. 43.2 Secondary empty sella. (**a**–**d**) Coronal T2WIs. (**a**) At diagnosis. Large T2-hyperintense RCC (*asterisk*) with intra- and suprasellar extension. (**b**) After cyst puncture. (**c**, **d**) Two and 12 months later. After cyst puncture (**b**), partial shrinkage of the cyst; flow artifacts (*white arrow*) in the subarachnoid spaces, not in the residual cyst (*asterisk*). Later on, after a second cyst puncture (**c**), complete cyst shrinkage; flow artifacts extend into the secondary empty sella. Partial recurrence at 12 months (**d**). The cyst wall (*curved arrow*) is floating at the upper surface of the recurrent cyst

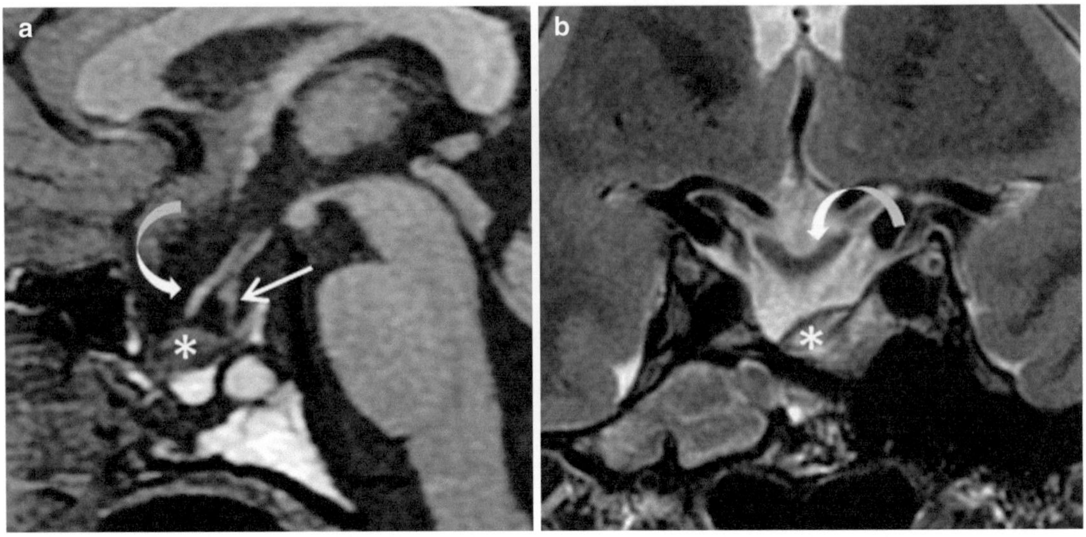

Fig. 43.3 Secondary empty sella 10 years after transsphenoidal pituitary surgery. (**a**) Sagittal T1 and (**b**) coronal T2WIs. Ptosis of the optic chiasm and optic nerves (*curved arrow*). Pituitary stalk (*straight arrow*). Small tumoral remnant (*asterisk*)

patients (not in the elderly) on incidental discovery of a primitive empty sella. Primitive or acquired sellar diaphragm incompetence is so frequent that it cannot be held responsible for all empty sellae. Chronic elevated CSF pressure secondary to obesity has been proposed as a risk factor, in addition to the rare occurrence of benign intracranial hypertension. The role of multiple pregnancies is fairly certain: at each pregnancy, both the pituitary gland and sella enlarge; the pituitary gland shrinks after delivery, but the sella remains slightly enlarged. Ultimately the sella is too large for the pituitary gland, permitting CSF to penetrate the sella. We have hypothesized that nonpneumatization of the posterior part of sphenoid sinus could be an adjunctive facilitating factor: deepening of the sella could be facilitated if the sellar floor is in contact with cancellous bone and not with the more resistant cortical bone bordering the sphenoid sinus. Finally, an empty sella can be found incidentally in asymptomatic patients with global enlargement of subarachnoid spaces such as the oculomotor nerve sheaths, the gasserian ganglion cistern, or the cerebellar cistern (Fig. 43.6).

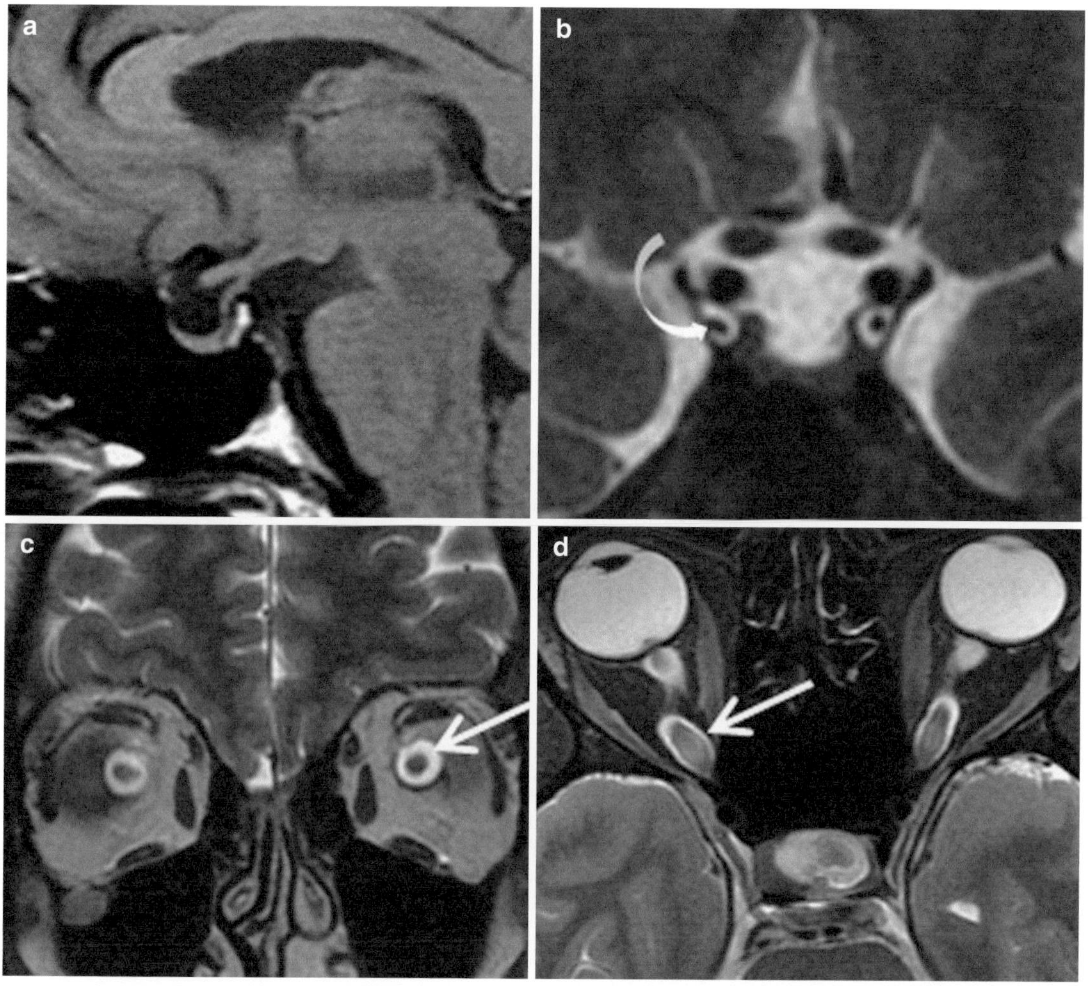

Fig. 43.4 Empty sella and benign intracranial hypertension. Chronic headache in a 28-year-old man. (**a**) Sagittal T1. (**b**, **c**) Coronal T2 and (**d**) axial T2 WIs. Enlargement of the oculomotor nerves sheaths (*curved arrow*) and optic nerve sheaths (*straight arrow*)

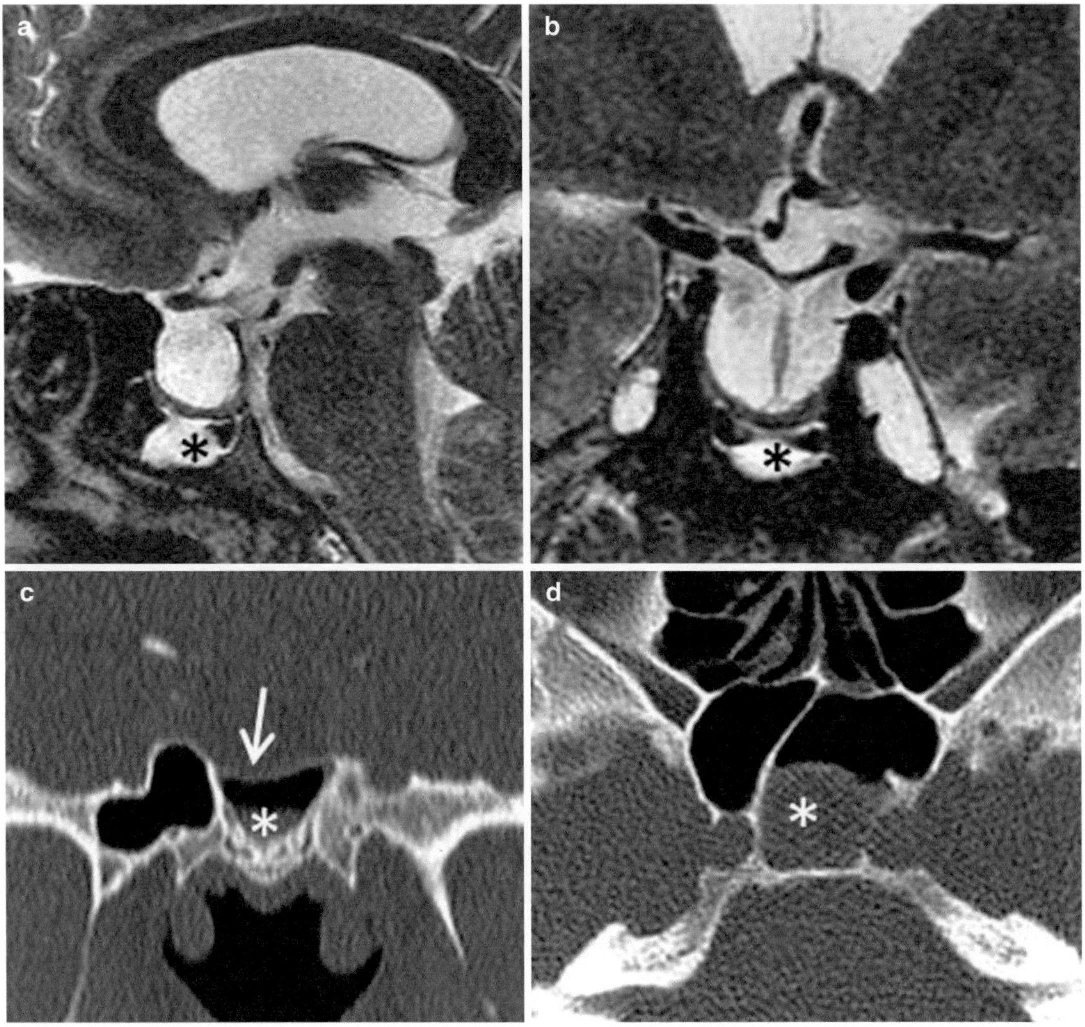

Fig. 43.5 Rhinorrhea, meningitis, and empty sella in a 49-year-old multiparous woman. (**a**, **b**) Sagittal and coronal T2WIs. (**c**, **d**) Coronal and axial CT, bone window. Extreme thinness of the sellar floor (*arrow*). CSF-like effusion in the sphenoid sinus (*asterisk*)

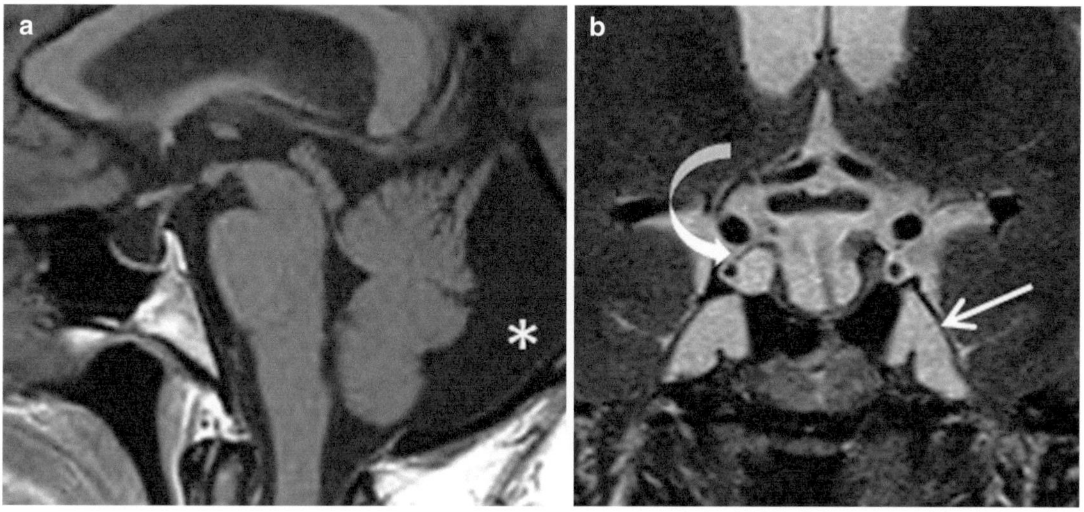

Fig. 43.6 Primary empty sella in a 36-year-old man with large subarachnoid spaces. (**a**, **b**) Sagittal T1 and coronal T2 WIs. Large retrocerebellar cistern (*asterisk*). Enlargement of oculomotor nerve sheaths (*curved arrow*) and gasserian ganglion cistern (*straight arrow*)

Further Reading

Aruna P, Sowjanya B, Reddy PA et al (2014) Partial empty sella syndrome: a case report and review. Indian J Clin Biochem 29(2):253–256

De Marinis L, Bonadonna S, Bianchi A et al (2005) Primary empty sella. J Clin Endocrinol Metab 90(9):5471–5477

Guitelman M, Basavilbaso NG, Vitale M et al (2013) Primary empty sella: a review of 175 cases. Pituitary 16:270–27

Sheehan Syndrome

44

Jean-François Bonneville

Sheehan syndrome corresponds to a pituitary necrosis following severe postpartum hemorrhage and hypovolemia. It has been suggested that a small sella may be a risk factor and play a role in the pathogenesis of the necrosis. Improvement in obstetric care, blood transfusion, and embolization of uterine arteries have permitted a drastic reduction in the frequency of this complication in Western countries. Sheehan syndrome may manifest itself very early after delivery, with headache and hypopituitarism responsible for lack of milk production immediately or some weeks later. Hyponatremia can also be observed. More usually, Sheehan syndrome is diagnosed years later.

Early neuroimaging is of uppermost importance, in particular to differentiate pituitary necrosis of Sheehan syndrome from lymphocytic hypophysitis, pituitary apoplexia, or other causes of postpartum headache such as cerebral thrombophlebitis, posterior reversible encephalopathy syndrome, or even intracranial hypotension following failed epidural anesthesia.

In the few days after the ischemic infarct, MRI typically shows an enlarged, nonhemorrhagic pituitary gland. However, this diagnosis of "enlarged" pituitary is not easy, the normal pituitary gland being possibly as high as 12 mm in the immediate postpartum period. On T1WI, the signal of the sellar content appears hypointense if compared with its normal reference, the cerebral white matter (Figs. 44.1 and 44.2). On T2WI, the pituitary gland can be heterogeneous with hyperintense foci, very similar to what is shown in hypophysitis. Gadolinium injection makes the difference: when the pituitary enhances strongly with hypophysitis, only a peripheral enhanced rim is observed in patients with Sheehan syndrome (Fig. 44.3). A dural enhancement is demonstrated in addition to thickening of the sphenoidal mucosa.

Diagnosis of Sheehan syndrome is usually made late, sometimes as late as 20 or even 30 years after the hemorrhagic event. For this reason, it has been suggested that an autoimmune process involving the pituitary gland and the hypothalamus may also contribute to late pituitary insufficiency. Pituitary hormone deficiencies involve almost always GH, followed by gonadotropins, ACTH, and TSH. Diabetes insipidus is rare.

The pituitary gland becomes atrophic, making possible irruption of CSF within the sella, and a so-called empty sella develops (see Chap. 43). It has been proposed that empty sella in Sheehan syndrome has the particularity of being of normal size (Fig. 44.4) and not enlarged, as is usually the case in empty sella related to sellar diaphragm incompetence or multiparity. This is debatable because it is not infrequent that Sheehan syndrome affects multiparous women in whom the sella has been progressively enlarged by successive pregnancies. On the other hand, long-term pulsating CSF in the empty sella, regardless of its pathogenesis, leads to a deepening of the sella.

J.-F. Bonneville et al., *MRI of the Pituitary Gland*, DOI 10.1007/978-3-319-29043-0_44

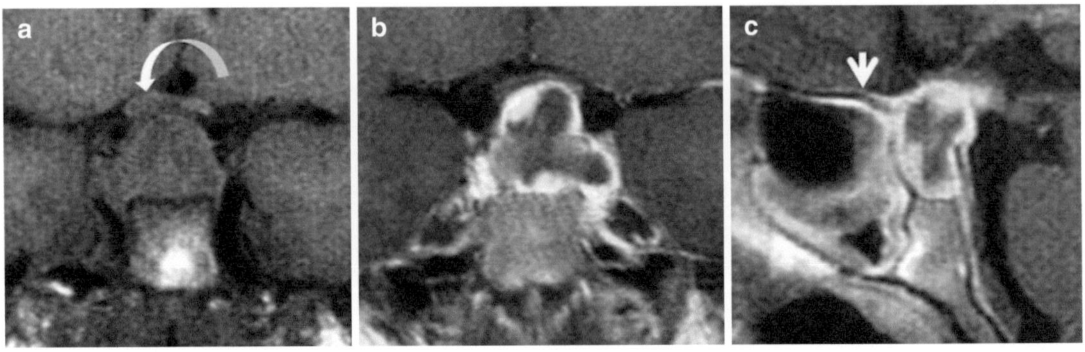

Fig. 44.1 Acute Sheehan syndrome in a 38-year-old woman with severe vaginal bleeding and collapsus 2 days after delivery. (**a**, **b**) Coronal T1 and CE T1 WIs. Enlarged T1-hypointense pituitary gland abutting the optic chiasm (*arrow*). Peripheral rim of enhancement in (**b**). (**c**) Sagittal CE T1WI. Rim enhancement associated with dural enhancement (*short arrow*) and thickening of sphenoid mucosa

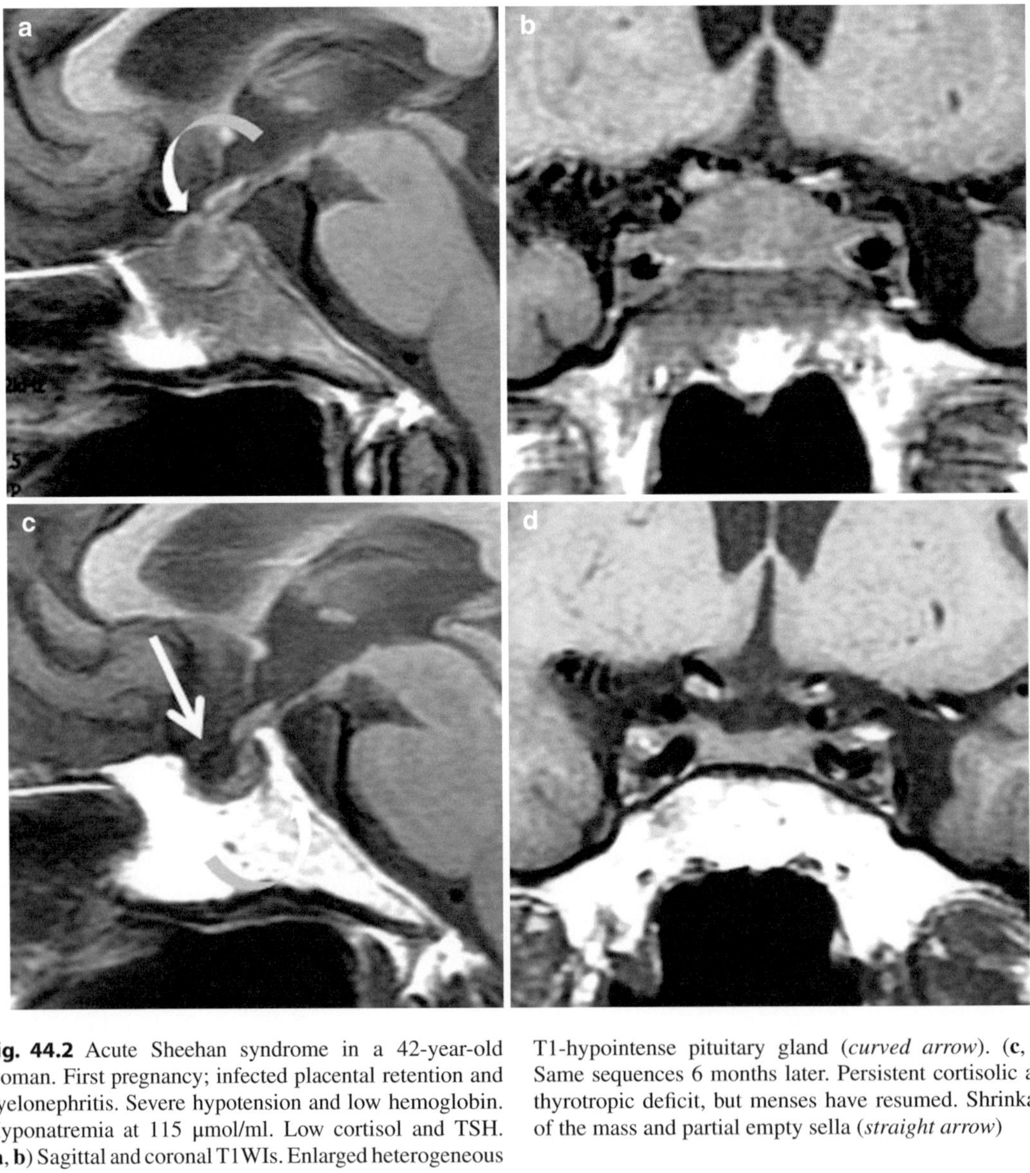

Fig. 44.2 Acute Sheehan syndrome in a 42-year-old woman. First pregnancy; infected placental retention and pyelonephritis. Severe hypotension and low hemoglobin. Hyponatremia at 115 μmol/ml. Low cortisol and TSH. (**a**, **b**) Sagittal and coronal T1WIs. Enlarged heterogeneous T1-hypointense pituitary gland (*curved arrow*). (**c**, **d**) Same sequences 6 months later. Persistent cortisolic and thyrotropic deficit, but menses have resumed. Shrinkage of the mass and partial empty sella (*straight arrow*)

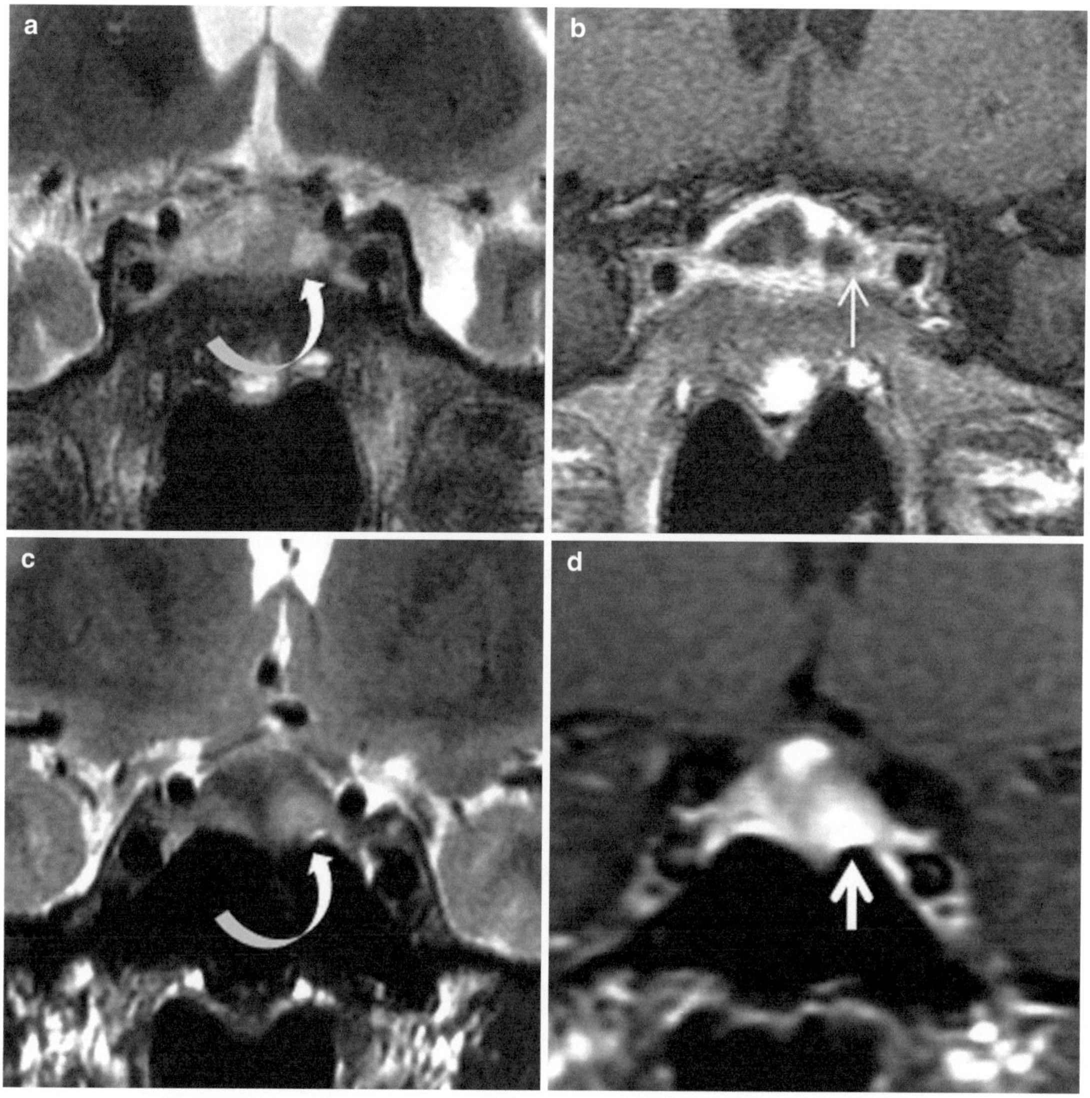

Fig. 44.3 (**a**, **b**) Coronal T2 and CE T1 WIs in same patient as Fig. 44.2 compared with (**c**, **d**) coronal T2 and dynamic CE T1 WIs in a patient with lymphocytic hypophysitis. In both patients, demonstration of areas of T2 hyperintensity (*curved arrows*) and corresponding areas of nonenhancement (*thin arrow*) in Sheehan syndrome (**b**), and strong enhancement (*thick arrow*) in hypophysitis (**d**)

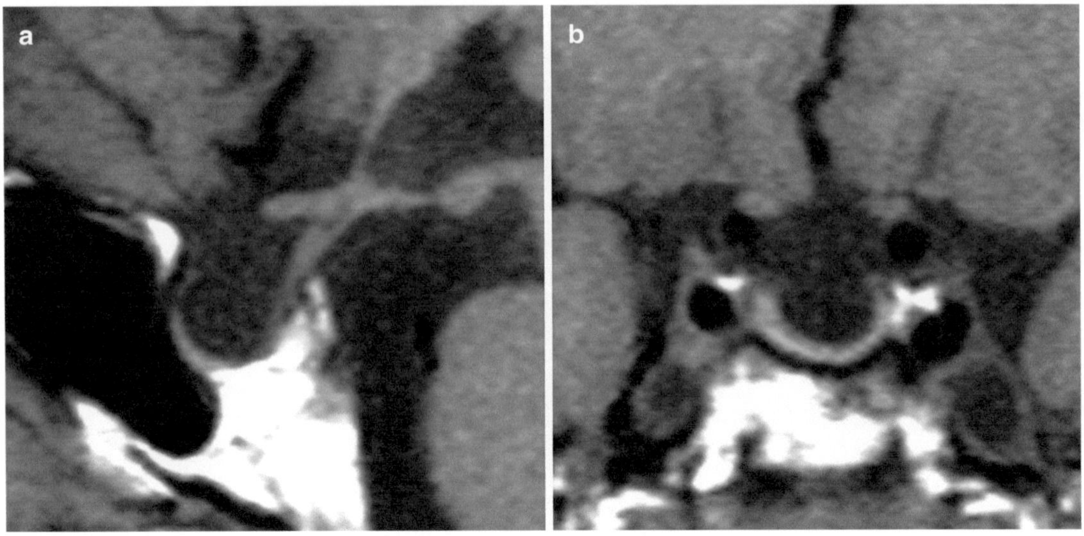

Fig. 44.4 Progressive hypopituitarism in a 57-year-old woman with history of massive hemorrhage at delivery 20 years previously. (**a**, **b**) Sagittal and coronal T1WIs. Partial empty sella. The sella turcica is not enlarged

Further Reading

Bakiri F, Bendib SE, Maoui R et al (1991) The sella turcica in Sheehan syndrome: computerized tomographic study in 54 patients. J Endocrinol Invest 14(3): 193–196

Keleştimur F (2003) Sheehan syndrome. Pituitary 6(4):181–188

Sert M, Tetiker T, Kirim S et al (2003) Clinical report of 28 patients with Sheehan syndrome. Endocr J 50(3):297–301

45 Pituitary Hyperplasia and Primary Hypothyroidism

Jean-François Bonneville

Pituitary enlargement in primary hypothyroidism in adults and children is rare, and can result from both acquired and congenital hypothyroidism. Children present with growth arrest, mental retardation, and slightly increased body weight; some with precocious or delayed puberty; and very few with visual field defects. Visual deficits are more frequently described in adults together with the classical symptoms of hypothyroidism; in females, the combination of amenorrhea, galactorrhea, and hyperprolactinemia can erroneously suggest a prolactin-secreting pituitary adenoma. Pituitary hyperplasia secondary to primary hypothyroidism must also be distinguished from TSH-secreting adenomas where T4 levels are increased. On imaging studies, secondary pituitary hyperplasia is characterized by a spherical or calabash-like enlargement of the gland with suprasellar extension; its height can reach 18 mm and the optic chiasm can be distorted. The T1W signal is unchanged and the T2W signal can be slightly hyperintense; enhancement is homogeneous after gadolinium injection (Fig. 45.1). Cavernous sinus invasion is never noted. Shrinkage of the mass occurs very quickly, as soon as some weeks, after thyroxine hormone replacement therapy (Fig. 45.2)

J.-F. Bonneville et al., *MRI of the Pituitary Gland*, DOI 10.1007/978-3-319-29043-0_45

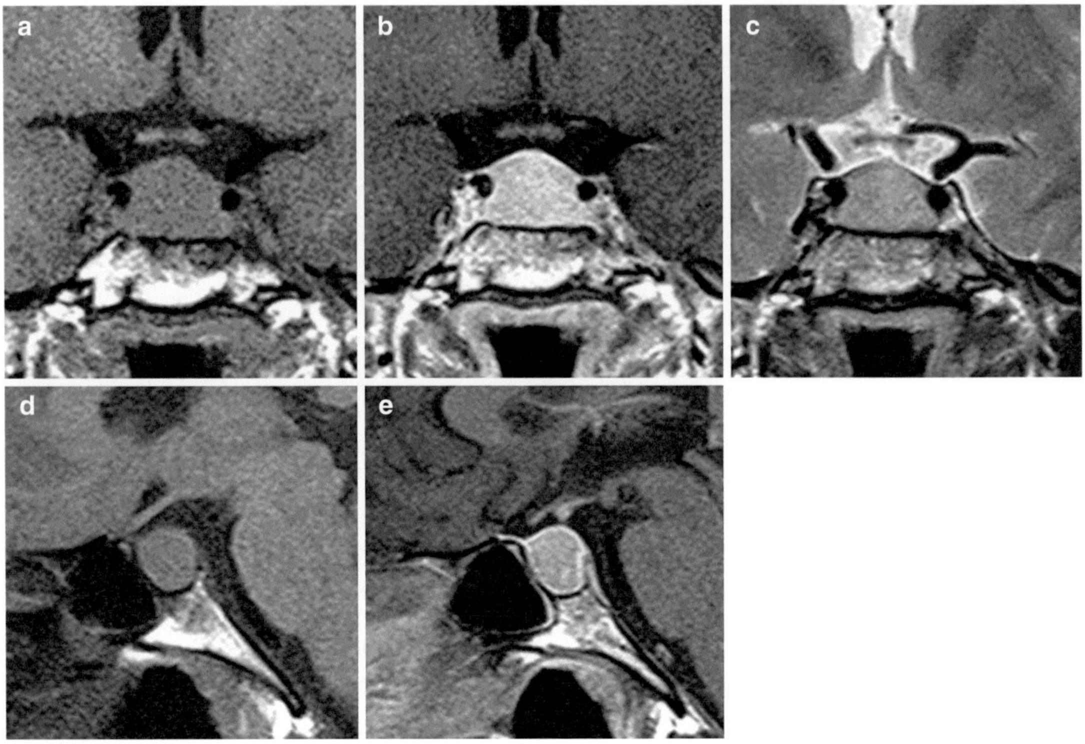

Fig. 45.1 Pituitary hyperplasia in a 46-year-old woman with primary hypothyroidism. Prolactin is 55 ng/ml. (**a**–**c**) Coronal T1, CE T1, and T2 WIs. (**d**, **e**) Sagittal T1 and CE T1 WIs. Diffuse enlargement of the pituitary gland which is slightly T2 hyperintense. Signal is homogeneous on all sequences

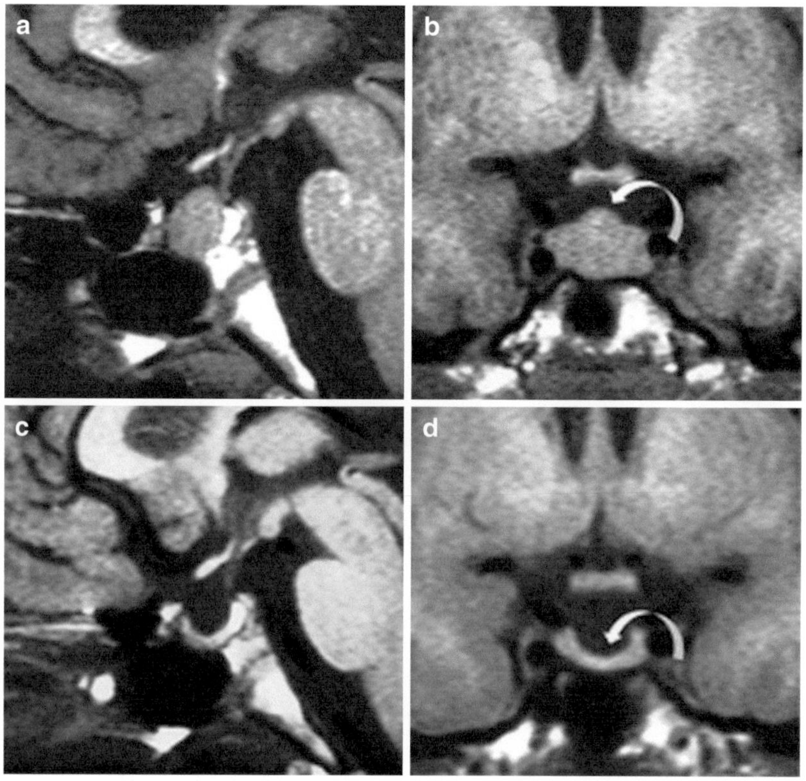

Fig. 45.2 Pituitary hyperplasia secondary to hypothyroidism in a 8-year-old girl with growth retardation. (**a**, **b**) Sagittal and coronal T1WI at diagnosis. Spherical enlargement of the pituitary gland. (**c**, **d**) Three months after replacement therapy. Shrinkage of the sellar content

Further Reading

Franceschi R, Rozzanigo U, Failo R et al (2011) Pituitary hyperplasia secondary to acquired hypothyroidism: case report. Ital J Pediatr 37:15

Joshi AS, Woolf PD (2005) Pituitary hyperplasia secondary to primary hypothyroidism. Pituitary 8:99–103

Kanza RE, Gagnon S, Villeneuve H et al (2013) Spontaneous ovarian hyperstimulation syndrome and pituitary hyperplasia mimicking macroadenoma associated with primary hypothyroidism. World J Radiol 5(1):20–24

46 Intracranial Hypotension Syndrome

Françoise Cattin

Intracranial hypotension syndrome is characterized by orthostatic headache and low CSF pressure and volume. Intracranial hypotension is either primary, also known as spontaneous intracranial hypotension, or secondary to cervical manipulation, lumbar puncture, or cranial/spinal surgery at the origin of a dural breach. Spontaneous intracranial hypotension can be observed in patients with dural weakness, e.g., in Marfan disease after mild trauma or in the presence of large Tarlov cysts. Sometimes the location of the dural breach can be demonstrated or suspected on spinal MR study. Invasive methods such as radionuclide cisternography are no longer carried out. An epidural blood patch provides the most efficient treatment for intracranial hypotension syndrome. MR findings in intracranial hypotension syndrome include dural thickening, dural enhancement, decreased ventricle size, subdural collections, tonsillar herniation, collapsed cisterns, venous distension signs and in the sellar region, bulging of the pituitary gland (Fig. 46.1). It is hypothesized that enlargement of the pituitary gland is related to hyperemia of the gland in the same way as venous hyperemia and enhancement occur in pachymeninges. We have observed that a prominent inferior intercavernous sinus is frequent in patients with intracranial hypotension syndrome, and probably reflects an engorgement of parasellar veins. Enlargement of inferior intercavernous sinus can also participate in the bulging of the pituitary gland. A prominent inferior intercavernous sinus is seen as a more or less thick T1-hypointense band doubling the sellar floor; the signal is variable on T2WI, either hyper- or hypointense depending on the flow velocity (Fig. 46.2). Thus, in the presence of an enlarged pituitary gland of unknown origin, demonstration of a prominent inferior intercavernous sinus leads one to consider the diagnosis of intracranial hypotension syndrome. After medical treatment and/or lumbar blood patch, shrinkage of the inferior intercavernous sinus is usually observed, simultaneously with clinical improvement (Fig. 46.3).

J.-F. Bonneville et al., *MRI of the Pituitary Gland*, DOI 10.1007/978-3-319-29043-0_46

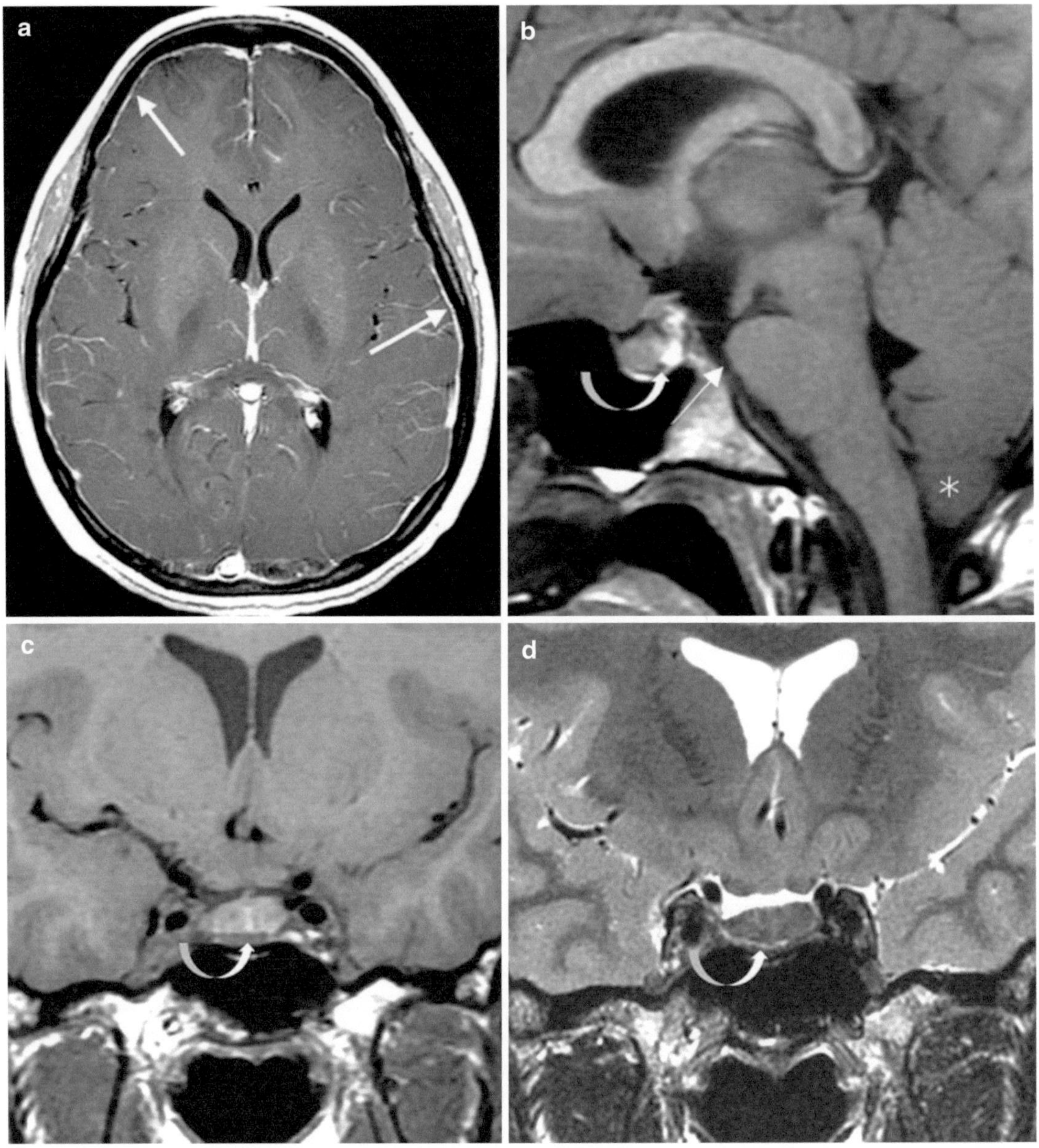

Fig. 46.1 A 21-year-old woman presenting with orthostatic headaches. (**a**) Axial CE T1WI shows small ventricles and diffuse thickening and enhancement of the dura (*arrows*). (**b**) Sagittal T1WI. Collapsed prepontine and suprasellar cistern (*thin arrow*) and tonsillar herniation (*asterisk*). A small round hypointense structure corresponding to the inferior intercavernous sinus is visualized below the posterior lobe of the pituitary gland (*curved arrow*). (**c**, **d**) Coronal T1 and T2 WIs demonstrating a bulging of the pituitary gland and a prominent inferior intercavernous sinus (*curved arrow*)

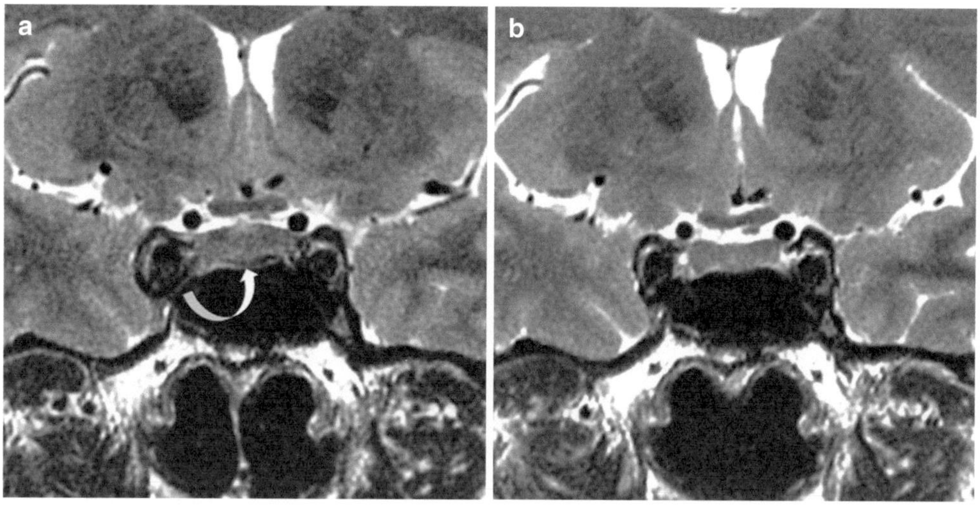

Fig. 46.2 A 58-year-old woman with spontaneous intracranial hypotension syndrome. (**a**) Coronal T2WI at diagnosis. Discrete bulging of the upper surface of the pituitary gland; unusual visualization in an adult of the inferior intercavernous sinus (*curved arrow*). Small lateral ventricles. (**b**) Coronal T2WI 1 month after lumbar blood patch. The patient is no longer symptomatic. Mild enlargement of lateral ventricles. The upper surface of the pituitary gland is planar and the inferior intercavernous sinus has vanished

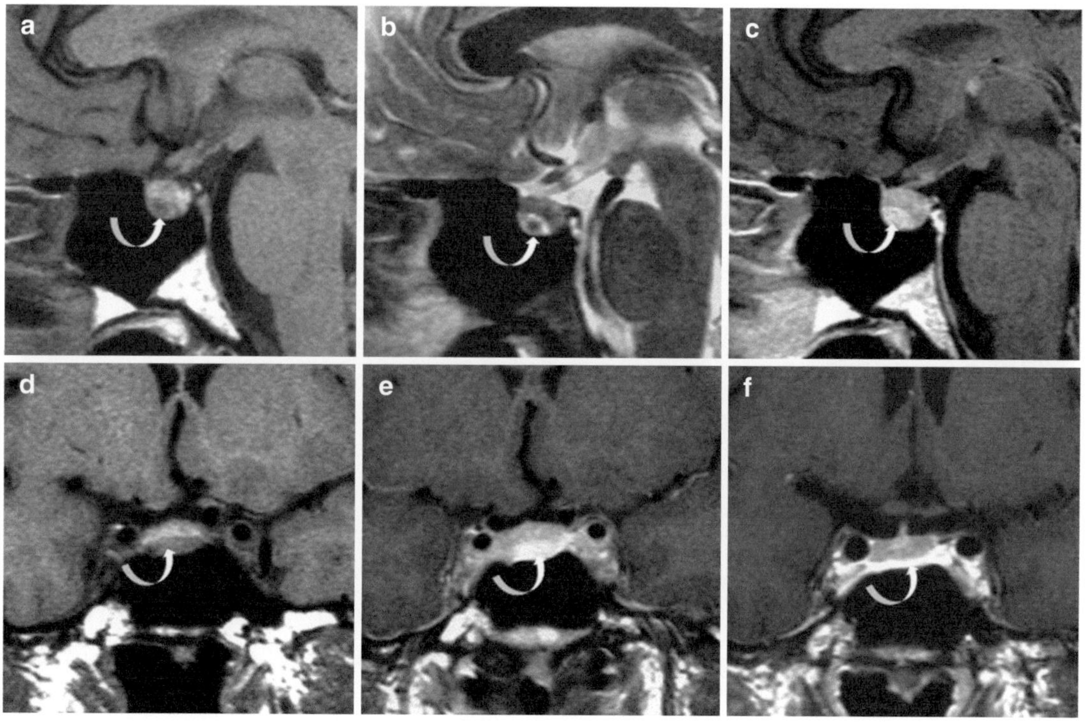

Fig. 46.3 A 45-year-old man with lymphoblastic leukemia. Intracranial hypotension syndrome secondary to iterative lumbar punctures. (**a–c**) Sagittal T1, T2, and CE T1 WIs. Bulging of the upper pole of the pituitary gland and impressive enlargement of the inferior intercavernous sinus (*curved arrow*), mimicking a pituitary lesion. The signal is heterogeneous on T2 with an eye-like appearance (*curved arrow*). Marked and homogeneous enhancement of the inferior intercavernous sinus. (**d**, **e**) Coronal T1 and CE T1 WIs. The inferior intercavernous sinus appears as a hypointense and markedly enhanced band parallel to the sellar floor (*curved arrow*), almost as thick as the pituitary gland. (**f**) Coronal CE T1WI 6 months later. Flattening of the pituitary gland and shrinkage of the inferior intercavernous sinus (*curved arrow*)

Further Reading

Bonneville JF, Cattin F, Bonneville F (2011) Enlargement of the inferior intercavernous sinus: a new sign for the diagnosis of craniospinal hypotension. AJNR Am J Neuroradiol 32(10):E194

Forghani R, Farb RI (2008) Diagnosis and temporal evolution of signs of intracranial hypotension on MRI of the brain. Neuroradiology 50(12):1025–1034

Spelle L, Boulin A, Tainturier C et al (2001) Neuroimaging features of spontaneous intracranial hypotension. Neuroradiology 43:622–627

47 Pituitary Hemochromatosis

Sonia Nagi and Cyrine Drissi

Hemochromatosis is a disorder caused by excess iron deposition in parenchymal cells that leads to cellular damage and organ dysfunction. There are two forms of hemochromatosis: genetic or primary hemochromatosis, and acquired or secondary hemochromatosis. The most common cause of secondary hemochromatosis is transfusional iron overload, encountered in patients with severe, chronic anemia such as β-thalassemia major or myelodysplasia. Excess iron is initially deposited in the reticuloendothelial system and then in all parenchymas, especially in the heart, liver, joints, skin, and endocrine glands. In the brain, structures lying outside the blood–brain barrier such as the choroid plexus, pituitary gland, and pineal gland are prone to elevated iron levels. The most common clinical manifestation of pituitary iron overload is hypogonadotropic hypogonadism. Hence, the diagnosis of pituitary hemochromatosis is usually made during adolescence or early adulthood. GH deficiency has also been reported. Iron deposition in the posterior lobe usually does not occur, and diabetes insipidus has not been reported.

The normal signal of the anterior pituitary gland is isointense to white matter on T1WIs and variable, usually close to the signal of gray matter on T2WI. The pathognomonic appearance of pituitary hemochromatosis is first demonstrated by T2WI showing reduced signal intensity of the anterior lobe resulting from ferritin deposition. Fast spin-echo sequences are less sensitive to such susceptibility effects as opposed to GE sequences. GE T2*W sequence is regarded as the most sensitive technique for the detection of parenchymal iron deposition. It shows marked decrease in the signal intensity of the anterior lobe of the pituitary gland (Fig. 47.1). With more severe disease, signal intensity is also reduced on T1WIs. MR signal reduction is followed by pituitary volume loss, explained by gonadotropin cell death owing to iron toxicity. GE T2*W sequence can also show hypointensity in the choroid plexus (Fig. 47.1) and pineal gland.

In patients with secondary hemochromatosis caused by chronic anemia, abnormal diploic thickening of the calvarium and skull base with abnormal hematopoietic bone marrow signal is seen on brain MRI scans (Fig. 47.1).

The cytotoxic effect of iron overload is considered to be dose dependent, and an initial reversible and a later irreversible phase of pituitary dysfunction has been suggested. Early MR detection of pituitary iron overload may be useful in preventing irreversible loss of pituitary function or in planning future treatment.

Other causes for decreased pituitary signal intensity on T2WIs should be discussed: hemorrhage, GH-secreting adenoma, melanoma, Rathke cleft cyst, amyloid deposition, craniopharyngioma, and colloid cyst. The lack of high signal intensity on T1WI and patient history help to narrow the differential diagnosis.

MRI of abdomen and chest in patients with hemochromatosis demonstrates low signal intensity in liver (Fig. 47.1), spleen, pancreas, and myocardium, indicating iron deposition in these organs.

J.-F. Bonneville et al., *MRI of the Pituitary Gland*, DOI 10.1007/978-3-319-29043-0_47

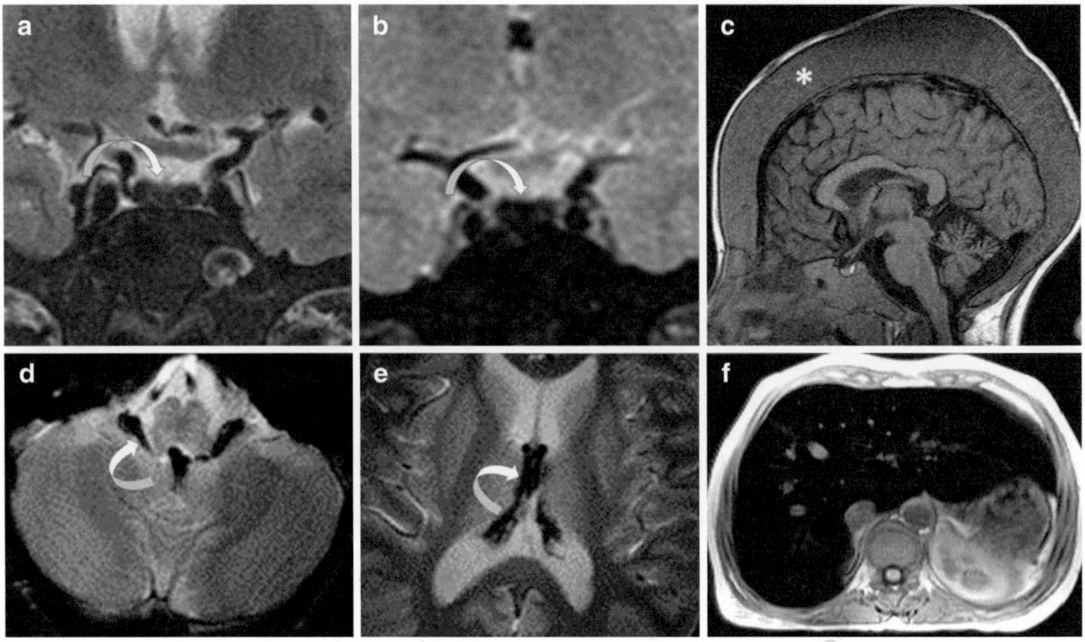

Fig. 47.1 Pituitary hemochromatosis in a 16-year-old girl with β-thalassemia major receiving monthly blood transfusions and iron chelation therapy. She presented with delayed puberty and short stature. (**a**, **b**) Coronal T2 and T2* WIs. Hypointensity of the anterior pituitary lobe (*curved arrow*). (**c**) Sagittal T1WI. Marked uniform thickening of diploic space of the calvarium and skull base with low signal of bone marrow (*asterisk*). (**d**, **e**) Axial T2*WIs. striking choroid plexus hypointensity (*curved arrow*). (**f**) Axial T1WI of an abdominal MRI scan. Liver hypointensity caused by iron overload

Further Reading

Adams PC, Barton JC (2007) Haemochromatosis. Lancet 370:1855–1860

Christoforidis A, Haritandi A, Perifanis V et al (2007) MRI for the determination of pituitary iron overload in children and young adults with β-thalassaemia major. Eur J Radiol 62:138–142

Hekmatnia A, Radmarda AR, Rahmani AA et al (2010) Magnetic resonance imaging signal reduction may precede volume loss in the pituitary gland of transfusion-dependent beta-thalassemic patients. Acta Radiol 51:71–77

48 Arachnoid Cyst

Fabrice Bonneville

Arachnoid cysts (ACs) are benign developmental CSF-like collections encased within an arachnoid membrane. They are randomly encountered at the surface of the brain, with a predilection for the middle cranial fossa or the cerebellopontine angle. ACs located in the sellar area represent slightly less than 10 % of all intracranial arachnoid cysts. There is no obvious sex ratio. ACs are described in the literature at all ages, but intrasellar ACs are reported more in adulthood while suprasellar ACs appear to be more frequent in the pediatric population.

Two different types of AC can be distinguished in the sellar region: intrasellar ACs, which often demonstrate a suprasellar extension that displaces the pituitary stalk posteriorly (Fig. 48.1), and suprasellar ACs, also called suprasellar-prepontine ACs, which push the floor of the third ventricle upward and the pituitary stalk forward (Fig. 48.2). The exact origin of intrasellar AC remains controversial, because there is no arachnoid membrane in the sella turcica. Therefore, an accepted hypothesis is an extension of a suprasellar AC cyst through the diaphragm aperture (Fig. 48.3).

If common intracranial ACs are typically clinically silent and almost never require surgical intervention, headache, visual disturbances, endocrine dysfunction, and hydrocephalus are frequent problems associated with AC in the sellar region. Thus, ACs may behave like any other nonsecreting sellar lesion but may also be asymptomatic and depicted randomly on brain CT or MRI.

Preoperative diagnosis of sellar AC looks simple on CT or MRI because such cysts are only filled with CSF-like fluid whose density and signal intensities are similar to those of CSF. They appear as well-defined, sharply marginated intra-/suprasellar or suprasellar purely cystic lesions with homogeneous T1-low signal intensity and T2-high signal intensity, with no solid portion, no contrast enhancement, and no calcification. However, on T1WI, intrasellar ACs have been reported to be slightly more intense than the CSF because of stagnation of the fluid or elevated protein concentration. FLAIR sequence is of great additional value by demonstrating signal suppression of the cyst content in ACs (Figs. 48.1, 48.2, and 48.4), while this content returns high signal intensity in other cystic lesions such as cystic pituitary adenoma, Rathke cleft cyst, craniopharyngioma, or neurenteric cyst.

Other MR features of sellar ACs are due to their mass effect. The sella turcica may be markedly increased in cases of large intrasellar component, with ballooning of its floor. Visual pathways, pituitary stalk, and gland may be displaced, while brain parenchyma and third ventricle can be compressed by large cysts. As mentioned earlier, the AC wall shows no enhancement after intravenous gadolinium

J.-F. Bonneville et al., *MRI of the Pituitary Gland*, DOI 10.1007/978-3-319-29043-0_48

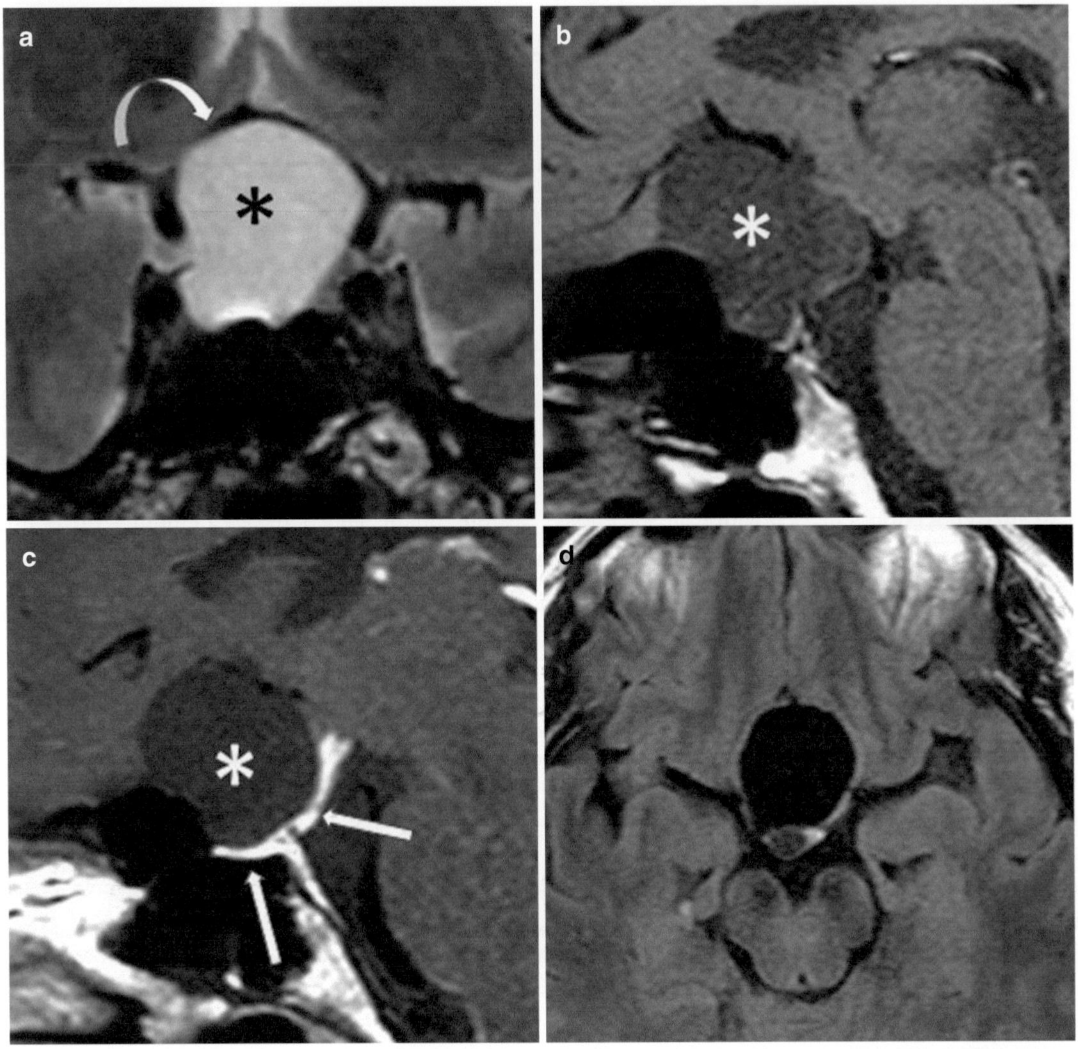

Fig. 48.1 Intra- and suprasellar AC. (**a**) Coronal T2WI shows a homogeneous intra-/suprasellar hyperintense cyst (*asterisk*) displacing the optic chiasm and anterior cerebral arteries (*curved arrow*) upward. (**b, c**) Sagittal T1WIs before and after gadolinium administration demonstrate no contrast uptake of the cyst walls. Only the normal adenohypophysis and pituitary stalk pushed posteriorly are enhancing (*straight arrows*). Note that cyst signal intensities are similar to those of CSF on all sequences, especially on (**d**) FLAIR image, on which the signal intensity is completely attenuated

administration. Peripheral and discontinuous gadolinium uptake may, however, be depicted at the edge of the cysts and is related to normal laminated adenohypophysis or pituitary stalk (Figs. 48.1 and 48.4).

Finally, the differential diagnosis between an AC and an empty sella may not be as easy as thought, because both entities have signal intensities similar to that of CSF. However, ACs have no communication with the surrounding subarachnoid space, which distinguishes them from an empty sella. In addition, high-resolution heavily T2W MRI sequences such as CISS, FIESTA, or DRIVE are able to

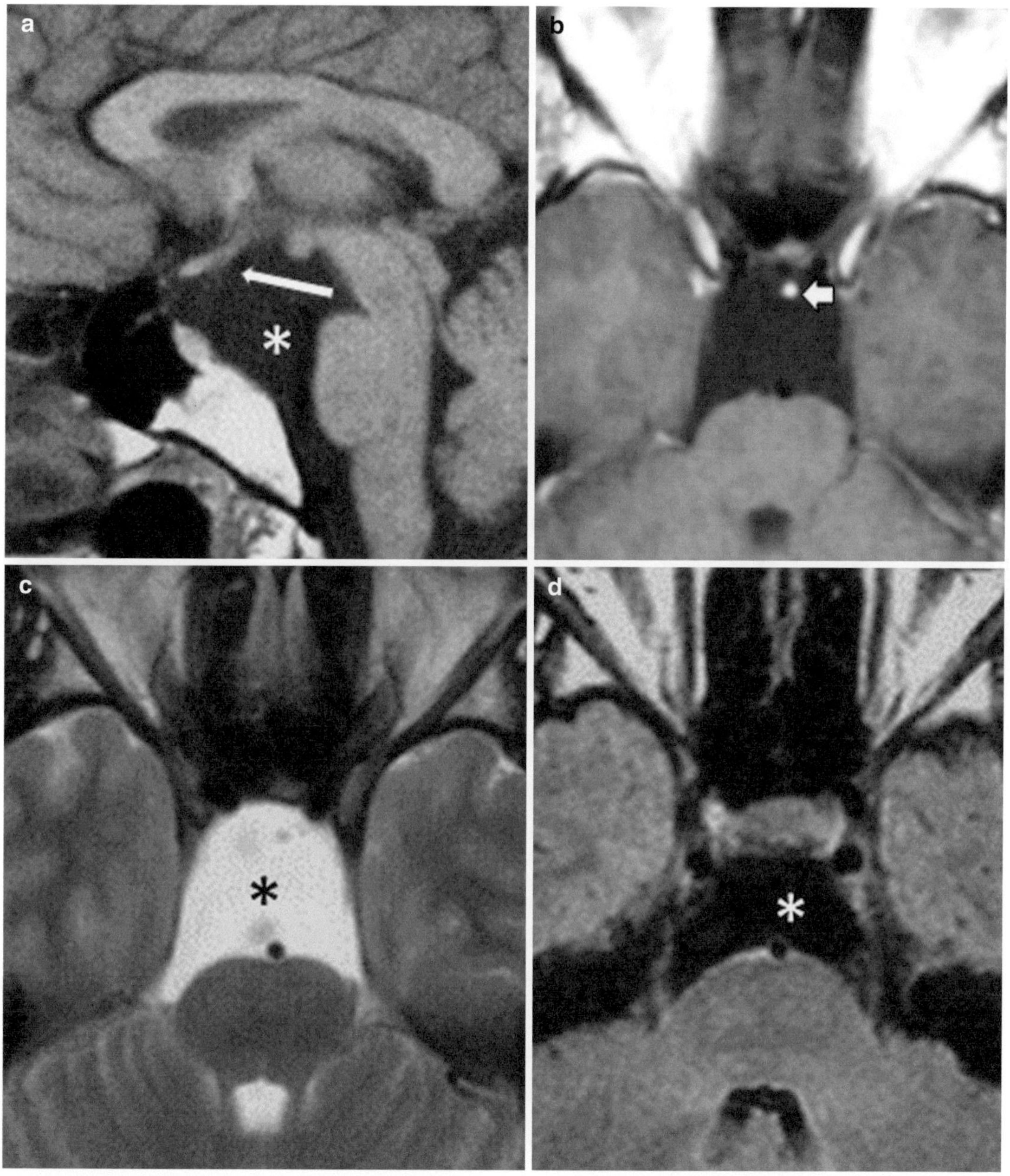

Fig. 48.2 Suprasellar AC. (**a**) Sagittal T1WI image illustrates the mass effect of a suprasellar-prepontine AC (*asterisk*) on pituitary stalk and floor of the third ventricle (*arrow*). The dorsum sellae is eroded. (**b**) Axial CE T1WI demonstrates no gadolinium uptake of the cyst wall. Only the pituitary stalk is normally enhancing (*small arrow*). (**c**, **d**) Axial T2WI and FLAIR images confirm the purely CSF-like nature of the cyst content, thus confirming the diagnosis of AC

delineate the membranous borders of the AC, which do not exist in empty sella. Moreover, the diagnosis of empty sella appears less likely in cases of mass effect by the cystic lesion and subsequent outer displacement of the parasellar structures, such as the optic nerve (Fig. 48.3), pituitary stalk, and floor of the third ventricle.

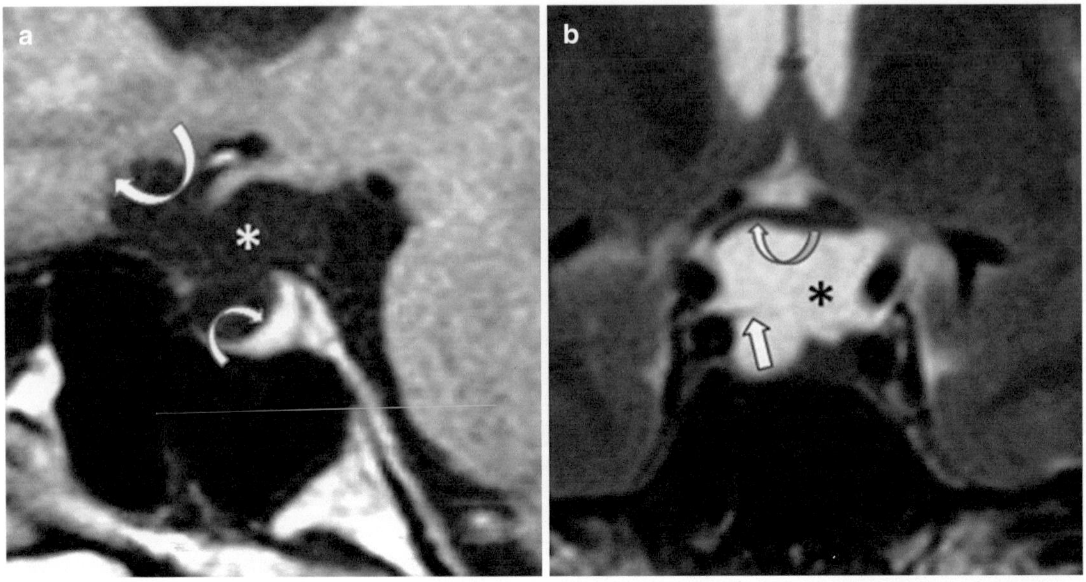

Fig. 48.3 Intra- and suprasellar AC (*asterisk*). (**a**) Sagittal T1WI shows a widening of the optochiasmatic cistern with mass effect on the superior aspect of the pituitary gland (*small curved arrow*) and orbitofrontal brain parenchyma (*long curved arrow*). (**b**) Coronal T2WI demonstrates the focal impingement of the inferior right aspect of the optic chiasm (*curved arrow*) and the intrasellar extension through a large aperture of the sellar diaphragm (*straight arrow*)

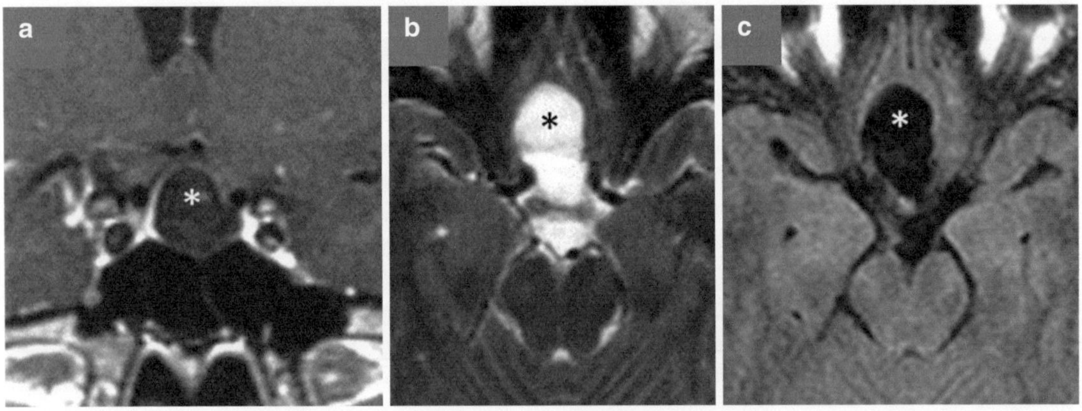

Fig. 48.4 Intra- and suprasellar AC. (**a**) Coronal CE T1WI shows a cystic lesion (*asterisk*) surrounded by a thin rim of normally enhancing pituitary tissue (*arrow*). (**b**) Axial T2WI image depicts the suprasellar component of this AC, only filled with CSF-like fluid completely attenuated on (**c**) FLAIR image

Further Reading

Dubuisson AS, Stevenaert A, Martin DH et al (2007) Intrasellar arachnoid cysts. Neurosurgery 61:505–513

Ozek MM, Urgun K (2013) Neuroendoscopic management of suprasellar arachnoid cysts. World Neurosurg 79(2 Suppl):S19.e13-8

Shim KW, Park EK, Lee YH et al (2013) Transventricular endoscopic fenestration of intrasellar arachnoid cyst. Neurosurgery 72:520–528

Epidermoid Cyst

49

Fabrice Bonneville

Epidermoid cysts are benign congenital lesions arising from the accidental inclusion of normal ectodermal epithelial tissue during neural tube closure in early embryogenesis. They grow from the slow accumulation of the products of the desquamation of the stratified keratinized epithelium that constitutes the cyst walls. Intracranial epidermoid cysts are ubiquitous, but about half of intracranial epidermoid cysts are located in the cerebellopontine angle. They are occasionally encountered in the sellar region, where they usually present in middle-aged patients with nonspecific neurologic symptoms rather than endocrine disturbances, such as headaches, visual impairment, or cranial nerve deficits. Intrasellar epidermoid cysts are extremely rare and have been reported as a cause of hypophysitis or mimicking pituitary apoplexy. In cases of trigeminal neuralgia, specific extension into Meckel cave should be meticulously sought. Epidermoid cysts are commonly large when symptomatic because these slow-growing malleable masses softly insinuate into pericerebral cisterns, where at first they gently encase and surround cranial nerves and vessels, and only later, when bigger, displace, stretch, and finally exert mass effect on cerebral structures.

On CT, epidermoid cysts appear hypodense with possible marginal calcifications. On MRI they have a fluid-like low-T1 signal intensity and high-T2 signal intensity, but are slightly brighter than CSF on both T1 and T2 WIs, and show no contrast enhancement after gadolinium administration. They may, however, be difficult to distinguish from arachnoid cysts based on the signal intensities only on those sequences. The shape and edges of these two cysts, however, are very different, as epidermoid cysts present with a unique irregular lobulated cauliflower-like outer surface (Fig. 49.1). With advances in MRI techniques, preoperative diagnosis of epidermoid cysts is now reliable and no longer poses a dilemma. On FLAIR sequence, epidermoid cysts can be easily differentiated from arachnoid cysts because the former show mixed iso- to hypersignal intensities, but with poor demarcation, while the signal of the latter is suppressed, like the signal of CSF. Heavily T2W 3D sequence, also called MR cisternography, demonstrates epidermoid cyst hypointense to CSF, and thus nicely demonstrates the lobulated margins of the tumor and clearly depicts its precise extent (Fig. 49.2). DWI offers a finding specific for extra-axial epidermoid cysts by showing a very high signal. Restricted ADC compared with CSF, almost comparable with that of the brain, and T2 shine-through effect both play an important role in the high signal intensity of epidermoid cyst at DWI. DWI is also crucial in the postoperative follow-up, as it allows confirmation of the presence of a possible residual tumor. Finally, MR spectroscopy may also be helpful, especially in cases of atypical epidermoid cysts, as it shows a unique pattern with only an elevated lactate peak.

J.-F. Bonneville et al., *MRI of the Pituitary Gland*, DOI 10.1007/978-3-319-29043-0_49

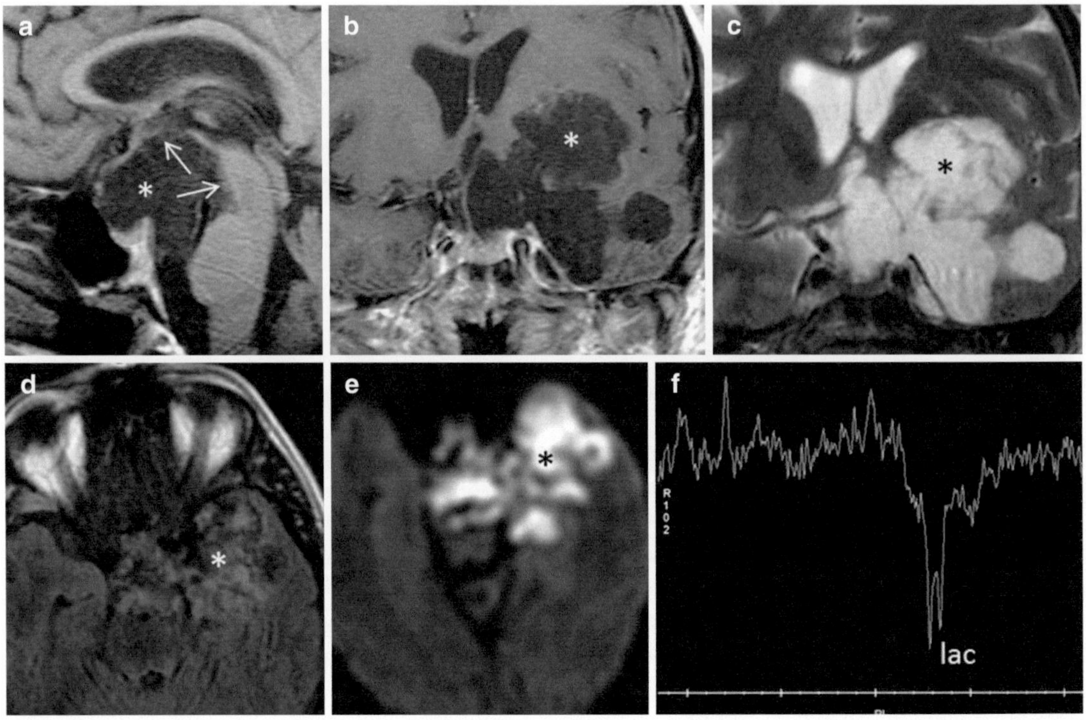

Fig. 49.1 Suprasellar epidermoid cyst (*asterisk*). (**a**) Sagittal T1WI shows large, suprasellar hypointense cyst with posterior extension impinging mesencephalon and pons, and upward displacement of the floor of the third ventricle (*thin arrows*). (**b**) Coronal CE T1WI demonstrates no enhancement of this suprasellar cyst with typical ill-defined borders indenting the brain parenchyma laterally. (**c**) Coronal T2WI demonstrates the very high signal intensity of the lesion that becomes characteristically isointense on (**d**) FLAIR image. (**e**) Diffusion-weighted axial image reveals very suggestive hyperintense signal. (**f**) Long echo-time MR spectroscopy depicts only lactate in epidermoid cyst, a metabolite that appears as a negative doublet at 1.3 ppm

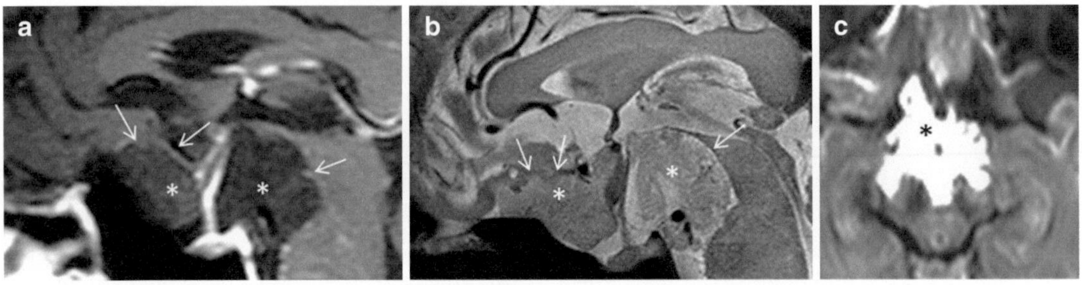

Fig. 49.2 Suprasellar epidermoid cyst. (**a**) Sagittal CE T1WI and (**b**) Sagittal T2WI show a large, nonenhancing nebulous cyst filling the optochiasmatic cistern, encasing the pituitary stalk, and displacing the floor of the third ventricle upward. (**c**) Axial DWI shows the characteristic hyperintense signal of the epidermoid cyst (Courtesy of J. Savatovsky, MD)

Further Reading

Bonneville F, Savatovsky J, Chiras J (2007) Imaging of cerebellopontine angle lesions: an update. Part 2: intra-axial lesions, skull base lesions that may invade the CPA region, and non-enhancing extra-axial lesions. Eur Radiol 17(11):2908–2920

Ren X, Lin S, Wang Z et al (2012) Clinical, radiological, and pathological features of 24 atypical intracranial epidermoid cysts. J Neurosurg 116(3):611–621

Tuna H, Torun F, Torun AN et al (2008) Intrasellar epidermoid cyst presenting as pituitary apoplexy. J Clin Neurosci 15:1154–1156

Zada G, Lin N, Ojerholm E, Ramkissoon S, Laws ER (2010) Craniopharyngioma and other cystic epithelial lesions of the sellar region: a review of clinical, imaging, and histopathological relationships. Neurosurg Focus 28(4):E4

Dermoid Cyst

50

Fabrice Bonneville

Intracranial dermoid cysts are rare congenital lesions resulting from the inclusion of ectodermal cells during the closure of the neural tube, which occurs between the third and fifth gestational week. They may be associated with dermal sinus tracts and other neural tube closure defects, although they are usually not present in the sellar region. The cyst wall is made of connective tissue, and they are filled with a heterogeneous mixture of fat, hair, dystrophic calcifications or teeth, and fatty products of sebaceous glands. The cyst growth results from the accumulation of these glandular secretions and epithelial desquamation. Dermoid cysts are intradural extra-axial lesions that tend to occur on the midline and particularly in the sellar/parasellar region. Exceptional extradural locations have also been reported, especially within the cavernous sinus. Common clinical symptoms include headaches, seizures, and suprasellar dermoid cysts often present with visual disturbances. Dermoid cysts are also well-known to cause chemical meningitis when they rupture and spill their content in the subarachnoid cisterns. Hydrocephalus is a rare presentation, and is subsequent to the trapping of the ventricular system rather than aseptic meningitis.

At imaging, a dermoid cyst appears as a well-circumscribed, fatty round mass with a peripheral capsule that may enhance or harbor calcifications. They are hypodense on CT, and possibly contain calcifications or teeth (Fig. 50.1). At MRI, dermoid cysts appear with characteristic fatty signal intensities on all sequences. Unlike lipomas, dermoid cysts are heterogeneous (Figs. 50.1 and 50.2) and have a capsule that may enhance (Fig. 50.2). The fatty content thus appears with T1- and T2-high signal intensities on spin-echo sequences, but demonstrate low GE T2 signal intensity. This point is crucial as it may mimic blood, like either a subacute parenchymal hematoma or a cavernoma. Therefore, T1WI with fat saturation is of precious help to confirm the fatty nature of the lesion and endorse the diagnosis of dermoid cyst when the lesion is heterogeneous (Figs. 50.1 and 50.4). Of course, in the absence of T1WI with fat saturation, one should consider that a simple nonenhanced CT scan easily demonstrates marked hypoattenuation in cases of fat and allows one to distinguish fatty from hemorrhagic lesions. Another clue to evoke the fatty origin of the signal is the presence of a chemical shift artifact that appears as a peripheral curvilinear hypointensity covering the lesion along the frequency-encoding direction (Fig. 50.3). In rare cases the fat floats on the rest of the liquid filling the cyst, giving a characteristic fat-fluid level, which we believe is pathognomonic of a dermoid cyst when observed in a well-defined intracranial lesion (Fig. 50.3). Finally, in cases of rupture in the subarachnoid space, the visualization of fatty T1-hyperintense droplets in the sulci or an anterior fat-fluid level in the ventricles is also highly suggestive of the diagnosis (Fig. 50.4).

J.-F. Bonneville et al., *MRI of the Pituitary Gland*, DOI 10.1007/978-3-319-29043-0_50

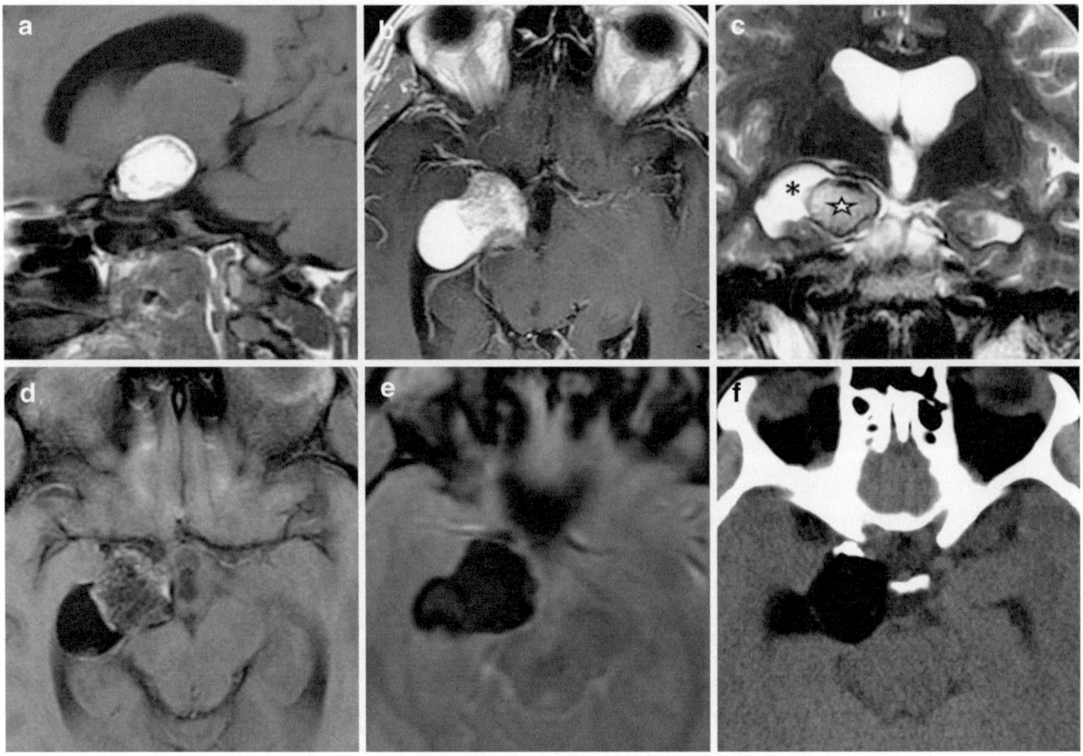

Fig. 50.1 Right parasellar dermoid cyst. (**a**) Sagittal T1WI depicts a hyperintense well-circumscribed right parasellar mass lesion that appears heterogeneous and nonenhancing on (**b**) axial CE T1WI. (**c**) Coronal T2WI nicely demonstrates that the lesion is composed of two distinct lobules, one being hyperintense (*asterisk*), the other isointense (*star*), a feature not present in lipoma. With decrease of both components signal intensities on (**d**) axial fat saturation T1WI, the fatty nature of the spontaneous T1 hyperintensity is confirmed. (**e**) Of note, fat content appears with low signal intensity on GE T2WI, as blood would. (**f**) Nonenhanced CT demonstrates marked hypoattenuation with no calcification

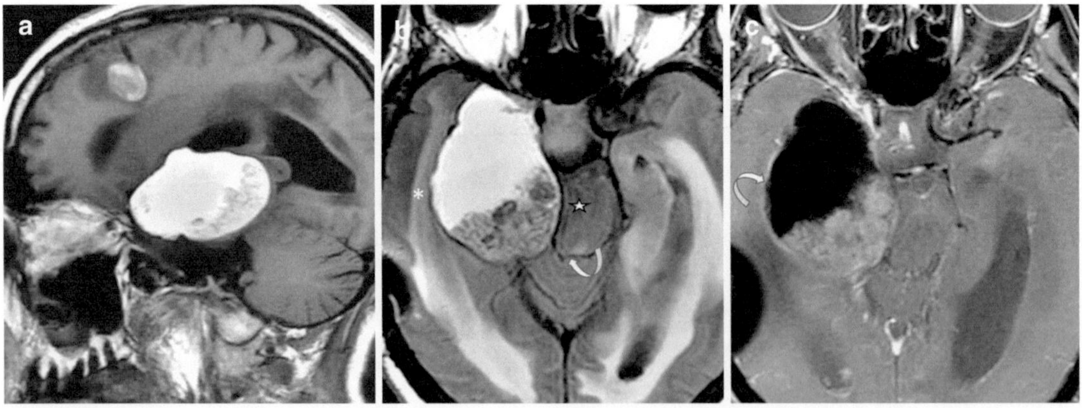

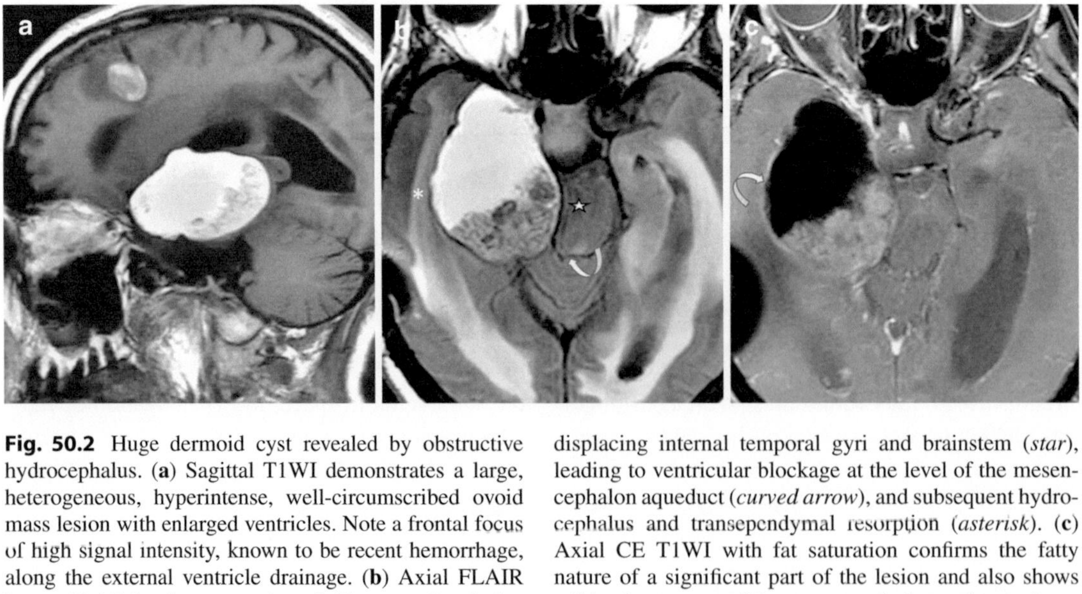

Fig. 50.2 Huge dermoid cyst revealed by obstructive hydrocephalus. (**a**) Sagittal T1WI demonstrates a large, heterogeneous, hyperintense, well-circumscribed ovoid mass lesion with enlarged ventricles. Note a frontal focus of high signal intensity, known to be recent hemorrhage, along the external ventricle drainage. (**b**) Axial FLAIR image highlights heterogeneity of this parasellar lesion displacing internal temporal gyri and brainstem (*star*), leading to ventricular blockage at the level of the mesencephalon aqueduct (*curved arrow*), and subsequent hydrocephalus and transependymal resorption (*asterisk*). (**c**) Axial CE T1WI with fat saturation confirms the fatty nature of a significant part of the lesion and also shows mild enhancement of the cyst capsule (*curved arrow*)

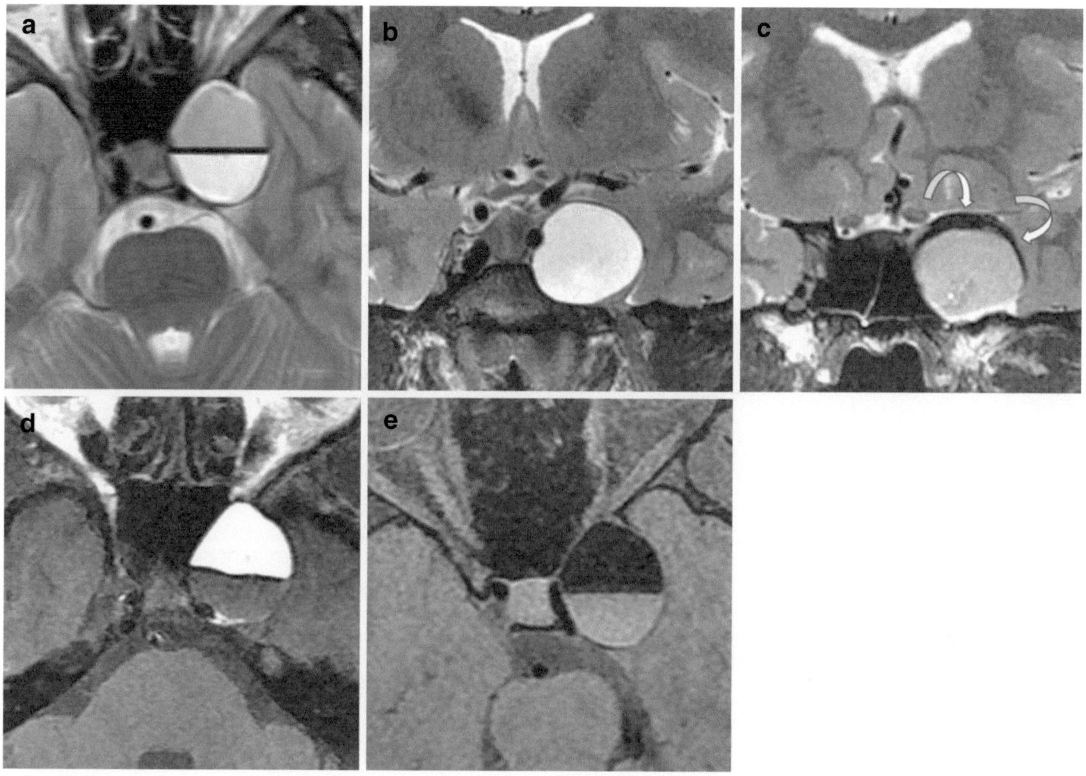

Fig. 50.3 Dermoid cyst of the left cavernous sinus. (**a**) Axial T2WI shows a round well-demarcated lesion within the left cavernous sinus, displacing the internal carotid artery medially. This axial slice reveals an obvious fluid-fluid level at mid-height of the lesion. On (**b**, **c**) Coronal T2WIs, the bottom part (**b**) appears with a homogeneous frankly hyperintense signal while the supernatant (**c**) appears less hyperintense, with a characteristic peripheral hypointense rim corresponding to a chemical shift artifact (*arrows*) along the frequency-encoding direction, as observed in the presence of fat. (**d**, **e**) Axial T1WIs without (**d**) and with (**e**) fat saturation confirm the fatty nature of the floating part of this cystic lesion. Such a fat-fluid level is a rare but very suggestive feature of dermoid cyst

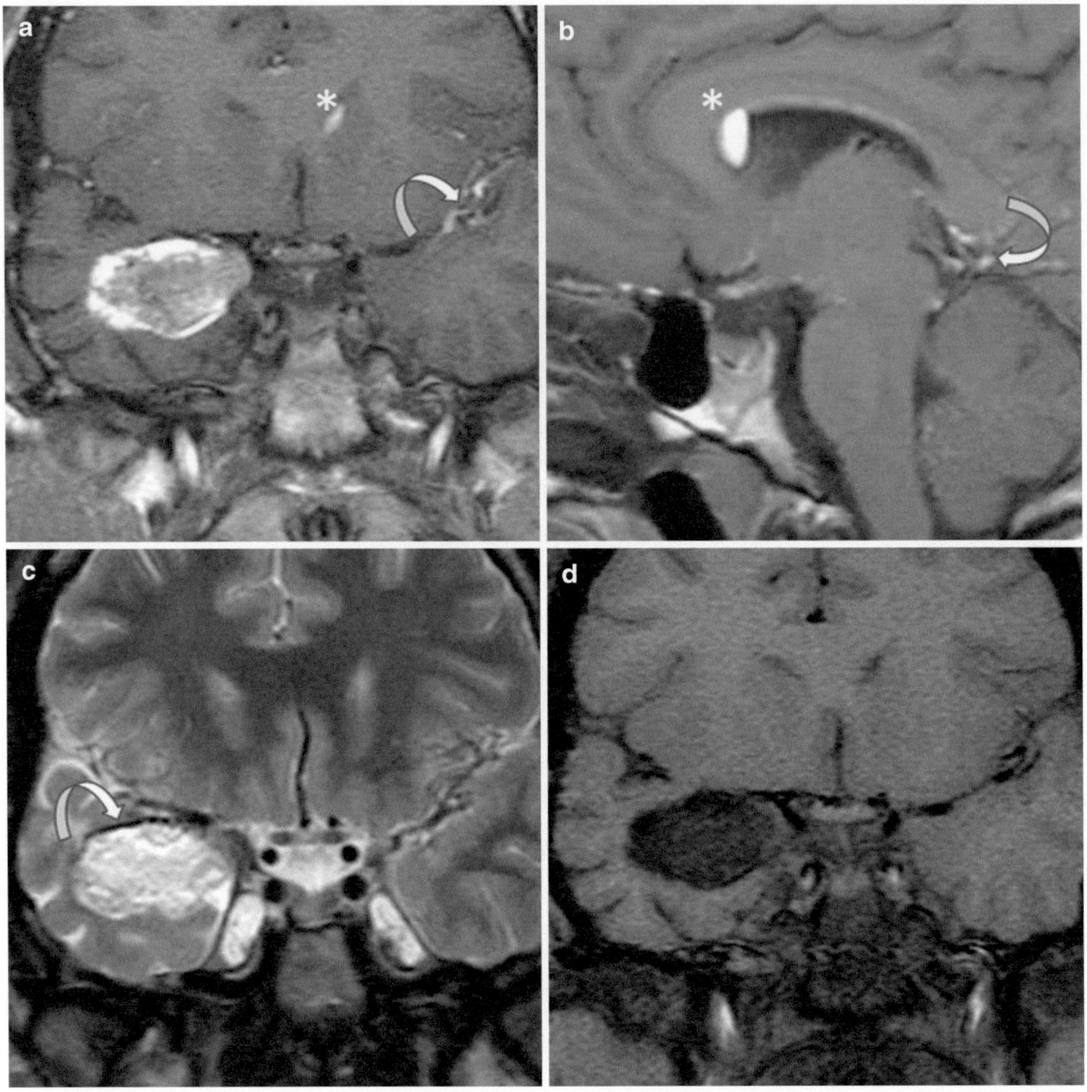

Fig. 50.4 Ruptured dermoid cyst with subarachnoid fatty droplets. (**a**) Coronal and (**b**) Sagittal T1WIs show a large ruptured right parasellar heterogeneous, hyperintense, well-demarcated mass and multiple foci of high signal intensity corresponding to lipid droplets scattered into the subarachnoid space and the left sylvian fissure (*curved arrow*), but also the left frontal horn, with a characteristic fat-fluid level (*asterisk*). (**c**) Coronal T2WI shows temporal/parasellar heterogeneous cyst covered by a hypointense rim consistent with a chemical shift artifact (*arrow*). (**d**) Coronal T1WI with fat saturation confirms the fatty component of this lesion by suppressing its spontaneous high signal intensity

Further Reading

Bonneville F, Cattin F, Marsot-Dupuch K et al (2006) T1 signal hyperintensity in the sellar region: spectrum of findings. Radiographics 26:93–113

Liu JK, Gottfried ON, Salzman KL et al (2008) Ruptured intracranial dermoid cysts: clinical, radiographic, and surgical features. Neurosurgery 62:377–384

Osborn AG, Preece MT (2006) Intracranial cysts: radiologic-pathologic correlation and imaging approach. Radiology 239:650–664

51 Neurenteric Cyst

Fabrice Bonneville

Neurenteric cysts (NCs) are endodermally derived lesions of the CNS, along with Rathke cleft cysts (RCCs) and colloid cysts. The exact etiology of NC is unknown, but may result from the incorporation of primitive endodermal cells of the foregut into the notochord during embryogenesis. NCs have several names, including enterogenous cyst, enteric cyst, and endodermal cyst. These cystic masses are lined by a mucin-producing cuboidal or columnar epithelium resembling gastrointestinal or respiratory tract mucosa. The cyst content is mainly mucoid in nature, with variable protein component. Most reported NCs occur within the spinal canal, usually ventral to the spinal cord. Intracranial cysts are rarer and mostly found in the posterior fossa. They are typically midline, anterior to the brainstem, or in the cerebellopontine angle. Supratentorial localizations are very rare. NCs have almost never been described in the sellar region. In fact, their mucoid content and their mucin-producing cell epithelium may appear very similar to those of RCCs or colloid cysts, two other endodermal cystic lesions frequently reported in the sellar region. However, RCCs and colloid cysts have different locations than NCs, which may be retrosellar, anterior to the mesencephalon (Fig. 51.1). Although final diagnosis of NC is based on histology, imaging characteristics are very suggestive of the preoperative diagnosis. NCs can be difficult to differentiate from arachnoid and epidermoid cysts because on imaging studies, NCs are well-circumscribed, nonenhancing cystic lesions, with round and smooth margins. However, their density and signal intensities are faintly different to those of normal CSF, but depend on their protein content. They are often iso-hypodense and iso-slightly hyperintense relative to brain parenchyma on T1WI and typically hyperintense on T2WI. NCs are also hyperintense on FLAIR imaging (Fig. 51.1). The lesions show mild or no restricted diffusion on diffusion-weighted sequence, a feature that enables differentiation from epidermoid cysts, which may exhibit similar intensities on spin-echo sequences but evocative high signal intensity on DWI.

J.-F. Bonneville et al., *MRI of the Pituitary Gland*, DOI 10.1007/978-3-319-29043-0_51

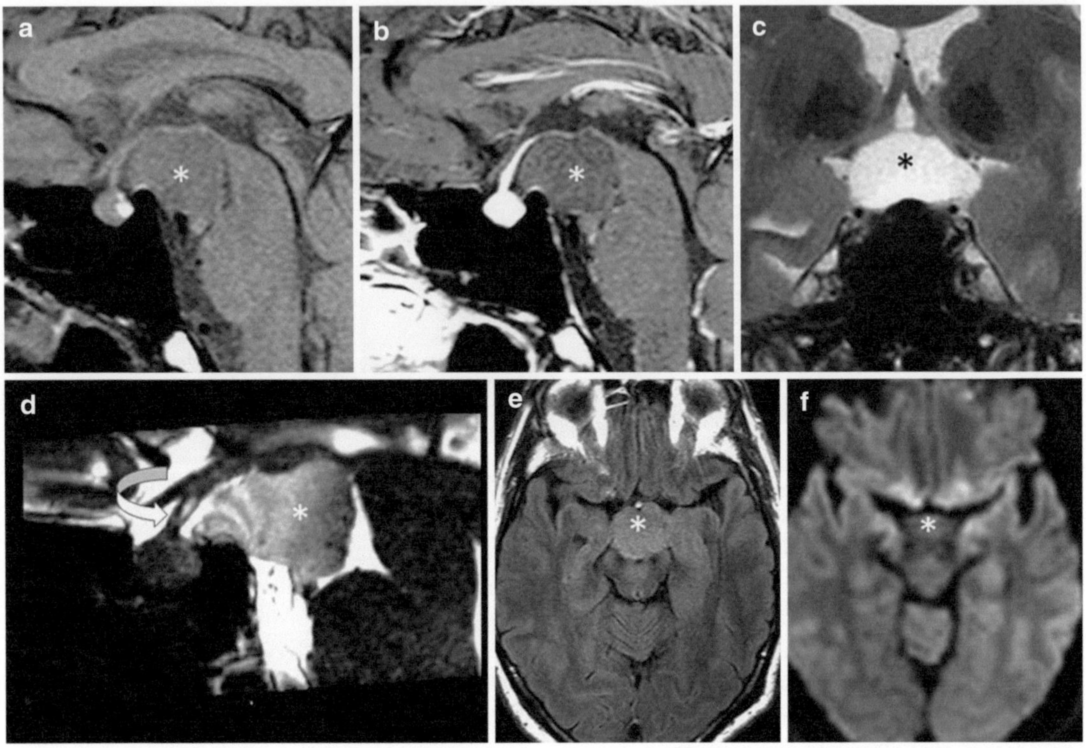

Fig 51.1 Retrosuprasellar neurenteric cyst. (**a**, **b**) Sagittal pre- and postcontrast T1WIs show a well-circumscribed retrosuprasellar lesion displacing the floor of the third ventricle upward. This nonenhancing cystic lesion appears with a homogeneous iso-hyperintense signal slightly different from CSF and hyperintense signal on (**c**) coronal T2WI (*asterisk*). (**d**) Sagittal reformatted CISS (constructive interference in steady state) image amplifies signal difference with CSF and accurately depicts cyst limits, especially behind the pituitary stalk (*curved arrow*). (**e**) Axial FLAIR image reveals a cystic mass with smooth margins isointense to brain parenchyma, anterior to the mesencephalon. (**f**) On DWI, the lesion does not show high signal intensity as epidermoid cysts do, but appears with isointensity, assuredly because of a T2 shine-through effect

Further Reading

Bonneville F, Savatovsky J, Chiras J (2007) Imaging of cerebellopontine angle lesions: an update. Part 2: intra-axial lesions, skull base lesions that may invade the CPA region, and non-enhancing extra-axial lesions. Eur Radiol 17(11):2908–2920

Gauden AJ, Khurana VG, Tsui AE et al (2012) Intracranial neuroenteric cysts: a concise review including an illustrative patient. J Clin Neurosci 19(3):352–359

Preece MT, Osborn AG, Chin SS et al (2006) Intracranial neurenteric cysts: imaging and pathology spectrum. AJNR Am J Neuroradiol 7:1211–1216

52 "Incidentalomas". Posterior Pituitary Cyst

Jean-François Bonneville and Fabrice Bonneville

The term "incidentaloma" is frequently used by radiologists and endocrinologists to describe the accidental discovery of an abnormal image of the sellar region on the brain MRI of an asymptomatic patient. However, a precise analysis of the MRI features permits one in the vast majority of cases to make a precise diagnosis, usually pituitary adenoma, Rathke cleft cyst (RCC), or anatomical variant. The management and follow-up of these "incidentalomas" being quite different, our suggestion is to replace the term "incidentaloma" by "pituitary adenoma—or RCC or anatomical variant—discovered by chance" in medical and radiological reports, keeping the term "incidentaloma" for those cases where the exact diagnosis is impossible. In front of "microincidentalomas" a precise diagnosis can be frequently made, for instance for the frequent T1-hyperintense RCC better demonstrated on axial T1WI than on sagittal T1WI, located strictly on the midline and in intimate contact with the posterior lobe (Figs. 19.1 and 52.1). Pituitary microadenomas are mostly laterally localized, mark an imprint on the sellar floor, and distort the upper surface of the pituitary gland (Fig. 5.1). T1-hypointense and T2-hyperintense images may also correspond to millimetric infarcts or hemorrhagic scars, as found regularly at autopsy of subjects with no pre-existing pituitary symptoms.

For "macroincidentalomas" the diagnosis also is often feasible, the main characteristics for RCC being midline location, characteristic T1 or T2 signal (mostly T1 hyperintense), absence of postgadolinium enhancement, hyperproteinic T2-hypointense micronodules, and low or absence of mass effect if compared with pituitary adenomas. This latter feature is particularly useful for the differentiation of mucoid RCC from hemorrhagic pituitary adenoma (Fig. 12.5), and for the diagnosis of concomitant lesions (Fig. 21.2).

Another good example of the so-called "incidentaloma" is the cyst or cleft of the posterior pituitary, rarely mentioned in autopsy reports or in the literature. Cysts of the posterior pituitary may be observed on axial T1WI without contrast as T1-hypointense clefts completely surrounded by a T1-hyperintense rim corresponding to vasopressin storage (Fig. 52.2). These cysts may coexist with other pituitary lesions and shrink or expand with time (Fig. 52.3). Multiple asymptomatic cysts of unknown origin are also sometimes encountered (Fig. 52.4). MRI follow-up may be recommended for the largest.

The extreme frequency of asymptomatic intrasellar images seen on MRI reinforces the absolute necessity of a close collaboration between endocrinologists, neurosurgeons, and neuroradiologists.

J.-F. Bonneville et al., *MRI of the Pituitary Gland*, DOI 10.1007/978-3-319-29043-0_52

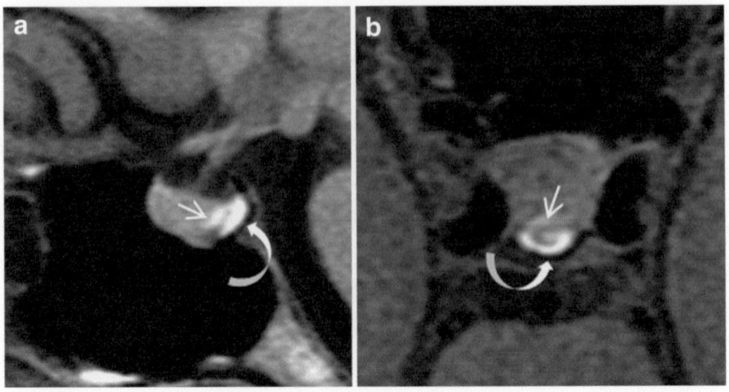

Fig. 52.1 Micro RCC. (**a**) Sagittal T1WI. (**b**) Axial T1 fat-saturated WI. The RCC (*thin arrow*) is just in front of the posterior lobe (*curved arrow*)

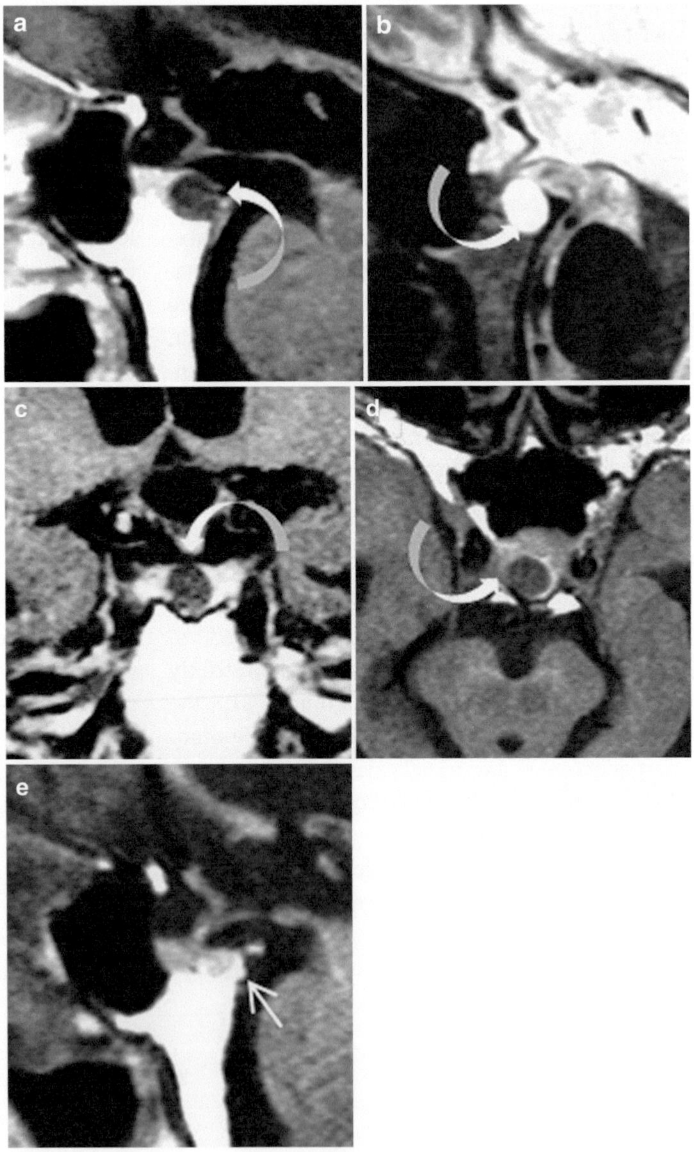

Fig. 52.2 Large asymptomatic posterior lobe cyst in a 63-year-old woman. (**a**, **b**) Sagittal T1 and T2 WIs. (**c**) Coronal T1WI. (**d**) Axial T1WI without contrast. (**e**) Sagittal follow-up 2 years later. The cyst is frankly T1 hypointense and T2 hyperintense. Characteristic T1 hyperintense rim in (**d**). Spontaneous shrinkage in (**e**) at 2 years

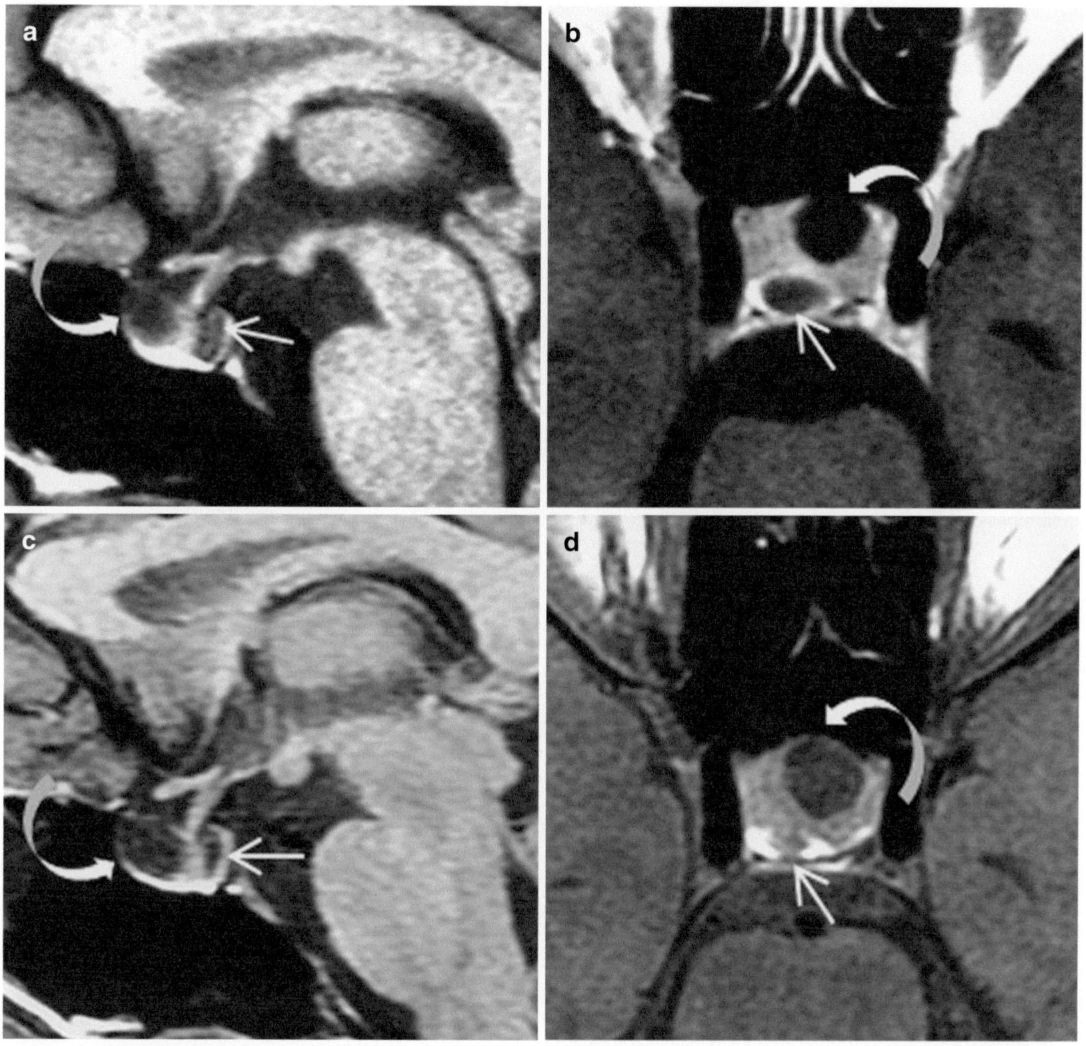

Fig. 52.3 Posterior lobe cyst and possible arachnoid cyst in an asymptomatic 37-year-old woman. (**a**, **b**) Sagittal T1 and axial CE T1 WIs. (**c**, **d**) Sagittal and axial T1WIs 6 years later. Characteristic location and signal of the posterior lobe cyst (*straight arrow*) is slightly compressed 6 years later, while the anterior cyst (*curved arrow*) increases in size and imprints more on the anterior wall of the sella

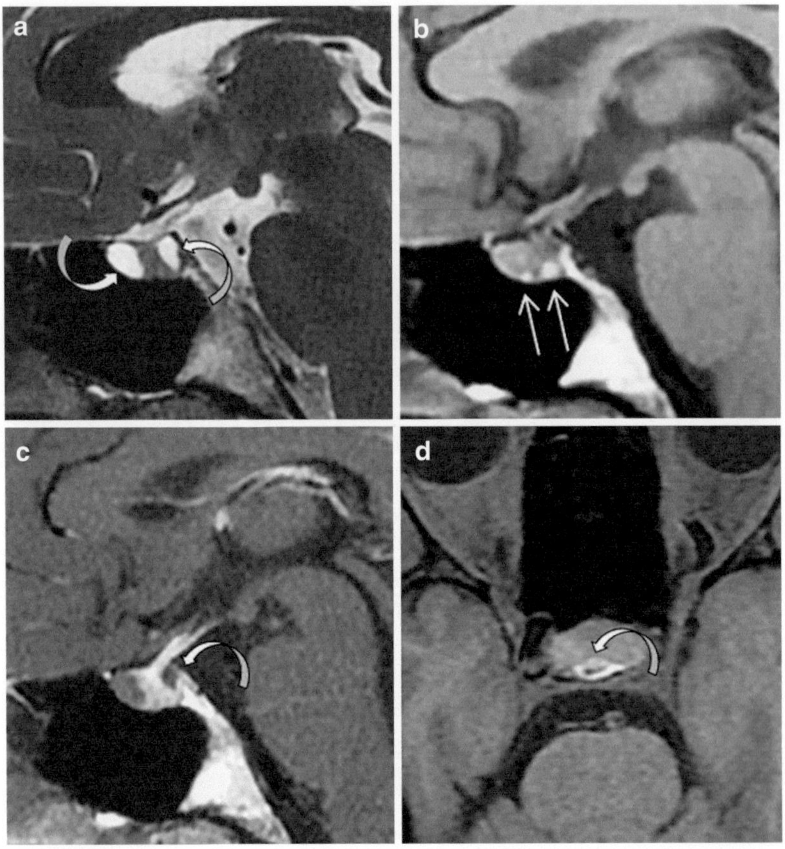

Fig. 52.4 Multiple intrasellar cysts in a 26-year-old asymptomatic woman with posttraumatic cervical pain. (**a**–**c**) Sagittal T1, T2, and CE T1 WIs. (**d**) Axial T1 fat-saturated WI. The more anterior cyst imprints on the anterior wall of the sella (*white arrow*). The more posterior cyst is surrounded by a hyperintense rim and is probably a posterior lobe cleft (*black* and *white arrow*). Two additional tiny cysts in contact with the sellar floor are T1 hyperintense and probably rich in proteins (*thin arrows*)

Further Reading

Meyrignac O, Idir IS, Cognard C, Bonneville JF, Bonneville F (2015) 3D TOF MR angiography to depict pituitary bright spot and to detect posterior pituitary lobe cyst: original description at 3T MR imaging. J Neuroradiol 42:321–325. pii: S0150-9861(15)00113-3. doi:10.1016/j.neurad.2015.04.009

Scangas GA, Laws ER Jr (2014) Pituitary incidentalomas. Pituitary 17(5):486–491

Shanklin W (1949) On the presence of cysts in the human pituitary. Anat Rec 104(4):379–407

Teramoto A, Hirakawa K, Sanno N, Osamura Y (1994) Incidental pituitary lesions in 1,000 unselected autopsy specimens. Radiology 193(1):161–164

53 The Ectopic Posterior Lobe

Jean-François Bonneville and Fabrice Bonneville

The biochemical nature of the T1-high signal intensity of the posterior lobe has been extensively discussed over time, but it is clear today that this MR signal characteristic is related to its secretory and metabolic activity, and reflects the antidiuretic hormone storage. An ectopic posterior lobe results from the impossibility for vasopressin synthesized in the hypothalamic nuclei to reach its storage place at the posterior part of the sella, the route being blocked by a nonfunctional pituitary stalk. Presence of an ectopic posterior lobe means that the upper part of the antidiuretic hormone system works normally, and is thus not consistent with central diabetes insipidus. Presence of an ectopic posterior pituitary bright spot associated with a pituitary stalk abnormality has been abundantly described with isolated GH or multihormonal deficiencies (Fig. 53.1), and in association with midline defects such as septo-optic dysplasia (Fig. 53.2) and Kallmann syndrome (Fig. 53.3). Kallmann syndrome is a neuronal migration disorder characterized by anosmia/hyposmia and hypogonadotropic hypogonadism. MRI shows absence of bilateral olfactory bulbs and sulcus with an apparently normal-appearing pituitary gland, and bilateral loss of distinction between the gyrus rectus and medial orbital gyrus.

GH deficiency is responsible for short stature and delayed skeletal maturation. It is often associated with reduced levels of gonadotropins, causing failure of sexual development. Idiopathic GH deficiency predominates in boys. It may be detected early in the first years of life, or even in the first days of life in cases of multihormonal deficits, and may be responsible for hypoglycemic attacks. The diagnosis can also be made later during childhood with growth deceleration, or even in adulthood. MRI demonstrates an ectopic posterior lobe, a missing or hypoplastic pituitary stalk, and a small anterior pituitary. Three-dimensional magnetic resonance volumetry of the pituitary gland has been proposed to complement the diagnosis of GH or multiple hormone deficiencies but is, in our opinion, not required to make the diagnosis.

Acquired ectopic posterior lobe has received much less attention.

An acquired ectopic posterior lobe occurs when the pituitary stalk function is disrupted: very rarely after severe head trauma; frequently after pituitary surgery; and usually in the case of large tumors of the sellar region pressing on the pituitary stalk. In the latter it has been shown that, in cases of pituitary macroadenomas, an ectopic posterior lobe is developing if the tumor height is more than 20 mm (Fig. 53.4) or less if a tumoral hemorrhage has suddenly compressed the pituitary stalk. With smaller pituitary adenomas, the posterior lobe is found in its usual or eutopic position, i.e., in front of the dorsum sellae. Presence of an ectopic posterior lobe above a sellar mass less than 20 mm high may evoke the diagnosis of a tumor of a firmer consistency than

J.-F. Bonneville et al., *MRI of the Pituitary Gland*, DOI 10.1007/978-3-319-29043-0_53

that of a pituitary adenoma such as a sellar meningioma. Furthermore, an ectopic posterior lobe can be observed in cases of hemorrhagic pituitary adenoma, as already stated, or with tumor recurrence after surgery (Fig. 53.5).

Topography of vasopressin storage within the stalk varies with the level of compression of the stalk. It has been speculated that the sellar diaphragm may play a role in the transportation blockade and the proximal accumulation

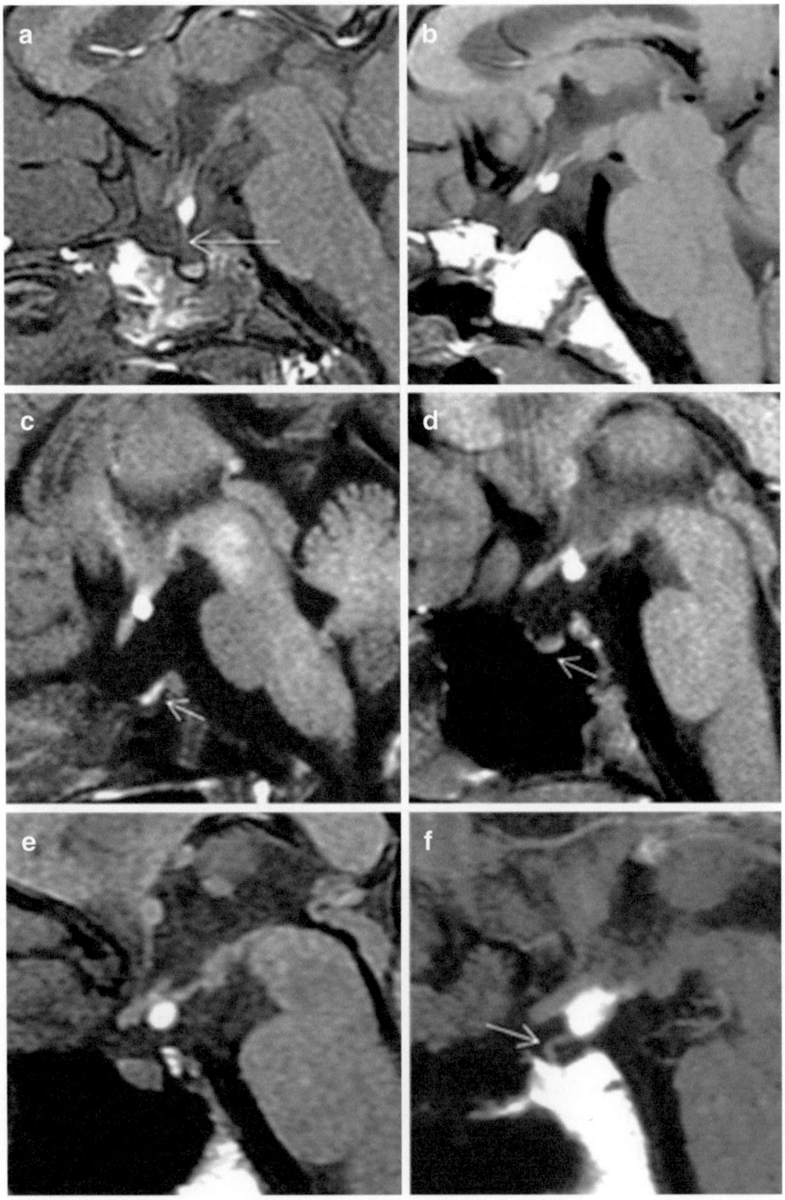

Fig. 53.1 Ectopic posterior pituitary gland in patients with GH hormone deficiency or multihormonal deficiencies. Sagittal T1WIs. (**a**) Three-year-old boy. A thin pituitary stalk is faintly visible (*arrow*). (**b**) Five-year-old boy. The pituitary stalk is not demonstrated. (**c**, **d**) Hypoglycemic attack in a newborn at 1 month (**c**) and MR follow-up at 9 years (**d**). The stalk is not seen. Note the hypoplastic anterior pituitary (*arrows*). (**e**, **f**) Congenital ectopic posterior pituitary gland detected in adulthood. Note the large size of the ectopic posterior pituitary and the hypoplastic pituitary stalk (*arrow*) in (**f**)

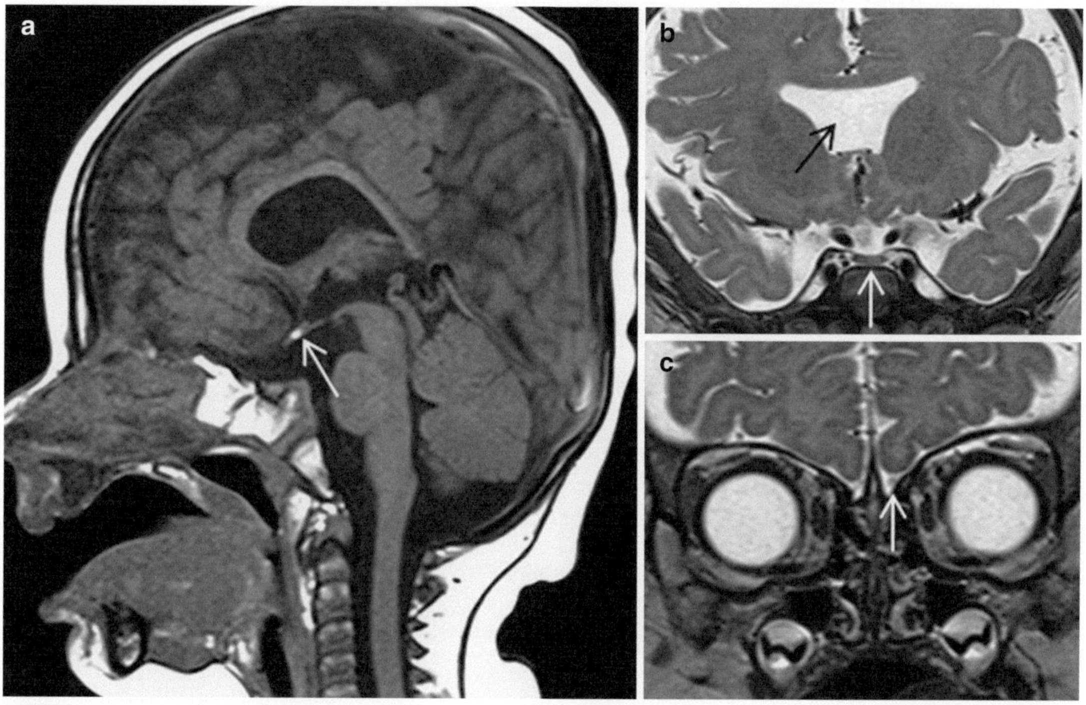

Fig. 53.2 Septo-optic dysplasia. (**a**) Sagittal T1WI. Ectopic posterior lobe (*arrow*). The pituitary stalk is not visible. (**b**) Coronal T2WI. Absent septum lucidum (*black arrow*); hypoplastic anterior pituitary (*white arrow*). The optic chiasm is not recognizable. (**c**) Coronal T2WI 2 cm in front of (**b**). The olfactory bulb is hypoplastic on the left (*arrow*) and not seen on the right; abnormal gyri and ptosis of the gyrus rectus on the right

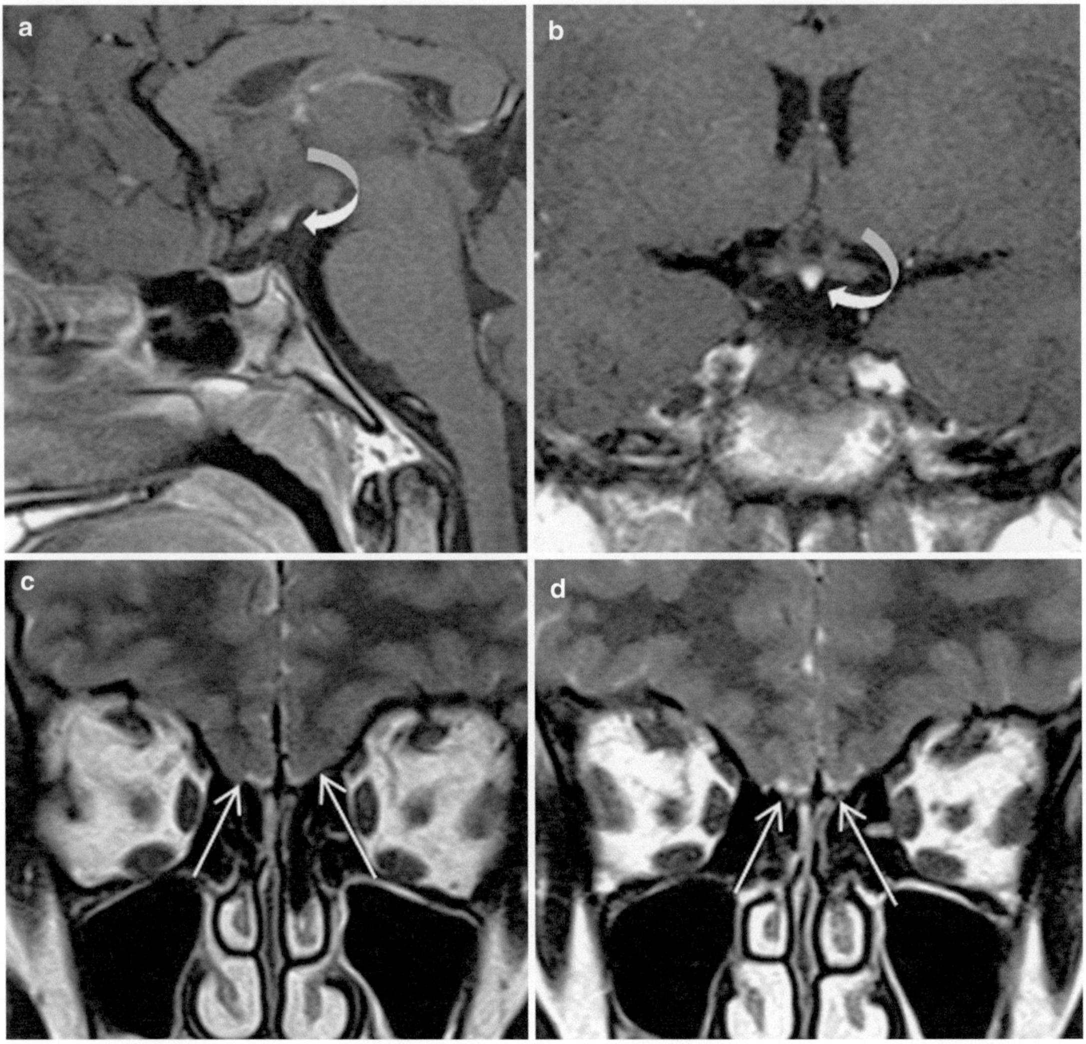

Fig. 53.3 Kallmann syndrome in an 18-year-old man with hyposmia and hypogonadotropic hypogonadism. (**a**) Sagittal CE T1WI. (**b**) Coronal T1WI. (**c**, **d**) Coronal T2WIs. Ectopic posterior lobe (*curved arrow*) and atrophic pituitary stalk. Hypoplastic olfactory bulbs (*small arrows*) and hypoplasia of olfactory sulci. Triangular shape of the inferior aspect of frontal lobes

of the vasopressin-containing neurogranules. The ectopic posterior lobe is usually located at the level of the median eminence with pituitary macroadenomas, and can be masked by the tumoral dome. Rarely, a bright spot can be demonstrated together in a eutopic and ectopic position in cases of partial blockage of the pituitary stalk (Fig. 53.3). After pituitary surgery or pituitary hemorrhage, reappearance of the ectopic posterior pituitary can be delayed for weeks to months or longer (Fig. 53.6); it is variably positioned along the pituitary stalk, most of the time at its lower visible end (Fig. 53.7). In the case of a large secondary empty sella after surgery, ptosis of the third ventricle can occur, bringing the pituitary stalk and ectopic posterior lobe down toward the bottom of the sella (Fig. 53.8). A potential relationship between the precise site of vasopressin storage and the occurrence of postoperative diabetes insipidus has been advanced but not proven.

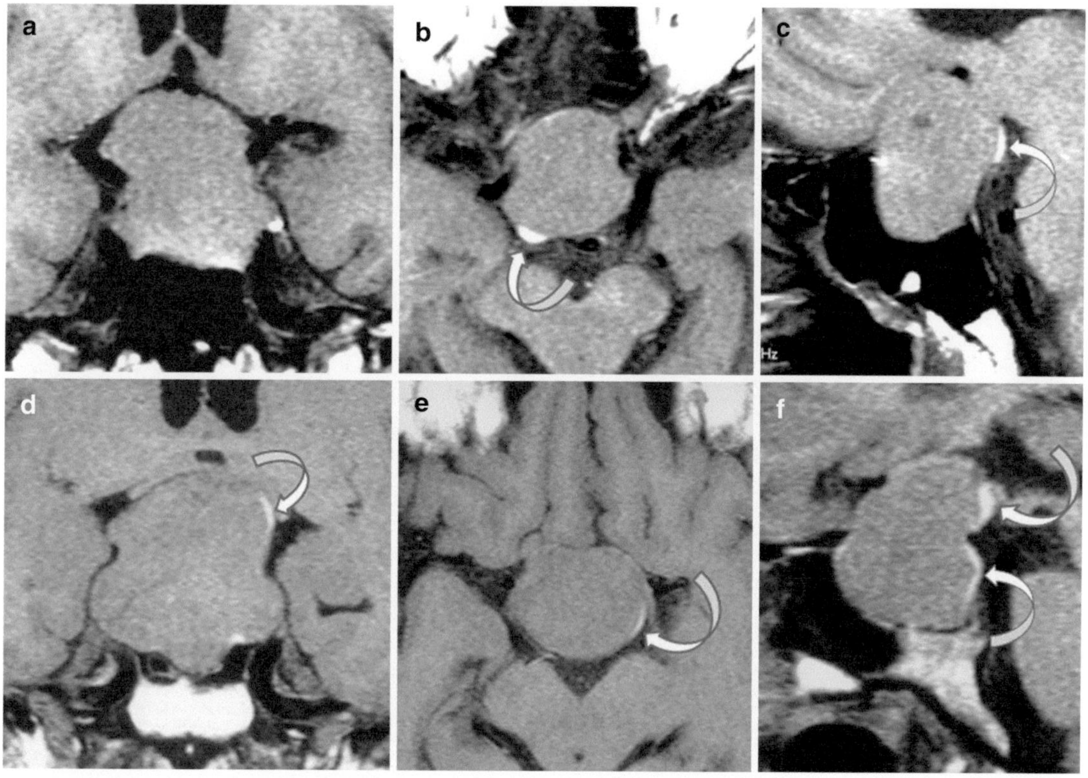

Fig. 53.4 Ectopic posterior pituitary (*arrows*) in three patients with pituitary macroadenomas. (**a–c**) Coronal, axial, and sagittal T1WIs in a nonsecreting adenoma. (**d**, **e**) Coronal and axial T1WIs in a large gonadotropic adenoma. The ectopic posterior pituitary (*arrow*), which is severely compressed, is frequently better demonstrated on axial view. (**f**) Sagittal T1WI in a pituitary adenoma with large suprasellar extension: eutopic and ectopic location of the posterior pituitary (*two arrows*)

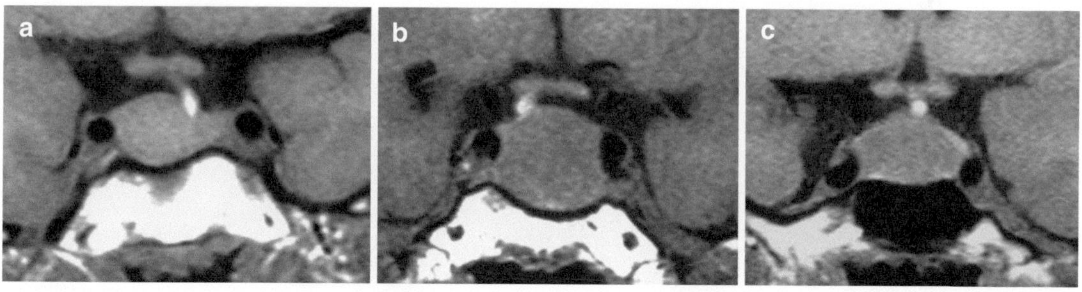

Fig. 53.5 (**a–c**) Coronal T1WIs in three patients. An ectopic posterior pituitary is unusual with pituitary adenomas less than 20 mm in height, except with hemorrhagic pituitary adenoma (**a**) and with recurrence of pituitary adenomas years after surgery (**b**, **c**)

Moderate spontaneous swelling of the ectopic posterior lobe is sometimes seen with time after surgery. More rarely its progressive enlargement is more pronounced, resulting in a potentially intriguing nodule in the suprasellar cistern (Fig. 53.9), especially if its T1W signal is weakly hyperintense. It must be borne in mind here that the signal intensity of the posterior lobe, in eutopic as well as ectopic position, varies with plasma osmolarity, and thus is less intense in various

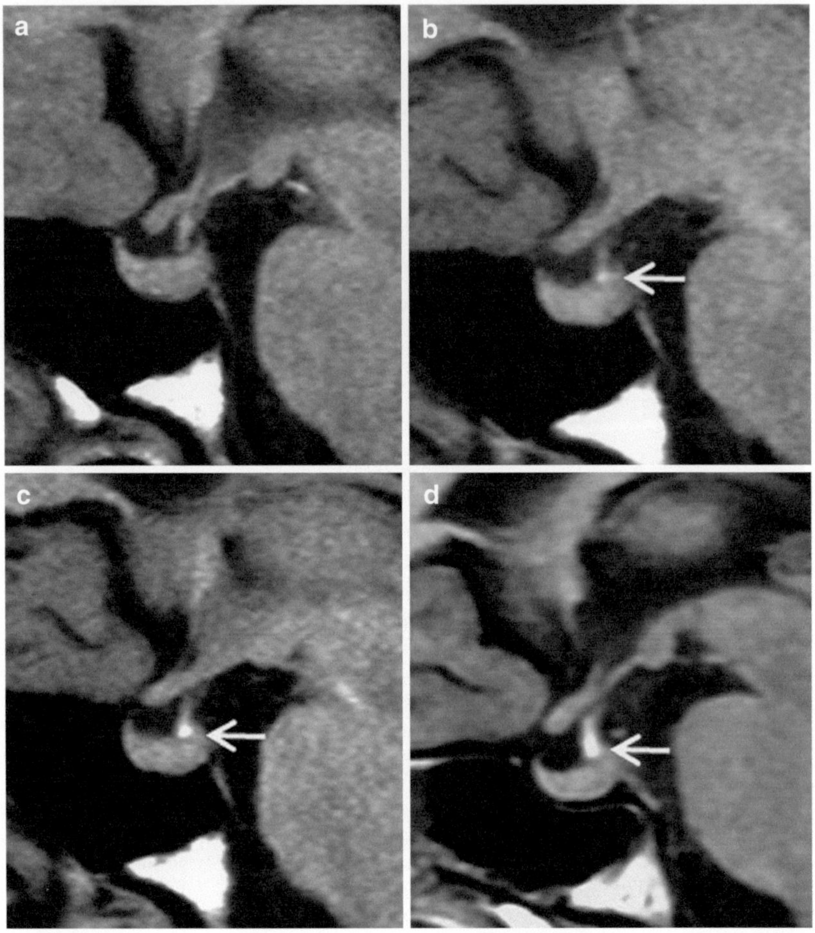

Fig. 53.6 Sagittal T1WIs. A 28-year-old hyperprolactinemic woman presenting with diabetes insipidus at the third trimester of an induced pregnancy. (**a**) Three months after delivery. Vasopressin storage is not demonstrated. (**b–d**) Progressive appearance and slow enlargement of an ectopic posterior lobe (*arrow*). Diabetes insipidus has resolved. (**d**) Nine years after (**a**)

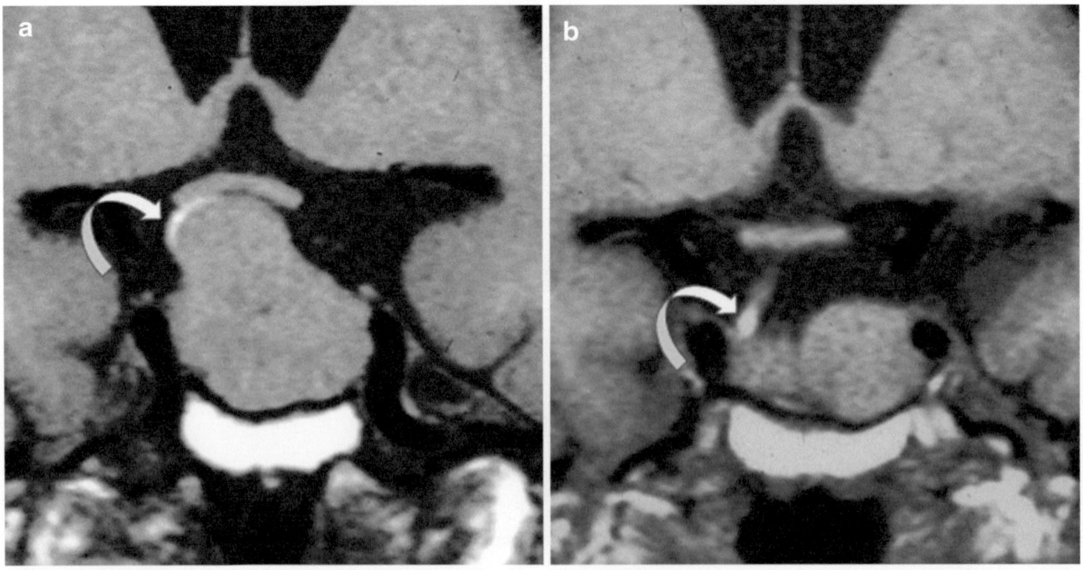

Fig. 53.7 Coronal T1WIs. Pituitary macroadenoma before surgery. (**a**) Vasopressin storage (*arrow*) at the dome of the adenoma. (**b**) Intrasellar recurrence 3 years later. Relocation of vasopressin storage at the inferior part of the pituitary stalk

conditions such as in the elderly, in stressful situations, during pregnancy, and with diabetes mellitus or renal dialysis. This nodular ectopic posterior lobe has been sometimes erroneously described as isointense intracisternal tumor at CT scan.

Differential diagnosis of ectopic posterior pituitary gland includes asymptomatic lipoma in contact with the tuber cinereum. Characteristic location, chemical shift artifact, and fat-suppression sequences make the diagnosis easy.

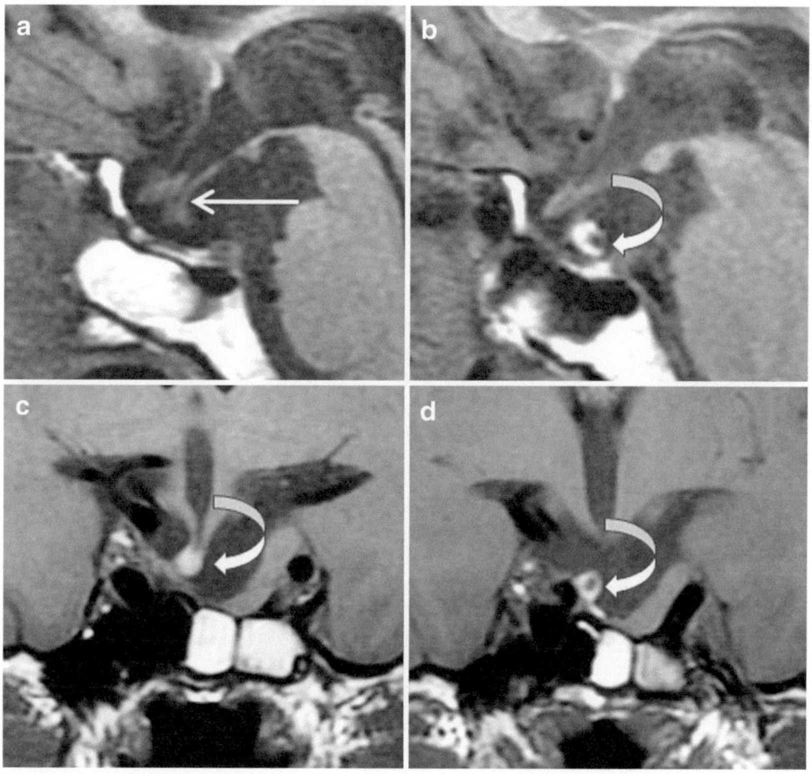

Fig. 53.8 Ectopic posterior pituitary and empty sella after surgery. Contiguous T1WIs in sagittal (**a**, **b**) and coronal (**c**, **d**) sections. A deep infundibular recess of the third ventricle (*straight arrow*) enters into the ectopic posterior lobe (*curved arrow*), which contains CSF in its center

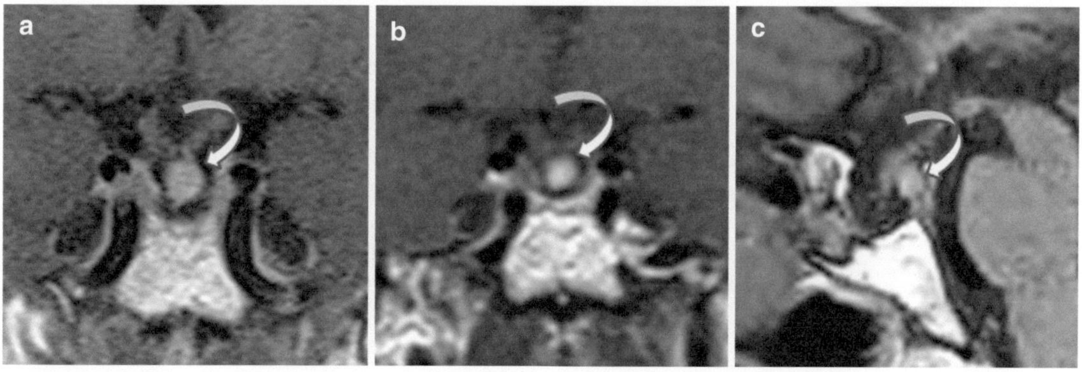

Fig. 53.9 Unusual large intrasellar ectopic posterior lobe (*curved arrow*) 15 years after pituitary surgery. Coronal and sagittal T1WIs (**a**, **c**) and dynamic imaging at the early phase (**b**). T1 hyperintensity of the ectopic posterior lobe is mild, the patient being 70 years old. Intense early enhancement on dynamic scanning

Further Reading

Bonneville F, Narboux Y, Cattin F et al (2002) Preoperative location of the pituitary bright spot in patients with pituitary macroadenomas. AJNR Am J Neuroradiol 23(4):528–532

Fujisawa I, Uokawa K, Hori N et al (2002) Bright pituitary stalk on MR T1-weighted images: damming up phenomenon of the neurosecretory granules. Endocr J 49(2):165–173

Han X, Xiu J, Huang Z et al (2014) Three-dimensional magnetic resonance volumetry of the pituitary gland is effective in detecting short stature in children. Exp Ther Med 8(2):551–556

54 Lipoma

Fabrice Bonneville

Rather than true neoplasms or hamartomas, intracranial lipomas are thought to represent congenital malformations that result from an abnormal persistence and maldifferentiation of the meninx primitiva. This embryologic concept explains the high frequency of callosal and other brain malformations associated with intracranial lipomas. Typically occurring in the midline, the most common locations for these lesions are the corpus callosum and the quadrigeminal cistern. In about 10–15 % of cases, intracranial lipomas are encountered in the suprasellar/interpeduncular region. Although intracranial lipomas are usually asymptomatic and often discovered incidentally on brain CT or MRI, symptoms related to intracranial lipomas have been reported. However, it cannot be excluded that symptoms might be related to an underlying associated brain malformation rather than to this congenital fat pad itself. Thus, so-called osteolipomas of the tuber cinereum have been reported in young girls with precocious puberty, but similar lesions have been found incidentally at autopsy in previously asymptomatic men (Fig. 54.1). In addition, in the rare reported cases of excision of tuber cinereum lipoma, no effect of the surgery was described on the precocious puberty itself. Finally, complete removal of intracranial lipomas by surgery is illusive because such lesions are intimately adherent to the surface of the brain, as explained by their embryogenesis. Diagnosis of lipomas is straightforward on brain imaging. On CT, they exhibit low density typical for fat and may harbor superficial calcification (Fig. 54.1). On MRI, lipomas are well-demarcated homogeneous lesions, hyperintense on T1WI and T2WI, and do not enhance following administration of gadolinium (Figs. 54.1 and 54.3). Of note, dermoid cysts are usually heterogeneous and demonstrate gadolinium uptake of their wall. It is also noteworthy that fat appears with a low-T2* signal intensity and may thus be misdiagnosed as hemorrhage. Additional T1 fat-saturation sequence makes it possible to confirm the presence of fat in the lesion and, subsequently, the diagnosis of lipoma. Such sequence rules out hemorrhage, high-protein content lesion, or any other source of T1 hyperintensity. In the sellar region, suprasellar lipoma may also be mistaken for ectopic pituitary posterior lobe, as observed in dwarfism. In the latter case, this T1 ectopic bright spot is seen at the infundibulum; this T1-high signal intensity is not attenuated on T1 fat-saturated sequence: the sella, anterior pituitary lobe, and stalk are hypoplastic, and overall, normal signal hyperintensity in the posterior aspect of the sella turcica is lacking (Fig. 54.2). If intracranial lipomas are frequently observed in midline, laterosellar lipomas might be encountered along cranial nerves (Fig. 54.3).

J.-F. Bonneville et al., *MRI of the Pituitary Gland*, DOI 10.1007/978-3-319-29043-0_54

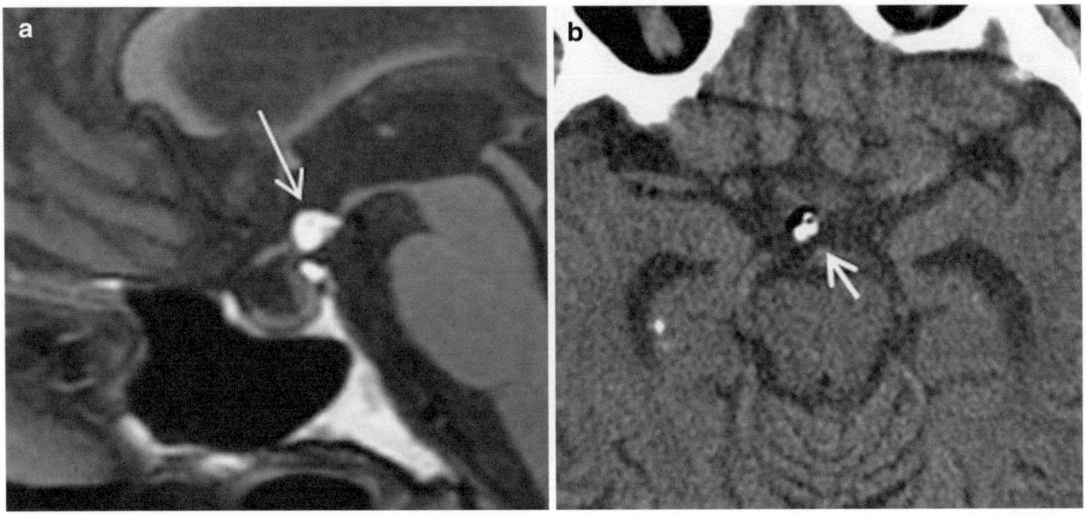

Fig. 54.1 Fortuitous osteolipoma in a 72-year-old man with gait disturbance. (**a**) Sagittal T1WI depicts a suprasellar round fat lesion of the tuber cinereum (*arrow*) with calcifications (*short arrow*), better demonstrated by (**b**) unenhanced CT scan

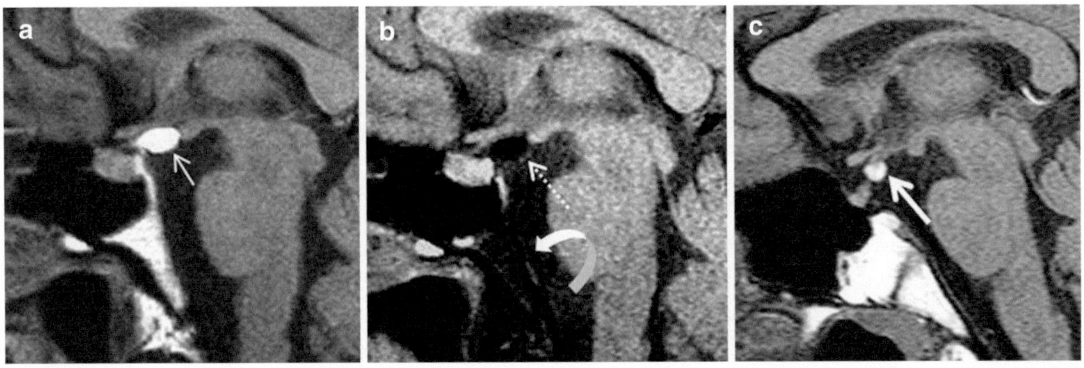

Fig. 54.2 Asymptomatic lipoma of the tuber cinereum in 49-year-old man with headaches. (**a**) Sagittal T1WI shows a typical suprasellar lipoma of floor of the third ventricle (*arrow*). The exclusive fatty nature of this lesion is confirmed on (**b**) T1WI with fat saturation, on which the hyperintense signal due to fat disappears (*dotted arrow*), as observed in the lesion and the fatty bone marrow of the clivus (*curved arrow*). This benign lipoma should not be misdiagnosed as an ectopic pituitary posterior lobe (*thick arrow*), as found in dwarfism and illustrated by (**c**) sagittal T1WI, which appears as a hyperintense bright spot at the infundibulum together with hypoplasia of the sella, anterior pituitary lobe and stalk, and absence of normal signal hyperintensity in the posterior aspect of the sella turcica

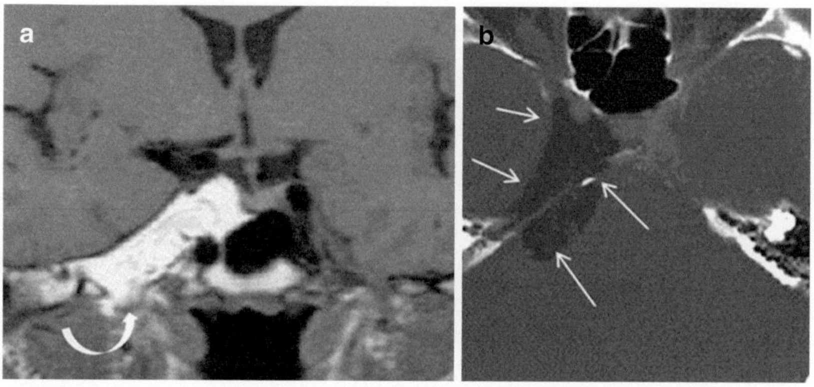

Fig. 54.3 Trigeminal lipoma in a 34-year-old woman with right-sided facial neuralgia. (**a**) Coronal T1WI depicts a right laterosellar hyperintense lesion that occupies the posterior aspect of the cavernous sinus and emerges through the foramen ovale (*curved arrow*). (**b**) Axial CT scan demonstrates the pure fatty nature of the lesion, which parallels the trigeminal nerve and its branches (*arrows*) (Reprinted with permission from Bonneville et al.)

Iatrogenic fatty substances may also be depicted in the sellar region. Iodinated lipiodol that has been used intrathecally may persist for decades and appear as fatty droplets with characteristic T1 hyperintensity (Fig. 54.4). After transsphenoidal resection of pituitary tumors, fatty materials may be used to fill the empty space after excised tissue at the bottom of sella turcica and prevent CSF leakage. In rare instances such fatty filling material may migrate within the subarachnoid space in the sellar region and be the source of subsequent infectious or vascular lesions (Fig. 54.5).

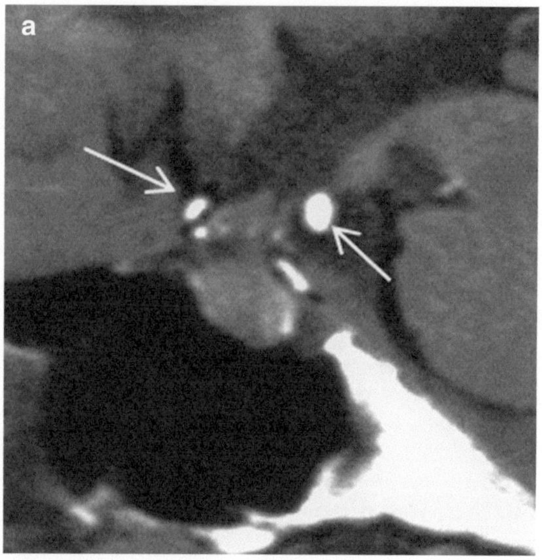

Fig. 54.4 Subarachnoid remnants of contrast material in a 79-year-old woman with a history of intrathecal injection of an iodinated lipid-containing contrast agent. (**a**) Sagittal T1WI shows multiple hyperintense nodules trapped in the chiasmatic cistern (*arrowheads*) (Reprinted with permission from Bonneville et al.)

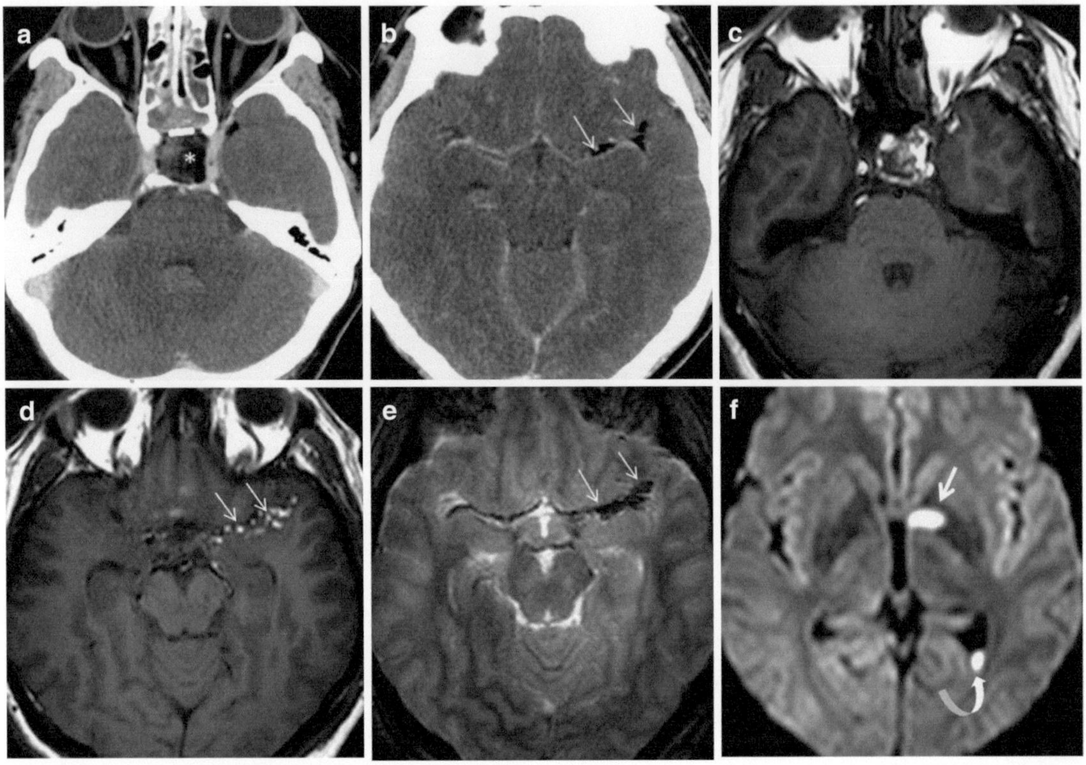

Fig. 54.5 Brain imaging of a 39-year-old man operated on for a macroadenoma via transsphenoidal approach 3 months previously and now suffering from febrile encephalomeningitis with right hemiparesis. (**a**, **b**) CE CT scan shows fat packing of the sellar surgical site (*asterisk*) with partial migration in the left sylvian fissure along the middle cerebral artery (*arrows*). (**c**, **d**) Axial unenhanced T1WIs confirm that the hypodense abnormalities observed on CT were not postoperative air, but true droplets of characteristic hyperintense fat (*arrows*). (**e**) GE T2WI illustrates how fat appears hypointense and can mimic blood on this sequence. (**f**) DWI depicts capsulolenticular ischemia (*thick arrow*). This lesion might be due to arteritis secondary to potential irritation of the left middle cerebral artery encased in the subarachnoid fat or the meningitis. Intracranial infection is established, with visualization of cellular debris and sedimentation in the left occipital horn (*curved arrow*)

Further Reading

Bonneville F, Cattin F, Marsot-Dupuch K, Dormont D, Bonneville JF, Chiras J (2006) T1 signal hyperintensity in the sellar region: spectrum of findings. RadioGraphics 26:93–113

Moschopulos M, Becheanu G, Stamm B (2006) Hypothalamic osteolipoma of the tuber cinereum. J Cell Mol Med 10:240–242

Vivanco-Allende A, García-González M, González-Jiménez D, Pérez-Guirado A, Fernández I, Gómez-Illan R (2012) Precocious puberty produced by an osteolipomas of the tuber cinereum. J Pediatr Endocrinol Metab 25:1165–1168

55 Rare T1 Hyperintensities of the Anterior Pituitary Gland

Jean-François Bonneville and Fabrice Bonneville

T1 signal hyperintensity of the sellar region has many different sources, summarized in Table 55.1. Apart from the normal T1 hyperintensity of the posterior pituitary lobe, the most frequent circumstances result from the presence of blood, such as in hemorrhagic pituitary adenomas, proteins, such as in craniopharyngiomas or Rathke cleft cyst (RCC), or fat, such as in lipomas or dermoid cysts. Another cause is melanin in pituitary primary or metastatic melanocytic tumors.

T1 signal hyperintensity of the anterior pituitary itself can be related to increased hormonal synthesis as seen in newborns and pregnant and lactating women. After pituitary surgery, a small remnant of normal pituitary tissue may in a few cases become T1 hyperintense, probably as a compensatory phenomenon, to increase hormonal production.

T1 hyperintensity of the anterior pituitary gland can also be related to deposition of paramagnetic substances in chronic liver diseases (Fig. 55.1), or of manganese in patients on long-term parenteral nutrition or some drug abusers. In these different conditions, T1 hyperintensity of the basal ganglia is also noted (Fig. 55.2). Endocrine assessment shows no significant abnormality.

Table 55.1 Sellar T1 hyperintensities

(A) Normal causes
Pituitary posterior lobe
Pituitary anterior lobe in newborns and pregnant or lactating women
Bone marrow in dorsum sellae, clinoid process, sellar spine
(B) Lesions with T1 hyperintensity
Due to blood
Pituitary apoplexy/Sheehan syndrome
Chronic hemorrhagic adenoma
Thrombosed aneurysm
Due to high protein content
Rathke cleft cyst
Craniopharyngioma
Mucocele
Abscess
Due to fat
Lipoma
Dermoid cyst
Due to calcification
Chondroid tumor
Chordoma
Other source
Manganese deposit (parenteral nutrition/chronic liver insufficiency)
Melanin in primitive or secondary tumor
Carotid-cavernous fistula

J.-F. Bonneville et al., *MRI of the Pituitary Gland*, DOI 10.1007/978-3-319-29043-0_55

T1 hyperintensity and associated bulging of the pituitary has been reported in high-flow carotid-cavernous fistula (Fig. 55.3). We hypothesized this pattern to be a reaction to the disrupted venous outflow of the pituitary, carotid-cavernous fistula increasing severely the intracavernous venous pressure. After embolization of these fistulas, shrinkage of the pituitary content occurs in a few days but T1 hyperintensity can persist some weeks; it is believed that the embolization material placed in the venous compartment of the cavernous sinus is temporarily responsible for a restriction of the pituitary venous drainage. Later on, cavernous sinus hemodynamics return to more physiologic conditions and the pituitary gland signal becomes again identical to that of the cerebral white matter (Fig. 55.4). The origin of T1 hyperintensity of the anterior pituitary gland observed with carotid-cavernous fistulas has not received any definitive explanation as yet, although pituitary hyperhydration is a possibility. Changes of the frequency of collision of protons or of the percentage of bound water versus free water have been evoked. A similar T1 hyperintensity of the anterior pituitary gland may be observed after therapeutic occlusion of intracavernous internal carotid artery aneurysm.

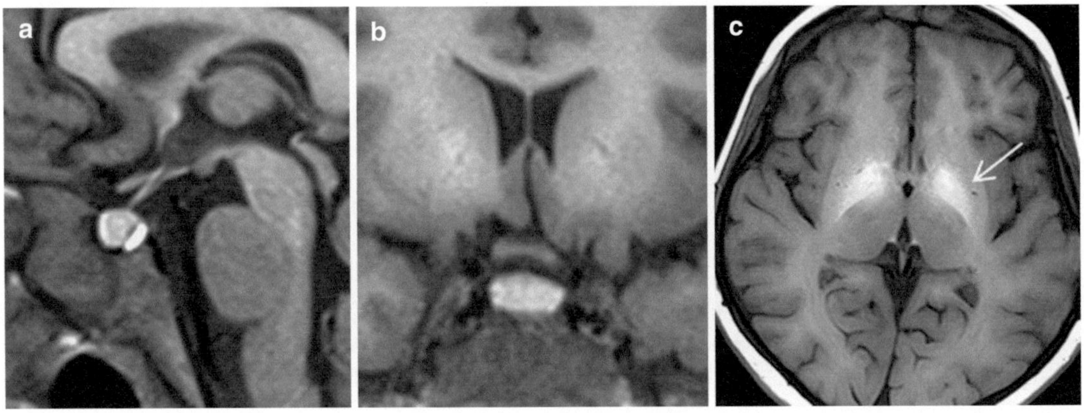

Fig. 55.1 Chronic liver disease in a 12-year-old boy. (**a–c**) Sagittal, coronal, and axial T1WIs. The anterior pituitary is bright, as is the pallidum (*arrow*)

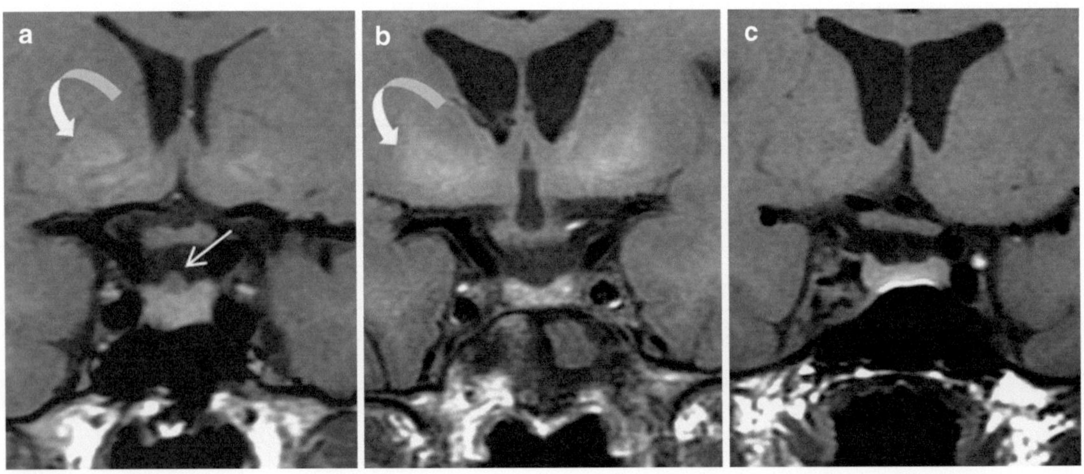

Fig. 55.2 Anterior pituitary hyperintensity on coronal T1WIs. (**a**) In a patient with Budd-Chiari syndrome. A small incidental RCC (*arrow*) is located on the upper surface of the hyperintense pituitary gland. (**b**) In a patient with long-term parenteral nutrition. In both patients, note the increase T1 intensity of the basal ganglia (*curved arrows*). (**c**) In a patient after treatment of a intracavernous internal carotid artery aneurism. In all three patients, the pituitary gland is more T1 hyperintense than the brain white matter

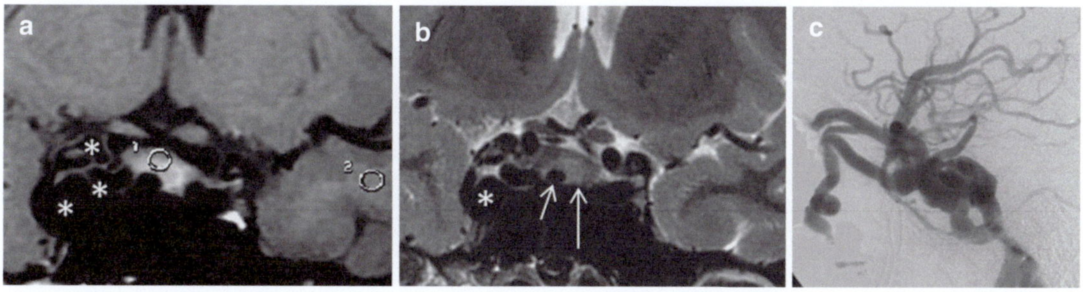

Fig. 55.3 High-flow carotid-cavernous fistula. (**a**) Coronal T1WI, Numerous high-flow vessels in right cavernous sinus (*asterisks*); the pituitary gland (*1*) is bulging and T1 hyperintense compared with the white matter (*2*). (**b**) Coronal T2WI slightly posterior to (**a**). Limited area of T2 hyperintensity (*long arrow*) centered by an intrasellar dilated vein (*short arrow*). (**c**) Right internal carotid artery angiography, sagittal view. The fistula is draining both anteriorly toward the ophthalmic veins and posteriorly toward the inferior petrosal sinus

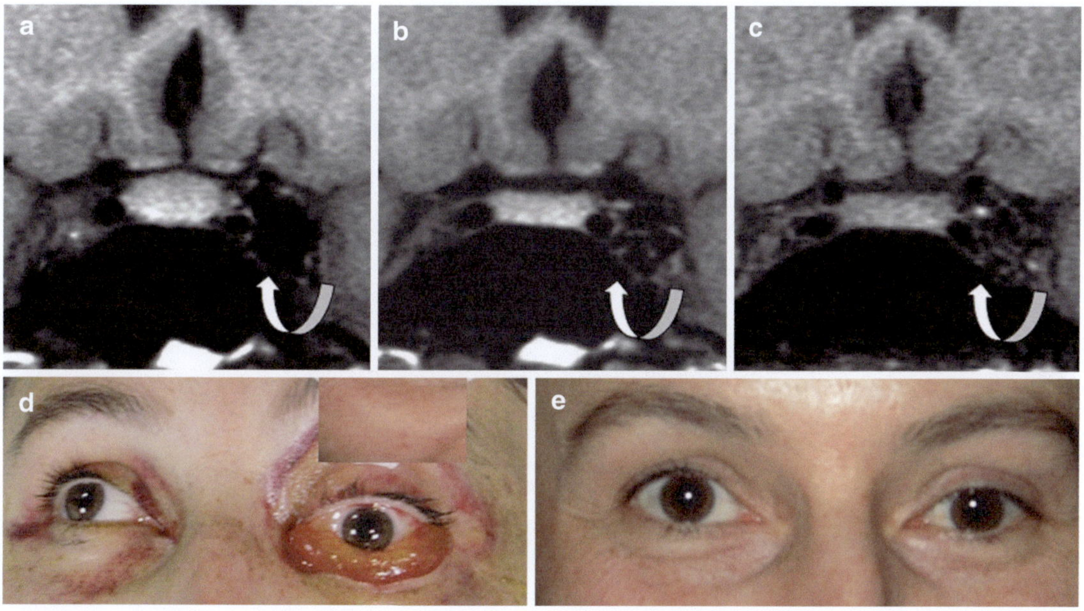

Fig. 55.4 Left carotid-cavernous fistula. (**a–c**) Coronal T1WIs. Before treatment (**a**), bulging of the pituitary gland is T1 hyperintense compared with the cerebral white matter. Enlarged parasellar veins (*arrow*). Left chemosis (**d**). (**b**) After embolization, rapid shrinkage of the pituitary gland, for which the signal is still bright. (**c**) At 1 month, shrinkage of the parasellar veins in left cavernous sinus. Shape and T1 signal of the pituitary gland are normalized. (**d**, **e**) Photographs before and after embolization. Left chemosis has vanished

Further Reading

Bonneville F, Cattin F, Marsot-Dupuch K et al (2006) T1 signal hyperintensity in the sellar region: spectrum of findings. Radiographics 26(1):93–113

Dietemann JL, Reimund JM, Diniz RL et al (1998) High signal in the adenohypophysis on T1-weighted images presumably due to manganese deposits in patients on long-term parenteral nutrition. Neuroradiology 40(12):793–796

Sato N, Putman CM, Chaloupka JC et al (1997) Pituitary gland enlargement secondary to dural arteriovenous fistula in the cavernous sinus: appearance at MR imaging. Radiology 203(1):263–267

Craniopharyngeal Canal and Meningocele

56

Sonia Nagi

Transsphenoidal meningoencephalocele is a rare congenital anomaly that consists of herniation of a CSF-filled cyst through a sphenoidal bony defect. It may be divided into two types: the intrasphenoidal type, extending into the sphenoid sinus and confined by its floor, and the true transsphenoidal type, traversing the floor of the sinus and protruding into the nasopharynx.

There are many theories regarding the formation of this basal meningoencephalocele, among which is incomplete closure of the neural tube and persistence of the craniopharyngeal canal (CPC), resulting in herniation of meninges and brain. CPC is a rare congenital skull defect oblique superiorly and posteriorly in the basisphenoid, extending from the sellar floor to the roof of the nasopharynx and containing a prolongation of dura and vascular structures (Figs. 56.1, 56.2, and 56.3). Transsphenoidal meningoencephaloceles represent less than 5 % of all basal meningoencephaloceles. In the true transsphenoidal type, the age of manifestation of disease ranges from newborn to about 60 years, while the intrasphenoidal type seems to manifest in the fifth or sixth decade of life. This malformation is usually associated with midfacial anomalies such as hypertelorism, broad nasal root, cleft palate, and cleft lip or high arch palate and nystagmus. Association with optic malformation such as optic disc

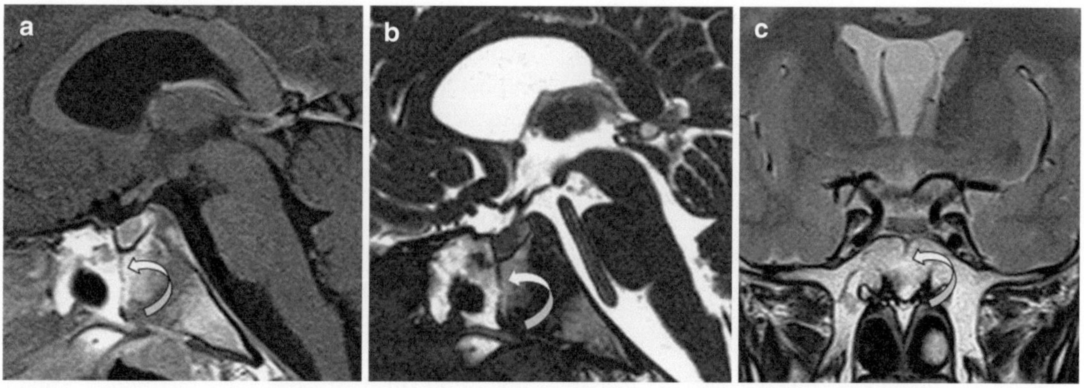

Fig. 56.1 Small incidental craniopharyngeal canal. (**a**, **b**) Sagittal CE T1 and T2 high-resolution WIs. (**c**) Coronal T2WI. Thin vertical hypointense line in the center of basisphenoid originating at the sellar floor level (*curved arrow*). Pituitary gland and stalk, suprasellar cistern, third ventricle, and optic chiasm are in normal position

J.-F. Bonneville et al., *MRI of the Pituitary Gland*, DOI 10.1007/978-3-319-29043-0_56

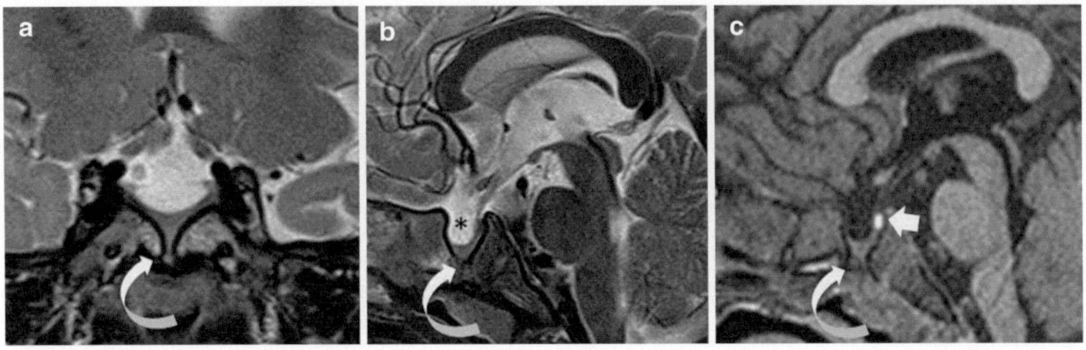

Fig. 56.2 Large persistent craniopharyngeal canal. (**a**) Coronal T2WI. (**b**, **c**) Sagittal T2 and T1 WIs. Well-corticated bone defect through the midline of the basisphenoid (*curved arrow*). Intrasellar arachnoidocele (*asterisk*). No transsphenoidal mass. Bright spot of posterior lobe (*arrow*)

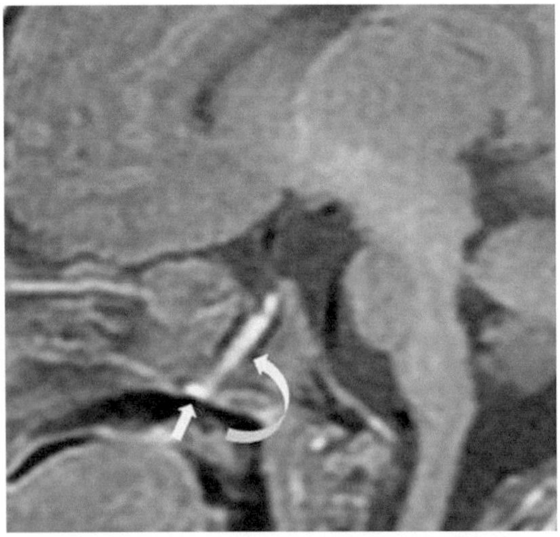

Fig. 56.3 Large persistent craniopharyngeal canal. Sagittal T1WI in a 2-day-old newborn. Defect in the center of basisphenoid (*curved arrow*) extends from the sellar floor to the roof of nasopharynx (*arrow*). Hyperintensity of canal content corresponds to displaced posterior lobe and anterior pituitary tissue in the canal (normal T1 hyperintensity of the anterior pituitary in the newborn)

coloboma, optic nerve coloboma, or microphthalmos has scarcely been reported.

The clinical presentation of patients with transsphenoidal meningoencephalocele is variable. Small meningoencephaloceles are usually asymptomatic. If larger with intrasellar or a transsellar extension, pituitary deficiency may be observed, from GH deficiency to panhypopituitarism. Other clinical manifestations may consist of progressive visual field defect, optic nerve hypoplasia, nasopharynx mass, respiratory distress caused by epipharyngeal obstruction, CSF rhinorrhea, or meningitis. However, intra- and transsphenoidal meningoencephaloceles can be seen in the absence of midfacial anomalies and pituitary dysfunction.

MRI is essential in evaluating the content of intra- and transsphenoidal meningoencephaloceles, the content of which is isointense to CSF. It usually contains the infundibulum, the optic chiasm, the recesses of the third ventricle and, less commonly, the hypothalamus. MRI will specify the type of meningoencephalocele by showing its extension into the sphenoid bone, above or through the sphenoidal floor. In the transsphenoidal type, the meningoencephalocele can cause hard palate scalloping (Fig. 56.4).

MRI allows visualization of the pituitary stalk and gland in medium-sized intrasphenoidal meningoencephaloceles. In large meningoencephaloceles, the pituitary gland and infundibulum are displaced within the nasopharyngeal cyst and, thus, not individualized. MRI will also show possible associated abnormalities such as agenesis of corpus callosum, abnormal cerebral vascularization, midline abnormalities, and posterior fossa malformation (Fig. 56.5).

The diagnosis of this condition is important in saving the patient from excision or biopsy, which may end in CSF leakage, meningitis, brain abscess, or death. Intrasphenoidal meningoencephalocele must be distinguished from cystic pituitary adenoma, Rathke cleft cyst, cystic craniopharyngioma, or hypophyseal duplication (see Chap. 57). Indications for treatment and choice of surgical approach remain controversial. The main indications for intervention are

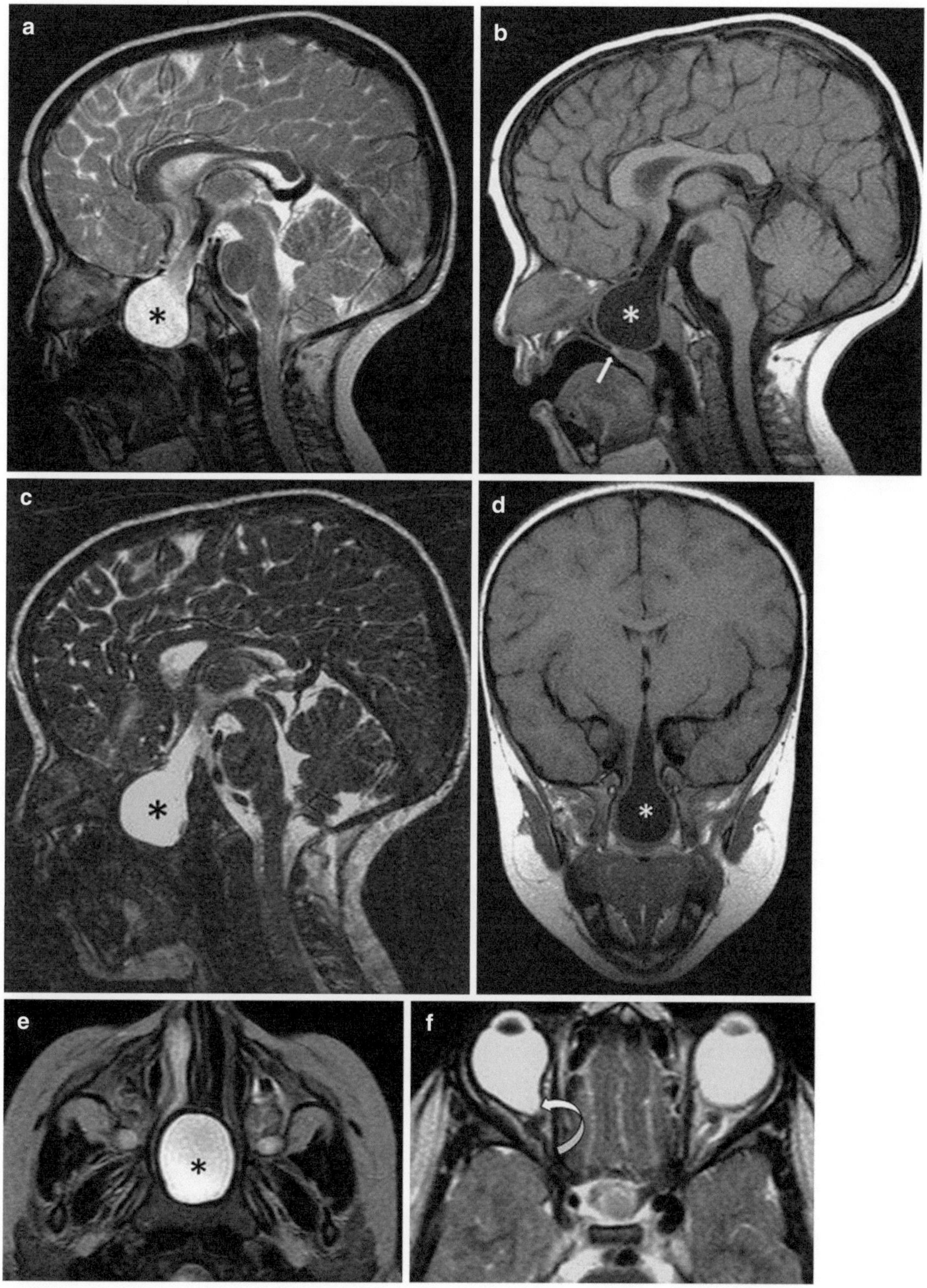

Fig. 56.4 Transsphenoidal meningocele. (**a–c**) Sagittal T2, T1, and T2 high-resolution WIs. Cystic lesion isointense to CSF on all sequences, in continuation with the third ventricle and extending to the nasopharynx through a large defect in the basisphenoid (*star*). Hard palate scalloping (*arrow*). Hypothalamus, optic nerves, and chiasm are displaced downward. Stalk and pituitary gland are not individualized because of lamination. (**e**, **f**) Axial T2WIs. Cystic nasopharyngeal mass (*asterisk*). Coloboma: cystic expansion of the right optic disc isointense with vitreous (*curved arrow*)

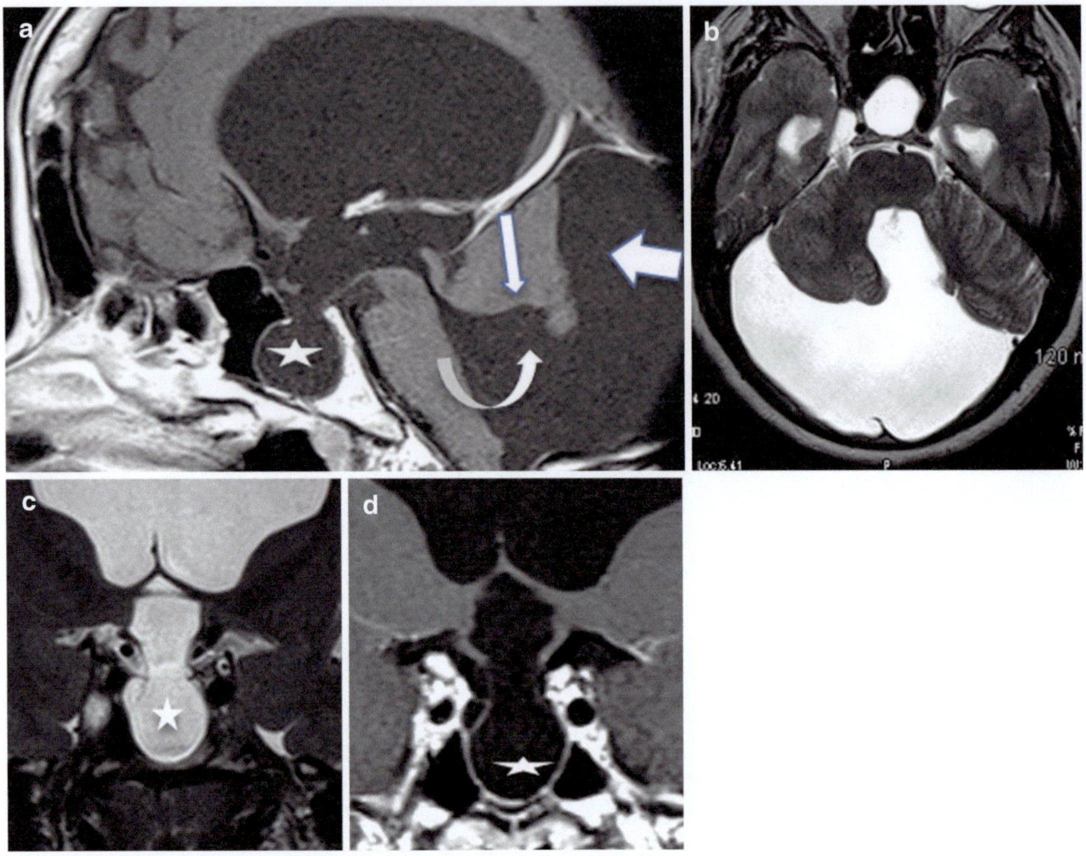

Fig. 56.5 Transsphenoidal meningocele in Dandy-Walker malformation. (**a**) Sagittal CE T1WI. Suprasellar, intrasellar, and transsphenoidal cystic lesion in continuation with the third ventricle and extending to the nasopharynx through the basisphenoid (*asterisk*). Dandy-Walker malformation with enlarged posterior fossa (*thick arrow*), hypoplasia of the vermis (*arrow*), cystic dilatation of the fourth ventricle extending posteriorly (*curved arrow*), and hydrocephalus. (**b**) Axial T2WI. Cystic dilatation of the fourth ventricle. (**c**, **d**) Coronal T2 and CE T1WIs. Intrasellar and transsphenoidal CSF-filled meningocele (*star*)

obstruction of the respiratory pathway, repeated meningitis, rhinorrhea, and progressive visual defect. The transnasal transsphenoidal endoscopic approach seems to be preferred.

Further Reading

Abele TA, Salzmann KL, Harnsberger HR et al (2014) Craniopharyngeal canal and its spectrum of pathology. Am J Neuroradiol 35:772–777

Currarino G, Maravilla KR, Salyer KE (1985) Transsphenoidal canal (large craniopharyngeal canal) and its pathologic implications. Am J Neuroradiol 6:39–43

Jabre A, Tabaddor R, Samaraweera R (2000) Transsphenoidal meningoencephalocele in adults. Surg Neurol 54:183–188

57 Pituitary Gland Duplication and Triplication

Sonia Nagi

Duplication of the pituitary gland is a rare malformation. It can be complete, involving both the pituitary gland and stalk, or incomplete, affecting the adenohypophysis or the pituitary stalk. Exceptionally the malformation consists in a triplication of the pituitary gland and stalk. The suggested pathogenesis is duplication of the prochordal plate and rostral end of the notochord during early embryologic development. When associated with severe abnormalities, this malformation often results in death within the neonatal period. In other cases, presenting signs are delayed puberty or precocious puberty. It is commonly associated with various midline craniofacial malformations such as hypertelorism, cleft palate, tongue anomalies, choanal atresia, pharyngeal mass protruding in the oral cavity, and persistence of the craniopharyngeal canal. Intracerebral anomalies include thickening of hypothalamus caused by tubomamillary fusion, corpus callosum agenesis, thalamic fusion resulting from mass intermedia agenesis, posterior cranial fossa malformations, olfactory nerve anomalies, circle of Willis anomalies, microcephaly, neuronal migration disorders, hydrocephalus, and spinal abnormalities. Incomplete duplication is considered a less severe malformation, usually not associated with other major anomalies and allowing patients to reach adulthood. Asymptomatic forms have been reported.

In complete duplication, the most constant sign on MRI is a midline elongated hypothalamic mass along the floor of the third ventricle, extending from the optic chiasm to the interpeduncular fossa. This characteristic sign is due to tubomamillary fusion, which is best seen on the midline sagittal image. Fusion of tuber cinereum and mammillary bodies is histologically consistent with an arrest of lateral migration in cells that would normally form the hypothalamic nuclei. This thickening of the hypothalamus leads one to perform thin-section images of the sellar region, which will show two infundibular recesses, two infundibular stalks, and two pituitary stalks extending to two small pituitary glands within two separated pituitary fossa. This is best demonstrated on coronal images (Fig. 57.1). A screening for all the aforementioned intracerebral anomalies should be performed on MR. MRA is recommended for the diagnosis of vascular anomalies, such as basilar artery fenestration. Cranial anomalies such as skull-base defects are better delineated on CT. Differential diagnosis of a mass of the floor of the third ventricle includes hypothalamic hamartoma and hypothalamic glioma. In cases of non-visualization of the pituitary gland or stalk on the midline sagittal MR image, pituitary gland agenesis or hypoplasia and transected pituitary stalk can be distinguished from

J.-F. Bonneville et al., *MRI of the Pituitary Gland*, DOI 10.1007/978-3-319-29043-0_57

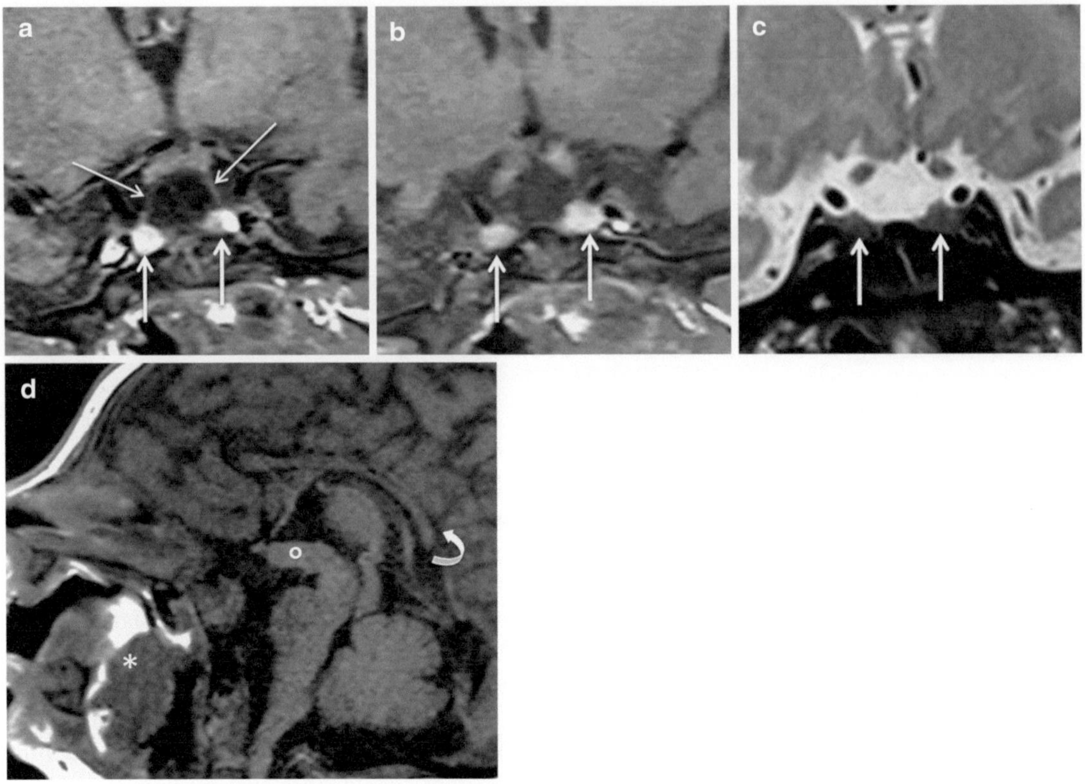

Fig. 57.1 7-day-old boy with mild facial dysmorphism. Duplicated pituitary gland and stalk; mass of the oral cavity. (**a**–**b**) Coronal T1WI and (**c**) T2WI: two pituitary stalks (*long arrows*) and two separate bright pituitary glands (*thick arrows*) within duplicated sella. (**d**) Midline sagittal T1WI: thickening of the floor of the third ventricle resulting from tubomamillary fusion (*circle*). Heterogeneous protruding mass in the oral cavity with fatty component (*asterisk*), the splenium of corpus callosum is thin (*curved arrow*)

complete pituitary duplication by findings in the coronal plane.

Unlike complete pituitary duplication, hypothalamus thickening is absent in incomplete duplication. In incomplete duplication that involves the pituitary stalk, there is a defect of the anterior aspect of the third ventricle floor, enlarging the infundibular recess. Two pituitary stalks, each arising from the floor of the third ventricle, are depicted. Adenohypophysis and sella are single and the posterior pituitary is normal. Anterior third ventricle defect may also suggest the diagnosis of meningocele. The best argument in favor of pituitary stalk duplication is absence of mass effect. Incomplete duplication involving the adenohypophysis is seen on MRI as a linear hypointensity on all sequences, splitting in two the adenohypophysis.

Triplication of the pituitary gland and stalk is exceptional. It can be incomplete with three separate pituitary stalks and a single pituitary gland (Fig. 57.2), or complete with two lateral pituitary glands and a midline gland, each with an independent stalk (Fig. 57.3).

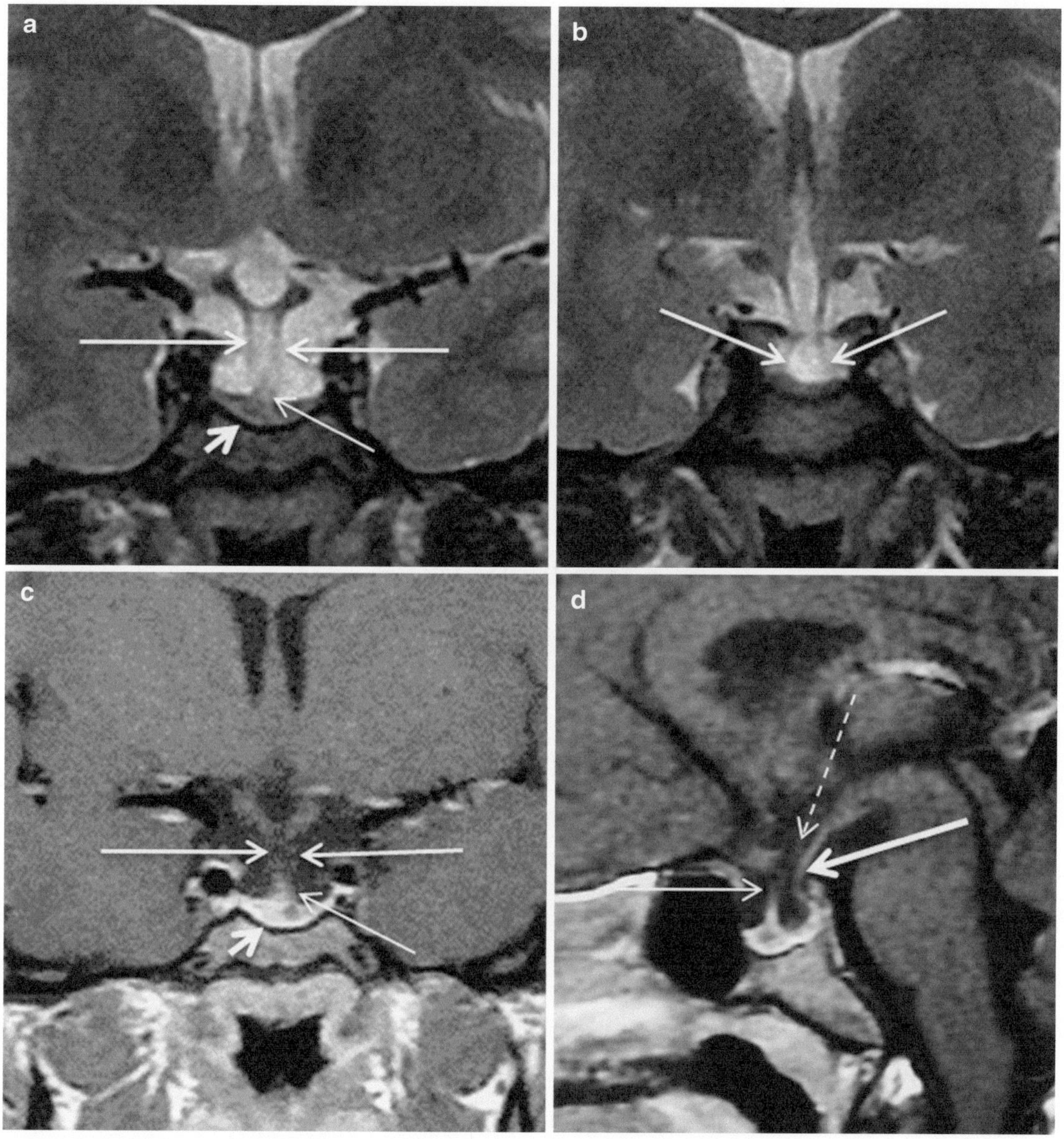

Fig. 57.2 A 20-year-old woman with harmonious dwarfism, spanomenorrhea, and dysmorphism. Pituitary stalk triplication. (**a**, **b**) Coronal T2WIs. Two separate parasagittal pituitary stalks, extending inferiorly to the lateral parts of the pituitary gland (*thick arrows*). Pituitary gland insertion of a median pituitary stalk (*thin arrow*). Single hypoplastic pituitary gland within a large sella (*short arrow*). (**c**) Coronal and sagittal CE T1WIs. Two separate parasagittal pituitary stalks (*thick arrows*). Enhancement of the median pituitary stalk (*thin arrow*) and pituitary gland (*short arrow*). (**d**) Midline sagittal CE T1WI. Defect at the anterior aspect of the floor of the third ventricle (*dotted arrow*) enlarging the infundibular recess without mass effect. Median anterior pituitary stalk (*thin arrow*). Left parasagittal pituitary stalk (*thick arrow*)

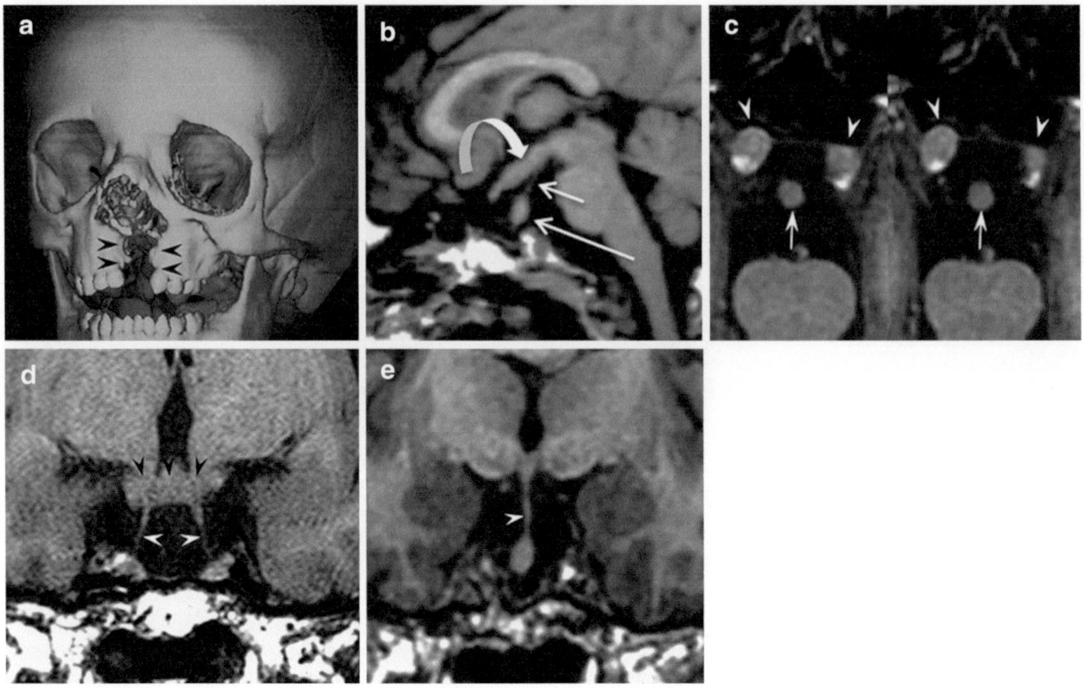

Fig. 57.3 7-y-old first child with midline palate cleft, occult spinal dysraphism, scoliosis. Hypophyseal triplication. (**a**) CT, 3D reconstructed image of the head : midline palate cleft (*black arrowheads*). (**b**) Midline sagittal multiplanar reconstruction T1WI. Thickened third ventricle floor (*curved arrow*). Homogeneous isointense median mass (*long arrow*) whith its independent stalk (*short arrow*). (**c**) Axial multiplanar reconstruction T1WIs: 3 pituitary glands are contemporaneously visible: two parasagittal each with a neurohypophyseal bright spot (*white arrowheads*) and a median one (*arrow*). (**d**) Coronal T1WI. Paired infundibula (*white arrowheads*) extending inferiorly to two pituitary glands fossa. The hypothalamus appears grossly thickened with two infundibula (*black arrowheads*). (**e**) Coronal multiplanar reconstruction T1WI : third medial pituitary stalk (*white arrowhead*). (Courtesy of R.Manara, MD)

Further Reading

De Penna GC, Pimenta MP, Drummond JB et al (2005) Duplication of the hypophysis associated with precocious puberty: presentation of two cases and review of pituitary embryogenesis. Arq Bras Endocrinol Metabologia 49:323–327

Kandpal H, Seith A, Philip J et al (2007) Partial duplication of the hypophysis in adult patients: report of 2 cases. J Comput Assist Tomogr 3:365–367

Manara R, Citton V, Rossetto M et al (2009) Hypophyseal triplication: case report and embryologic considerations. Am J Neuroradiol 30:1328–1329

The Sellar Spine

58

Françoise Cattin

The sellar spine is a bony intrasellar spine arising on the midline from the inferior portion of the anterior aspect of the dorsum sellae and protruding into the pituitary fossa. The sellar spine corresponds to the ossified remnant of the cephalic tip of the notochord. If unrecognized, the sellar spine can lead to misinterpretation of MRI of the pituitary region.

Identification of the sellar spine is easy on thin CT slices: it appears as a bony spur, more or less thick with variable length. Axial and sagittal images and 3D reconstructions demonstrate the spine arising from the lower part of the dorsum sellae (Fig. 58.1).

Visualization of the sellar spine is often more difficult on MRI. In the coronal plane it appears as a small midline intrasellar round image hypointense on T1 and T2 sequences, frequently bordered by a susceptibility magnetic artifact (Fig. 58.2). In the sagittal plane the sellar spine is very difficult to identify, and mostly only the presence of a stocky dorsum sellae attracts attention. It can be the source of a deformity and upward extension of the pituitary gland, mimicking a pituitary enlargement (Fig. 58.3).

J.-F. Bonneville et al., *MRI of the Pituitary Gland*, DOI 10.1007/978-3-319-29043-0_58

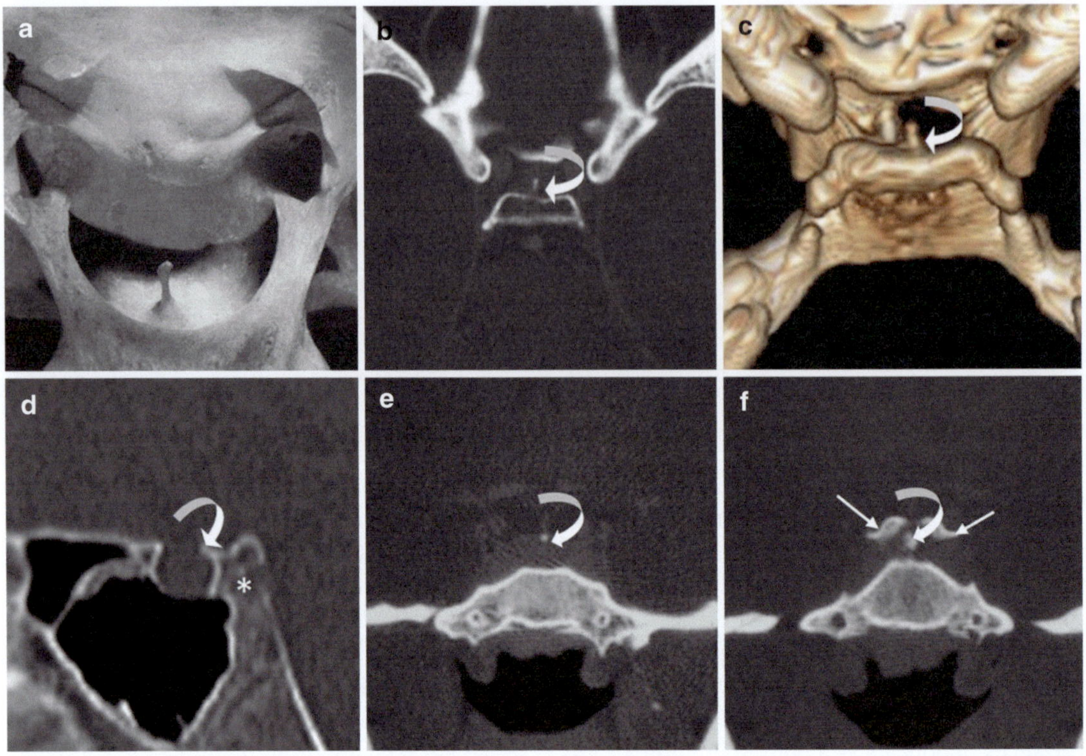

Fig. 58.1 (**a**) Anatomic specimen (Courtesy J Lang). (**b**) Axial CT scan, bone window and (**c**) 3D reformatted image. Thin spur arising from the anterior surface of the dorsum sellae (*curved arrow*). (**d**) Sagittal CT scan, bone window. The sellar spine (*curved arrow*) is associated with a stocky dorsum sellae (*asterisk*). (**e**, **f**) Coronal CT scan. The sellar spine appears as a small intrasellar hyperdense structure, very thin distally and thicker close to the dorsum sellae (*curved arrow*), between the posterior clinoid processes (*arrows*)

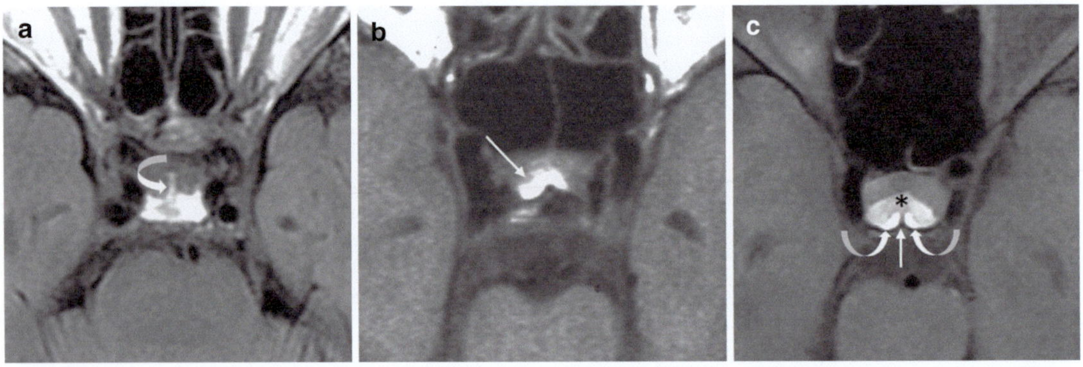

Fig. 58.2 Three different patients. (**a**) Axial T1WI. Thin spur (*curved arrow*) arising from a large fatty dorsum sellae. (**b**) Axial T1WI. Marked susceptibility magnetic artifact (*arrow*) in front of a short sellar spine, hiding the posterior lobe of the pituitary gland (**c**) CE T1W with fat-saturated MR images. Association of a sellar spine (*straight arrow*) and a Rathke cleft cyst (*asterisk*). The sellar spine transfixes the posterior lobe (*curved arrows*)

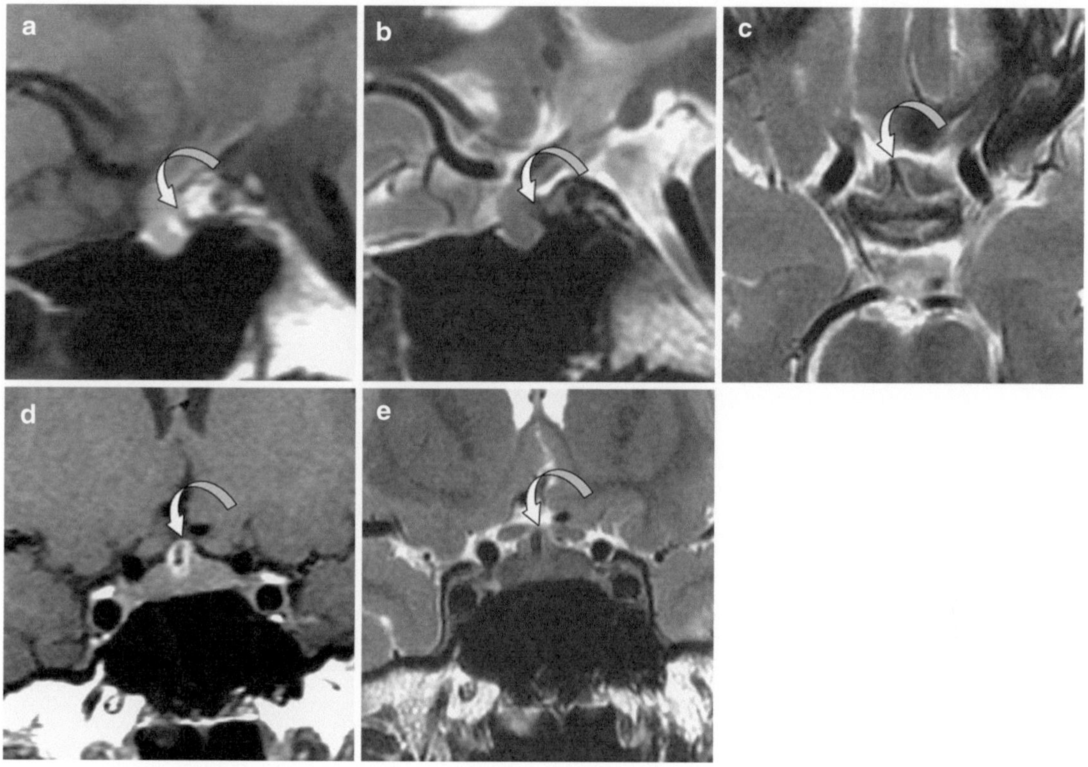

Fig. 58.3 (**a**, **b**) Sagittal T1 and T2 WIs. The sellar spine (*curved arrow*) is difficult to identify on sagittal plane. The small size of the sella turcica and the sellar spine are responsible for the bulging of the pituitary gland. (**c**) The sellar spine (*curved arrow*) is well demonstrated on axial T2WI. (**d**) On coronal T1WI (3 T), the sellar spine induces a susceptibility magnetic artifact. (**e**) On coronal T2WI, the sellar spine appears hypointense

Further Reading

Dietemann JL, Bonneville JF, Cattin F, Poulignot D (1983) Computed tomography of the sellar spine. Neuroradiology 24:173–174

Matsumoto K, Uchino A, Kato A, Kudo S, Kuno T (1997) CT and MRI of sellar spine with upward extension of the pituitary gland: case report. Eur Radiol 7:287–288

59 Vascular Variants of the Sellar Region

Françoise Cattin

59.1 Persistent Trigeminal Artery

The persistent trigeminal artery is the most common persistent fetal carotid-basilar anastomosis (0.1–0.2 %).

In the lateral type, the trigeminal artery arises from the lateral aspect of the intracavernous internal carotid artery, and runs caudally, passing round the bottom of the dorsum sellae to join the basilar artery (Fig. 59.1). In this case, the persistent trigeminal artery is easily identified and does not perturb the analysis of the sellar content.

In the medial type the trigeminal artery arises from the medial aspect of the internal carotid artery, runs caudally through the sella turcica, and pierces the dorsum sellae to join the basilar artery (Fig. 59.2). In this case, the unusual intrasellar vessel can be the source of traps. On coronal T1 and T2 WIs, it appears as a lateralized round hypointense structure in contact with the sellar floor. Sagittal and axial MR images and axial CT demonstrate the channel piercing the dorsum sellae. 3D time-of-flight (TOF) MRA helps to confirm the

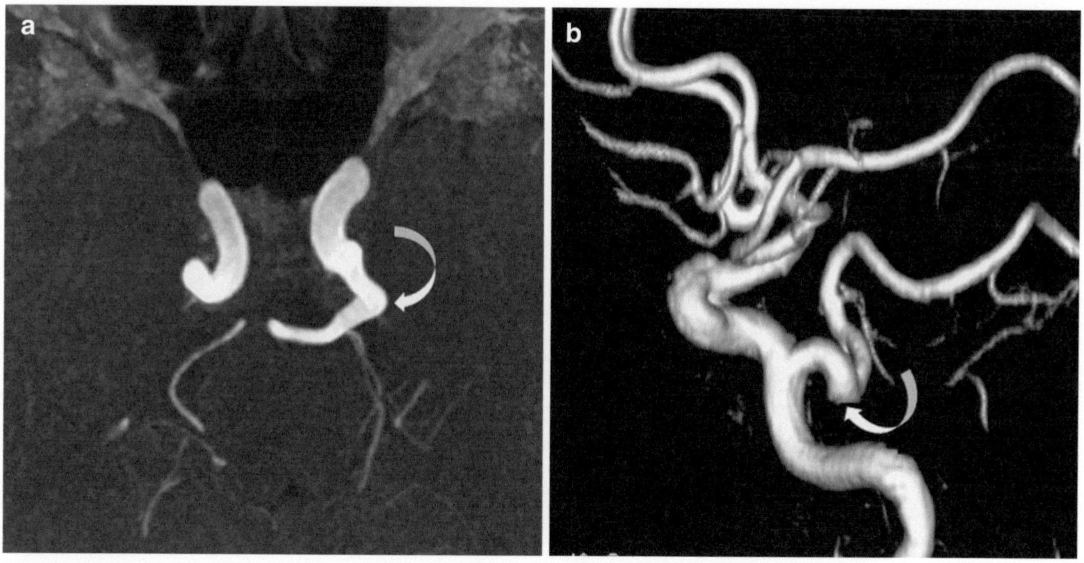

Fig. 59.1 MRA 3D TOF. (**a**) Axial maximal-intensity projection (MIP) reconstruction and (**b**) Volume-rendered sagittal view demonstrating a lateral persistent trigeminal artery (*curved arrow*) passing around the dorsum sellae to join the basilar artery

J.-F. Bonneville et al., *MRI of the Pituitary Gland*, DOI 10.1007/978-3-319-29043-0_59

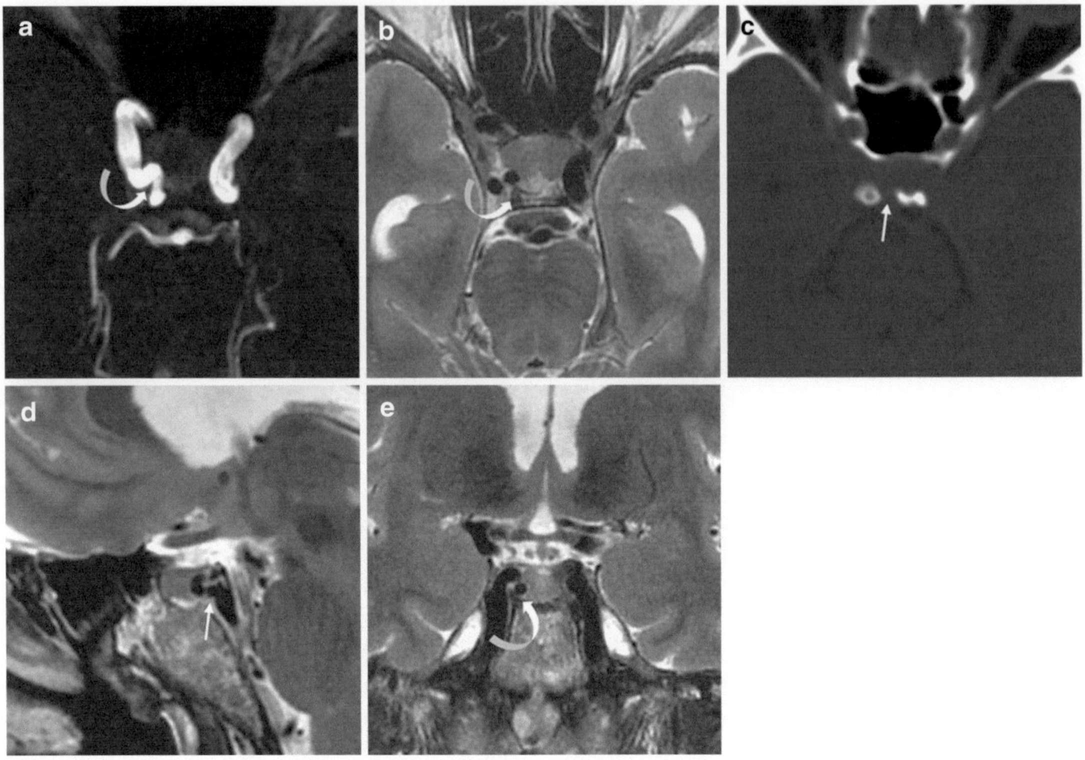

Fig. 59.2 Medial type of persistent trigeminal artery. (**a**) Axial MIP reconstruction of 3D TOF MR angiography. The persistent trigeminal artery (*curved arrow*) arises from the medial aspect of the intracavernous internal carotid artery. (**b**) Axial T2WI showing the posterior direction of the abnormal artery (*curved arrow*). (**c**) CT axial image, bone window and (**d**) sagittal T2WI showing the channel in the dorsum sellae (*arrow*). (**e**) Coronal T2WI. The trigeminal artery appears as an intrasellar round image close to the sellar floor, in contact with the pituitary gland (*curved arrow*)

diagnosis. Association of persistent trigeminal artery and pituitary adenoma has been reported. In this case, recognition of an intrasellar persistent trigeminal artery is crucial if transsphenoidal surgery is scheduled.

59.2 Intrasphenoidal Internal Carotid Artery

Transsellar intercavernous anastomosis is a rare congenital vascular anomaly, seen in the case of unilateral internal carotid artery agenesis. In the case of internal carotid artery agenesis, arterial insufficiency is usually compensated by the contralateral internal carotid artery and the vertebrobasilar system via the circle of Willis. Infrequently, the cerebral hemisphere with internal carotid artery agenesis is supplied by a transsellar intercavernous vessel connecting both internal carotid arteries. Transsellar intercavernous anastomosis is recognized on all MR sequences as a large, high-flow vessel with flow void running into the sella.

59.3 Inferior Intercavernous Sinus

The cavernous sinuses are interconnected by four venous structures: the anterior intercavernous sinus, the posterior intercavernous sinus, the inferior intercavernous sinus, and the basilar plexus. The inferior intercavernous sinus can be plexus-like, venous lake, or mixed. In its venous lake form, it is demonstrated on coronal images as a band doubling the sellar floor, usu-

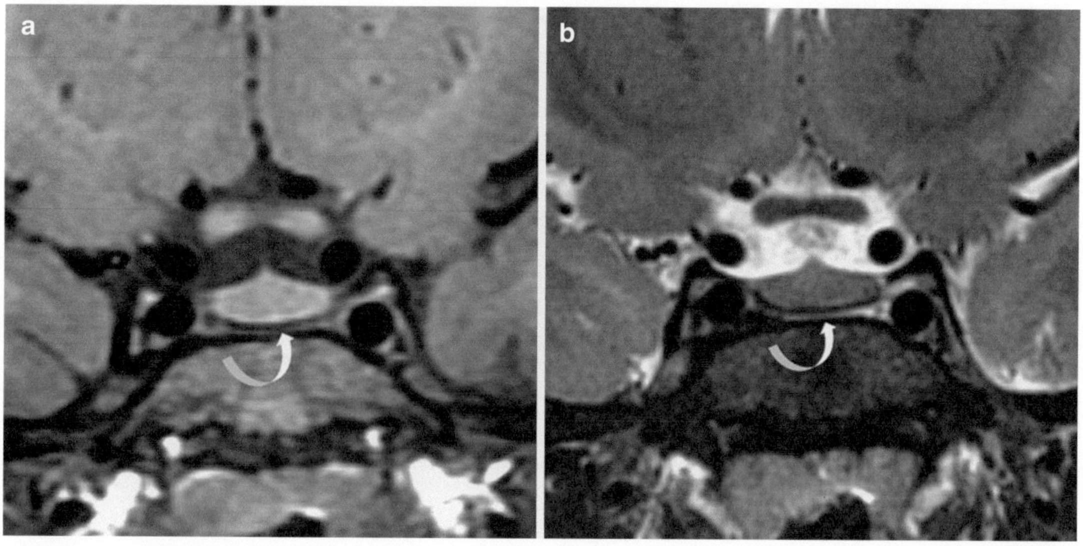

Fig. 59.3 (**a**, **b**) Coronal T1 and T2 WIs. Normal inferior intercavernous sinus in a 5-year-old boy. Its appears as a band doubling the sellar floor, hypointense on T1WI and hyperintense on T2WI (*curved arrow*)

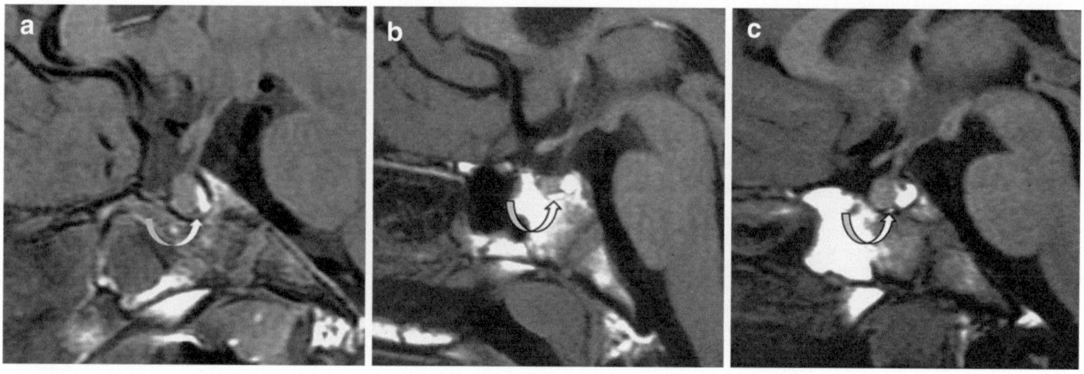

Fig. 59.4 (**a**–**c**) Sagittal T1WIs depicting inferior cavernous sinus in three children (*arrows*)

ally hypointense on T1WI and hyperintense on T2WI (Fig. 59.3). On sagittal images it appears as a small round image in contact with the sellar floor (Fig. 59.4). It is observed in about one in three normal children. In adults, its visualization is less common; demonstration of a large inferior intercavernous sinus can be observed in intracranial hypotension syndrome, cavernous sinus meningioma, and arteriovenous fistula of the sellar region. Anterior and posterior intercavernous sinuses are infrequently seen on MRI.

59.4 Intrasellar Internal Carotid Artery

Dolichoectatic internal carotid arteries are encountered in the elderly, in patients with atheromatous disease, in patients with chronic arterial hypertension, in acromegaly, and in various arterial wall diseases. Dolichoectatic siphons can penetrate into the sella turcica and reduce the space for the pituitary gland.

Medially located internal carotid arteries may reduce the sellar volume and lead to a convex

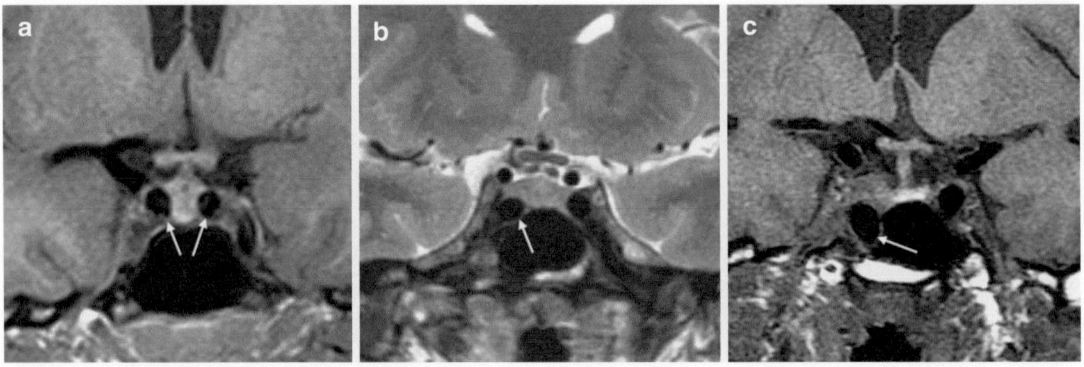

Fig. 59.5 (**a**) Coronal T1WI. Medially located intracavernous internal carotid arteries (*arrows*) decrease the sellar volume. The pituitary gland is cramped into the sella turcica. (**b**) Coronal T2WI. Unilateral medially located internal carotid artery (*arrow*). (**c**) Coronal T1WI. Prolapse of the right internal carotid artery in the sphenoid sinus (*arrow*)

pituitary gland (Fig. 59.5). Prolapse of the internal carotid artery into the sphenoid sinus may be the source of hemorrhagic complications during transsphenoidal surgery.

Further Reading

Aquini MG, Marrone ACH, Schneider FL (1994) Intercavernous venous communications in the human skull base. Skull Base Surg 4(3):145–150

Cattin F, Bonneville JF, Tang YS (1990) The convex pituitary gland. Diagn Interv Radiol 2:107–114

Piotin M, Miralbes S, Cattin F et al (1996) MRI and MR angiography of persistent trigeminal artery. Neuroradiology 38(8):730–733

Aneurysms

60

Fabrice Bonneville

Intracranial aneurysms are focal outpouchings of the wall of the cerebral arteries. They mainly develop close to the circle of Willis, an anastomotic network linking the internal carotid arteries and the vertebrobasilar system, which surrounds the sellar region. Therefore, intracranial aneurysm may present as an intra-, supra-, or laterosellar mass lesion. In this area, unruptured aneurysms may exert mass effect on the pituitary gland or the stalk or the cranial nerves, or may be discovered incidentally on brain or sellar MRI. They might be misdiagnosed or missed on preoperative MRI, but it is important to be aware that intracranial aneurysms may coexist with a pituitary adenoma (Fig. 60.1). They may be fortuitously associated with any nonsecreting or secreting pituitary adenoma, but acromegaly carries an increased risk of harboring intracranial aneurysms, with a reported incidence ranging from 4 to 17 %. In this setting, development of intracranial aneurysm might be due to the arterial hypertension frequently observed in this disease . Aneurysms in acromegalic patients are said to be usually located on the anterior circulation, are small (mean diameter <7 mm), and seem not to be more prone to rupture than aneurysms observed in the general population. It is of critical importance to evoke the diagnosis of sellar aneurysm preoperatively, because unruptured aneurysms should benefit from dedicated care and also because cases of aneurysms accidentally discovered during transsphenoidal surgery have been reported, with variable outcomes. Management of intracranial unruptured aneurysms principally depends on their risk of spontaneous rupture, which is influenced by the size and location of the aneurysm. First, the larger the aneurysm, the higher the risk of rupture. Risk is considered minimal, <1 % per year, when aneurysm diameter is smaller than 7 mm, while it may reach 30 % at 5 years for giant aneurysms larger than 25 mm. Second, the location is crucial because it is fundamental in determining whether an intracranial aneurysm is intradural or extradural, especially in the sellar region. The origin of the ophthalmic artery divides the two subgroups. On one hand, extradural aneurysms rise before the origin of this artery. They are intracavernous and thus virtually never cause subarachnoid hemorrhage, but behave as would any cavernous lesion, compressing the adjacent structures or destroying the bony skull base. On the other hand, intradural aneurysms arise after the origin of the ophthalmic artery and may rupture in the subarachnoid space. In the sellar region, such aneurysms precisely arise from the superior hypophyseal artery and extend medially, from the supraclinoid segment of the internal carotid artery (so-called carotid-ophthalmic aneurysm) and usually develop upward, or grow downward from the anterior communicating artery. Note that intracranial aneurysms are multiple in about 20 % of cases and that carotid-ophthalmic aneurysms are often bilateral.

On MRI, intracranial aneurysms appear as well-delineated, round, hypointense lesions on

J.-F. Bonneville et al., *MRI of the Pituitary Gland*, DOI 10.1007/978-3-319-29043-0_60

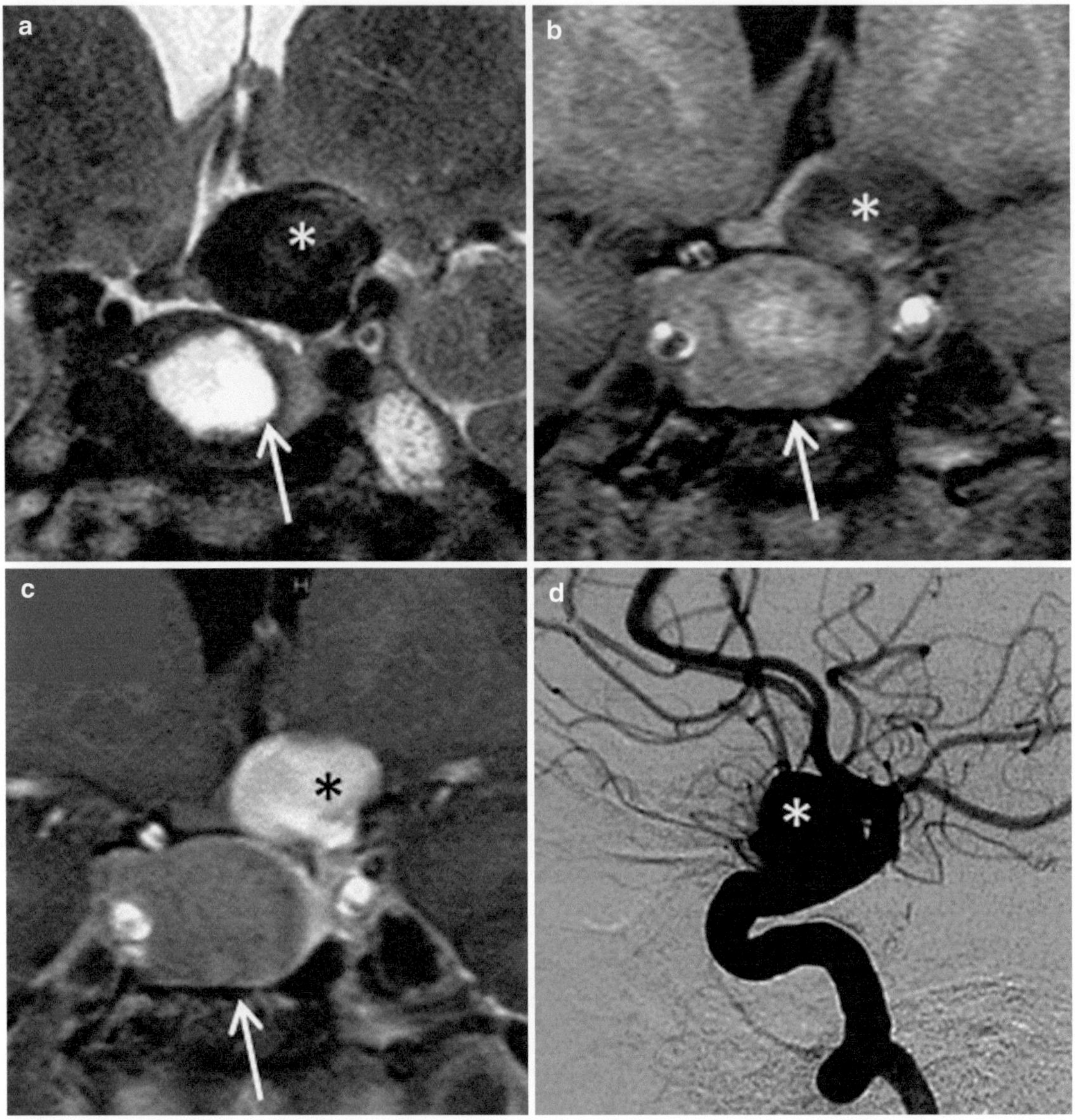

Fig. 60.1 Large supraclinoid left internal carotid artery aneurysm in a 60-year-old woman with acromegaly. (**a**) Coronal T2WI shows a large heterogeneous hyperintense pituitary adenoma (*arrow*) and a suprasellar aneurysm with characteristic flow void (*asterisk*) impinging on the left aspect of the optic chiasm. Coronal GE T1WIs (**b**) before and (**c**) after gadolinium injection clearly depict the adenoma invading laterally the right cavernous sinus, and a separate aneurysm that enhances after gadolinium administration, a feature usually observed in patent aneurysm on GE sequences. (**d**) Lateral view of left internal carotid artery angiogram confirms the nature and the location of this supraclinoid aneurysm

all spin-echo sequences. The signal intensity is so low that, in fact, they present with signal void or flow void (Fig. 60.2). This is obvious on T2WI, which is the best sequence to depict an aneurysm on MRI of the pituitary region. They usually lack contrast enhancement after gadolinium administration on spin-echo sequences, but may enhance on GE sequences (Fig. 60.2). In cases of small intrasellar aneurysm, this lack of enhancement may mimic pituitary microadenoma, particularly on contrast-enhanced T1WI (Fig. 60.3). Close attention should be paid to the other sequences, and especially MRA if needed. Similarly, midline suprasellar aneurysm may

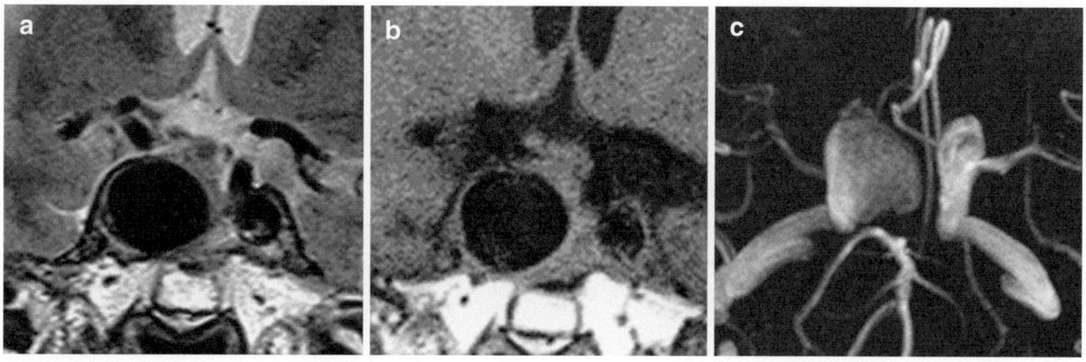

Fig. 60.2 Typical intracavernous internal carotid artery aneurysm in a 65-year-old woman with right ocular palsy. The aneurysm appears as a well-demarcated lesion within the right cavernous sinus and demonstrates marked hypointensity on (**a**) T1WI and (**b**) T2WI. (**c**) MRA confirms the arterial nature of this patent aneurysm

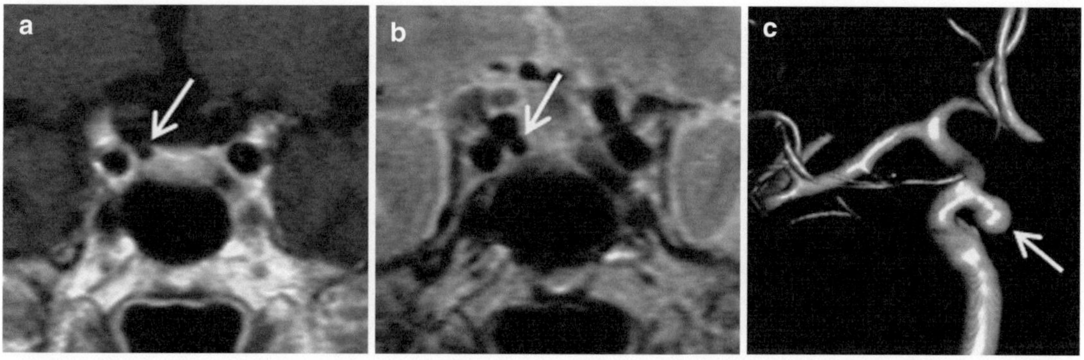

Fig. 60.3 Small intrasellar superior hypophyseal aneurysm in a patient with Cushing syndrome. (**a**) CE T1WI depicts a tiny nonenhancing lesion in the right part of the pituitary gland that may mimic a pituitary adenoma (*arrow*). The lesion appears very dark on (**b**) T2WI, a feature very suggestive of an aneurysm, as confirmed on (**c**) 3D volume rendering reformatted MRA. Note that no adenoma is demonstrated in this pituitary gland

mimic proteinaceous Rathke cleft cyst (RCC), which sometimes appears with marked homogeneous T2-low signal intensity (Fig. 60.4). Of note, flow turbulences are often observed within large aneurysms, and appear as signal heterogeneities on spin-echo sequences, giving a marble-like pattern. Similarly, repetition artifacts resulting from intrasaccular arterial pulsations may sometimes be depicted beside large aneurysms along the phase axis. When an aneurysm is suspected, it should be confirmed by adjunctive MRA. Aneurysms may also be partially thrombosed, mainly when large, thus giving different signal intensities according to the age of the clotting. Such thrombosed aneurysms appear with characteristic heterogeneous iso- to hypersignal intensities on both T1 and T2 WIs (Fig. 60.5). While the noncirculating clotted parts of the aneurysm sac do not enhance after contrast media administration, the aneurysm walls do enhance on GE 3D T1WI. Differential diagnosis may be difficult with other nonenhancing hemorrhagic lesions such as pituitary apoplexy. Because a giant aneurysm with partial internal clotting may mimic a solid destructive tumor of the skull base, MRA or conventional angiography should definitely be performed in doubtful cases before biopsy or surgery is considered. The finding of a residual patent lumen on images helps confirm the diagnosis of aneurysm. Other sellar lesions returning T1 hyperintensity may also be mistaken for partially thrombosed aneurysm. Signal heterogeneity, especially on T2WI, is a key feature of thrombosed aneurysm, a sign usually not observed in a protein-rich content lesion such as, for example, RCC.

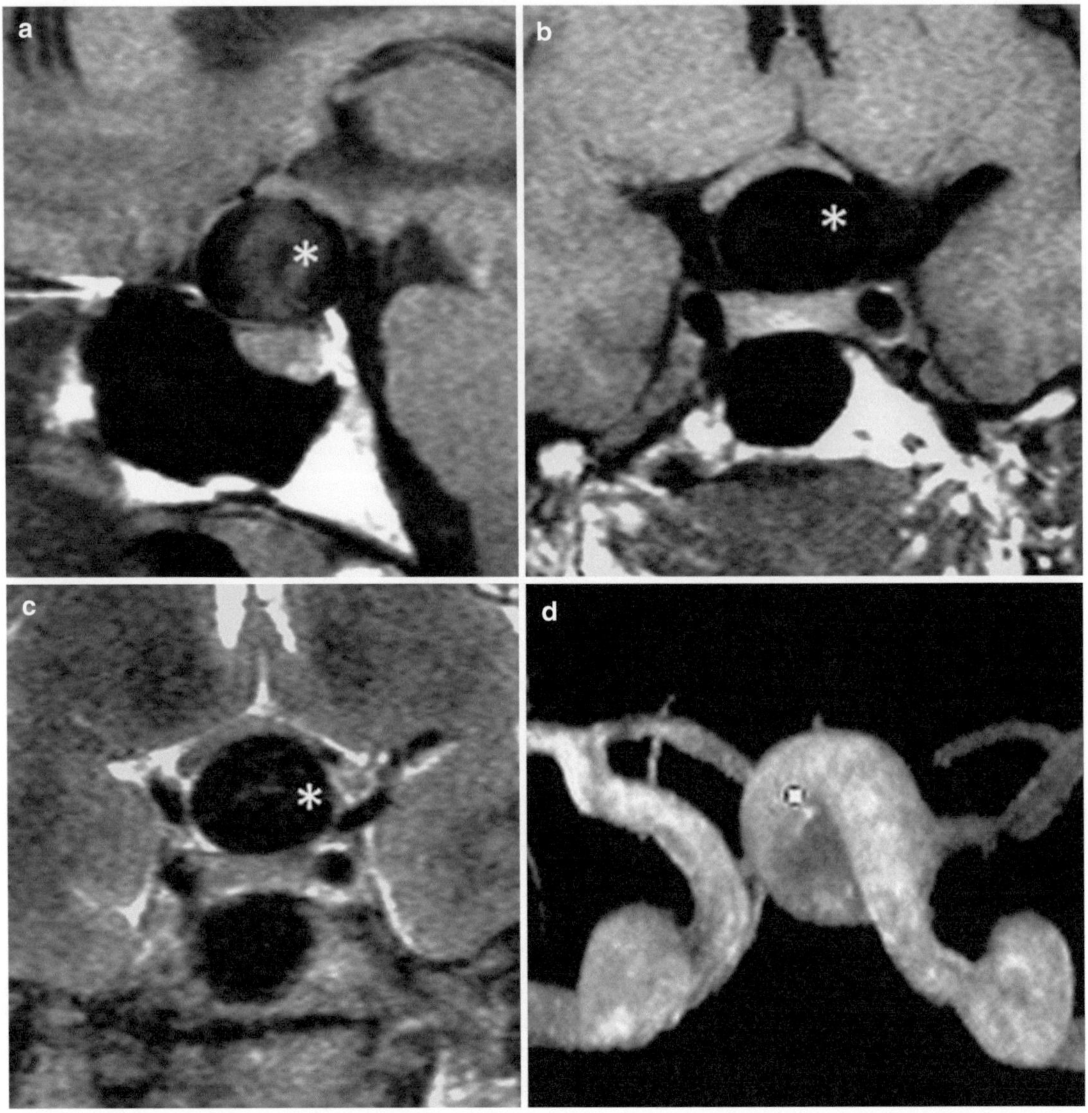

Fig. 60.4 Midline suprasellar aneurysm. (**a**, **b**) Sagittal and coronal T1WIs show a large, well-demarcated suprasellar hypointense lesion impinging on the optic chiasm that appears with a homogeneous hypointense signal on (**c**) T2WI, thus mimicking a suprasellar mucoid RCC. (**d**) MRA rules out this hypothesis by confirming the flow in this aneurysm

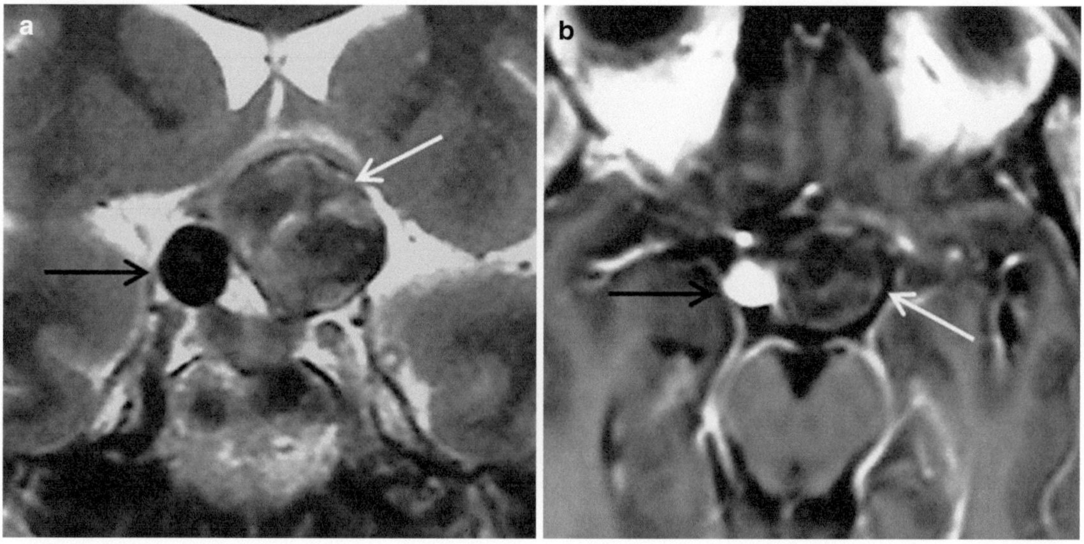

Fig. 60.5 Bilateral carotid-ophthalmic aneurysms in a 58-year-old woman with vertigo. (**a**) Coronal T2WI and (**b**) axial GE CE T1WI illustrate two different aneurysms in the same patient: a small patent aneurysm (*black arrow*) on the right side, appearing as a flow void on T2WI and enhancing on GE CE T1-WI, and a large thrombosed aneurysm on the left side (*white arrow*), impinging the optic chiasm, demonstrating heterogeneous isointense signal on T2WI and not enhancing on (**b**) (Reprinted with permission from Bonneville et al.)

Further Reading

Bonneville F, Cattin F, Marsot-Dupuch K, Dormont D, Bonneville JF, Chiras J (2006) T1 signal hyperintensity in the sellar region: spectrum of findings. RadioGraphics 26:93–113

Hanak BW, Zada G, Nayar VV et al (2012) Cerebral aneurysms with intrasellar extension: a systematic review of clinical, anatomical, and treatment characteristics. A review. J Neurosurg 116:164–178

Oshino S, Nishino A, Suzuki T et al (2013) Prevalence of cerebral aneurysm in patients with acromegaly. Pituitary 16:195–201

61 Trauma of the Pituitary Region

Jean-François Bonneville

The frequency of pituitary hormone deficiency after head trauma has been debated for a long time. Nevertheless, today it has become accepted that traumatic brain injury (TBI) can generate gonadotropin and somatotropin deficiency. Diabetes insipidus is frequent in the early phase, but permanent diabetes insipidus is much rarer than anterior pituitary dysfunction. Diagnosis is confirmed by axial T1WI, which best demonstrates the absence of posterior pituitary bright spot (Fig. 61.1). Severity of TBI seems to be an important risk factor for developing post-traumatic hypopituitarism, which has also been described. Post-traumatic pituitary deficiency is more frequently observed in young adults, involved mainly in motor vehicle accidents, than in the elderly, who are more commonly involved in falls. Pathophysiology of post-traumatic pituitary deficiency includes pituitary or hypothalamus hemorrhage or necrosis, vascular damage to the long hypophyseal portal system, hypoxic insult, shearing axonal injury, or direct mechanical insult to the pituitary gland, the pituitary stalk, or the hypothalamus.

Literature dealing with MRI aspects of pituitary trauma is scarce. Focal changes in the pituitary gland (hemorrhage/hemorrhagic infarction), swollen gland with bulging superior margin, and heterogeneous signal intensities in the anterior lobe have been described. Section of the pituitary stalk is rarely visible. Recently, it has been proposed that DWI could be interesting for the evaluation of the pituitary gland after trauma and that the ADC could be a marker to predict pituitary function.

Demonstration of basal skull fractures, particularly of the sellar region, must draw attention to and prompt the search for a pituitary dysfunction (Fig. 61.2). A long delay between initial trauma and development of hormone deficiencies is not infrequent. For medicolegal reasons, the peculiar pattern of some skull-base fractures seen as late as 20 years after brain injury must be recognized. Fractures of the planum sphenoidale, for instance, heal with a blistering appearance of the sphenoid sinus, mimicking a meningioma osteoma. In such cases it could be of the utmost importance to be able to analyze the initial radiological files (Fig. 61.3). The most common late radiological pattern of post-traumatic hypopituitarism is shrinkage of the sellar content and, consequently, a partial or complete empty sella. T1 hypointensity of the pituitary gland can been observed (Fig. 61.4). Fibrotic tissue may occupy the bottom of the sella: marked T2 hypointensity and strong postgadolinium enhancement differentiate fibrosis from residual normal pituitary tissue (Fig. 61.5). Pituitary failure may coexist with apparently normal pituitary MRI.

J.-F. Bonneville et al., *MRI of the Pituitary Gland*, DOI 10.1007/978-3-319-29043-0_61

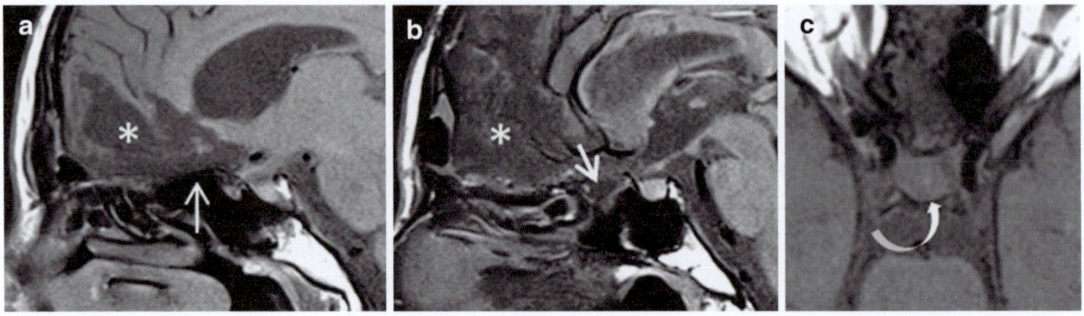

Fig. 61.1 Post-traumatic diabetes insipidus and gonadotropic deficit in a 17-year-old girl persisting 2 years after a severe traffic accident. (**a**, **b**) Mid- and parasagittal T1WIs. Severe post-traumatic alterations of the frontal lobe (*asterisk*). Post-traumatic blistering (*thin arrow*) and displaced fracture (*thick arrow*) of the planum sphenoidale on two consecutive sections. (**c**) No ADH storage demonstrated on axial T1WI (*curved arrow*)

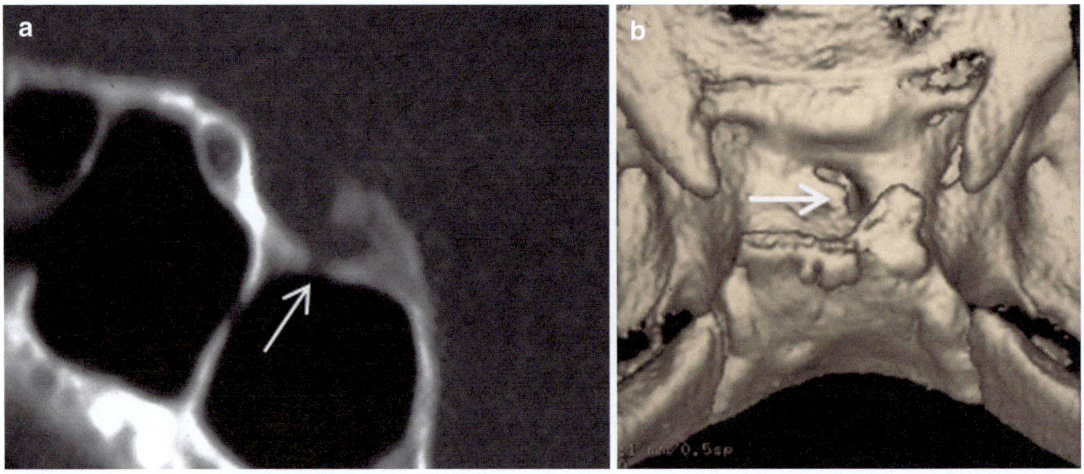

Fig. 61.2 Sella turcica fracture (*arrow*) diagnosed 1 year after head trauma in an 18-year-old patient with gonadotropin deficiency. (**a**) Sagittal CT. (**b**) 3D reformatted image

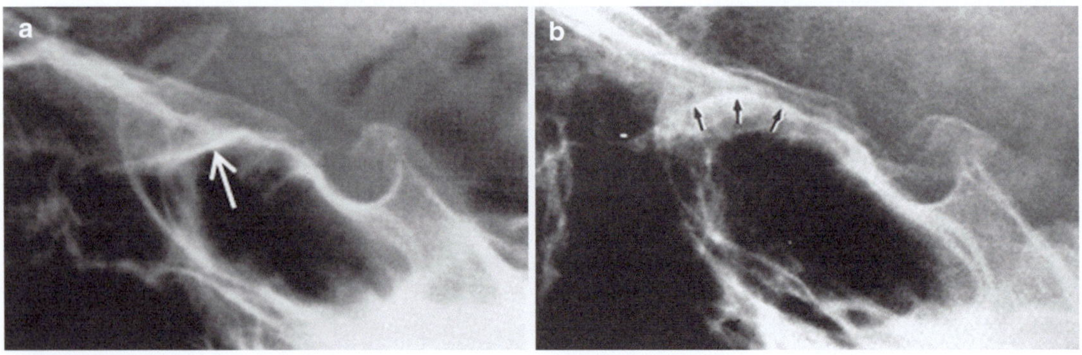

Fig. 61.3 Post-traumatic blistering of the planum sphenoidale in a 25-year-old man. (**a**, **b**) Sagittal radiographs. At the time of trauma (**a**), the fracture of the planum was not recognized and the planum was flat (*arrow*). Seven years later (**b**), the patient presents with transient blunt vision. A blistering of the planum sphenoidale (*small arrows*) is described and a presellar meningioma is first suspected, then eliminated by further examinations. Final diagnosis was post-traumatic blistering mimicking an osteoma of a meningioma of the planum sphenoidale

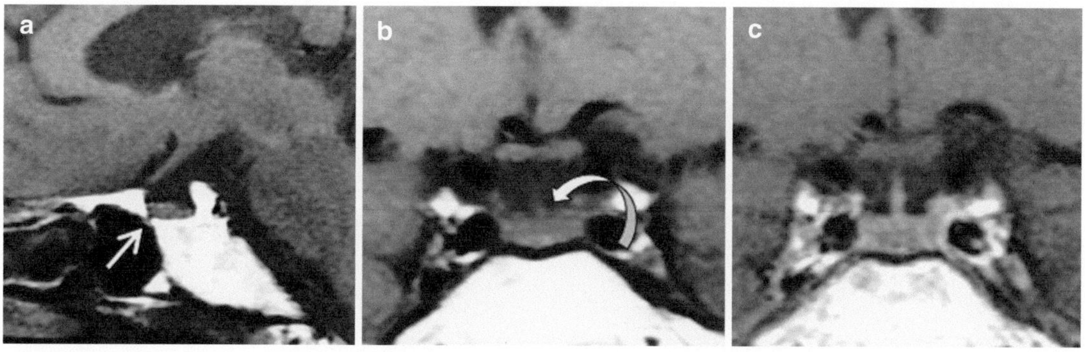

Fig. 61.4 GH deficiency seen 35 years after severe head trauma in a 45-year-old-man. (**a**) Sagittal T1WI. Fracture of the sella turcica; the sphenoid sinus is weakly pneumatized. (**b**, **c**) Coronal T1 and CET1WIs. T1 hypointensity of the pituitary gland; normal postgadolinium enhancement

Fig. 61.5 Anterior pituitary deficit in a 38-year-old woman 3 years after traumatic brain injury. No diabetes insipidus. (**a**) Sagittal CT at the time of the accident. Fracture of the tuberculum sellae and effusion of the sphenoid sinus. (**b–d**) Sagittal T1, T2, and CE TIWIs 3 years later. The sella is quite empty; ADH ectopic storage at the stalk level (*arrow*). T2 hypointense fibrotic tissue at the sellar floor with strong enhancement after contrast (*curved arrows*)

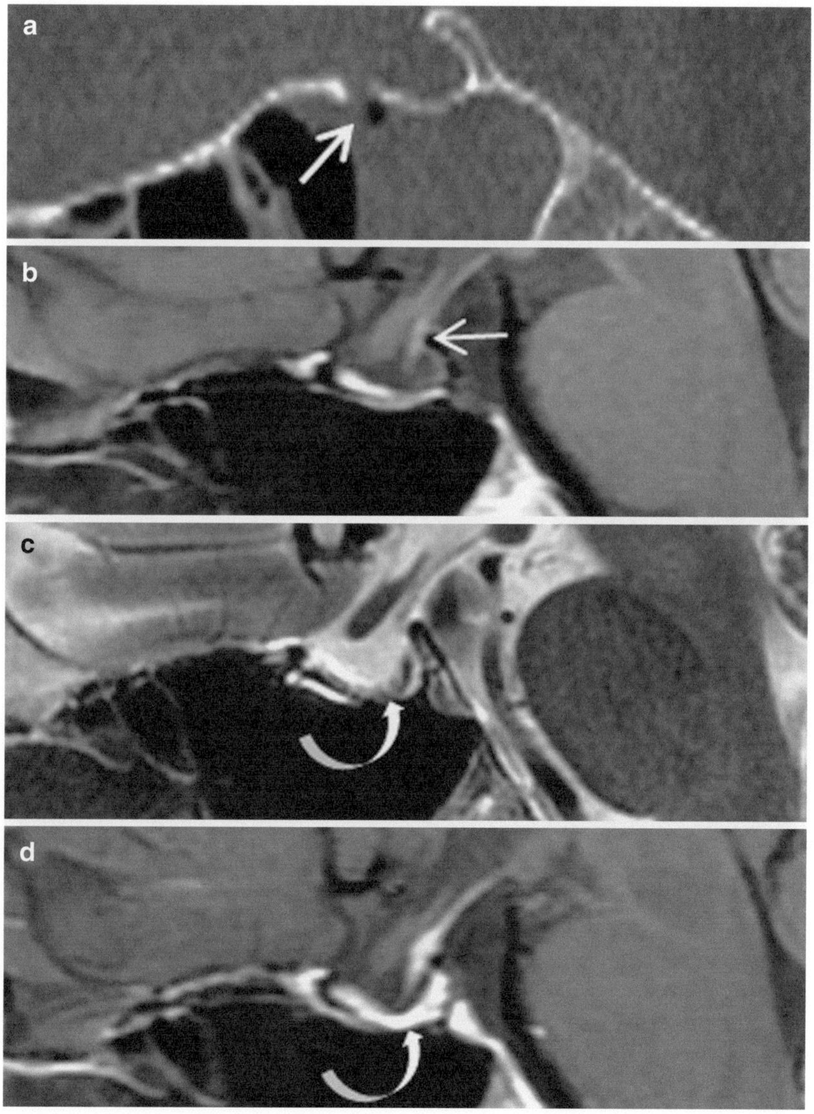

Further Reading

Klose M, Stochholm K, Janukonyté J et al (2015) Patient reported outcome in posttraumatic pituitary deficiency: results from. The Danish National Study on posttraumatic hypopituitarism. Eur J Endocrinol 172(6):753–762

Maiya B, Newcombe V, Nortje J et al (2008) Magnetic resonance imaging changes in the pituitary gland following acute traumatic brain injury. Intensive Care Med 34(3):468–475

Popovic V, Aimaretti G, Casanueva FF et al (2005) Hypopituitarism following traumatic brain injury. Growth Horm IGF Res 15(3):177–184

Index

J.-F. Bonneville et al., *MRI of the Pituitary Gland*, DOI 10.1007/978-3-319-29043-0

MIX
Papier aus verantwortungsvollen Quellen
Paper from responsible sources
FSC® C105338

If you have any concerns about our products,
you can contact us on
ProductSafety@springernature.com

In case Publisher is established outside the EU,
the EU authorized representative is:
Springer Nature Customer Service Center GmbH
Europaplatz 3, 69115 Heidelberg, Germany

Printed by Libri Plureos GmbH
in Hamburg, Germany